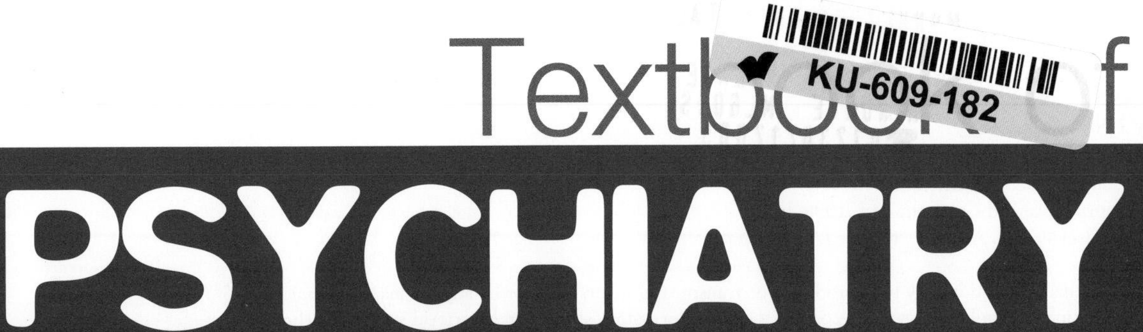

Basant K. Puri MA PhD MB BChir FRCPsych BSc (Hons) MathSci PG Dip Maths DipStat MMath

Professor and Consultant, Hammersmith Hospital, London, UK

Ian H. Treasaden MB BS LRCP MRCS FRCPsych LLM

Consultant Forensic Psychiatrist, Three Bridges Unit, West London Mental Health NHS Trust, London and Honorary Clinical Senior Lecturer in Psychiatry, Imperial College, London, UK

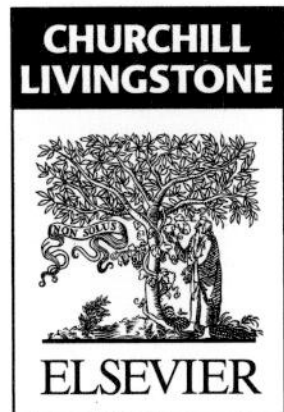

CHURCHILL
LIVINGSTONE
ELSEVIER

First edition 1996
Second edition 2002
Third edition 2011

ISBN 978-0-7020-3157-1

British Library Cataloguing in Publication Data
A catalogue record for this book is available from the British Library

Library of Congress Cataloging in Publication Data
A catalog record for this book is available from the Library of Congress

Notices

Knowledge and best practice in this field are constantly changing. As new research and experience broaden our understanding, changes in research methods, professional practices, or medical treatment may become necessary.

Practitioners and researchers must always rely on their own experience and knowledge in evaluating and using any information, methods, compounds, or experiments described herein. In using such information or methods they should be mindful of their own safety and the safety of others, including parties for whom they have a professional responsibility.

With respect to any drug or pharmaceutical products identified, readers are advised to check the most current information provided (i) on procedures featured or (ii) by the manufacturer of each product to be administered, to verify the recommended dose or formula, the method and duration of administration, and contraindications. It is the responsibility of practitioners, relying on their own experience and knowledge of their patients, to make diagnoses, to determine dosages and the best treatment for each individual patient, and to take all appropriate safety precautions.

To the fullest extent of the law, neither the Publisher nor the authors, contributors, or editors, assume any liability for any injury and/or damage to persons or property as a matter of products liability, negligence or otherwise, or from any use or operation of any methods, products, instructions, or ideas contained in the material herein.

The Publisher's policy is to use **paper manufactured from sustainable forests**

Dedication

Dr Paul J. Laking (1955–2005)

It is with deep sadness and regret that we relate the death of our co-author of the first two editions of this textbook, Dr. Paul Laking.

Paul trained in psychiatry at St. George's Hospital, London, and then in child and adolescent psychiatry in Oxford. He practised as a Consultant in Child and Adolescent Psychiatry in Suffolk from 1987 until just before his death in 2005. It was during Paul's time as a Consultant that the first author of this textbook, BP, received excellent junior doctor training in child and adolescent psychiatry in Paul's department. As a result, BP had no hesitation in asking Paul to join with us as a co-author. Paul readily agreed and, as expected, brought his considerable expertise and holistic humane approach to this textbook as a whole.

Paul died in January 2005 as a result of choroid melanoma, at the age of 49, survived by his wife and three children. A full obituary appeared in the *British Medical Journal*, together with a photograph: www.bmj.com/content/330/7489/483.4/suppl/DC1.

Paul's expertise as a clinician and teacher, together with his excellent writing ability, helped establish the reputation of the first and second editions of this book. His vision for this textbook to bring together the latest clinically relevant findings with a solid foundation of the fundamentals of the principles and practice of psychiatry in an accessible manner was shared by the surviving co-authors; we have tried to continue this approach with this new edition and we hope that he would approve of it.

BK Puri and IH Treasaden
Cambridge and London
December 2010

Preface

The passing of eight years since the publication of the second edition of this book has once again given us the opportunity to update the new edition by rewriting all the chapters. Like the first edition, the second edition was well received, and we trust that the same will be true of this new third edition.

We should like to thank those medical students and junior doctors who kindly provided detailed comments on the second edition. We have taken on board the suggestion that this book would benefit from the inclusion of self-assessment multiple-choice questions. Accordingly, about one hundred 'best of five' multiple-choice questions, together with answers, have been written by us and placed towards the end of the book. There was a minority opinion that Chapter 3, on classification, aetiology, management and prognostic factors, might be better being split up, with management perhaps appearing as a separate chapter much later on in the book. After much consideration of the advantages and disadvantages of such an option, we decided to stay with the *status quo*; the present order of coverage of material, we feel, provides a more logical and better foundation for the reader.

It is with regret that we mark the death, since the second edition, of both Dr. Paul Laking, our co-author on the first two editions, and Mrs. Gwen Stock. A separate tribute to Paul appears in this book. Gwen was the personal assistant to Dr. Ian Treasaden for many years and offered him invaluable assistance in the preparation of the first and second editions. She is much missed.

BP and IT
December 2010

Contents

Introduction

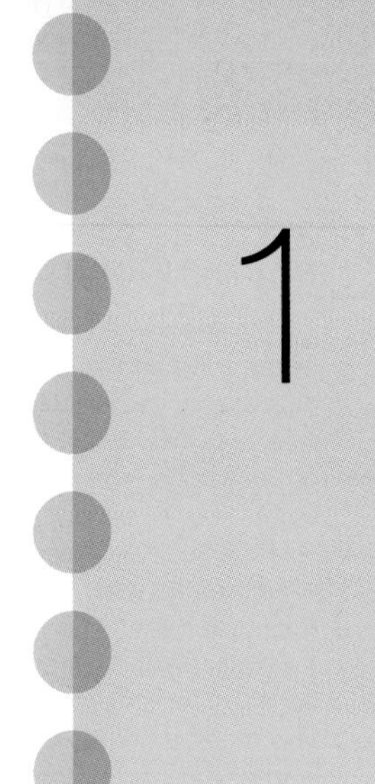

Psychiatry is that branch of medicine dealing with mental disorder and its treatment. The word is derived from *psyche*, the Greek word for soul or mind, and *iatros*, which is Greek for healer. In Greek mythology Psyche was a mortal woman made immortal by Zeus (see box, p. 01).

Psychiatry is also sometimes called psychological medicine. A psychiatrist is a medical doctor who has undergone postgraduate specialist training, gained experience and obtained qualifications in the area of mental disorders, for example illness and emotional disorders. Whenever there is something relating to the mind or soul, 'psyche' is included in the title (e.g. psycholinguistics, the study of the psychology of language). Common confusions associated with psychiatry are summarized in Table 1.1.

Why study psychiatry?

As this is an introductory text, many students reading this book will not go on to become psychiatrists. However, the principles in the general chapters and the specific information about mental illness in the other parts of the book are essential for all doctors and potential health professionals.

Consideration of the psychological aspects of the doctor–patient relationship may well affect its outcome (Chapter 4). Many complaints about doctors do not concern technical mistakes (although these may be involved), but originate because of a patient's or relative's dissatisfaction with the way psychological aspects have been managed. For example, a family complained not about the caring, compassionate GP who delayed making a diagnosis of deep vein thrombosis in their father, but were vociferous in berating the technically perfect intensive care unit doctors who treated the family in a busy, but brusque manner, while managing the subsequent pulmonary embolus.

Eros and Psyche

Psyche was the youngest and most beautiful daughter of a Greek king. The local populace began to neglect worship of the local goddess Aphrodite, preferring instead to flock round Psyche whenever she appeared in public. Although Psyche tried to avoid the adulation, Aphrodite was furious and resolved to punish Psyche.

The king, at a consultation with the oracle at Delphi, was told that he must sacrifice his daughter on a mountainside where she would be consumed by a monster, or nothing would be right in his kingdom. He did this. Eros, the son of Aphrodite, had meanwhile fallen in love with Psyche, and bade the West Wind, Zephyrus, lift her from the mountainside and take her to a beautiful palace in a valley.

At the palace, all Psyche's needs were attended to by invisible hands. At night Psyche was joined in her comfortable bed by a mysterious lover. He instructed her never to look at his face, threatening that terrible things would happen and he would never see her again. This was, of course, Eros who, captivated by Psyche's gentle ways and beauty, had disobeyed Aphrodite's instructions to punish Psyche.

After some time at the Palace, Psyche heard in the distance the wails of her sisters who were mourning her loss. Psyche made her way over the mountain and brought them back to the palace. The sisters were extremely envious of the rich palace and Psyche's invisible lover. They urged her to look at the lover's face, saying he must be a monster to hide it away from her.

Continued

Eros and Psyche—cont'd

Psyche eventually gave way to the teasing and lit an oil lamp, to find the handsome Eros by her side. Eros berated her for her lack of trust and disappeared. Psyche was extremely upset and tried to kill herself on a number of occasions, on each occasion being saved by the continuing invisible watchfulness of Eros.

Psyche's searching eventually took her to the palace of Aphrodite, who, still jealous, set her a series of tasks, hoping she would fail them. Psyche, however, passed all the trials (usually with the help of some entity who felt sorry for her). She was eventually reunited with Eros and made immortal by the intercession of Zeus, the king of the Gods.

Table 1.1 Common confusions within psychiatry

Psychology	A non-medical discipline; a science that investigates behaviour, experience and the normal functioning of the mind (e.g. memory, learning, development)
Psychotherapy	The treatment of psychological issues by non-physical means. This usually refers to the 'talking therapies', but in the wider sense of the word can include art, drama, music therapies, etc. Practitioners do not need to be medically qualified
Psychoanalysis	A particular sort of psychotherapy, or means of exploring the unconscious mind, derived by Sigmund Freud, but elaborated by many others since. A psychoanalyst must undergo a training analysis and is not necessarily a psychiatrist
Psychodynamics	The study of the way in which past experiences and current ways of relating result in present symptoms (sometimes shortened to 'dynamics')
Psychiatric nursing	A specialist nursing training (also known as 'mental nursing') for those professional nurses caring for people with mental health problems on a day-to-day basis, both in hospital and (increasingly) in the community
Psychobabble	Jargon used by any of the above, and others, to communicate with each other, but often confusing to patients

It has been estimated that up to one in five people at any one time may suffer from unwanted psychological symptoms such as anxiety, despondency, irritability and insomnia. One in six of the UK population receive treatment from their GP each year for primarily psychiatric disorders. In a further one-sixth, psychological factors are important contributors to illness.

At any one time, one in 20 people is suffering from depression. One in 25 women and one in 50 men are admitted to hospital with depression at some time in their lives (Chapter 9). The lifetime incidence of schizophrenia is one in 100 (Chapter 8). The prevalence of dementia (Chapters 6 and 20) in those over the age of 65 is one in 20, and over the age of 80 is double that. If one also includes admissions to hospital for deliberate overdoses of medication and other episodes of self-harm, and psychological problems as a result of physical disorder and delirium, then it is clear that a large part of a doctor's work in most fields may be concerned with psychological or psychiatric problems.

In physical conditions, performing a competent mental state examination can be an essential part of an assessment and reveal problems in other organ systems. For example, a London medical student was surprised to be asked in his medical exam to examine the mental state of a woman with mitral valve disease. When he did so, he discovered a significant impairment in cognitive functioning, which was resolved with judicious use of extra oxygen to deal with her hypoxia.

In general hospital practice, a junior doctor in training may be the most likely to be called to see a disturbed, confused patient at night. The doctor will need to be well aware of the myriad causes of such a state (from alcohol withdrawal to infection or a 'silent' myocardial infarct).

Whereas the busy orthopaedic surgeon may be concerned mainly with healing of fractures, mobility and so on, the psychological effects of trauma and chronic debility are being increasingly recognized.

There is a considerable influence of psychoactive substance use disorders (most notably alcohol dependence) on medical practice. The 1998 General Household Survey in England recorded that 27% of men and 14% of women drink alcohol at a level known to be harmful. The 1993 Health Survey (England) found that 7.5% of males and 2.1% of females reported symptoms indicative of alcohol dependence. Six out of 10 people admitted to hospital with serious head injuries have raised blood alcohol levels, on average two and a half times the legal limit. Alcohol consumption is implicated in 20% of deaths by drowning and 40% of deaths by fire.

Although a developmental perspective is useful in dealing with patients at all stages of the life cycle (Chapter 2), this is particularly the case for children and adolescents. In a UK questionnaire study of 7- to 12-year-old general practice attenders, 22% were found to be suffering from a child psychiatric disorder. The figure for frequent attenders in the same age range rose to 29%. Similar figures were produced in a WHO study in four 'developing' countries and in an American study in 'pediatric primary care'. Disorders of the brain increase the frequency of child psychiatric disorders by five times.

Knowledge of psychiatric treatments and their side-effects is also important. In the UK, psychotropic drugs are the most commonly prescribed group of medication.

Models of mental illness

Table 1.2 summarizes the various models of mental illness. It must be emphasized that these are different theoretical frameworks, which are by no means mutually exclusive. Their usefulness depends on their respective abilities to predict outcome, prognosis and response to treatment. Each approach has, to a large extent, derived from modes of treatment. For example, an organic approach may be more associated with drug or physical treatments, and a psychodynamic approach in psychotherapy. However, it is important to note that research is increasingly showing that combinations of approaches are most helpful in treating mental illness. An example would be the combination of working with the family of a person with schizophrenia and providing appropriate medication: each reduces the risk of relapse, but a combination has an additive effect.

Table 1.2 lists current models, and it must be remembered that these are the currently acceptable approaches and many others have fallen by the wayside throughout history.

The history of psychiatry

It is impossible to say when exactly psychiatry 'began', as it is apparent that 'mental illness' or its equivalent has been recognized as long as there have been records, and possibly before. Archaeological evidence of skull burr holes in early man could be 'releasing noxious humors' or an effective treatment for subdural haematoma.

Biblical references to mental maladies are often equated with possession by evil spirits (e.g. Saul, the Gadarene swine). Greek writings began to propose mental aberrations as disease. Plato proposed that the behaviour of a grown man could be affected by childhood experiences.

Aristotle labelled emotions and suggested people were drawn to positive experiences and avoided pain. Hippocrates classified mental illness into mania, paranoia, melancholia and epilepsy. He also coined the term 'hysteria', but was then referring to a condition of women in which the womb wandered in the pelvis until cured by sexual intercourse! The writings were generally charitable towards those afflicted by mental illness. Roman treatments were more punitive, advocating whipping or ducking to purge the body of ghosts.

In the Middle Ages, the Christian Church in the West took over speculation on mental illness and its management. (This may have been because the Church was a repository of learning, healing and knowledge.) Equating insanity with alienation produced the extremes of charity and cruelty to those afflicted. It is interesting to note that the term 'alienist' was used at a later date to refer to those concerned with mental ill health.

Islamic psychiatry in the Middle Ages used hospital treatment for the mentally ill. Revered as messengers from God, mentally ill people were housed in commodious buildings in some of the big cities of the Middle East.

During the Renaissance there were few benefactors of the insane. Indeed, art and literature suggest that the prevailing attitude was of ridicule (insane seen as buffoons) or fear (ill seen as being possessed by demons).

In the 17th century, medical writers, philosophers and anatomists searched for a physical site for psychological and spiritual entities. There was still a strong belief in demonic possession. From the 17th century onwards, institutions for the insane such as London's Bethlem Hospital and Bicêtre and Salpetrière in Paris did exist. However, many accounts refer to unpleasant conditions and treatment.

From the 18th century there arose physicians such as Chiarugi in Italy, Pinel in France and Tuke in England, who advocated kinder treatments and the removal of chains. Pinel began the definition of

Table 1.2 Models of mental illness

Model	Main characteristics
*Organic/biological/neuropsychiatric	Theories based on biochemistry, genetics and brain function
	Strong association with general medicine
	Physical treatment emphasized (e.g. drugs, ECT, psychosurgery)
	Risk of medicalizing problems: impersonal approach
	Good model for dementia, organic mental disorders caused by physical illness, brain tumours, drug- and alcohol-induced psychoses and (probably) schizophrenia and bipolar (manic–depressive) disorder
	Less useful for neurosis but holds that all emotion has a biochemical basis in the brain
*Psychotherapeutic/dynamic (e.g. psychoanalysis of Freud, Jung)	Emphasizes early childhood disturbance and difficulties as cause of later problems in adjustment
	Importance of therapist's self-knowledge in treatment, which is based on interpersonal relationships and relationship of patient to therapist
	Unconscious motives and impulses are analyzed and unravelled
	Advantage of patient appreciating opportunity to talk
	Risk of not attributing symptoms to physical disease
	Can explain anything (e.g. behaviour, emotion, etc.)
	Has not fulfilled treatment expectations
*Sociotherapeutic	Emphasizes social functioning of patient and circumstances, place in family and society (e.g. poverty, politics)
	Treatment aimed at relationship between patient's social adequacy and the demands of society
	Therapeutic community approach
	Sometimes wrongly confused with community psychiatry, i.e. psychiatric rehabilitation within the community
*Cognitive–behavioural	Treatment aimed at removal at conscious level of symptom/problem behaviour or cognition (thought, belief, attitude), not its original cause in the past
	Most useful for neurosis and behavioural disturbances
	Treatment can be undertaken by non-medically trained professionals (e.g. psychologists)
Conspirational	Mental illness is only in the eye of the beholder (society) and the patient is a victim of labelling and institutionalization
	Most applicable to delinquency and personality disorder
Family interaction	Entire family deemed sick and patient may even be the healthiest
	Especially useful in child psychiatry and family/marital problems

Continued

Table 1.2 Models of mental illness—cont'd

Model	Main characteristics
Moral	Mental illness is identical with deviancy, and the mentally ill should be held responsible for their actions
	More applicable to personality disorder
Psychedelic (e.g. theories of Laing)	Mental illness is a metaphysical trip for those too sensitive to a harsh world, which leads to enlightenment and self-awareness

*Can be regarded as a medical model in which diagnosis (label) of a disease is made on symptoms, the disease has a cause (organic and/or environmental) and the diagnosis leads to specific treatment. Does not have to be impersonal.
ECT, electroconvulsive therapy.

psychological phenomenology by describing mood swings, hallucinations and flight of ideas.

Hypnosis was introduced by Franz Mesmer and explored further in the 19th century, most famously by Charcot and Freud. The preoccupation with classification also continued with seminal texts by Kraepelin and Bleuler. This built on works by prominent European psychiatrists such as Esquirol.

The rapid rise of the asylum or mental hospital in Western countries is documented in archives and accounts by their proprietors (who may have overemphasized their benefits). The balance of private and public asylums both in the USA and the UK was strongly influenced by social and funding policy. The balance of funding available between local community or parish, and county or state determined where those with mental incapacity were placed. When the balance transferred more centrally (e.g. when the Poor Law was abolished in the UK), this led to large county or state institutions (i.e. the patient followed the money). The stereotype of the enlargement of mental hospitals because of the non-discharge of patients was really only true when the elderly were included among the inmates. Early asylums had a rapid turnover and expected people to leave and return to their parishes when better (there was also pressure from the parishes who were paying).

As mentioned above, the use of physical restraint such as manacles and strait-jackets decreased over time. It has been argued that, subsequently, other methods of treatment took their place as restraining methods. All of these treatments have, in their time, been promoted as therapeutic methods rather than modes of control. Nevertheless, historical research has unearthed examples of official inquiries into, for example, the use of hydrotherapy (immersion in water of different kinds and temperatures), which have striking parallels with more modern day inquiries into mental hospital procedures. Other treatments that were advocated but later abandoned have included malaria fever therapy (to halt the progression of neurosyphilis), and, in the 20th century, induced insulin coma and continuous modified narcosis (both induced unconsciousness).

Other physical treatments, which are still in use, were once used much more widely and with less specificity than today. The most notable examples are psychosurgery and electroconvulsive therapy (ECT) (Chapters 3 and 10). Whereas psychosurgery was formerly a gross procedure involving the ablation or cutting of connections to large areas of brain (the frontal lobotomy or leucotomy), it is now a rarely used and very specific procedure employing fine 'stereotactic' techniques. Similarly, ECT has progressed from induction of unmodified seizures, which ran the severe risk of fracture, to a modified procedure performed under anaesthesia. These old techniques have added notoriety because of their prominent appearances in films such as 'One Flew Over The Cuckoo's Nest'.

Although the widespread use of psychotropic medication, beginning in the 1950s, may have accelerated the shift in emphasis to care in the community from inpatient-based care, the emptying of the mental hospitals had begun before this. The swing back to community- or locality-based treatment and services has continued to the present day, despite the inevitable backlashes promoted by widespread publicity surrounding people with mental illness harming themselves or others.

Antipsychotic-containing plants have been known in India for centuries for their efficacy in treating mental illness. Indeed, the reserpine-containing shrub *Rauwolfia serpentina* was known in India as the 'insanity herb'. Although initially investigated for its hypotensive effects, a paper from India on the use of *Rauwolfia* in psychosis was followed up by Western researchers. The other class of antipsychotics introduced in the 1950s was the phenothiazine group of compounds, including chlorpromazine. These were synthesized derivatives from the dye industry, which were initially studied for their antihistaminic effects in avoiding surgical shock.

At first, the main interest in the antipsychotics was their tranquillizing effect, rather than their effects on the positive symptoms of psychosis. In this respect they largely replaced earlier tranquillizers such as paraldehyde and chloral. (Senior psychiatrists still can remember the sweet smelling 'pall' of the volatile paraldehyde, which emanated from some wards of large mental hospitals.) For many years they were classified as 'major' tranquillizers, in comparison with the 'minor' tranquillizers such as diazepam. Neither term has been found to be particularly useful; each has dropped out of use.

Reserpine was not as effective as the phenothiazines and so is now rarely used. The adverse side-effects of the phenothiazines (especially restlessness and parkinsonism) have made compliance with continuing treatment a problem. This has only been partially circumvented by the use of concurrent administration of antiparkinsonian medication, and the development of long-acting ('depot') injections.

There has been more recent interest in the class of compounds related to clozapine. This group was also an early discovery, but fell into disrepute because of the high (1–2%) risk of associated agranulocytosis. Modern usage of clozapine requires extremely regular blood monitoring. Other 'atypical' antipsychotics (second-generation antipsychotics) do not present such difficulties (see Chapter 3).

Community psychiatry

It could be argued that the wheel has turned full circle, with the move in most of the Western world to local community-based services. However, the emphasis on 'cost' and 'who pays' is still there. Although arguments have been made that community psychiatry is cheaper than hospital-based care, the requirement for a wide range of service options to be made available to those with mental health problems means that the converse could be true.

Some lessening of the stigma of mental disorder has also led to a widening of the remit of psychiatric and psychological services to encompass those suffering from the stresses of everyday living (rather pejoratively termed 'the worried well'). The debate still rages over whether this is a justifiable use of resources to tackle extensive and expensive morbidity or a diversion of funds from those chronically mentally ill people in greatest need. The difficulty in expressing such a need by chronically ill people has led to the development of advocacy services in which (usually) volunteers speak up for and promote the interests of individuals with mental disorders.

The special needs of people with mental illnesses are wide and multifarious and may include supported residential placements, as well as the range of acute and supportive treatments. Rehabilitation needs to occur in all activities of daily living, from self-care to work.

All the above means that mental health care is a *multiagency* task, which may involve *multidisciplinary* teams of workers developing, in conjunction with the patient/client and their carers, a programme of treatment and support to meet their needs. This may be simply good clinical practice or may be more formalized (e.g. in the UK 'the Care Programme Approach'). The main agencies that may be involved are summarized in Table 1.3, but this list may vary with the individual, their problems and their culture (used in the widest sense of the word to include government policy, available services and so on).

Table 1.3 Possible agencies concerned with mental health

Health
Psychiatry service
Psychology service
Internal medicine service (including geriatrics and paediatrics)
General practice
Community health
Social Services
Housing
Probation
Voluntary agencies
Education
Night shelters
Prison service

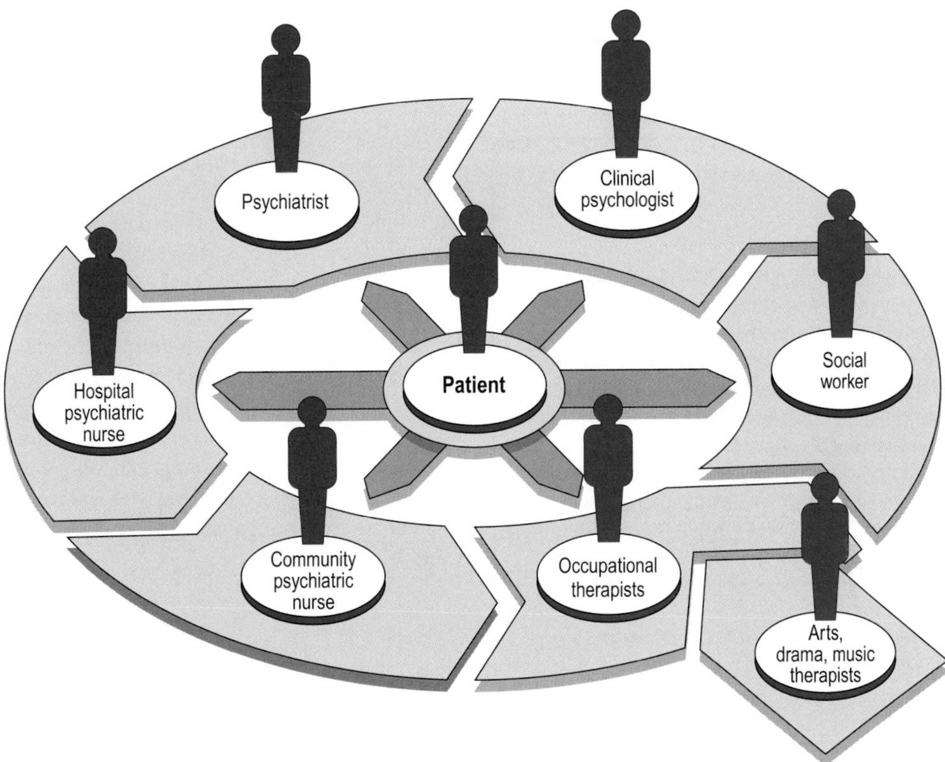

Figure 1.1 • The multidisciplinary team. • A 'key worker' could be any member of the team.

Similarly, possible members of the multidisciplinary team are shown in Figure 1.1. The management of such teams (which may include members of more than one agency) is a matter of local variation, and may be a source of tension. Such issues certainly require careful attention, if professional rivalries are not to cause splitting of the team to the detriment of the patient. Included in this may be the question of 'leadership' and 'models' of working. Members in such teams need to be clearly aware of their core roles and responsibilities, especially as, paradoxically, the less sure professionals are of their boundaries, the more difficult it is to overlap and cooperate with other roles.

The patient can suffer from an 'overload' of professionals if a *keyworker* system is not worked out, which encompasses the above considerations. This arrangement (which may go under a number of titles, e.g. case worker, core professional) allows the resources and expertise of other members of the multidisciplinary team to be available to the patient, while maintaining a consistent individual to whom the patient relates. The keyworker is also able to continue an overall holistic management view.

For the most difficult-to-reach and disturbed individuals, the concept of the assertive community team has been developed. Such patients frequently default from treatment and are often admitted to hospital 'in crisis'. They are also at increased risk of harming themselves or others. Assertive community outreach requires frequent, proactive involvement with clients and a low caseload for the practitioner. The approach is only successful in reducing emergency admissions when these conditions pertain.

The medical/psychiatric overview of an individual patient may remain with the general practitioner and primary health care team or may involve the psychiatrist. In some teams the consultant is involved as a matter of course, whereas in others this only occurs on specific referral, either from the original referrer or from another member of the team with the original referrer's permission.

Multiagency involvement can complicate matters as a number of teams may be involved, as well as the patient's own supportive network. Clear communication is, more than ever, essential in these circumstances and may require regular planning meetings or interactions, which, these days, almost always involve the patients themselves.

Indeed in some countries (e.g. the UK) and in certain circumstances, such meetings are enshrined in legislation (Chapter 21).

Introduction

- Like all specialties psychiatry has developed gradually with fits and starts, some accidental discoveries and latterly the application of science.
- The rise and fall of the mental hospital were influenced by the development of community treatments, but bore greater relation to changes in social and funding policy.
- The complex needs of people suffering with psychological disturbance require well-organized, multidisciplinary and multiagency approaches with excellent communication between professionals and organizations.

Conclusion

The development of psychological medicine has involved the move from community to hospital to community again. Major changes have occurred in who is responsible for those with mental illness and how such illness is regarded. Fear and ignorance are still present. However, it is these human characteristics, together with curiosity, that produce the developments that have occurred and continue the search for more and better ways of helping those who suffer from mental disorders and their effects. Although this book hopes to aid the student in beginning an understanding of the current level of knowledge in psychiatry, such a beginning can only be enriched and enhanced by consulting the greater textbook of clinical experience and, of course, the patients themselves.

The life net

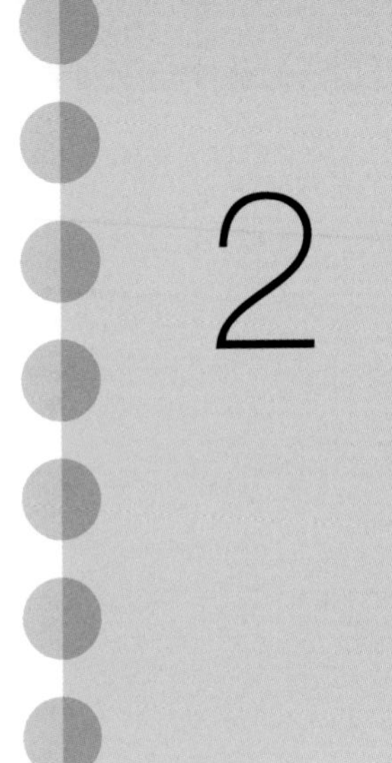

Introduction

It is usual, when discussing animal development, to refer to the 'life cycle'. In many ways this is appropriate. One could argue that human beings start from dependency and develop through to dependency again. However, the average human being also goes through periods of dependency throughout life, at times of weakness, illness and catastrophe. Furthermore, apart from the odd hermit, it could be said that the human condition is one of *mutual* dependency.

In another sense the perpetuation of the species is a 'cycle' of birth and death. In the following this notion is extended to consider a series of interlocking and interrelated life scripts or lines, which trace human development (Figure 2.1). These are punctuated by life events, some significant, some less significant depending on context, but at many of which doctors are present or involved. At each consultation the doctor sees only a snapshot of a person, family or community and their predicament. However, each predicament has its history and influences, which must be taken into account in determining, first, a formulation of the most prominent problem at that time, second, the most appropriate intervention, and, third, the likelihood of change in a wanted direction.

All psychiatric disorder occurs in a developmental context. There are characteristic life events, interactions with the lives of others and psychiatric disorders at each developmental stage. Some behaviours may be considered within the normal range at one age but as evidence of disorder at another (e.g. belief in Santa Claus would, in some Western cultures, be normal at age 4, but thought very strange at age 24). This example also illustrates the importance of context: if the 24-year-old was professing the belief in an infant school classroom, it would be less worrying than if it was reported in all seriousness in a consulting room (Figure 2.2).

That patterns of behaviour and interaction are repeated in successive generations has been frequently observed, and has led to theories and controversies about the relative contributions of nature and nurture. Clearly, this is only a question of focus of interest. It is not possible to be without a genetic inheritance, nor is it possible to avoid upbringing and environmental influences, and it is important to consider these different influences when determining the appropriateness and possibility of intervention. Genetics and environment continually interact, as, for example, when an individual genetically at increased risk of epilepsy has a seizure when hypoxic for some reason; or a woman with a strong family history of mood disorder becomes depressed when isolated looking after young children.

Since Descartes, Westerners have got used to considering the mind and body as separate entities. Macroscopically and microscopically this is spurious. All disorders – indeed all of life – have both psychological and physical components: even a fracture is determined by the psychological 'set' that led to the activity in which the fracture occurred, and the care that was taken over the activity. Similarly, the speed and circumstances of recovery and any subsequent disability may be determined as much by psychological as physical factors. Conversely, one cannot have a 'thought' without a corresponding

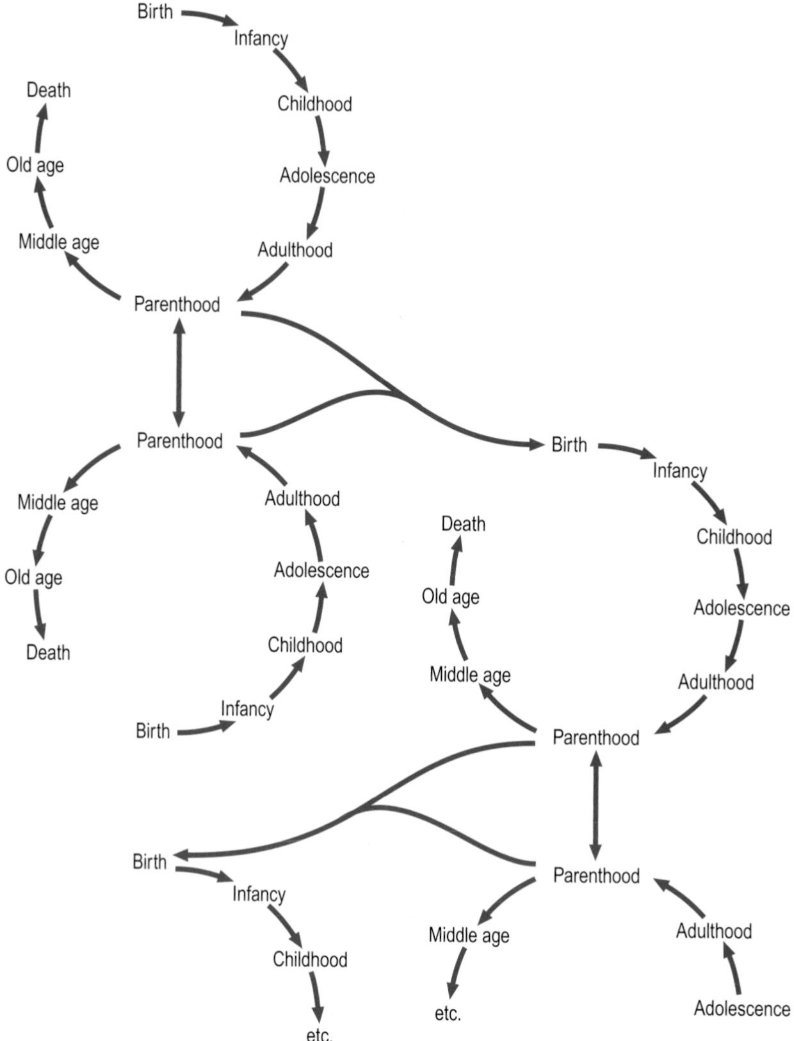

Figure 2.1 • The 'chain-link' net of interrelating and interlocking life cycles.

parallel electrical and biochemical configuration in the brain. A *multilevel developmental approach* is illustrated schematically in Figure 2.3.

Where to start?

Even before conception there are influences on an individual's likely life script. 'Assortative' mating determines one's parents, their respective genetic inheritances and life experiences. This concept suggests that there is not a random distribution of genes in society. One's parents are usually joined by similar and/or complementary lifestyles, backgrounds, interests, levels of education, personalities and outlooks on life. Cultural considerations will determine how much, if at all, individuals may choose their own partner. Depending on the above, conception may have resulted from circumstances that range from a single encounter to a lengthy courting ritual followed by a careful choice of time, place and social setting.

Expectations of the pregnancy, birth, delivery and subsequent development, together with the degree to which these are fulfilled, can have a profound influence on the future of an individual. A 14-year-old who becomes pregnant after losing her virginity when drunk at a party has rather different expectations (and will experience different environmental pressures) from a 32-year-old professional woman, in a stable relationship for six years, who decides in

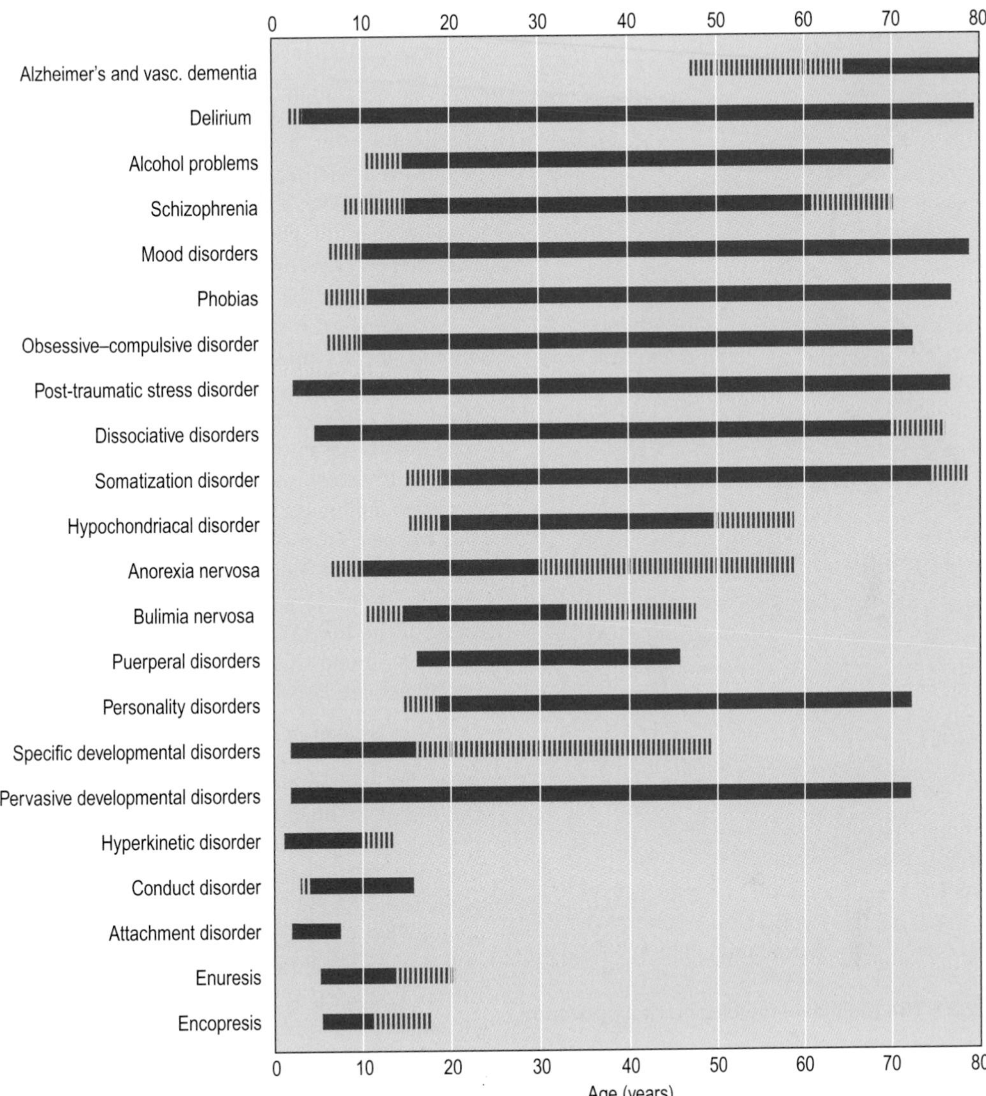

Figure 2.2 • The occurrence of psychiatric disorders according to age.

consultation with her partner that 'the time is right to start a family'.

Pregnancy may be marked by careful attention to preventing adverse influences on fetal development ('good antenatal care') or not ('lacking in antenatal care'). This will in turn influence birthweight and the likelihood of perinatal complications. The presence or absence of such complications, apart from determining the risk of brain injury, will have an effect on the bonding of parent and child. A sick neonate may have reduced contact with its parents because of treatment, or indeed because of possible parallel sickness of the mother. Whether the child's father is present can result from a number of factors, and his continued involvement will also affect the child's future circumstances. An ill neonate is likely to present different responses from those presented by a healthy baby, being less responsive or more twitchy, for example. A twitchy baby may be disconcerting for parents, who may reduce their handling of the child and become more tense, thereby increasing the child's jumpiness.

Studies of large cohorts of infants also show that there are wide variations, from birth, in the behaviour of individuals. The temperament of an infant, its 'fit' with the expectations of its parents and their

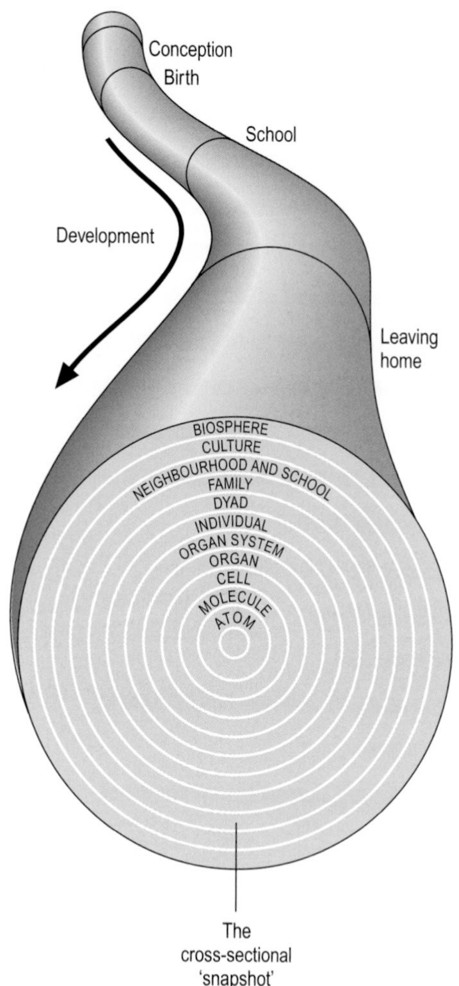

Figure 2.3 • The multilevel developmental approach.

capacity to manage the child may be crucial in determining a person's future, or indeed their survival. Researchers in New York have shown a spectrum of infant temperaments ranging from 'difficult' to 'easy'. A 'difficult' infant is not easy to cuddle, is irregular in its routines and cries frequently. In contrast, an 'easy' baby is regular in its routine, smiles frequently and is cuddly. An intermediate cluster of characteristics was labelled 'slow to warm up'. Such infants appear 'difficult' at first, but after a little time come to resemble the 'easy' child.

Postnatal or puerperal depression occurs in 10–20% of women, depending on the criteria used. In some this will develop into a psychosis (see Chapter 12). The rapidity or otherwise with which this resolves will have an effect on the whole family, but in particular on the developing infant. It has been shown that there is poor coordination in the interactions between a depressed mother and her child, as though the 'give and take' is 'out of step'. The infant becomes distressed and avoids interaction, which, in turn, affects the mother's approaches, and their frequency and type. It has even been observed that maternal depression is associated with subsequent delays in the cognitive development of the infant. Also of later concern may be problems of attachment, although these may be mitigated by the availability of other carers.

'Attachment' is the quality of interaction between a child and its principal carer. It can be disrupted or altered by life events or disorders affecting the child, its carer or both. Clinical evidence suggests that quality of initial attachment is a template for future relationships. Also, the type of attachment experienced in early life will influence the speed and manner with which the various levels of independence are achieved. Both of these can influence the risk of developing a psychiatric disorder at a later stage in the life cycle (see Chapter 16).

In childhood the sorts of problems presenting to psychiatry are largely dictated by the stage of development and the expectations of the child's carers. For example, most parents expect to be woken at night by a newborn infant, but they also expect the infant gradually to develop a sleep–wake cycle that resembles that of the rest of the family. If this does not occur and there are problems settling or night-time waking, then a sleep disorder may be presented (see Chapter 16). Similarly, when there are delays, abnormalities or excesses in behaviours at different stages of childhood, which cause suffering and/or handicap, then other child psychiatric disorders may be present.

The widening social world

Before birth the child has its mother and the influences on her as its social sphere (a fetus may 'jump' if the doorbell rings). Postnatally there is a predominant relationship with a single carer, usually the mother. Winnicott used the term 'primary maternal preoccupation' to describe the mother's extreme involvement with her infant in the first few weeks of life. There are various 'design features' that emphasize this close social relationship: the peculiarly evocative infant cry is designed to cause a response in adults (including lactation in the mother); the infant's visual focus is initially limited to almost exactly the distance to its mother's eyes when cradled in the feeding position;

infants show a preference for the timbre of a female voice (note how, when speaking to babies, adults often make their voices 'higher' in pitch); infants also show a preference for face-like patterns. Normal babies are 'programmed' to imitate facial expressions.

As the child develops extended visual focus and some manipulative skills, its social world widens to include objects and a wider range of people. This extends further with introduction to the extended family. The child begins to notice events and activities outside the home. As it becomes older, children from other families are introduced and these relationships are then formalized in nursery, kindergarten or playgroup. The introduction to school produces a further social milieu. This, together with television and other media, will present knowledge of the wider world. Nowadays in Western cultures such knowledge is assumed at an early age (Figure 2.4).

Research shows that peer interactions are important for normal development as a means of developing social skills, practising future relationships and developing self-esteem. Children of similar ages show higher levels of conflicting interactions than do those of differing ages. A normal child will show more nurturing and protective behaviour to a younger child than to a same-age child. Conversely, the younger child will show more submissive and following-type behaviour when with the older child. Developmental anomalies and psychiatric disorders can interfere with this scheme of things to produce secondary difficulties in relationships, which, in turn, can confer greater disability. This is expanded on in individual chapters, but examples are the personality problems seen in early-onset schizophrenia (Chapter 8) and the higher rates of mental illness in those with learning disabilities (Chapter 17).

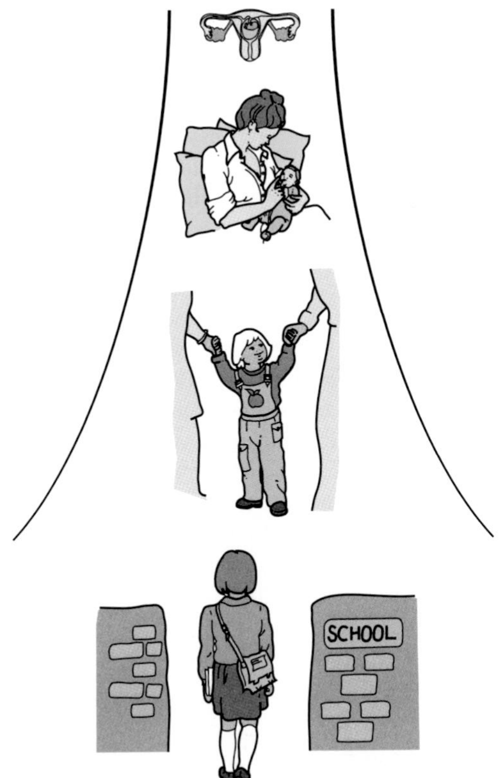

Figure 2.4 • The widening social world.

With increasing age, the relative importance of social milieu alters. In adolescence and young adulthood, involvement with peers usually overtakes involvement with the immediate family. The family is still extremely influential but this is not always admitted! Young people interviewed separately from their families show considerable conformity of views with those families. The 'adolescent turmoil' often assumed in Western society does not occur in the majority of teenagers. When it does, there have usually been previous difficulties.

With the transition from school or college to the workplace there is often a constriction in social contacts to a smaller group of people. Most people do not operate regularly in groups of say 20–30 others of the same age, as can occur at school.

With courtship, and the establishment of a stable relationship with a partner, there may be a further constriction of the sphere of friends. This may occur particularly if and when a child is born. With increasing age, the likelihood is of an even smaller social sphere, although this will, of course, depend on individual circumstances. Divorce may also result in a widening or a narrowing of social sphere, depending on demography. Bereavement in later life is a further progressive narrowing of one's group of acquaintances (see below).

For women in later adulthood in recent Western society, there may arise a combination of circumstances sometimes referred to as the 'empty nest syndrome'. This is a combination of children having left home; the partner being less available because of career demands; the menopause, with its loss of fertility and symbolic loss of 'womanhood'; and the sense of lacking money or a career for oneself. Social changes (later pregnancy with prior career advancement, hormone replacement therapy, male unemployment) are reducing the relevance of this notion but it is mentioned here as an example of the coterminosity of a number of life events that may lead to increased mental health problems.

The 'life events' literature is now extensive and research relating life events to most mental health problems has been carried out, although the initial work was in depression. It is important to remember, for example, that subjects rate a house move as only slightly less significant, mentally, than the death of a spouse.

Ageing

Growing older involves negotiating changes at all levels of functioning, including coping with attitudes that may caricature the aged person as a 'burden on society'. Much has been written about the increase in proportion of populations in Western countries who are 'aged'. Although there is certainly an increased risk of mental and physical infirmity in old age, only a minority of elderly people experience the extreme dependency of senility and physical incapacity. The 1993 Health Survey for England showed that, of those over the age of 65, 14% of women and 7% of men required daily help to maintain independent living (these figures rise over age 85 to 40% of women and 21% of men). This is, however, a large total number, and is likely to grow larger with the increase in the proportion of elderly in the population of the Northern hemisphere. (Reduction in morbidity in the elderly in the USA has been associated with 'healthier lifestyles' and prompt medical care.)

Media images often portray elderly people 'enjoying retirement' in seaside resorts. Although this may be true for some, on the whole there is still a significant relationship between ageing and poverty. The financial position of an older person will reflect prior socioeconomic position, age, gender and marital status. Married couples are better off than unmarried, men better off than women, spinsters better off than widows, and the younger elderly better off than the older.

The experience of ageing is also likely to be heavily dependent on the social amenities available, including the presence or absence of companionship and family support. It is essential to consider these aspects when assessing the mental health of elderly people, as statistically they are more likely to be lacking. The interaction of individual and environmental factors is as important for older people as it is for neonates (see Chapter 20).

Bereavement

Bereavement is a term that can apply to any loss event, from the loss of a relative by death to unemployment to divorce or even the loss of a family pet. The effects of bereavement may be modified by the significance of the loss; its suddenness; the degree of anticipation; the support available before, during and after the loss; the degree to which appropriate mourning occurs; and the material and social consequences of the loss.

Grief can be defined as those psychological and emotional processes, expressed both internally and externally, that accompany bereavement. Uncomplicated grief follows a fairly consistent course. Initially there is shock and disbelief, often described as a feeling of numbness, followed by a period of increasing awareness of loss with accompanying painful emotions of sadness and anger. Individuals may deny the anger they feel, especially if there is ambivalence concerning the object of their grief (see pathological grief, below). This may intensify the increased irritability seen with other symptomatology, which can be indistinguishable from that seen in depression. Symptoms can include sleep disturbance, early morning waking, tearfulness, loss of appetite, weight and libido, reduction of performance and interest in everyday activities and so on. The differential diagnosis of depression should include a grief reaction (see Chapter 9).

Mourning, although sometimes used as a synonym for grieving, may helpfully be considered as referring to those culture-bound social and cognitive processes through which one must pass in order to return to more normal functioning. This is necessarily a lengthy period, with regressions at the times of anniversaries and in response to other reminders of loss. One may hear such comments as 'She seems to have got over it quite well', but it is a mistake to assume that this is so. It is more likely that the individual concerned is responding to social pressures not to share her grief. Those who have experienced significant bereavement, even after many years, will, if asked, say something like: 'The hole in my life is still there. It's just that I don't come across it so often. When I do the pain is just as intense' (Figure 2.5).

Pathological grief occurs when there is disruption of the mourning process. The expression of grief may be delayed or become chronic. Pathological grief may occur for a large number of reasons, depending

Figure 2.5 • The effects of grief.

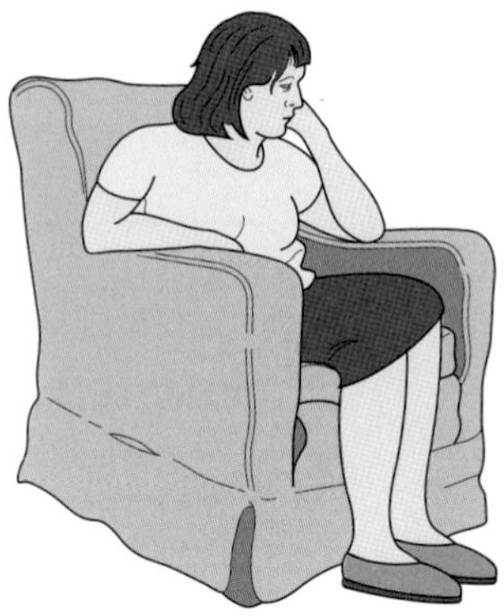

- Social avoidance
- Depressive ideation
- Lack of sleep
- Anorexia
- Increased mortality
- Somatic symptoms of pain or discomfort
- Constipation
- Loss of libido
- Impairment of performance
- Lack of energy
- Emotional numbness
- Preoccupation with deceased, e.g. vivid imagery
- Perceptual disturbances, e.g. transient hallucinations
- Mummification (preservation of possessions)

on the life stage of the person concerned and the nature of the bereavement.

Children are particularly vulnerable to problems with bereavement, not necessarily because of the loss itself but because of their extreme dependence on their carers to provide an appropriate environment in which to grieve. Children's adaptation to loss is mediated by family and cultural attitudes and styles. In their own grief, parents or other carers may miss the grief of the children. Uncharacteristic behaviour in a child may well be their expression of grief, depending on developmental level, and may be misinterpreted by observers. This may be further complicated by the grieving process being delayed in children, who, being sensitive to the adults' distress, hide their own.

Conversely, grieving may be disrupted when other activities, such as caring for children or other dependants, take precedence over individual concerns. This may be particularly problematic in pregnancy, when bereavement may be overshadowed by the concerns for the developing life. Grief for the loss may well then arise unexpectedly in the puerperium, and be confused with or complicate postnatal depression. If the loss at this time is of an infant, then the grief reaction may be further complicated (e.g. when a twin is lost). Dealing with the practical consequences of the loss may well be a barrier to proper mourning, so that delay in the expression of grief occurs.

Social or family disapproval of the expression or sharing of emotion may inhibit mourning. Such disapproval may, in individual cases, be associated with inadequate mourning of previous losses and the consequent avoidance of the reawakening of painful emotions. To some extent, all experiences of bereavement can resonate with prior instances of loss, and some separations, such as early miscarriage or death in wartime, may be seen as so frequent an occurrence that mourning is not thought appropriate and no space is allowed, by either family or professionals. However, in these cases surveys and clinical experience confirm that the level and intensity of grief felt is by no means insignificant. (Reactions will always be modified by circumstances: for example, the use of ultrasound imaging in early pregnancy may intensify the reality of the loss felt after a miscarriage, but may also facilitate the grieving process.)

Separation from the reality of loss may interfere with adequate mourning. This is particularly highlighted in the West by the increased involvement of hospitals and associated technological paraphernalia with death and dying, thus separating a large portion of the population from contact with the reality of death. The depiction of death by the media may promote unhelpful fantasies that further deter a realistic appraisal of death and dying. The use of psychoactive medication by the bereaved may also separate them from the bereavement experience. Mental or physical illness at a time of loss may be a reason for delayed grief. If the loss is due to traumatic circumstances, then reactions to the trauma including post-traumatic stress disorder (see Chapter 10), are likely to interfere with normal mourning.

It is only when grief becomes pathological in its intensity or length that mental health services may need to be involved. In particular, depression itself may occur in the context of grieving (although, as mentioned above, care must be taken as normal grief may include all the symptoms of depression). Normal grieving may be facilitated by the extended family, by the primary health care team (general practitioner, health visitor, etc.) where available, by religious organizations and by specialist voluntary sector organizations such as CRUSE.

Specialist treatments include bereavement counselling and guided mourning. Drugs may be used if mental illness supervenes, but care must be taken that these themselves do not interfere with the grieving process.

Conclusion

Much as it may be tempting to separate or disregard psychological issues, they are always present. They will have an influence on and be influenced by other aspects of life. Although sometimes it may be necessary to ignore psychological ramifications, for example when there is immediate threat to life, a health professional will not be taking a 'complete' approach without bearing them in mind.

The life cycle

- An individual's life cycle interacts with, interrelates with and is modified by the life cycles of others.
- A cross-sectional view is only a snapshot of an individual and their predicament.
- For optimum intervention a longitudinal or historical perspective must be taken.
- Changes can, and do, occur at all levels, from the molecular to the societal; intervention at one level will have implications for all other levels.

Classification, aetiology, management and prognostic factors

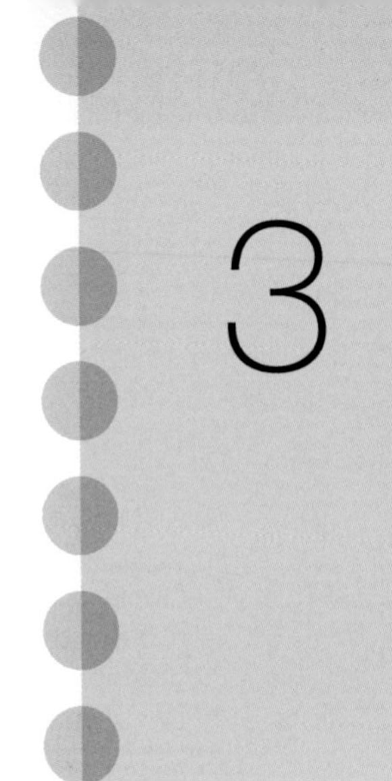

Introduction

This chapter begins with a discussion of the classification of psychiatric disorders. This includes two major internationally used classifications: the International Classification of Diseases, 10th Revision (ICD-10) of the World Health Organization and the Diagnostic and Statistical Manual of Mental Disorders, 4th edition, Text Revision (DSM-IV-TR) of the American Psychiatric Association. Factors that cause psychiatric disorders are considered next, followed by a look at the main ways in which such disorders can be treated. The chapter ends by considering prognostic factors.

Classification

Types of psychiatric disorder

As shown in Figure 3.1, most psychiatric disorders can be divided into organic psychiatric disorders, which are secondary to known physical causes, and 'functional' disorders. As research in the neurosciences progresses, the underlying physical causes of the functional disorders are being discovered, for example at a neuronal, genetic and biochemical level. Therefore, it could be argued that the traditional dichotomy between organic and functional disorders is gradually becoming less appropriate.

Organic psychiatric disorders

Psychiatric symptoms can be caused by *organic disorders*, such as cerebral tumours and endocrine disorders. For example, depressed mood may result from hypothyroidism or from primary hypoadrenalism (Addison's disease). Psychiatric symptoms can also result from the abuse of alcohol and drugs, that is, *psychoactive substance use disorders*. For example, soon after injecting amphetamine intravenously, a drug abuser may experience and exhibit symptomatology indistinguishable from that seen in acute schizophrenia.

Functional disorders

Psychoses

In psychoses there is loss of contact with reality. The symptoms that occur are not readily understandable and can include:

- hallucinations
- delusions
- several abnormalities of behaviour, e.g.
    - gross excitement and overactivity
    - marked psychomotor retardation
    - catatonic behaviour
- lack of insight.

The major psychotic disorders are schizophrenia and mood disorders.

Neuroses/psychoneuroses

In neuroses, or psychoneuroses, the symptoms that occur are understandable and it is possible to empathize with them. The symptoms differ from normal in a quantitative but not a qualitative way. For example, most normal people have experienced anxiety; the more severe neurotic counterpart of this is an anxiety disorder (of which there are several types).

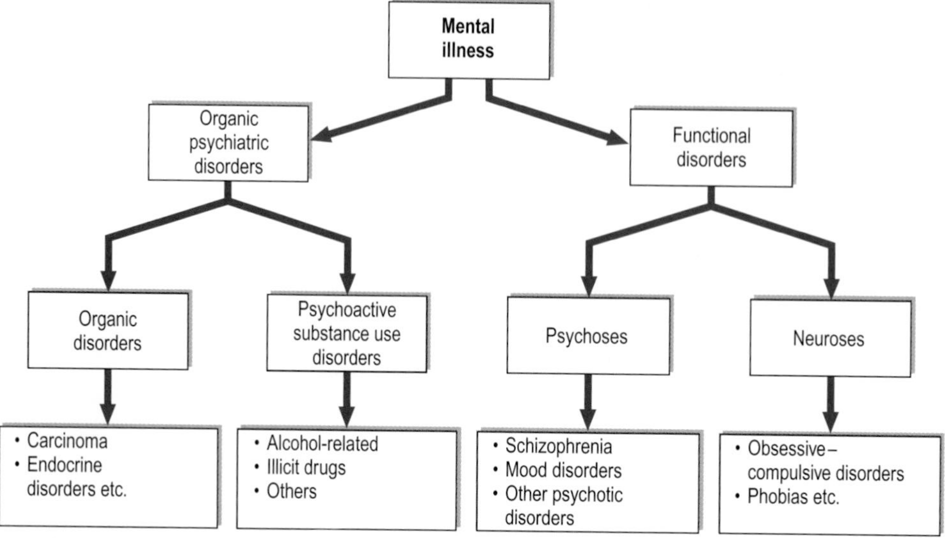

Figure 3.1 • Classification of psychiatric disorders.

Similarly, most normal people will have rechecked something once or twice, for example that their front door is locked or that they have switched off the iron. In the more severe neurotic counterpart of this, obsessive–compulsive disorder, rechecking may occur repeatedly many times.

Diagnostic hierarchy

Figure 3.2 shows the diagnostic hierarchy used for the above types of disorder. The highest level in this hierarchy takes precedence over those below it when a diagnosis is being made. For example, if an otherwise well patient presents with symptoms seen in acute schizophrenia, which turn out to be secondary to intravenous amphetamine abuse, then the diagnosis is psychoactive substance use disorder and not schizophrenia. Similarly, if a patient with chronic schizophrenia has depressive symptoms, the diagnosis is schizophrenia rather than a mood disorder.

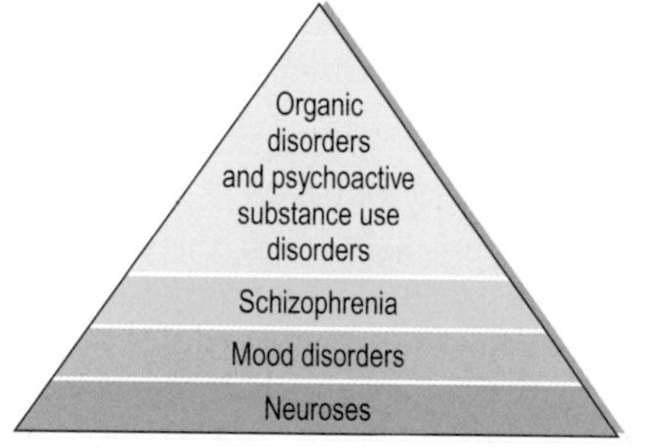

Figure 3.2 • Diagnostic hierarchy. • A given diagnosis takes precedence over those below it.

Developmental and behavioural disorders

There are a number of developmental and behavioural disorders that are not usually classed under the organic psychiatric disorders, psychoses or neuroses. These include personality disorders, learning disability (mental retardation), eating disorders and psychosexual disorders. It is possible to see both a developmental or behavioural disorder and an organic, psychotic or neurotic disorder in the same patient. In such cases both diagnoses are given. For example, a patient with a personality disorder may also suffer from a depressive disorder. A patient with a learning disability may in addition suffer from schizophrenia.

ICD-10

The International Classification of Diseases (ICD) of the World Health Organization (WHO) contains clinical descriptions and diagnostic guidelines for psychiatric disorders. In 1992 the WHO published the 10th revision of the ICD, named ICD-10. For each psychiatric disorder, ICD-10 provides a description of the main clinical features, associated features, and usually also diagnostic guidelines. A supplement for providing diagnostic criteria for research is also available, which gives more structured ('operationally defined') criteria for psychiatric diagnoses. Reference is made to ICD-10 diagnoses throughout this book, and the appendix contains a summary of the ICD-10 classification.

DSM-IV-TR/DSM-5

DSM-IV refers to the 4th edition of the Diagnostic and Statistical Manual of Mental Disorders, published by the American Psychiatric Association in 1994. The text accompanying the classification was published in revised form in 2000, giving the Diagnostic and Statistical Manual of Mental Disorders, 4th edition, Text Revision (DSM-IV-TR). DSM IV-TR is a multiaxial classification system. A multiaxial evaluation entails the assessment of each patient on several axes, each of which refers to a different class of information, such as the psychiatric disorder, a description of personality features, physical disorders and the severity of any psychosocial stressors. Although primarily intended for use in the USA, the previous versions of DSM – DSM-III (1983) and DSM-III-R (1987) – have been used in many other countries. This is partly because, unlike the ICD, they gave operational definitions for diagnoses, so making them very useful in research.

The next edition of the DSM will be named DSM-5 and is due to be published in 2013.

Aetiology

In this section a chronological classification of causes of psychiatric disorders is first outlined, followed by a description of individual causes.

Chronological classification

A psychiatric disorder in a single patient can have multiple causes. These can usefully be classified chronologically into predisposing, precipitating and perpetuating factors for a given patient (Figure 3.3).

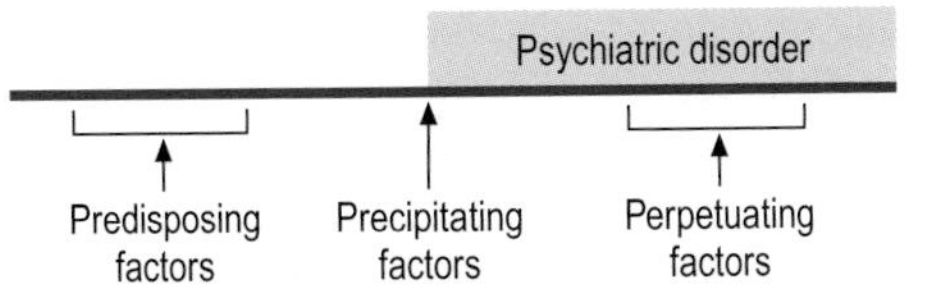

Figure 3.3 • Chronological classification of causes of psychiatric disorders.

Classification

- Organic disorders and psychoactive substance-use disorders take precedence over all other diagnostic classes.
- Psychoses are severe psychiatric disorders in which there is loss of contact with reality.
- Neuroses are less severe psychiatric disorders, which are understandable and with which it is possible to empathize.
- Psychoses take precedence diagnostically over neuroses, with schizophrenia taking precedence over mood disorders.
- The above disorders can occur in the presence of developmental and behavioural disorders.
- ICD-10 is the international classification of the WHO.
- DSM-IV-TR/DSM-5 is an American classification of psychiatric disorders that is multiaxial and highly structured.

- *Predisposing factors* are those predisposing a person to being vulnerable to suffering from a psychiatric disorder. Examples include the person's genetic makeup and personality, and obstetric complications.
- *Precipitating factors* are those arising just before a psychiatric disorder starts and which appear to have precipitated it. Examples include life events, such as the death of a parent.
- *Perpetuating factors* are those causing an existing psychiatric disorder to continue. An example is social withdrawal, which itself is often a result of psychiatric disorders (such as depression and schizophrenia).

Individual causes

Psychiatric disorders usually have a multifactorial aetiology. Some individual causes include:

- genetic
- biochemical and neurotransmitter changes
- psychoneuroendocrinological
- psychoimmunological
- electrophysiological
- neuropathological and neuroanatomical
- prenatal and perinatal factors
- infections
- psychosocial stressors

- personality
- psychological
- psychodynamic.

Note that in some cases, for example biochemical and endocrine factors, the changes may contribute to symptoms of the psychiatric disorder and/or may also be secondary to the disorder itself. Further details of the biopsychosocial approach are given in Chapters 1 and 2.

Genetic causes play an important role in many psychiatric disorders, including schizophrenia, mood disorders, Huntington's disease and a number of individual causes of learning disability such as Down's syndrome.

For some disorders caused by chromosomal abnormalities, such as Down's syndrome, the abnormalities can be determined directly by *karyotyping*.

In the case of Huntington's disease, the genetic cause is an increased number of CAG repeats at a locus on chromosome 4p16. Therefore, patients with this disorder, and indeed also presymptomatic gene-positive subjects, can be identified by measuring the CAG triplet repeat number at this genetic locus.

Studies in *molecular genetics* aim to characterize causative genes (as was successfully managed in the case of Huntington's disease in 1993).

For many psychiatric disorders, the main causative or contributing genes are not currently known. In such cases, the role of genetic factors can be investigated through family studies, twin studies, adoption studies and studies in molecular genetics. Consider the case of a psychiatric disorder in which genetic factors play an important part. In such a case, *family studies* are likely to show that the lifetime risk for developing the disorder is greater in the biological relatives of an affected individual, or *proband*, than in the general population. Moreover, the risk is likely to be greater in first-degree relatives, such as full siblings and parents (who have on average 50% of the genome in common with the proband), than in second-degree relatives, such as aunts and uncles (who share 25% of the genome, on average, with the proband). In the case of twins, *twin studies* would be likely to show that when one twin has the disorder, then the rate of concurrence (the *concordance rate*) of the disorder in the sibling twin (or *co-twin*) is greater if the twins are monozygotic (identical) than if they are dizygotic (fraternal). This is because monozygotic twins are genetically identical, whereas dizygotic twins are simply first-degree relatives sharing, on average, 50% of the genome.

Adoption studies look at the rates of occurrence of the disorder in the children of affected biological parents, when these children have been brought up by adoptive parents who either do or do not suffer from the disorder. (Other variants of adoption studies, such as looking at the rate of illness in the children of unaffected biological parents brought up by affected adoptive parents can also be carried out.)

An important cause of some psychiatric symptoms is *epilepsy*, particularly that affecting the temporal lobe (complex partial seizures of the temporal lobe or temporal lobe epilepsy). For example, complex partial seizures can give rise to features typical of schizophrenia.

Prenatal infection can affect the developing brain *in utero* and may cause or predispose an individual to certain psychiatric disorders, such as learning disabilities and possibly schizophrenia, (similarly with *perinatal head injury* during a prolonged forceps delivery, for example, and *prolonged hypoxia*).

Major *stressful events* are sometimes associated with the onset of psychiatric disorders. Examples include marriage, divorce, the death of a loved one and losing one's job. They are known as *life events*. Another psychosocial stressor that can be important is *migration*.

Long-term unemployment can lead to low morale, poor self-esteem, social isolation and depressed mood. These, in turn, can act as perpetuating factors not only for depression but also for other psychiatric disorders such as schizophrenia.

There is often a relationship between the incidence and prevalence of psychiatric disorders and *social class* and *marital status*. The direction of causality is not necessarily from social class to the disorder. In schizophrenia, for example, the disorder can lead to *social drift* downwards.

Psychological causes may play an important role in the development of certain psychiatric disorders, such as phobias and psychoactive substance use disorders, and in the development of modes of behaviour in pre-existing psychiatric disorders such as chronic schizophrenia and learning disabilities.

One important group of psychological causes involves *behavioural (learning) theory*. Learning can be defined as a relatively permanent change in behaviour brought about as a result of prior experience. It may occur through associations being made between two or more phenomena. Two forms of such *associative learning* are recognized: classical conditioning and operant conditioning. *Cognitive learning* is a more complex process in which current perceptions are interpreted in the context of previous information in order to solve unfamiliar problems. *Social learning theory* is based on evidence that learning can also take place through the observation and imitation of others (*modelling*).

Psychodynamic factors are concerned with unconscious processes that can lead to such psychiatric disorders as hysterical conversion disorders.

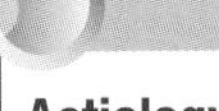

Aetiology

- Causes can be considered chronologically in terms of predisposing factors, precipitating factors and perpetuating factors.
- Genetic causes can be studied using karyotyping (for gross chromosomal changes), molecular genetic studies, family studies, twin studies and adoption studies.
- Complex partial seizures can cause psychiatric symptoms.
- Prenatal and perinatal causes include head injury during forceps delivery and hypoxia.
- Psychosocial stressors include life events and migration.
- Psychological causes can give rise to psychiatric disorders through associative learning and modelling.
- Psychodynamic causes arise from unconscious processes.

Management

When considering the management of a new patient, it is important to determine whether this should take place in the community or in an inpatient setting. The types of treatment available can be considered to fall into the following three groups: physical, psychological and psychosocial. Forms of treatment from these three groups are not mutually exclusive for any given patient. Rather, an integrated approach, in the setting of the multidisciplinary team approach, is required.

Hospitalization

Most patients with psychiatric disorders can be assessed and managed as outpatients. However, there are cases in which hospitalization is necessary. Such cases include first episodes of disorders such as schizophrenia in which appropriate investigations need to be carried out. Hospitalization is also necessary when the patient's life is at risk, for example because of suicidal thoughts in depression and schizophrenia, and in cases of severe weight and electrolyte loss in anorexia nervosa. In some cases compulsory admission may be necessary under the appropriate mental health legislation.

For patients who are recovering from a psychiatric disorder and who require some help during the day, but who do not need full inpatient care, day hospital places can be used. Day patients attend a particular ward on an agreed number of days each week, enabling monitoring of their mental state and response to medication. Day patients are often offered therapeutic activities such as occupational therapy.

The most appropriate setting for the management of individual disorders is given in the corresponding chapters later in this book.

Physical treatments

The most important type of physical treatment currently in use is *pharmacotherapy* (drug treatment). Individual classes of the most widely used psychotropic drugs are considered in this section. This is followed by details of other types of physical treatment.

Antipsychotic drugs (neuroleptics)

Antipsychotic drugs are also called neuroleptics. Their main uses are in the treatment of schizophrenia, the acute symptoms of mania and psychotic symptoms resulting from organic disorders and psychoactive substance use. Figure 3.4 shows a classification of some of the main antipsychotic drugs according to whether they are typical (conventional or first-generation) or atypical (second-generation).

Typical or first-generation antipsychotics

These block postsynaptic dopamine D_2 receptors in the central nervous system. The main central dopaminergic systems are the:

- mesolimbic system
- tuberoinfundibular system
- nigrostriatal system
- retinal pathways.

The *antidopaminergic action* on the mesolimbic system is the effect required, as this is thought to be largely responsible for the antipsychotic activity of the typical antipsychotics.

The antidopaminergic action on the tuberoinfundibular system results in unwanted hormonal side-effects. Dopamine is prolactin inhibitory factor, so typical antipsychotics cause *hyperprolactinaemia*. This, in turn, results in galactorrhoea, gynaecomastia, menstrual disturbances, reduced sperm count and reduced libido.

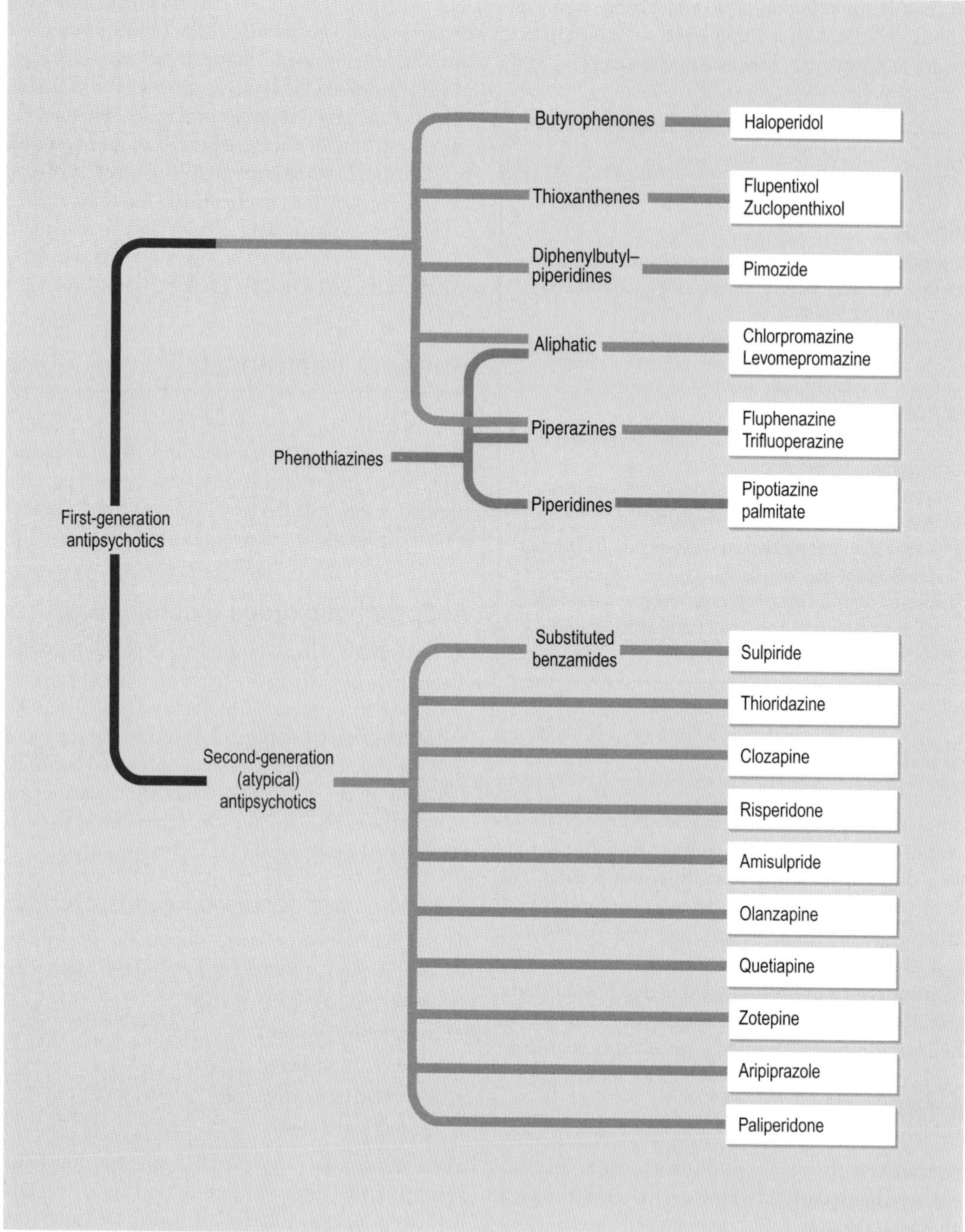

Figure 3.4 • Types of antipsychotic drugs.

The antidopaminergic action on the nigrostriatal system results in the following unwanted *extrapyramidal side-effects*:

- parkinsonism
- dystonias
- akathisia
- tardive dyskinesia.

Details of these drug-induced movement disorders are given in Chapter 8.

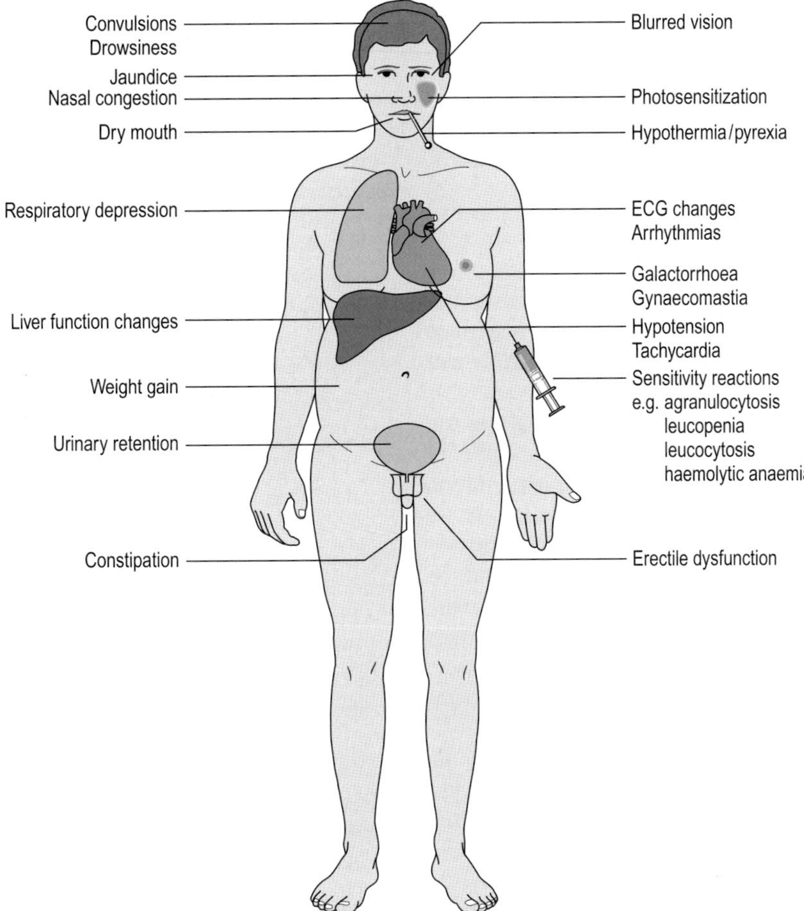

Figure 3.5 • Side-effects of chlorpromazine. • Effects are not shown (see text).

Other side-effects of *chlorpromazine*, the archetypal antipsychotic, are shown in Figure 3.5. Most of these side-effects also occur, in varying degrees, with other typical (first-generation) antipsychotics. Many of these side-effects are the result of antagonist action on the following neurotransmitters:

- dopamine
- acetylcholine (muscarinic receptors)
- adrenaline/noradrenaline
- histamine.

The effects of the central antidopaminergic actions have been mentioned above. Peripheral *antimuscarinic* (anticholinergic) symptoms include:

- dry mouth
- blurred vision
- urinary retention
- nasal congestion
- constipation.

Central antimuscarinic actions can lead to convulsions and pyrexia. *Antiadrenergic* effects include postural hypotension and failure of ejaculation. Drowsiness is an *antihistaminic* effect.

The most serious unwanted action of antipsychotics is a rare but potentially fatal toxic delirious state called the *neuroleptic malignant syndrome*. It is characterized by:

- autonomic dysfunction: hyperthermia; tachycardia; labile blood pressure; pallor; sweating
- fluctuating level of consciousness
- muscular rigidity
- urinary incontinence

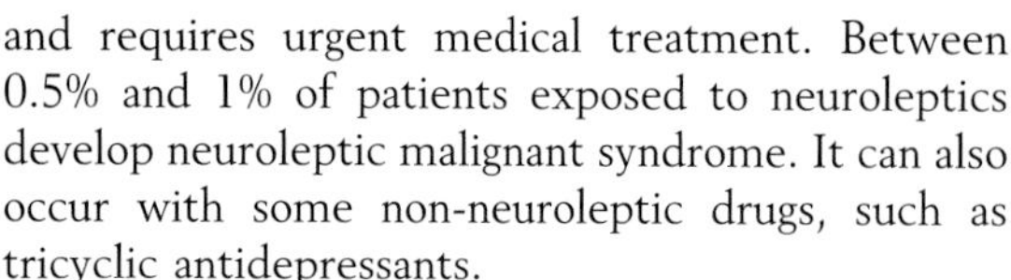

and requires urgent medical treatment. Between 0.5% and 1% of patients exposed to neuroleptics develop neuroleptic malignant syndrome. It can also occur with some non-neuroleptic drugs, such as tricyclic antidepressants.

Laboratory investigations commonly, but not always, show:

- increased serum creatinine kinase
- increased white blood cell count.

Chlorpromazine can also lead to photosensitivity. Patients should be warned about this and may need to be offered a topical preparation to block ultraviolet light, especially on sunny days.

Long-term pharmacotherapy with high doses can lead to eye and skin changes, including opacities of the lens and cornea, and a purplish pigmentation of the skin, conjunctiva, cornea and retina.

Typical antipsychotics are available in the form of slow-release *depot* preparations. These should be administered by deep intramuscular injection, usually at intervals of two to eight weeks. Their advantage over the oral forms is one of improved compliance. Examples of commonly administered depot preparations are given in Table 3.1.

Owing to their sedative side-effects, patients on typical antipsychotics, particularly phenothiazines, should, in general, be advised not to drive. (In Britain, the Driver and Vehicle Licensing Agency requires that: 'Drugs having anticholinergic side-effects should be avoided in drivers. These include tricyclic antidepressants and phenothiazines.')

Atypical or second-generation antipsychotics

Atypical or second-generation antipsychotics (see Figure 3.4) have a lower propensity to cause extrapyramidal symptoms (although, in general, they do have potential to cause tardive dyskinesia). This results from the fact that their primary action is not dopaminergic D_2 receptor blockade, although most do bind to these receptors. Instead, they have a greater action than typical antipsychotics on other receptors, such as other dopaminergic receptors and serotonergic (5-HT) receptors. As with typical antipsychotics, neuroleptic malignant syndrome can occur with atypical antipsychotic treatment.

The archetypal atypical antipsychotic is *clozapine*, which has a higher potency than typical antipsychotics on 5-HT_2, D_4, D_1, muscarinic and α-adrenergic receptors. Important side-effects of clozapine are neutropenia and potentially fatal agranulocytosis. As a result, patients taking this medication must undergo regular haematological monitoring. This should be weekly for the first 18 weeks and then at least fortnightly during the first year of treatment. After one year, if treatment with clozapine is continued and the blood count is stable, the haematological monitoring should be at least four-weekly. It should also be carried out four weeks after discontinuation. Clozapine treatment should be withdrawn permanently if the leucocyte count falls below 3000 mm^{-3} or the absolute neutrophil count falls below 1500 mm^{-3}. Other side-effects are given in Table 3.2 and also include hypersalivation, ECG changes, impaired temperature regulation and hypertension.

The atypical antipsychotic *risperidone* is indicated for psychoses in which both positive and negative symptoms (see Chapter 8) are prominent. Risperidone is an antagonist at 5-HT_{2A}, 5-HT_7, D_2, α_1- and α_2-adrenergic and histamine H_1 receptors, but not at cholinergic receptors. Side-effects are shown in Table 3.2 and also include gastrointestinal disturbances and hyperprolactinaemia (which may be associated with galactorrhoea, menstrual cycle changes, amenorrhoea and gynaecomastia). In order to avoid

Table 3.1 Commonly administered antipsychotic depot preparations

First-generation antipsychotics
Flupentixol decanoate
Fluphenazine decanoate
Haloperidol decanoate
Pipotiazine palmitate
Zuclopenthixol decanoate
Second-generation antipsychotics
Risperidone

Table 3.2 Side-effects of second-generation (atypical) antipsychotic drugs

Weight gain, dizziness, postural hypotension (particularly during initial dose titration)
Hyperglycaemia and possibly type 2 diabetes mellitus (particularly with clozapine, olanzapine and risperidone). Therefore, body mass and plasma glucose should be monitored regularly
Neuroleptic malignant syndrome may occur rarely

initial orthostatic hypotension, treatment should begin with a three-day escalating dose titration: usually 2 mg in one to two divided doses on the first day, followed by 4 mg in one to two divided doses on the second day, with the usual dose range of 4–6 mg daily being achieved on the third day; a slower titration may be appropriate in some patients. The atypical antipsychotic *paliperidone* is a metabolite of risperidone. Risperidone is the first second-generation (atypical) antipsychotic to be made available in the form of a long-acting depot injection (see Table 3.1).

The atypical antipsychotic *quetiapine* is indicated for the treatment of both positive and negative symptoms of schizophrenia. It has a higher affinity for cerebral 5-HT_2 receptors than for cerebral D_1 and D_2 receptors. It also has high affinity for histaminergic and α_1-adrenergic receptors, but not for cholinergic receptors. As it may cause QT interval prolongation, quetiapine should be used with caution in patients with cardiovascular disease. Other side-effects are outlined in Table 3.2.

The atypical antipsychotic *olanzapine* is effective in maintaining the clinical improvement during continuation therapy in patients who respond to initial treatment. Olanzapine has a similar structure to clozapine. It has a binding affinity to D_2 receptors that is less than that of typical antipsychotics but greater than that of clozapine. It is an antagonist at several 5-HT receptor subtypes (including 5-$HT_{2A/2C}$, 5-HT_3 and 5-HT_6), and α_1- and α_2-adrenergic, histamine H_1 and muscarinic receptors. Side-effects are given in Table 3.2.

The atypical antipsychotic *amisulpride* is indicated for the treatment of both positive and negative symptoms of schizophrenia. It is a highly selective antagonist at D_2 and D_3 receptors, and therefore produces mild extrapyramidal side-effects and hyperprolactinaemia, which may manifest as galactorrhoea, amenorrhoea, gynaecomastia, breast pain and sexual dysfunction. Other side-effects are given in Table 3.2.

Aripiprazole has high affinity for D_2 (as a partial agonist), D_3, 5-HT_{1A} (as a partial agonist) and 5-HT_{1B} receptors. Side-effects are given in Table 3.2.

Zotepine has a molecular structure similar to that of clozapine. It has high affinity for 5-HT_{2A} receptors. Before treatment and each time the dose of zotepine is increased, the patient's plasma electrolytes and ECG (to check for QT interval prolongation) should be monitored. Other side-effects are given in Table 3.2.

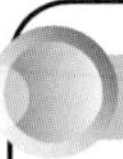

Antipsychotic drugs

- Antipsychotic drugs (neuroleptics) are used to treat schizophrenia, mania and psychotic states resulting from organic illnesses and psychoactive substance use.
- Typical (first-generation) antipsychotics (e.g. chlorpromazine, haloperidol and fluphenazine decanoate) block D_2 receptors and therefore affect central dopaminergic systems: they also block muscarinic, adrenergic and histaminergic receptors.
- Atypical (second-generation) antipsychotics (e.g. clozapine, amisulpride, aripiprazole, olanzapine, paliperidone, quetiapine, risperidone and zotepine) have a low propensity to cause extrapyramidal side-effects.
- Both typical and atypical antipsychotics may, rarely, cause the potentially fatal toxic delirious state neuroleptic malignant syndrome (hyperthermia, fluctuating level of consciousness, muscular rigidity and autonomic dysfunction).
- Compliance with antipsychotic treatment can be improved by using depot preparations.

Antimuscarinic drugs used in parkinsonism

When antipsychotic drug treatment causes parkinsonian symptoms, these may be amenable to treatment with antimuscarinic (anticholinergic) drugs (see Table 3.3).

Antimuscarinic drugs should not routinely be prescribed to patients being treated with typical antipsychotics. They should only be considered when such patients are affected by parkinsonism, because:

- not all patients develop parkinsonism while being treated with typical antipsychotics
- antimuscarinic drugs can clearly cause antimuscarinic side-effects
- antimuscarinic drugs can worsen tardive dyskinesia.

Table 3.3 Antimuscarinic drugs used in the treatment of parkinsonism resulting from pharmacotherapy with antipsychotics
Procyclidine
Trihexyphenidyl (benzhexol)
Orphenadrine

The use of these drugs is discussed further in Chapter 9.

One type of extrapyramidal side-effect of typical antipsychotics is an abnormal involuntary movement caused by slow and continuous muscle contraction or spasm. The collective name for such movements is *dystonias*. Types of acute drug-induced dystonic reactions include:

- tongue protrusion
- grimacing
- opisthotonos – involving most of the body
- torticollis – involving the neck
- oculogyric crisis – the eyes move superiorly and laterally.

The treatment for an acute dystonic reaction is the parenteral administration of an antimuscarinic (such as procyclidine).

Lithium

Lithium salts are used in the:

- prophylaxis of bipolar mood disorder
- treatment of mania/hypomania
- treatment of resistant depression
- prophylaxis of recurrent depression
- treatment of aggression
- treatment of self-mutilation.

The commonest lithium salts used in clinical psychiatry are lithium carbonate and lithium citrate. Lithium is simply a cation (Li^+), which is, therefore, not metabolized. It is excreted mainly by the kidneys. Therefore, before starting lithium therapy, the patient's renal function must be checked. In most patients this involves assessing the plasma urea, electrolytes and creatinine levels. However, if there is any suggestion of poor renal function, full renal function studies must be carried out.

Lithium has a low therapeutic index (the ratio of toxic dose to therapeutic dose). Therefore, regular monitoring of plasma lithium levels is required once a patient is started on lithium therapy. Plasma levels are estimated 8–12 hours after the preceding dose. The lithium dose is adjusted to achieve a lithium level of between 0.4 and 1.0 mmol L^{-1} for prophylactic purposes (the lower levels are required in the elderly). Plasma lithium concentrations are checked up to twice weekly when the drug is first started. In established maintenance lithium therapy, the frequency of plasma monitoring can be reduced to once every three months. Plasma urea, electrolytes and creatinine levels can be checked at the same time to monitor renal function. Thyroid function tests should be carried out every six months because thyroid function disturbances can result from long-term lithium treatment.

Side-effects are shown in Figure 3.6. Oedema should not be treated with diuretics because thiazide and loop diuretics reduce lithium excretion and so could cause lithium intoxication. Figure 3.7 shows signs of lithium intoxication. At plasma levels of above 2 mmol L^{-1} the following effects can occur:

- hyperreflexia and hyperextension of limbs
- toxic psychoses
- convulsions
- syncope
- oliguria

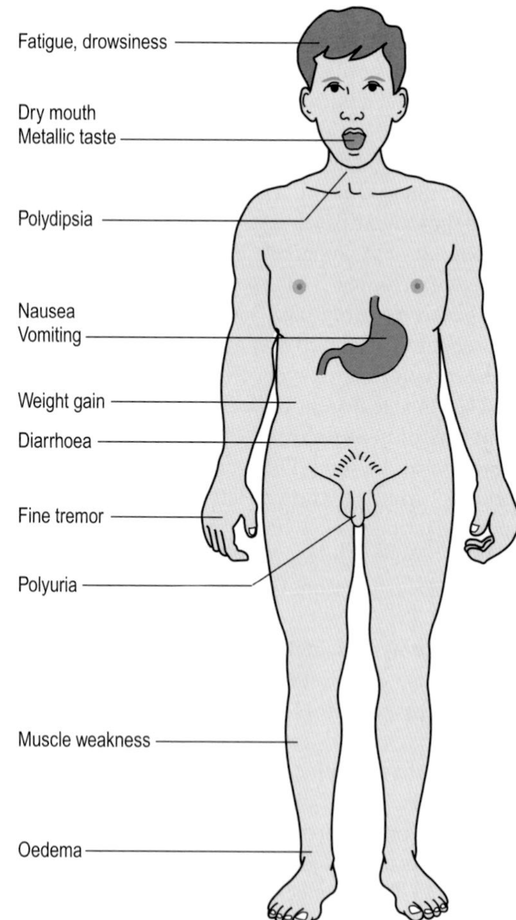

Figure 3.6 • Side-effects of lithium.

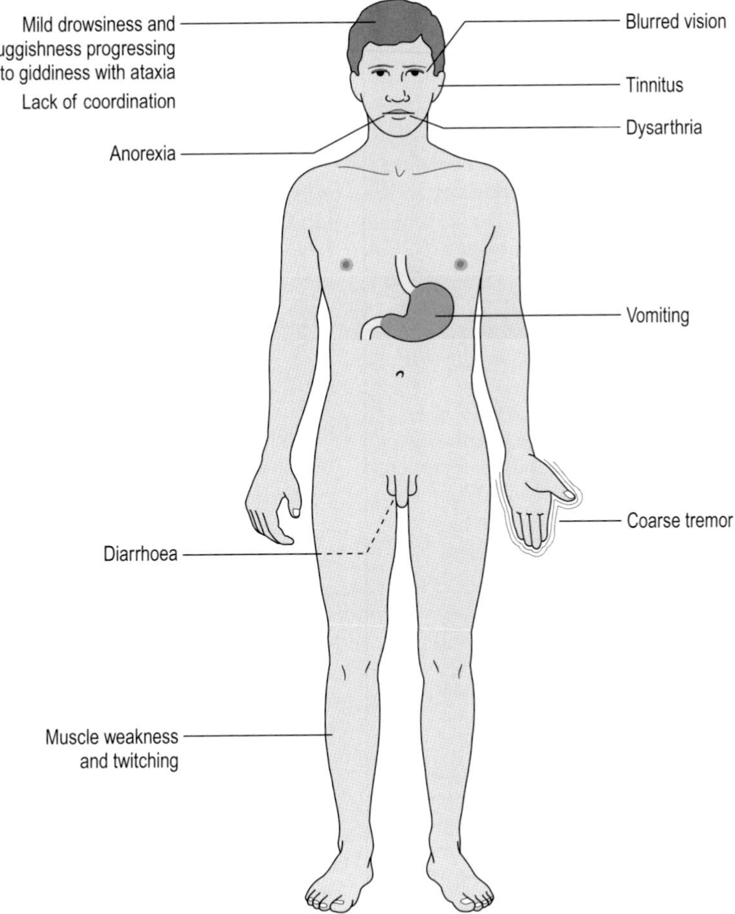

Figure 3.7 • Signs of lithium intoxication.

- circulatory failure
- coma
- death.

Side-effects following long-term treatment include:

- thyroid function disturbances
  - goitre
  - hypothyroidism
  - hyperthyroidism
- memory impairment
- nephrotoxicity
- cardiovascular changes
  - T wave flattening on the ECG
  - arrhythmias.

In view of these side-effects and the low therapeutic index, it is useful to give patients a *lithium card*. This describes the side-effects, how to take the medication and the need for regular blood checks. It is important to explain that an adequate fluid intake must be maintained. In hot weather, the patient should increase his fluid intake. Also, explain that dietary changes that may cause sodium intake alterations should be avoided.

Carbamazepine

Carbamazepine is used instead of, or in combination with, lithium in cases of:

- bipolar mood disorder resistant to lithium
- resistant mania
- resistant depression.

Carbamazepine is also used as an antiepileptic and in the treatment of the paroxysmal pain of trigeminal neuralgia. Carbamazepine may depress the white cell count and therefore regular monitoring of plasma carbamazepine levels is necessary.

Prophylaxis of bipolar mood disorder

- Lithium salts are used in the prophylaxis of bipolar mood disorder and recurrent depression, and in the treatment of (hypo)mania, resistant depression, aggression and self-mutilation.
- Before starting treatment with lithium, renal functioning must be checked (lithium is excreted by the kidneys).
- Once on lithium therapy, regular monitoring is required of the lithium level and renal and thyroid function.
- Signs of lithium intoxication include blurred vision, anorexia, vomiting, diarrhoea, muscle weakness, drowsiness and sluggishness, giddiness with ataxia, coarse tremor, lack of coordination and dysarthria.
- Lithium overdosage leads to hyperreflexia and hyperextension of the limbs, toxic psychoses, convulsions, syncope, oliguria, circulatory failure, coma and death.
- Side-effects following long-term lithium treatment include thyroid function disturbances, memory impairment, nephrotoxicity and cardiovascular changes.
- Carbamazepine, in addition to its use as an antiepileptic and in the treatment of the paroxysmal pain of trigeminal neuralgia, may be used instead of, or in combination with, lithium, in cases of bipolar mood disorder resistant to lithium, resistant mania, and resistant depression; regular monitoring of plasma carbamazepine levels is required as it may depress the white cell count.

Tricyclic antidepressants

Tricyclic antidepressants are used in the treatment of depression, obsessive–compulsive disorder, generalized anxiety disorder, panic disorder and phobic disorders. Owing to their antimuscarinic action, leading to urinary retention, they are also used in low doses in treating nocturnal enuresis (bedwetting) in children.

Some of the different types of tricyclic antidepressants are shown in Figure 3.8, which also shows other types of antidepressants. The two original tricyclic antidepressants – imipramine and amitripyline – are still used clinically. *Imipramine* is less sedating and therefore more useful in patients who are slowed down, withdrawn and apathetic. *Amitriptyline* is more sedating and therefore more useful in those who are agitated or anxious. In those who suffer from initial insomnia, the more sedating tricyclic antidepressants such as amitriptyline are often given as a night-time dose to aid the onset of sleep.

In the CNS, tricyclic antidepressants inhibit the reuptake of the monoamines noradrenaline and 5-HT. Therefore, these antidepressants are also called MARIs (monoamine reuptake inhibitors). *Clomipramine* is a more selective inhibitor of 5-HT reuptake. Obsessive–compulsive disorder is associated with brain changes in 5-HT; clomipramine is often used in the treatment of this disorder. (As discussed below, the SSRIs are even more selective in inhibiting 5-HT reuptake.)

The main side-effects of tricyclic antidepressants, when taken in therapeutic doses, are shown in Figure 3.9. Some of these side-effects are caused by an antimuscarinic action. The peripheral and central antimuscarinic side-effects include:

- dry mouth
- blurred vision
- constipation
- urinary retention
- sedation
- nausea.

Postural hypotension is an antiadrenergic effect. Another important cardiovascular side-effect is arrhythmias. Owing to these side-effects, the use of tricyclic antidepressants is contraindicated in patients who have suffered a recent myocardial infarction and in those who have heart block.

As tricyclic antidepressants may impair alertness and also potentiate the CNS depressant effects of alcohol, patients should be warned not to drive or operate machinery.

Tricyclic antidepressants are toxic in overdose, causing cardiac conduction defects, arrhythmias, convulsions, respiratory failure, coma and death. This is an unfortunate property of a class of drug prescribed for the treatment of depression. Indeed, many successful cases of suicide have resulted from patients taking an overdose of their prescriptions of tricyclic antidepressants. Moreover, the troublesome side-effects of these drugs at therapeutic doses, such as postural hypotension and antimuscarinic effects, often lead to poor compliance. The result is that depressed patients may have large amounts of unused tricyclic antidepressants, which can then be taken in one go if they wish to commit suicide. Fortunately, these side-effects and toxicity in overdose are not features of newer classes of antidepressants, such as the SSRIs, SNRIs, NARIs and NaSSAs (see below).

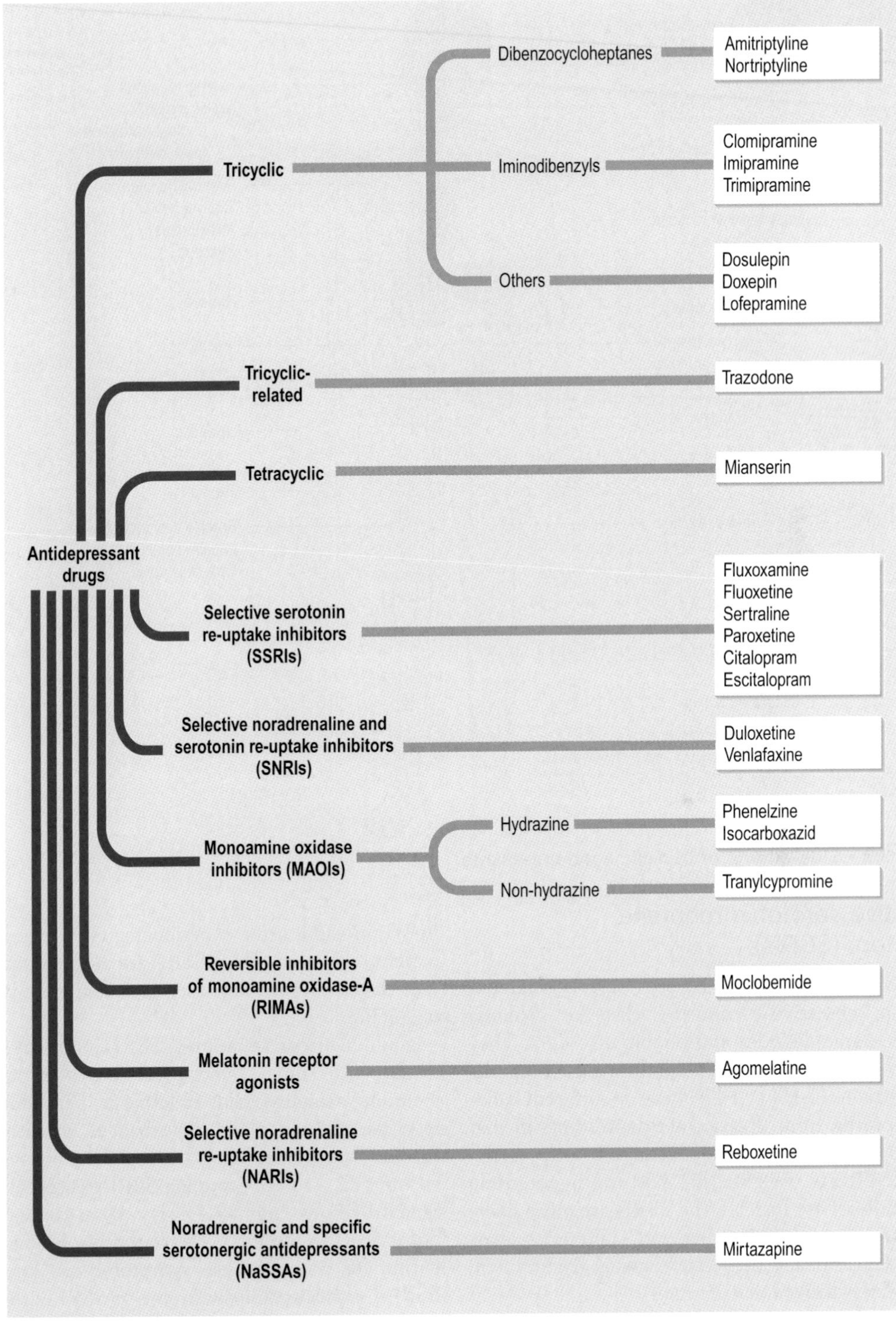

Figure 3.8 • Types of antidepressant drugs.

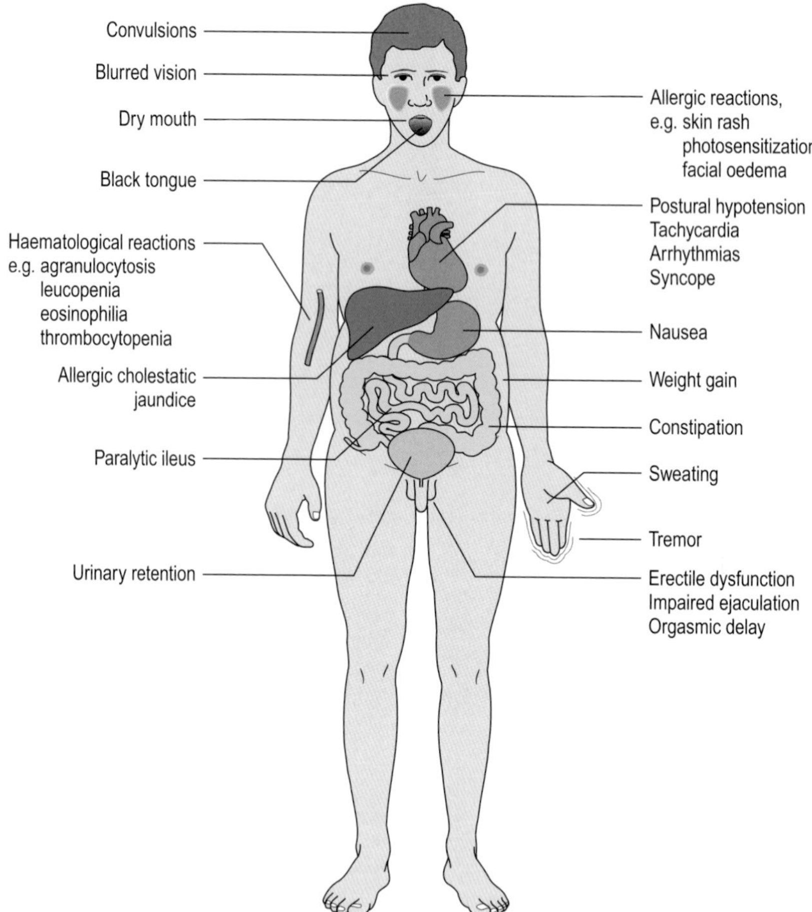

Figure 3.9 • Side-effects of tricyclic antidepressants.

Selective serotonin reuptake inhibitors (SSRIs)

The SSRIs (see Figure 3.8) are used to treat depression, obsessive–compulsive disorder, bulimia nervosa, panic disorder and phobic disorders. They act in the CNS by selectively inhibiting the reuptake of serotonin (5-HT). They have a different side-effect profile from tricyclic antidepressants in that SSRIs rarely cause significant sedation, antimuscarinic side-effects, weight gain, postural hypotension or cardiotoxicity. Instead, the SSRIs are more likely to cause nausea and vomiting, and, sometimes, diarrhoea. Occasionally they cause sexual dysfunction, particularly delayed ejaculation.

In overdose the SSRIs are safe. For example, in one case a patient swallowed the equivalent of approximately three months' supply of fluvoxamine and survived. Similarly, in another case, a patient is believed to have ingested 150 times the recommended dose of fluoxetine and, after experiencing two seizures, the patient recovered. Thus, SSRIs are a safer antidepressant than tricyclics to prescribe when there is a risk of suicide.

Sudden discontinuation of SSRI treatment is associated with somatic and psychological symptoms, including dizziness, nausea, lethargy, headache, anxiety, paraestheia, sleep disturbances, sweating and flu-like symptoms. They are usually mild and start within one week of stopping SSRI treatment. They tend to resolve spontaneously within three weeks, but if SSRI treatment is reinstated resolution occurs within 48 hours. These symptoms are known as SSRI discontinuation syndrome or SSRI withdrawal syndrome. Therefore, SSRI treatment should be withdrawn gradually. The dose can gradually be tapered over several weeks. (In general, it is good clinical practice to withdraw any antidepressant gradually rather than abruptly.)

Selective noradrenaline and serotonin reuptake inhibitors (SNRIs)

The SNRIs *duloxetine* and *venlafaxine* are indicated for the treatment of major depression and generalized anxiety disorder. SNRIs selectively inhibit reuptake of noradrenaline and serotonin in the brain. They might have better efficacy than the SSRIs in some cases. SNRIs have similar side-effects to the SSRIs.

Selective noradrenaline reuptake inhibitors (NARIs)

The NARI *reboxetine* is indicated for the treatment of major depression. NARIs selectively inhibit reuptake of noradrenaline in the brain. Side-effects include nausea, anorexia, insomnia, increased sweating, dizziness, vasodilation, postural hypotension, headache, chills, vertigo, paraesthesia, impotence, dysuria, urinary retention (mainly in men), dry mouth, constipation, palpitation and tachycardia. Reboxetine has a very low toxicity with a wide safety margin.

Noradrenergic and specific serotonergic antidepressant (NaSSA)

The NaSSA *mirtazapine* is indicated for the treatment of major depression. It is an antagonist at 5-HT_2 and 5-HT_3 receptors and central α_2-adrenoceptors. It increases central noradrenaline release by antagonizing inhibitory presynaptic α_2-adrenoceptors. It also increases serotonin release by both enhancing a facilitatory noradrenergic input to serotonergic cell bodies and antagonizing inhibitory presynaptic α_2-adrenoceptors on serotonergic neuronal terminals. Side-effects include increase in appetite and weight gain, and drowsiness and sedation (generally occurring during the first few weeks of treatment).

Mirtazapine is relatively safe, with no serious adverse effects being associated with overdose. Symptoms of acute overdosage are confined to prolonged sedation.

Agomelatine

Agomelatine acts as an agonist at melatonin MT1 and MT2 receptors, and also as a selective 5–HT_{2C} receptor antagonist. As indicated by its name, its molecular structure is close to that of melatonin. Agomelatine is indicated for major depression. Its more common side-effects include nausea, diarrhoea, constipation, abdominal pain and increased levels of serum transaminases. Liver function tests should be monitored before treatment and, initially, after six, 12 and 24 weeks of treatment. If serum transaminases are higher than three times the upper reference range limit, then agomelatine treatment should be discontinued.

Monoamine oxidase inhibitors (MAOIs)

The MAOIs (see Figure 3.8) are used less often these days than in the past. One reason for this is that they interact dangerously with tyramine-containing foods (see below). Another reason is that tricyclic, tricyclic-related and tetracyclic antidepressants should not be given until at least two weeks have elapsed after stopping a MAOI. It is therefore easier to give a MAOI to a patient who has first been found to be resistant to a tricyclic antidepressant. In the case of a SSRI or related antidepressant (such as a NARI, SNRI or NaSSA), two weeks must also elapse after stopping a MAOI before a SSRI can be started. However, for a patient first treated with an SSRI, the length of time that must elapse after stopping the SSRI before a MAOI can be started varies from two weeks to, in the case of fluoxetine, five weeks.

The main uses nowadays of MAOIs are in the treatment of:

- depression refractory to treatment with other antidepressants
- depression with severe anxiety, atypical, hypochondriacal or hysterical features
- phobic disorders with atypical, hypochondriacal or hysterical features
- agoraphobia
- obsessive–compulsive disorder.

MAOIs act by inhibiting the metabolic degradation of monoamines by monoamine oxidase. The inhibition of the peripheral metabolism of pressor amines, particularly dietary tyramine, can lead to a hypertensive crisis (the 'cheese reaction') in patients being treated with MAOIs who eat foodstuffs rich in tyramine. Examples of foods that should, therefore, be avoided are given in Table 3.4. Indirectly acting sympathomimetic amines such as amphetamine, ephedrine, fenfluramine and phenylpropanolamine must be avoided. Sympathomimetics are also present in many cough mixtures and nasal decongestants available without prescription; these must also be avoided. L-Dopa and pethidine must also be avoided. Tricyclic antidepressants can also interact dangerously with MAOIs; for example, deaths have resulted from the combination of tranylcypromine with clomipramine.

Table 3.4 Foods that may interact with MAOIs

Table 3.4 Foods that may interact with MAOIs
Cheese (*except* cottage cheese and cream cheese)
Meat extracts and yeast extracts (e.g. Bovril, Marmite, Oxo)
Alcohol (particularly Chianti, fortified wines and beer)
Non-fresh fish, meat or poultry (e.g. seasoned game)
Offal
Avocado
Banana skins
Broad bean pods
Caviar
Herring (pickled or smoked)

Although it is good practice always to check drug interactions before prescribing any medication, this is particularly important in the case of MAOIs. MAOI treatment cards listing precautions that need to be taken should be given to patients by the prescribing doctor or dispensing pharmacy.

After stopping MAOI treatment, at least two weeks should elapse before it is safe to take any of the forbidden foodstuffs and medicines.

Other side-effects include antimuscarinic actions, hepatotoxicity, appetite stimulation and weight gain. Tranylcypromine may cause dependency.

Overdosage is extremely serious and should lead to immediate hospitalization. Death may not occur immediately following the overdose. For example, symptoms and signs may be absent or minimal during the initial 12-hour period following ingestion of an overdose of phenelzine.

Reversible inhibitor of monoamine oxidase-A (RIMA)

In the CNS, type A monoamine oxidase (MAO-A) acts on noradrenaline, serotonin, dopamine and tyramine, whereas type B MAO (MAO-B) acts on dopamine, tyramine, phenylethylamine and benzylamine (Figure 3.10). The RIMA *moclobemide* is a selective and reversible inhibitor of MAO-A. Therefore, it acts preferentially to reduce the metabolism by MAO of the monoamines noradrenaline and serotonin, which are implicated in depression. As its inhibition is reversible, moclobemide can be displaced by other substances, such as tyramine, and therefore it is much less likely to cause a food or drug interaction

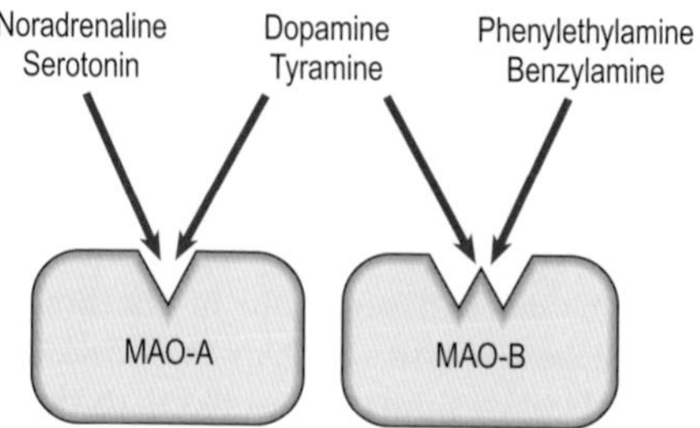

Figure 3.10 • Metabolism of monoamines by MAO-A and MAO-B.

leading to a hypertensive crisis. In contrast, conventional MAOIs are irreversible inhibitors of MAO-A and MAO-B. This is shown diagrammatically in Figures 3.11 and 3.12. (Because the inhibition is irreversible, after stopping MAOI treatment the synthesis of new MAO has to be awaited before it is safe to take forbidden foodstuffs and medicines; this is not the case with a RIMA.) A few patients may be

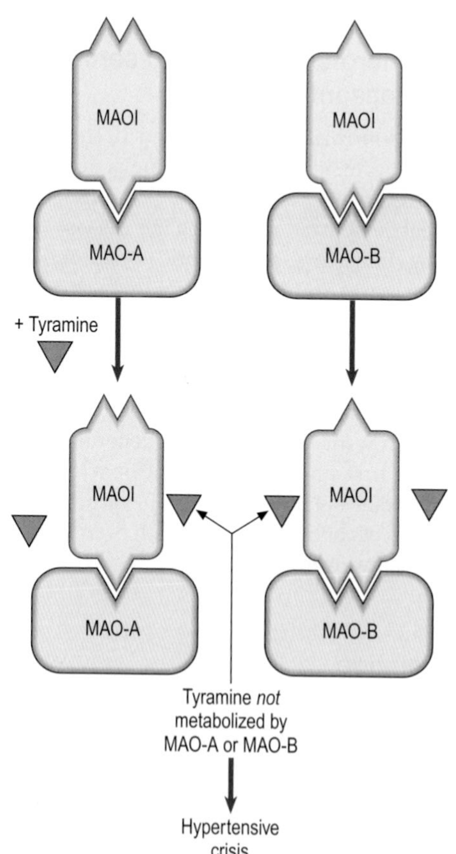

Figure 3.11 • Non-selective and irreversible inhibition of MAO-A and MAO-B by MAOIs.

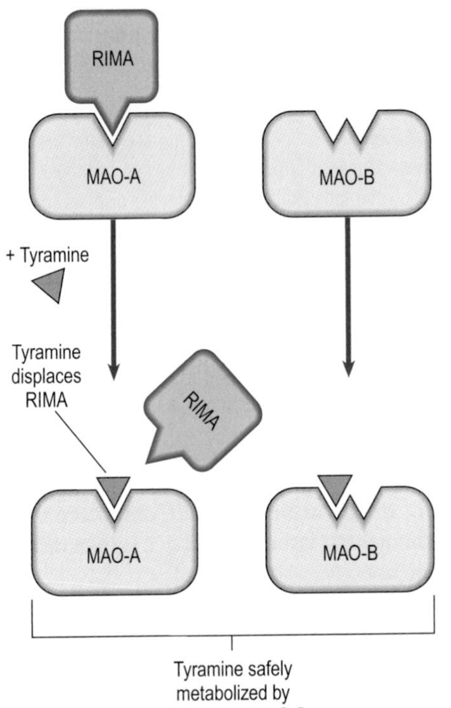

Figure 3.12 • Selective and reversible inhibition of MAO-A by RIMAs.

especially sensitive to tyramine and, therefore, all patients are advised not to consume large quantities of tyramine-rich foodstuffs in one go (see Table 3.4). Similarly, the medicines avoided by patients taking MAOIs are also generally avoided in those taking moclobemide.

The indications of moclobemide are depressive illness and social anxiety disorder.

Antidepressants

- Antidepressants are mainly used to treat depression, obsessive–compulsive disorder, generalized anxiety disorder, panic disorder, phobic disorders and, in certain cases, nocturnal enuresis (tricyclic antidepressants) and bulimia nervosa (fluoxetine).
- Tricyclic antidepressants (e.g. amitriptyline, imipramine, clomipramine and dosulepin (dothiepin)) act as monoamine reuptake inhibitors and cause numerous side-effects; they are potentially fatal in overdose.
- SSRIs (fluvoxamine, fluoxetine, paroxetine, sertraline, citalopram and escitalopram) selectively inhibit the

Antidepressants—cont'd

reuptake of serotonin and may cause gastrointestinal side-effects and delayed orgasm; they are relatively safe in overdose.
- Like the SSRIs, the 5-HT_2 antagonist (nefazodone), SNRIs (venlafaxine and duloxetine), NARI (reboxetine), and NaSSA (mirtazapine) classes of antidepressant also cause fewer side-effects than tricyclic antidepressants, and are also relatively safe in overdose.
- Agomelatine acts as an agonist at melatonin MT1 and MT2 receptors, and also as a selective 5–HT_{2C} receptor antagonist.
- MAOIs (e.g. phenelzine and tranylcypromine) irreversibly inhibit the metabolic degradation of monoamines by binding irreversibly to MAO types A and B, and thereby can lead to a potentially fatal hypertensive crisis ('cheese reaction') owing to inhibition of the peripheral metabolism of pressor amines. Foods rich in tyramine, indirectly acting sympathomimetic amines, L-dopa and pethidine should all be avoided by patients taking MAOIs. MAOIs are potentially fatal in overdose.
- The RIMA moclobemide is a reversible inhibitor of MAO type A. It does not cause sexual dysfunction and is relatively safe in overdose.

Benzodiazepines

Benzodiazepines may be used for the short-term relief of anxiety or insomnia. Their use as anxiolytics and hypnotics has steadily declined since the 1980s. This is because patients can develop physical and/or pharmacological dependence and tolerance to their effects. A withdrawal syndrome (described below) may occur when trying to discontinue treatment. They are also used as anticonvulsants, muscle relaxants, as premedication in anaesthesia, in the immediate treatment of aggressive behaviour, and in the treatment of alcohol dependence.

Table 3.5 lists some commonly used benzodiazepines, divided according to the length of action. Those having a long action are likely to cause hangover-like effects if used as hypnotics. In contrast, those having a relatively short action are more likely to give rise to withdrawal effects.

Benzodiazepines bind to benzodiazepine receptors that are linked to γ-aminobutyric acid type A ($GABA_A$) receptors in a complex involving $GABA_A$ and benzodiazepine receptors and a chloride channel. (Binding of GABA to a postsynaptic $GABA_A$

Table 3.5 Examples of benzodiazepines

Long-acting	Short-acting
Alprazolam	Loprazolam
Chlordiazepoxide	Lorazepam
Diazepam	Lormetazepam
Flurazepam	Oxazepam
Nitrazepam	Temazepam

receptor leads to opening of the associated chloride channel, which, in turn, allows passage of chloride ions into the neurone and therefore hyperpolarization of the latter.)

A side-effect of all benzodiazepines is psychomotor impairment; the performance of complex tasks involving psychological and motor functioning, such as driving and operating machinery, may therefore be impaired. In general, it is safest to advise patients to avoid driving; as the Driver and Vehicle Licensing Agency in Britain has pointed out: 'Benzodiazepines are most dangerous, and are over-represented in drivers involved in road traffic accidents.'

If benzodiazepines are taken regularly for four weeks or more, dependence may develop. This manifests itself mainly as the occurrence of the benzodiazepine withdrawal syndrome when regular benzodiazepine intake is stopped suddenly, and by the occurrence of tolerance to the drug. The main features of the benzodiazepine withdrawal syndrome are:

- anxiety symptoms, e.g. palpitations, tremor, panic, dizziness, nausea, sweating, other somatic symptoms, depressed mood
- low mood
- abnormal experiences, e.g. depersonalization, derealization, hypersensitivity to sensations in all modalities, distorted perception of space, tinnitus, formication, a strange taste in the mouth
- influenza-like symptoms
- psychiatric/neurological symptoms, e.g. epileptic seizures, confusional states, psychotic episodes
- insomnia
- loss of appetite and weight.

The withdrawal from regular benzodiazepine use should be very gradual in order to avoid these effects. This should be explained carefully to the patient, who may benefit from counselling while withdrawal takes place. In order to avoid dependence on this group of drugs, in Britain the Committee on Safety of Medicines has issued the advice shown in Table 3.6 on their use.

Table 3.6 Advice on the prescribing of benzodiazepines issued by the Committee on Safety of Medicines (London)

Benzodiazepines are indicated for the short-term relief (2–4 weeks only) of anxiety that is severe, disabling or subjecting the individual to unacceptable distress, occurring alone or in association with insomnia or short-term psychosomatic, organic or psychotic illness
The use of benzodiazepines to treat short-term 'mild' anxiety is inappropriate and unsuitable
Benzodiazepines should be used to treat insomnia only when it is severe, disabling or subjecting the individual to extreme distress

The symptoms of a mild to moderate overdose are mainly an intensification of the therapeutic actions (sedation, muscle weakness and profound sleep) or paradoxical excitation. In most cases observation of vital functions is all that is required. Extreme overdosage, however, may cause coma, areflexia, cardiorespiratory depression and apnoea and, therefore, requires hospitalization.

Zopiclone, zolpidem, zaleplon

These (non-benzodiazepine) drugs are benzodiazepine agonists that bind to neuronal $GABA_A$ receptors. They are all indicated for short-term use in insomnia (up to four weeks in the case of zopiclone and zolpidem, and up to two weeks in the case of zaleplon).

Zopiclone is a cyclopyrrolone that has an elimination half-life of approximately five hours, and causes little or no hangover effect. Side-effects include a bitter or metallic taste. Overdose is usually manifested by varying degrees of CNS depression (from drowsiness to coma) related to the quantity of zopiclone ingested. Overdose should not be life-threatening unless combined with other CNS depressants (including alcohol). The benzodiazepine antagonist flumazenil may be a useful antidote in cases of overdose.

Zolpidem is an imidazopyridine that has an elimination half-life of around 2.4 hours, and causes little or no hangover effect. A dose relationship for some CNS and gastrointestinal side-effects may occur, most frequently in the elderly. The most common side-effects include drowsiness, dizziness, diarrhoea, headache, nausea and vomiting, vertigo and asthenia. Patients have fully recovered from zolpidem overdoses of up to 400 mg (40 times the recommended dose). Flumazenil may be a useful antidote in cases of overdose.

Zaleplon is a pyrazolopyrimidine that has an elimination half-life of approximately one hour, and so can be administered during the night (up to four hours before morning rising), without causing significant adverse effects on awakening in the morning. Side-effects include drowsiness, paraesthesia, dysmenorrhoea and amnesia.

Melatonin

The hormone melatonin is available for the short-term treatment of insomnia in those aged over 55 years. Reported side-effects include pharyngitis, back pain, headache and asthenia.

Buspirone

Buspirone is an azaspirodecanedione that is used in the short-term management of anxiety disorders and for the relief of anxiety symptoms with or without associated depressive symptoms. Unlike the benzodiazepines, buspirone does not cause dependence. It acts as a central 5-HT_{1A} partial agonist. Its main side-effects are dizziness, headache, lightheadedness, excitement and nausea. Buspirone appears to be relatively safe in overdose.

β-Adrenoceptor blocking drugs

β-Blockers (e.g. propranolol) act by blocking peripheral β-adrenoceptors, for example in the heart and peripheral vasculature. They are used rarely in psychiatry, for the treatment of anxiety symptoms – for example performance anxiety such as may occur in public speaking or in interviews. They do not directly help psychological symptoms of anxiety, such as worry, fear and tension.

Drugs used in alcohol dependence

Long-acting *benzodiazepines* (e.g. chlordiazepoxide and diazepam) and *clomethiazole* can be used in the management of alcohol withdrawal symptoms. A reducing regimen is administered to lessen withdrawal symptoms.

Disulfiram is used in prophylactic adjunctive pharmacotherapy to prevent alcohol intake in alcohol dependence. Disulfiram is taken regularly and causes acetaldehyde (ethanal) to accumulate in the body if alcohol (ethanol) is taken. The ingestion of even small amounts of alcohol (including that in, for example, aftershave lotions) leads to very unpleasant systemic reactions including facial flushing, headache, palpitations, tachycardia, nausea and vomiting. Large amounts of alcohol can lead to air hunger, arrhythmias and severe hypotension. One of the difficulties with this treatment is that in the community patients may refuse to take the disulfiram in order to drink alcohol without suffering these unpleasant effects.

Acamprosate, in combination with counselling, may be used in the maintenance of abstinence in alcohol dependence. The recommended treatment period is 1 year. Treatment should be initiated as soon as possible after abstinence has been achieved (after the withdrawal period) and should be maintained if the patient relapses. However, continued alcohol abuse negates the therapeutic benefit of acamprosate. Side-effects tend to be mild and transient and are predominantly gastrointestinal (diarrhoea, nausea and vomiting, and abdominal pain) and dermatological (pruritus and maculopapular rash).

Drugs used in opioid dependence

Methadone, an opioid agonist, can be used to lessen withdrawal symptoms in opioid dependence by substituting for an opioid such as heroin (diamorphine). As methadone is itself dependency-forming it should only be used in those who are physically dependent on opioids. It should not be used during labour, as its prolonged duration of action increases the risk of neonatal respiratory depression. The ability to drive or operate machines may be severely affected during and after treatment. It also has the potential to increase intracranial pressure, particularly when it is already raised. Serious overdosage is a medical emergency, being characterized by respiratory depression, extreme somnolence progressing to stupor or coma, maximally constricted pupils, skeletal muscle flaccidity, cold and clammy skin, and sometimes bradycardia and hypotension.

Lofexidine is used for the alleviation of symptoms in patients undergoing opioid withdrawal. It appears to act centrally (on α-adrenergic receptors). As lofexidine may, therefore, have a sedative effect, affected patients should be advised not to drive or operate machinery. Other side-effects include dryness of mucous membranes (especially the mouth, throat and nose), hypotension and bradycardia.

Naltrexone is an opioid antagonist that is used as an adjunct to prevent relapse in detoxified formerly opioid-dependent patients (who have remained opioid-free for at least seven to ten days). Treatment should be initiated in a drug addiction centre under appropriate medical supervision. Naltrexone is extensively metabolized by the liver and should not be given to patients with acute hepatitis or liver failure. As it is not uncommon for opioid-abusing individuals to have impaired hepatic functioning, and as liver function test abnormalities have been reported in obese and elderly patients taking naltrexone who have no history of drug abuse, liver function tests should be carried out before and during treatment. Side-effects include difficulty in sleeping, anxiety, nervousness, abdominal pain or cramps, nausea and vomiting, low energy, joint and muscle pain, and headache.

Buprenorphine may be administered sublingually as an adjunct in the treatment of opioid dependence. It is an opioid that has both agonist and antagonist actions; it may precipitate withdrawal in patients dependent on high opioid doses owing to its partial antagonist properties – in such patients the daily opioid intake should be gradually reduced before administering buprenorphine. Side-effects include drowsiness, nausea and vomiting, dizziness, sweating and hypotension. Sublingual buprenorphine has a wide safety margin.

CNS stimulants

Caffeine is a CNS stimulant found in coffee, cola and tea (see Figure 7.9),which is not usually prescribed in clinical psychiatric practice

Methylphenidate is indicated as part of a comprehensive treatment programme for attention-deficit hyperactivity disorder (ADHD) when remedial measures alone prove insufficient. Treatment must be under the supervision of a specialist in childhood behavioural disorders. It has a stimulant effect on the CNS but its mode of action is not understood. Although it is licensed for use in children with ADHD, it should be borne in mind that methylphenidate, being related to the amphetamines, may retard growth; *height and weight should be monitored carefully* in children prescribed this drug.

Dexamfetamine is indicated for narcolepsy and also for children with refractory ADHD under the supervision of a physician specializing in child psychiatry. As in the case of methylphenidate, the amphetamine dexamfetamine may retard growth; height and weight should be monitored carefully in children prescribed this drug. Symptoms of overdosage include excitement, hallucinations, convulsions leading to coma, tachycardia and cardiac arrhythmias, and respiratory depression.

Atomoxetine is a non-stimulant indicated for ADHD (initiated by a specialist physician who is experienced in managing this disorder). Side-effects include anorexia, dry mouth, vomiting, constipation, dyspepsia, abdominal pain, flatulence, sleep disturbance, palpitation, tachycardia, hot flushes, lethargy, depression, aggression, hostility and psychotic symptoms.

Modafinil is used for the treatment of daytime sleepiness associated with narcolepsy, obstructive sleep apnoea and chronic shift work.

Cyproterone acetate

Cyproterone acetate is an antiandrogen, the actions of which are detailed in Figure 3.13.

It can be used to control the libido in severe hypersexuality and/or sexual deviation in the adult male. For example, it has been used in the control of adult males who repeatedly carry out paedophilic offences. However, its use in forensic psychiatry is controversial. It is also used in the treatment of patients with prostate cancer.

Side-effects include inhibition of spermatogenesis, tiredness, gynaecomastia, weight change, improvement of existing acne vulgaris (related to a reduction in sebum production), increased growth of scalp hair and female pattern of growth of pubic hair. As there

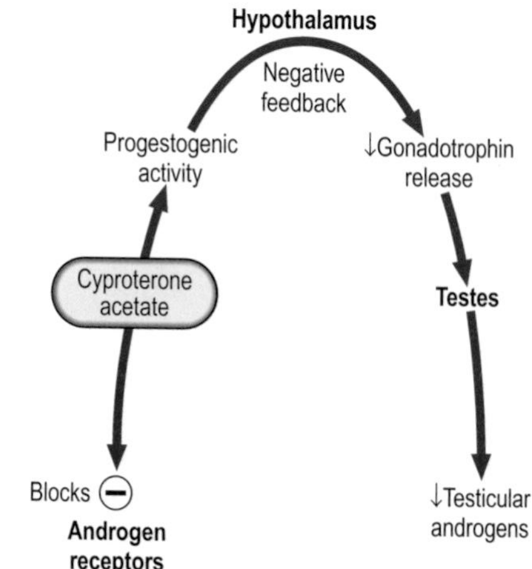

Figure 3.13 • Antiandrogen actions of cyproterone acetate.

is a theoretical risk to the liver, liver function tests should be carried out regularly. High-dose treatment may lead to dyspnoea.

Drugs to treat erectile dysfunction

Drugs that may be used for treating erectile dysfunction (after excluding treatable organic causes) include alprostadil (prostaglandin E_1) and phosphodiesterase type-5 inhibitors.

Alprostadil is administered by intracavernosal injection or intraurethral application. In addition to treating erectile dysfunction, it may also be used as a diagnostic test. Important side-effects include changes in blood pressure, penile pain and priapism, as well as reactions at the injection site.

The phosphodiesterase type-5 inhibitors *sildenafil*, *tadalafil* and *vardenafil* are orally administered. They enhance the action of nitric oxide on smooth muscle and increase penile blood flow. The more common side-effects include dyspepsia, headache, flushing, dizziness, visual disturbances, nasal congestion, nausea and vomiting. Headaches can include migraine. Treatment should be stopped if the patient complains of sudden visual impairment, as non-arteritic anterior ischaemic optic neuropathy has been reported. They should not be administered to those receiving nitrates. Other contraindications include recent stroke, myocardial infarction, systolic blood pressure $<$90 mmHg, unstable angina and a history of non-arteritic anterior ischaemic optic neuropathy. Sildenafil and vardenafil are also contraindicated in hereditary degenerative retinal disorders.

Drugs for dementia

Treatment with these drugs should be started and supervised by an experienced specialist in this area. Cognitive assessment is repeated at around three months and, if the patient is not responding, the drug should be discontinued. Many specialists repeat the cognitive assessment four to six weeks after discontinuation to confirm lack of deterioration. Acetylcholinesterase inhibitors may cause unwanted cholinergic side-effects.

Donepezil is a reversible acetylcholinesterase inhibitor, which is metabolized by the liver. Its indications are mild to moderate dementia in Alzheimer's disease. Common side-effects include nausea, vomiting, diarrhoea, fatigue, insomnia, headache, agitation, aggression and muscle cramps.

Rivastigmine is a reversible non-competitive acetylcholinesterase inhibitor (preferentially inhibiting acetylcholinesterase G1). Its indications are mild to moderate dementia in Alzheimer's disease and in Parkinson's disease. Side-effects include nausea, vomiting, diarrhoea, asthenia, anorexia, weight loss, abdominal pain, dizziness, agitation and drowsiness.

Galantamine is a reversible acetylcholinesterase inhibitor, which also allosterically modulates nicotinic receptors thereby potentiating their response to acetylcholine. It is a botanical alkaloid extracted from daffodil bulbs. Its indications are mild to moderate dementia in Alzheimer's disease. Common side-effects include nausea, vomiting, diarrhoea, abdominal pain, fatigue, sleep disturbance, headache and depression.

Memantine is a non-competitive NMDA antagonist affecting glutamate neurotransmission. Its indications are moderate to severe dementia in Alzheimer's disease. Common side-effects include constipation, hypertension, dizziness, drowsiness and headache.

Highly unsaturated fatty acids (HUFAs)

Certain HUFAs, such as the *n*-3 fatty acid eicosapentaenoic acid (EPA), may be of therapeutic benefit in a range of neuropsychiatric disorders including depression, Huntington's disease, schizophrenia and ADHD. Naturally occurring fatty acids such as EPA have the advantage that their side-effects are, in general, beneficial rather than adverse; they include, for example, beneficial actions on the cardiovascular system, skin, hair and joints.

Electroconvulsive therapy (ECT)

ECT involves the induction of fits by briefly electrically stimulating the brain. Its main indications include:

- major depression, e.g. when there are strong suicidal plans or the patient's life is threatened because of a refusal to eat and drink
- severe mania associated with life-threatening exhaustion or treatment resistance
- catatonia when treatment with lorazepam has been ineffective
- puerperal depressive illness (postpartum-onset major depressive episode).

It can work rapidly and effectively in the above cases. A course of ECT of around six fits is usually sufficient to cause remission of a severe depressive illness. The ECT is usually given twice per week. A patient receiving ECT in the morning should not eat or drink anything ('nil by mouth') before the ECT from midnight. Atropine and a muscle relaxant are given. The muscle relaxant prevents the body of the patient moving violently during the convulsion; otherwise there would be a risk of sustaining injury, such as a bone fracture. The atropine reduces secretions and prevents the muscarinic actions of the muscle relaxant. If there is any possibility that the patient may have low or atypical plasma pseudocholinesterase enzymes, the anaesthetist must be informed as this could lead to prolonged muscle paralysis with the muscle relaxant. The ECT is administered under a short-acting general anaesthetic, given by the anaesthetist. A bite is placed in the patient's mouth to prevent damage from biting during the convulsion.

There are two ways of administering ECT: bilateral and unilateral. *Bilateral ECT* is given by placing one electrode on each side of the skull at the points marked 'A' in Figure 3.14. ('A' is 4 cm perpendicular to the midpoint of the imaginary line joining the external angle of the orbit to the external auditory meatus.) *Unilateral ECT* is given by placing both electrodes on the side of the head containing the non-dominant cerebral hemisphere. In most right-handers the non-dominant hemisphere is the right one. In determining cerebral dominance, it is not sufficient simply to ask which hand the patient writes with. There are cases, for instance, of people who are naturally left-handed, but who write with the right hand because they were forced to do so in childhood. A handedness questionnaire or the way in which the patient holds a pen while writing will usually give an accurate indication of cerebral dominance. The electrode placements in unilateral ECT (usually given to the right side) are the points marked 'A' and 'B' in Figure 3.14. ('B' lies 10 cm away from 'A' and vertically above the external auditory meatus.) If unilateral ECT is accidentally given to the dominant side, the patient may appear very confused for at least five minutes afterwards. Furthermore, as Broca's area is in the dominant hemisphere, the patient may also suffer temporarily from dysphasia during this time. If these features are observed following unilateral ECT, from then onwards either the opposite side, or bilateral placement should be used; bilateral placement is used if cerebral dominance is uncertain.

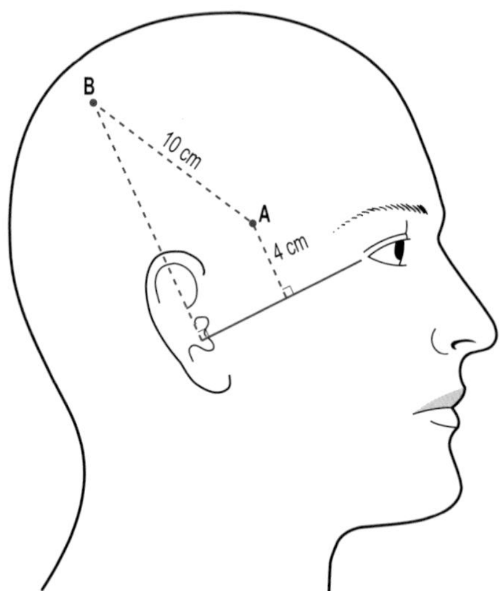

Figure 3.14 • Placement of electrodes during electroconvulsive therapy. • Point A is 4 cm perpendicular to the middle of the line joining the angle of the orbit to the external auditory meatus. Point B is 10 cm from A.

The mechanism of action of ECT is not known. Changes occurring during a course of ECT that might play a role include central neurotransmitter and receptor changes, release of hormones, and a change in the seizure threshold.

The main early side-effects of ECT are headache, temporary confusion and some loss of short-term memory. The loss of short-term memory is more marked after bilateral ECT. Depressed patients with bipolar mood (affective) disorder may become manic as a result of the treatment.

Contraindications include: increased intracranial pressure; recent cerebral infarction; severe cardiovascular disease; severe pulmonary disease; aneurysms and vascular malformations which may rupture during increased blood pressure; physical disorders that make anaesthesia risky, for example cardiac disease and chest infection.

Phototherapy

Phototherapy involves exposure to high-intensity light for patients suffering from seasonal affective disorder or SAD (see Chapter 9), in whom the onset of depression is in the autumn or winter months.

Sleep deprivation

Here, the patient may be fully deprived of sleep for at least one night or deprived of only rapid eye movement (REM) sleep. A variant involves altering the time at which the patient goes to sleep. The major indication is severe depressive episodes. It is thought that it leads to a change in the phase relationships of endogenous circadian rhythms that may be out of phase in severe depression.

Psychosurgery

Psychosurgery is the selective surgical removal or destruction of central neural tissue in order to influence behaviour. The cerebral tissue removed may be intrinsically normal. It is now used very rarely indeed. It is a last resort treatment, which is considered in certain disorders, such as chronic severe intractable depression and obsessive–compulsive disorder, when all other treatments have failed.

Stereotaxic lesions are made in a variety of ways, such as electrocautery, the implantation of radioactive yttrium and thermocoagulation. Specific operations have been used for different disorders; for example, frontal lobe lesions in chronic severe intractable depression and cingulotomy in chronic severe intractable obsessive–compulsive disorder.

Other physical treatments

- Benzodiazepines (e.g. diazepam, chlordiazepoxide and temazepam) are indicated for the short-term relief (two to four weeks only) of anxiety that is severe, disabling or subjecting the patient to unacceptable distress; they should be used to treat insomnia (short-term use only) only when it is similarly severe, disabling or subjecting the patient to unacceptable distress.
- The non-benzodiazepine drugs zopiclone, zolpidem and zaleplon are benzodiazepine agonists that are indicated for short-term use in insomnia.

  Melatonin is available for the short-term treatment of insomnia in those aged over 55 years.
- Buspirone, which acts as a central 5-HT_{1A} partial agonist, can be used in the short-term management of anxiety disorders and the relief of anxiety symptoms.
- Drugs used in alcohol dependence include long-acting benzodiazepines, clomethiazole, disulfiram and acamprosate (in combination with counselling).
- Drugs used in opioid dependence include methadone, lofexidine, naltrexone and buprenorphine.
- CNS stimulants may be used, under strict psychiatric supervision, for the treatment of ADHD (methylphenidate and dexamfetamine) and also in narcolepsy (dexamfetamine and modafinil). Atomoxetine is a non-stimulant indicated for ADHD.

Other physical treatments—cont'd

- Cyproterone acetate is an antiandrogen, which can be used to control the libido in severe hypersexuality and/or sexual deviation in the adult male.
- Drugs that may be used for treating erectile dysfunction (after excluding treatable organic causes) include alprostadil (prostaglandin E_1) and the phosphodiesterase type-5 inhibitors sildenafil, tadalafil and vardenafil.
- The anticholinesterase inhibitors donepezil, rivastigmine and galantamine may be used for cognitive enhancement in mild to moderate Alzheimer's disease; the NMDA antagonist memantine may be used for cognitive enhancement in moderate to severe Alzheimer's disease.
- Certain HUFAs, e.g. EPA, may be of therapeutic benefit in a range of neuropsychiatric disorders including depression, Huntington's disease, schizophrenia and ADHD.
- Other physical treatments include:
  - ECT
  - phototherapy (for treating SAD)
  - sleep deprivation
  - psychosurgery.

Psychological treatments

Psychotherapy is a form of giving help, which differs from informal help, such as guidance and advice from friends, in that:

- the help is given by a person (the therapist) who is specially trained
- the therapy is administered within a theoretical framework.

Various forms of psychotherapy are available, and some of these are now outlined.

Behaviour therapy

Behaviour (or behavioural) therapy is a brief, goal-directed psychological treatment that deals with the current features of the disorder, rather than considering its previous development. It is based on behavioural learning theory, which, in turn, is based on classical and operant conditioning. A continuing objective assessment of the patient's progress is made. Examples of the use of behaviour therapy follow.

Phobic disorders can be treated by *systematic desensitization*. The patient is exposed, in a graded way, to the phobic stimulus. This is coupled with anxiety management in the form of *relaxation training*. The graded exposure can take place in reality or in the patient's imagination. Figure 3.15 shows an example of how a simple phobia – fear of spiders (arachnophobia) – may be treated.

An alternative way of treating phobic disorders is by *flooding*, in which the patient is subjected to the phobic stimulus all at once, and not in a graded way.

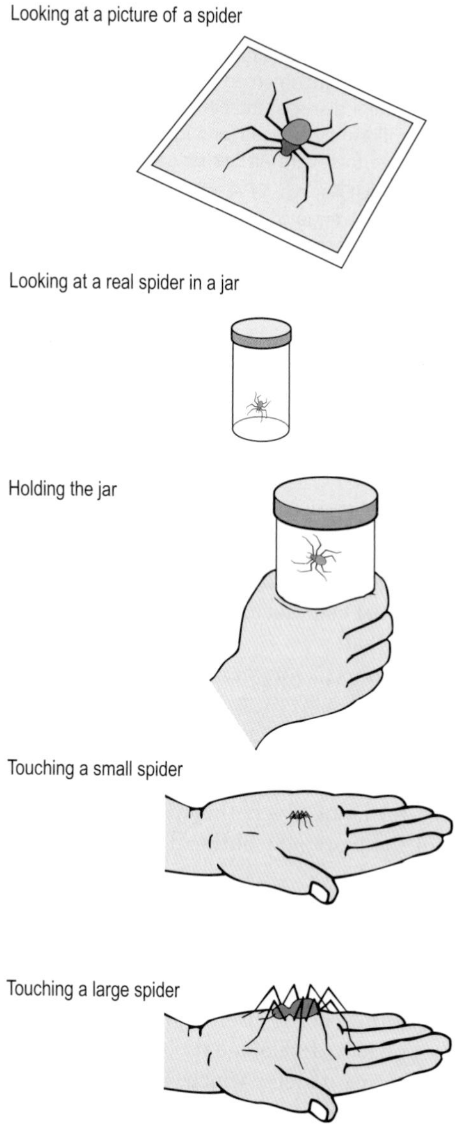

Looking at a picture of a spider

Looking at a real spider in a jar

Holding the jar

Touching a small spider

Touching a large spider

Figure 3.15 • Treatment of arachnophobia by systematic desensitization. • At each stage of the hierarchy of stimuli causing increasing anxiety, the subject practises the techniques of relaxation training.

This is repeated until the patient no longer feels anxious.

The motor compulsions of obsessive–compulsive neuroses can be treated using *response prevention*, in which the patient is prevented from carrying out the rituals. The associated distress gradually diminishes as response prevention is repeated. If the ritual involves obsessional thoughts about cleanliness, for instance repeated hand-washing to get rid of germs, then the patient is asked to touch a 'contaminating' object (such as the sole of a shoe) and then refrain from hand-washing. This can be demonstrated by the therapist, who might, for example, touch a 'contaminating' object and then refrain from hand-washing. The patient is then expected to begin to follow the example of the therapist through the process of *modelling*.

In *thought stopping* the patient is instructed to interrupt recurring obsessional thoughts. Here the patient can think or say out loud the word 'STOP' whenever the obsessional thought occurs. At first it may also be helpful to wear a rubber band around the wrist and snap this against the wrist whenever the thought occurs.

In those who have difficulty coping with social situations, such as those who are shy or suffer from social phobia, *assertiveness training* can be used. This involves acting out roles in imaginary situations that replicate circumstances found difficult, using role playing, role reversal, modelling and coaching. A similar technique, *social skills training*, can be used in those with poor social skills. Video feedback can be a helpful additional method in such training.

Changes in the behaviour of long-stay patients in hospitals and hostels, for example those with chronic schizophrenia or learning disability, can be effected by implementing a system in which desired behaviours are rewarded with tokens. These tokens are saved up and can then be used to buy goods or privileges. This technique of a *token economy* is based on operant conditioning in which the tokens become a secondary reinforcer.

In the *pad and bell method* of treating enuresis, described in Chapter 18, a bell rings whenever the child starts to wet the bed. The child then has to arise and use the lavatory. In time, the child may stop bedwetting and thereby have uninterrupted sleep.

The technique of *aversion therapy*, in which negative reinforcement is used to stifle unsuitable thoughts or behaviour, is now rarely used in clinical psychiatry. In the past, aversion therapy was used to treat sexual deviancy and alcohol dependency.

Unpleasant sensations, such as mild electric shocks or apomorphine-induced nausea, were associated with images of inappropriate foci of sexual desire or the taste and smell of alcohol, for example.

Biofeedback is an application of operant conditioning in which patients are given feedback on the functioning of their autonomic nervous system (e.g. sweating) or motor system (e.g. muscle tension), and can be trained to exert some control over this – for example to lower blood pressure.

Cognitive therapy

This is based on an information-processing model of disorders. It differs from behaviour therapy in that the processing of information, of internal and external origin, by the individual is considered to be of central importance. An attempt is made to change this in certain psychiatric disorders.

Psychiatric disorders that have been found to respond to cognitive therapy include depression, phobic disorders, anxiety disorders and bulimia nervosa. Concepts used in the cognitive therapy of depression are given as an example.

In depression the patient is considered to have a negative bias based on the cognitive triad shown in Figure 3.16. This negative outlook is maintained by errors in thinking, such as:

- *selective abstraction* – the patient selectively focuses on negative aspects of any situation, e.g. 'My child isn't doing well at school so I must be a bad parent'
- *arbitrary inference* – the worst negative inferences are arbitrarily made from situations, e.g. 'He didn't say good morning to me so he must hate me'

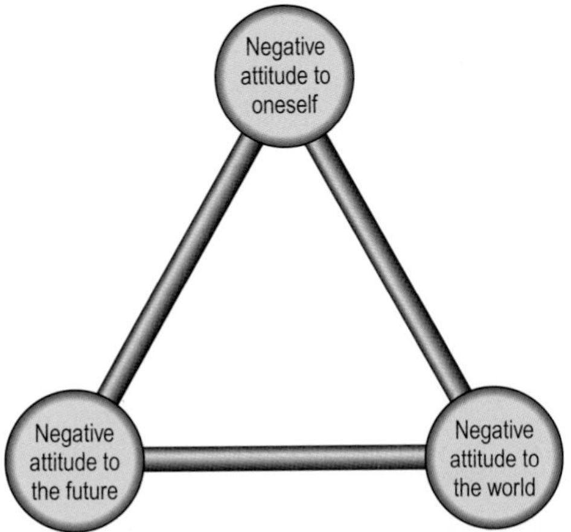

Figure 3.16 • The cognitive triad in depression.

- *overgeneralization* – overgeneralized inferences are made from one negative occurrence, e.g. 'He didn't say good morning to me so everyone must hate me'
- *dichotomous thinking* – things are seen in a dichotomous, 'black and white' way, e.g. 'If he doesn't love me, he must hate me'
- *personalization* – negative occurrences are personalized to oneself, leading to guilt, e.g. 'My friend didn't get a good mark in her exam. It's because I'm depressed. It's my fault'
- *catastrophizing* –errors are turned, cognitively, into catastrophes, e.g. 'I'm convinced that the mistake I made is going to mean I'll lose my job'
- *minimization* – the significance of positive occurrences is minimized, e.g. 'I passed that exam by pure chance'
- *maximization* – the significance of negative occurrences is maximized, e.g. 'I didn't get the answer to that exam question right so I'm going to fail all my exams.'

Examples of these maladaptive thoughts are elicited. In a collaborative manner, evidence for and against is then sought in order to expose possible maladaptive beliefs.

Cognitive-behavioural therapy

Cognitive-behavioural therapy (CBT) marries useful aspects of behaviour therapy to cognitive therapy. Its primary goal is to help individuals achieve the changes they wish for in their lives. The basic assumptions underlying CBT include:

- patients respond according to their interpretations rather than the reality
- thoughts, behaviour and emotions are interrelated
- therapeutic interventions need to clarify and change the way the patient thinks
- the benefits of changing both cognitive processes and behaviour are likely to be greater than the benefits of changing just one or the other.

For example, behaviour therapy may be married with prior hypothesis testing, in which the patient predicts the likely outcomes (in terms of the emotions that will be felt, for instance) from following the new behaviours.

CBT is time-limited. Goals are agreed by the patient and therapist. Important features of CBT include problem solving and new adaptive learning, and focusing on bringing about desired changes outside the therapy sessions. CBT has been found to be of benefit in anxiety states (panic and generalized anxiety), phobic disorders, obsessive–compulsive disorder, depression, somatic problems, eating disorders, chronic psychiatric handicaps, marital problems, sexual dysfunction and problem solving.

Individual psychotherapy

Individual long-term psychodynamic psychotherapy takes place within the theoretical framework of the school of psychotherapy to which the therapist belongs. These include schools based on the work of pioneers such as Freud and Jung. The essential elements of therapy are discussed above and include:

- free association
- dream analysis
- analysis of the transference
- analysis of the countertransference
- working with the resistance and defence mechanisms of the patient
- using clarification, linking, reflection, interpretation and confrontation.

The main aims are symptom relief and personality change. It is generally not used with psychotic patients.

Individual therapy can take a very long time, for example five sessions per week over many years, with each session lasting approximately 50 minutes. An alternative is a shortened and more focused therapy called brief focal psychotherapy. In contrast to long-term psychodynamic psychotherapy, brief focal psychotherapy has the following features:

- it is much briefer (say between one and 40 sessions)
- a focus is selected to be worked on
- the ending of the therapy may have to be worked with much sooner.

Group psychotherapy

Group psychotherapy has similar aims to individual psychotherapy but is carried out by one therapist with a group of patients.

Family therapy

This is a special form of group psychotherapy in which the group consists of members of one family, together with either one therapist or two co-therapists. It is useful in treating family psychopathology. The difficulties in the family often become known because one member of the family, a child say, is referred initially.

As with the other therapies, different styles and approaches have been used (see Chapter 16). A key component is the willingness to consider all components of the family system (even if not all family members are present) and their interactions. An extension of this, which encompasses the wider system impinging on the individual and family, is *systemic therapy*.

In all disorders the family and wider system should be acknowledged. Components and goals of family intervention programmes include:

- education about the disorder
- education about the treatment of the disorder
- communication training
- facilitation
- problem-solving training.

Marital therapy

Marital therapy is offered to couples who require and seek help with difficulties in their relationship. It is sometimes sought as a last resort by married couples who wish to avoid getting divorced. Behavioural models and contracts may be used by the therapist.

Sex therapy

This is used in the treatment of a couple who present with sexual dysfunction. Its goals are to:

- enable individuals to feel at ease with their sexuality
- improve the quality of the sexual relationship enjoyed by the couple.

Both behavioural and psychotherapeutic techniques are used. Examples of behavioural techniques are those of Masters and Johnson for treating premature ejaculation. Further details are given in Chapter 13.

Art and music therapies

Other therapies that can be helpful include art therapy and music therapy. These are two of the arts therapies, which consist of:

- art therapy
- music therapy
- dance therapy.

Various modalities can be used in art therapy, including painting, collage, clay pottery and sculpture.

An emphasis may be put on the production of the artwork and no formal interpretation is given. This is art therapy proper. In art psychotherapy, the therapist does analyze the artwork. In analytical art psychotherapy there is greater emphasis on psychoanalytical theories and an emphasis on the transference.

In music therapy the patient either makes live music or listens to music with therapeutic intent. The music therapist is a musician trained in this form of therapy. Music therapy can be individual or group. Live music-making can involve a musical instrument, percussion and/or the patient's voice.

Psychological treatments

- Psychotherapy is a form of help administered by a specially trained therapist within a theoretical framework.
- Behavioural therapy is a brief, goal-directed psychological treatment, based on behavioural learning theory, dealing with the current features of the disorder.
- Behavioural therapies are available for the treatment of phobic disorders (systematic desensitization with relaxation training, flooding), obsessive–compulsive disorder (exposure and response prevention, thought stopping, paradoxical injunction), social phobia (assertiveness training), poor social skills (social skills training), abnormal behaviour in long-stay patients with chronic schizophrenia or learning disability (token economy) and functional nocturnal enuresis (star chart, pad and bell method).
- Cognitive therapy is based on an information-processing model of disorders and attempts to alter the processing of information by patients suffering from psychiatric disorders such as depression, phobic disorders, anxiety disorders and bulimia nervosa.
- CBT aims to help patients achieve their explicitly stated goals through time-limited sessions that include problem solving and new adaptive learning, and that focus on bringing about desired changes outside the therapy sessions. CBT has been found to be of benefit in anxiety states, phobic disorders, obsessive–compulsive disorder, depression, somatic problems, eating disorders, chronic psychiatric handicaps, marital problems, sexual dysfunction and problem solving.
- Individual psychodynamic psychotherapy uses free association, dream analysis, analysis of transference and countertransference, working with resistance and

Psychological treatments—cont'd

defence mechanisms, clarification, linking, reflection, interpretation and confrontation.

- Sex therapy aims to enable individuals to feel at ease with their sexuality and to improve the sexual relationship of the couple being treated.
- Art and music therapies allow patients to express themselves in art and music.

Psychosocial aspects

Occupational therapy

Some patients, e.g. those with chronic schizophrenia, may lose or never develop the skills required for daily living. These are sometimes called activities of daily living (ADL). In occupational therapy the patient is taught skills such as shopping and cooking, and how to organize his life better. He may be taught how to write a shopping list and then be taken to the shops and taught how to buy appropriate goods, which may then be used to cook a meal. Sometimes patients in long-stay inpatient wards or in hostels in the community may take it in turn to cook communal meals for the other patients and staff.

Psychoeducation

The goals of psychoeducational interventions are to provide patients and/or their relatives/carers with information relating to the psychiatric disorder and its treatment.

Social skills training

The main goals of social skills training are to enable the patient to:

- achieve better interpersonal behaviour
- achieve improved self-care
- adapt to life in the community.

Approaches used include behavioural techniques (positive reinforcement, modelling, role play), videotapes and psychoeducational material.

Rehabilitation

Rehabilitation programmes are used in treating chronically ill patients, e.g. those with chronic schizophrenia who find it difficult to live outside hospital.

A detailed assessment of the patient's disabilities and potential abilities is conducted. Objectives are then set. A plan is designed to reach them using professional, voluntary and family input. The response to this input is monitored and allows the programme to be modified accordingly.

Sheltered workshops

These are specially set up places of employment, which allow chronically ill patients to gain work experience and an increased sense of self-worth. Some patients may then go on to compete successfully for employment in the open market.

Accommodation

Some chronically ill patients cannot cope with living on their own in the community but do not require full inpatient care. In some cases they benefit from being placed in special hostels run by psychiatrically qualified staff (e.g. nurses with expertise in psychiatry). This enables their mental state, physical health and medication to be monitored. It also allows the patient gradually to acquire the ADL under careful supervision.

In some countries the old-style large asylums are being closed down, with chronically ill patients, such as those with chronic schizophrenia and learning disability, being moved into the community. These patients may be placed in such hostels.

Community mental health services

Early intervention and crisis management services enable patients to be seen and treated rapidly in the community or as daypatients. This can help to pre-empt their need for admission as inpatients. These services are offered by multidisciplinary teams, including psychiatrists and community psychiatric nurses. They provide a cost-effective form of treatment, which is particularly useful in those countries where there is a move away from hospital-based treatment to care in the community.

In most developed countries the most important route of referral to psychiatric care is via the general practitioner (family doctor). However, this route may disadvantage certain groups of patients, such as married women, the elderly and those with poor education. Community mental health services may, therefore, operate an open referral system, allowing any agency, including patients, to contact the service by letter or telephone, giving priority to cases of serious psychiatric disorder. An open referral system is likely to be sensitive to the needs of patients in the community, particularly in inner-city areas.

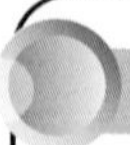

Psychosocial aspects

- The social aspects of treatment include the use of occupational therapy, psychoeducation, social skills training, sheltered workshops and hostels; these can all be part of a rehabilitation programme.
- Patients in the community can be treated by early intervention and crisis management services which may thereby pre-empt the need for inpatient admission.

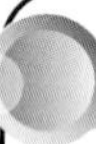

Prognostic factors

- The prognosis of a psychiatric disorder is influenced by compliance with treatment, the disorder itself and support in the community and/or from the family.
- For an ill patient the prognosis can be given in terms of the prognosis for the current episode and the long-term prognosis.

Prognostic factors

The prognosis of a psychiatric disorder is a prediction of the likely course of the disorder. It is influenced by a number of factors.

Compliance with treatment is important. For example, a patient with a bipolar mood disorder who has been prescribed lithium prophylaxis is much more likely to relapse if the lithium therapy is stopped against medical advice. Similarly, a phobic patient who stops attending behavioural therapy sessions is unlikely to fare as well as when a full course of sessions is attended.

Another important factor is the actual disorder itself. Some disorders tend to respond very well to treatment, whereas others tend to be associated with a poor outcome. In the following chapters the outcome for individual disorders is given.

The support received in the community and from the family can also influence the prognosis. Sometimes the patient actually does better if *less* time is spent with the family, as in the case of patients with schizophrenia and high expressed emotion families (see Chapter 9).

Medical students and novice practitioners of psychiatry should not use their lack of experience as an excuse not to give a prognosis. Instead, they should carefully weigh up all the factors relevant to the individual patient and then give a considered prediction of the outcome. This can be checked against the actual progress of the patient in due course.

Further reading

British Medical Association and Royal Pharmaceutical Society of Great Britain, 2011. British National Formulary (BNF 61). British Medical Association and Royal Pharmaceutical Society of Great Britain, London [Always refer to the latest edition of a formulary].

Puri, B.K., 2006. Oxford handbook of drugs in psychiatry. Oxford University Press, Oxford.

Puri, B.K., Treasaden, I. (Eds.), 2010. Psychiatry: an evidence-based text. Hodder Arnold, London.

Doctor–patient communication

Introduction

Consideration of the relationship between doctor and patient is essential in all fields of medical specialization, even in those where there is no direct patient contact.

Patients construe a bad consultation as one in which there is inaccurate medical assessment. For patients to construe a doctor contact as 'good', however, there must additionally be good communication. Doctors need to include communication in their training to ensure clarity, precision, completeness and lack of ambiguity in their interactions with patients. Good communication improves patient satisfaction, memory for information provided, adherence to treatment plan and patient outcome.

This chapter considers the general issue of doctor–patient communication for medicine in general and specifically for psychiatry. Various theoretical aspects of the workings of the mind are described that provide a basis for understanding patient and doctor functioning ('dynamic psychopathology'). Chapter 5 describes the content of the psychiatric interview and assessment.

First contact

Even before meeting, the patient and the doctor will have expectations of each other, based on culture (including media portrayal), prior experience and the accounts of others. These will determine the initial presentation, which will be modified by the degree to which the contact fulfils these expectations. This applies to all levels of interaction, from posture and degree of body and limb movement, through accent and vocabulary used, to mood and level of familiarity; and of course the *content* of the information presented. This applies as much to the patient as it does to the doctor. There are always going to be differences between the doctor and patient: sometimes there is an enormous cultural divide, sometimes communication is limited by impairments in one or other participant. These factors do not lessen the need for accuracy, efficiency and supportiveness.

As is often emphasized, doctors should be treating patients, not diseases. This may be lost in the fascination of MRI scan results or EEG traces, but if forgotten entirely will increase the likelihood of doing harm, or at least lessen the potential to be of benefit.

A distinction has been made between *disease*, the pathological abnormality occurring as a result of some specific noxious insult, and *illness*, the subjective interpretation of problems that are perceived as related to health. These are related to each other but can occur independently. Illness without disease can, for example, be malingering, hypochondriasis or somatization (the distinctions are covered in Chapter 11). In other 'non-psychiatric' disorders there may be a strong psychological contribution with varying levels of pathological or physiological change (e.g. tension headache, irritable bowel syndrome). A similar distinction has been made between:

- 'health behaviour' – actions taken by people who see themselves as healthy in order to prevent disease or detect it while it is still asymptomatic
- 'illness behaviour' – actions of people who see themselves as ill, for the purpose of defining their health state and finding a remedy

- 'sick-role behaviour' – activity by individuals who consider themselves as ill for the purpose of getting well.

The first doctor–patient contact may not be this simple. The patient's initiation of contact may, for example, be to gain support for a housing application, to plead mitigation in criminal proceedings, or to put pressure on an ex-partner in divorce. The doctor may be gaining experience, being trained, carrying out research or working out their time until retirement. The only assumption the doctor can make about the patient is that a 'message' is being transmitted, which is a combination of *informative* (giving information), *promotive* (intended to make the doctor do something) and *evocative* (intended to make the doctor feel something). The doctor must be careful to pay attention to 'illness' information as well as 'disease' information in order to have a clearer idea of the patient's perspective.

In most circumstances the doctor sets the rules of interaction, including the venue. This being the case, the doctor has a duty to pay explicit attention to the rules so the contact has an optimum outcome.

Appearance

The doctor must feel comfortable with his or her general appearance, but should be aware that jeans and a T-shirt give a different impression from a suit with or without white coat, stethoscope and so on. It is recommended that the doctor is neat, tidy and reasonably smartly dressed, at the very least to demonstrate a businesslike and organized attitude. Patients will vary according to whether the psychiatrist looking reasonably nondescript reassures them, or whether they prefer the 'wacky' image beloved of media representations. In general it is better to err on the side of caution.

Setting

The facilities available to the psychiatrist will vary in their level of formality and comfort. The aim should be to provide comfort and informality at a level that encourages but does not deter the disclosure of important information or emotion. For example, a patient may, paradoxically, feel more able to disclose intimate details in a formal consulting room, where there is adequate provision of freedom from interruption and being overheard, than at home, where this is not so certain. Thus a balance must be struck between 'homeliness' and clinical atmosphere. The increase in the practice of community psychiatry in Western countries means that it is more than likely that the consultation will occur outside the office setting.

The layout of all settings should try to ensure that patient and doctor are at a similar height, that there is no barrier to communication (e.g. a desk) and that eye contact is possible but not forced. Placing similar chairs at an angle of 90° to each other usually achieves this, possibly with a low table to one side. If the doctor requires a writing surface, the doctor sitting to one side of the desk (Figure 4.1) can achieve a similar effect. Lighting should be adequate but not too bright, and should not shine in the patient's eyes.

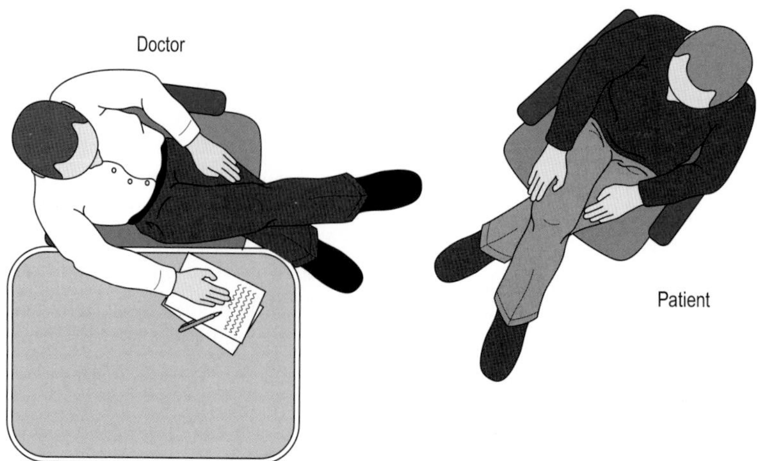

Figure 4.1 • The clinical setting.

(The antithesis of this emphasizes the power differential: one professor of psychiatry, a big man, sat in a large 'airline'-type chair behind a large empty desk, in front of the window; his hapless trainee was perched on a low small chair facing the desk.)

Behaviour

The sequence of 'smile, touch, question' (where touch is a handshake or gentle direction to the consulting room) is fine for general medical consultations, but may be less straightforward in psychiatric assessment. The paranoid patient may interpret a smile as mocking. A touch may produce a flashback or unpleasant memories for the patient with post-traumatic stress syndrome following assault. Thus, a neutral but welcoming stance is advised.

Note-taking during the interview is a matter of personal preference. It is argued that taking notes reduces the potential for observation and the amount of attention given to the patient. On the other hand, many patients regard it as indicative of the doctor taking what they say seriously. Judicious note-taking can greatly aid formulation and is particularly useful where there are mental state abnormalities to record verbatim, for example the speech in thought disorder or delirium.

Looking interested also facilitates disclosure. It is important for the doctor to examine personal attitudes at the outset of the interview, as a jaded or bored state of mind will be picked up by the patient and will interfere with the quantity and quality of the information derived by the doctor. (Non-verbal communication is continuous and on the edge of consciousness. Where there is an inconsistency between verbal and non-verbal communication the latter takes precedence.) Leaning forward, nodding and slightly inclining the head tend to encourage further disclosure. Looking at the patient also gives the impression of listening. In normal circumstances, while patients are talking, they will not maintain eye contact all the time but will keep checking that the listener is paying attention, and may fix their gaze at important junctures (Figure 4.2). If the doctor is looking at the notes while the patient is talking, the quality of the communication deteriorates significantly.

Questioning should progress from open ('Can you tell me of your concerns?' ... 'Tell me more about that' ...) to more specific closed questions ('When did your father die?'). Different types of question will tend to produce different responses (Figure 4.3).

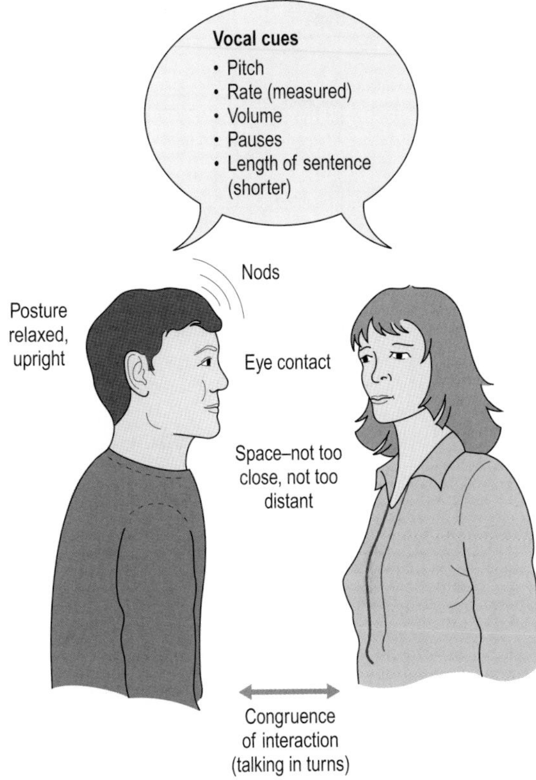

Figure 4.2 • Non-verbal communication.

Studies have shown that doctors tend to interrupt opening statements from their patients, and as a result do not hear the full reasons for attendance. This may explain the phenomenon of 'important topics' being introduced later in the consultation (perhaps when there is insufficient time to explore them).

Attentive listening is an active process that improves the efficiency of doctor–patient communication. There are four core skill areas:

- *Wait time.* Allowing longer for responses before interruption increases the amount and quality of information volunteered.
- *Facilitative response.* A short, non-verbal cue that encourages continued response from the patient is more effective at the beginning of a meeting. Later in the interview echoing, paraphrasing and interpretation are more useful.
- *Non-verbal skills.* The most important of these is eye contact.
- *Picking up patient cues.* These are verbal and non-verbal hints of other information that are seen more at the beginning of the interview, and need appropriate acknowledgement.

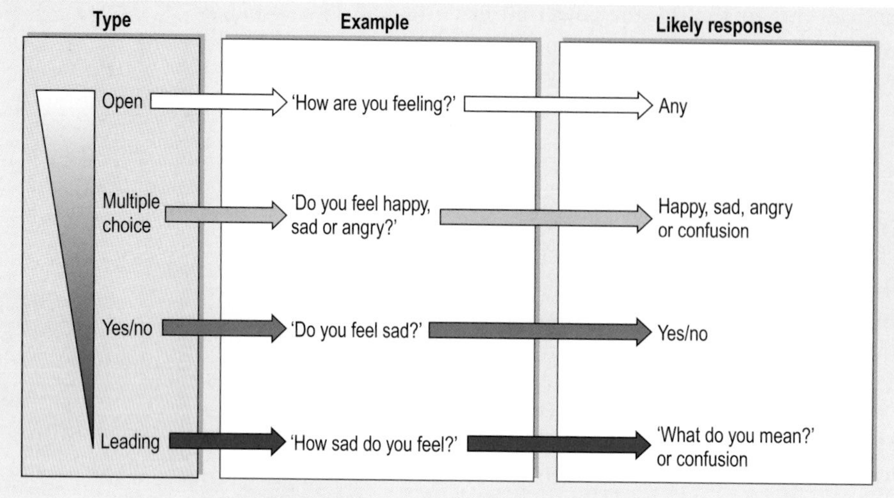

Figure 4.3 • Type of question (in order of decreasing openness and increasing chance of limited response).

Carl Rogers identified three therapist characteristics most associated with successful therapy outcome:

- empathy
- non-possessive warmth
- unconditional positive regard (this is not the same as liking or always agreeing with the patient).

These further emphasize the need for an attitude of truthfulness and honesty, remembering that truthfulness is not the same as bluntness.

All the doctor's senses will be necessary for an accurate and effective diagnosis and treatment:

- *hearing* to hear the symptoms, breath sounds, heart sounds, etc.
- *sight* to see the signs, read the non-verbal signals, etc.
- *smell* to detect diabetic ketoacidosis on the breath, fetor, etc.
- *touch* to palpate the abdomen
- *taste* to taste the cups of tea offered on home visits (has salt replaced the sugar?).

A further vital sixth sense has been proposed: the emotional response evoked in the doctor by the attitude and bearing of the patient. Most experienced psychiatrists will report rather quizzically the 'feeling' that a patient is psychotic or that a condition is organic, which amounts to more than a confluence of the signs and symptoms. Trainees would do well to cultivate such 'feelings'. Perhaps more straightforwardly, the emotions of anger, depression, anxiety, admiration and sexual arousal may arise in the context of the doctor–patient relationship and influence actions, particularly the decision to refer on. These themes will be developed further below.

Boundaries

Boundaries to the consultation are essential to provide sufficient safety and familiarity with the setting and circumstances for the patient to use the session appropriately, and are best made explicit in the introductory phase. In style, this is a collaboration, but the degree of leeway available should be clear (and will vary with setting). Following introductions, the doctor should outline what is understood about the purpose of the interview. The time available and the availability of further appointments should be noted. The form of the interview (family, individual, etc.), the areas to be covered and the likely outcomes to be considered at the end of the interview are outlined. Questions, concerns or clarifications should be invited. A longer discussion or negotiation of the purpose of the interview may well be merited. Explanation and planning are key skills to foster, particularly when a series of meetings is required.

In therapy, and to some extent in assessments, behaviours that are expected and not expected should be laid down, together with clear statements of the doctor's response if these boundaries are breached, and what the patient should expect in return for respecting the limits. In therapy, no alcohol or drug intoxication, no smoking and no physical violence are reasonable minimal requirements. (The lighting of a cigarette can inhibit talk and often occurs at times of tension, when verbal communication would be more fruitful.) Chapter 5 considers further the matters of individual safety in interviewing.

General relationship issues

Confidentiality

Confidentiality is an important characteristic of the doctor–patient relationship, and indeed of all interactions between patient and health professional. (Doctors, nurses and others can lose their jobs and/or their professional registration by betraying confidentiality.) On the face of it this seems a simple principle, but there are complications and limitations when the issues are examined critically. These are depicted in Figure 4.4.

Legal responsibility

Doctors, and particularly psychiatrists, are responsible for enacting the mental health legislation according to the law, and knowledge of this, particularly for experienced patients, is a potent influence on the doctor–patient relationship and can evoke intense emotion in the patient and the family. Mental health legislation makes medical power explicit, but in Western countries at least it also encompasses safeguards to prevent abuse of that power (see Appendices re mental health legislation).

Compulsion/persuasion

Many writers have drawn attention to elements of persuasion and compulsion inherent in the doctor–patient relationship, both in the doctor's wish to encourage more healthy behaviour ('compliance') and in the patient's wish for effective health care. This is something of a barter. It is recommended that the doctor's professional skills and knowledge are placed at the disposal of the patient – within limits (see below). The power of the doctor is something of which each should be aware. Browne and Freeling have pointed out that the doctor should 'resist the temptation to prove oneself all-powerful and all knowing, especially since he is neither but is often asked to be'.

Balint referred to the 'apostolic function' of the doctor in his classic treatise *The doctor, his patient and the illness*. By this he meant that:

> In the first place . . . every doctor has a vague, but almost unshakeably firm, idea of how a patient ought to behave when ill . . . and further [behaves] as if he had a sacred duty to convert to his faith all the ignorant and unbelieving among his patients.

A GP might refer to this as 'training his patients'. In psychiatry too, patients quickly learn the way to behave – institutionalization is an extreme example of this. While this smoothes the wheels of the interaction, it also narrows the repertoire of responses of both doctor and patient, and may miss key

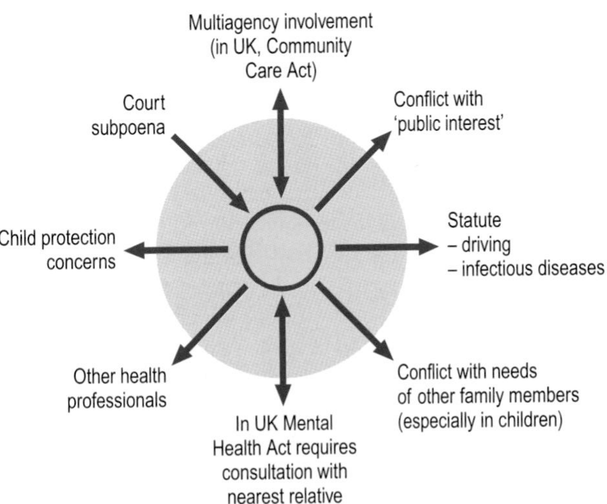

Figure 4.4 • The boundaries of confidentiality.

aetiological and possible remedial factors. The apostolic function cannot be avoided, but if the clinician is aware of it the negative attributes can be minimized.

The illness iceberg

The psychiatrist and patient usually only meet following the intervention of a third party: the referrer. It is always useful for the doctor to consider why has *this* patient been referred with *this* problem at *this* time? The term 'illness iceberg' refers to the fact that the majority of illness symptoms are ignored or receive non-medical attention. In one study, medical consultation occurred only once in 18 'illness episodes'. Similarly, most psychiatric and psychological symptoms are not referred on to the specialist services. The decision to refer is a key point in the illness process, and is determined by many factors other than the severity of the presenting disorder.

The treatment alliance

Once the link between patient and doctor is made, the question of 'treatment' will arise. It may be argued that not all doctor–patient interactions lead to treatment, but the very conclusion of 'no treatment' is in itself an intervention, and may or may not be acceptable to the patient. The treatment alliance is a consequence of the rapport between them and has been described as 'conscious commitment'. Trainees can learn skills to enhance this (see Further reading). Erikson used the term 'basic trust' to cover the early development of a sense of reliability about carers and the environment. If this is not achieved, there may be problems in developing an effective working alliance between doctor and patient. Previous experiences of doctors can also strongly colour a patient's subsequent reactions to the medical profession.

The treatment alliance must be distinguished from the 'wish to get better'. The latter can often have a magical quality, which means that a patient may start a course of treatment or action but then break it off (the 'function of the symptom' in the patient's life is often important here). Theories of behaviour change emphasize the normality of ambivalence about change and the repeated cycle between stages of precontemplation, contemplation, preparation and action.

The privations of illness can often be associated with the doctor or the medical setting and affect the attitude of the patient. The purveyor of bad tidings can be tainted with the unwelcome news, and the patient may initially take out anger and frustration on the doctor.

Modulation of sympathy and reassurance

In the doctor–patient relationship the 'comfort always' aphorism emphasizes the importance of empathy for the patient. It has been suggested that modern medicine is losing sight of the benefits of empathy as a treatment in its own right. Part of this means putting oneself on the 'same side of the fence' as the patient, and will modify a doctor's wish to bring a patient abruptly face to face with their anxieties (in any case this is likely to produce 'resistance' in the patient with anger and rejection).

On the other hand, sympathy – seeing things from the 'outside' – may prevent the patient from expressing negative feelings (e.g. about the loss of a relative or friend). Tears induced by sympathy may also prevent a patient discussing a key topic. In marital disputes, sympathy for one party's account may be confused by hearing the usually equally valid account of the other party.

Reassurance is often provided by doctors, but paradoxically the effect of excessive reassurance is frequently not appreciated, particularly when it is accompanied by actions that suggest the opposite: 'I'm sure there's nothing seriously wrong but we'll just do this scan to be sure.' The more a person is reassured, the more they can become concerned that there *is* something wrong: otherwise, why would people keep saying there wasn't?

When to stop

The importance of 'boundaries' has already been mentioned. It may be thought that the more listening the better, and that continuing interviews as long as possible can only be a good thing. However, it is important to maintain a balance between leaving a patient feeling understood and relieved, and leaving them feeling somehow robbed, humiliated or empty, which can occur if contact goes on too long. A continuous interview of an hour is usually plenty (the psychoanalyst traditionally allows 50 minutes, to give time for note-writing and change of tack to the next patient). This may be increased in group and family interviews to allow more space for others' contributions, but the same principle applies.

Dynamic psychopathology

This refers to the theoretical structure of the mind first developed by Sigmund Freud and subsequently by other *psychoanalysts*. According to psychoanalytic theory, the *mental apparatus* is the existence of a stable or relatively stable psychological organization involved in behaviour and subjective experiences such as dreaming. Concepts of dynamic psychopathology can be useful in conceptualizing issues arising in the relationship between doctor and patient. Such *hypothetical constructs* may be further used in therapy.

Structure of the mental apparatus

The *id* is an unconscious part of the mental apparatus, made up partly of inherited instincts and partly by acquired, but repressed, components. The *ego* is at the interface of the perceptual system and the internal demand system. Its functions include the control of voluntary thoughts and actions and, at an unconscious level, defence mechanisms (see below). The *superego* derives from the ego and exercises self-judgement and holds ethical and moralistic values.

Functions of the mental apparatus include:

- the control and discharge of excitation
- defending the individual against affects and ideas that may be distressing, such as those that are unacceptable to their conscious standards and wishes
- laying down associative memory traces
- attention
- perception
- development of the ego.

One way in which *the unconscious* can be studied is by using *free association*, in which the patient is encouraged to articulate all thoughts that come to mind without censorship, thus allowing the unconstrained linking of thoughts. A second way is by studying so-called *Freudian slips* (slips of the tongue or of writing), more formally known as *parapraxes*, in which unconscious thoughts slip through to the surface when the censorship function of the mind is temporarily off guard. The censor is not as vigilant while dreaming as during the waking hours, so that a third way is through the analysis of dreams. Indeed, Freud called dreams 'the royal road to the unconscious'. Dreams may be based on one's unconscious wishes. Characteristics of the unconscious, according to Freud (who did not like the term subconscious) include:

- the *absence of contradictions and negation*: in the unconscious there is no 'either' or 'or', only 'and'
- *timelessness*
- subjection to the *pleasure principle*, i.e. a dominating principle that aims to avoid pain and maximize pleasure
- *censorship*: an unconscious process that protects the consciousness from an awareness of instincts and unconscious wishes that would be threatening if allowed to reach consciousness
- *disregard of reality* of the conscious world
- *psychical reality*: memories of real and imagined events are not distinguished.

Resistance is the term used for everything that prevents the ego of a person from gaining full access to the unconscious.

Defence mechanisms

Consciousness is described as being protected from the affects, ideas and desires of the unconscious by means of *defence mechanisms*. These are summarized in Table 4.1.

Repression is the pushing away of unacceptable affects, ideas and wishes so that they remain in the unconscious. For example, a 22-year-old male

Table 4.1 Defence mechanisms
Repression
Denial
Reaction formation
Isolation
Introjection and identification
Undoing (what has been done)
Projection and splitting
Projective identification
Displacement
Rationalization
Sublimation
Regression

graduate, who had been the head of the Christian Union at university, gave in to his sexual feelings for his girlfriend and had sexual intercourse with her, something that he then immediately regretted deeply and considered sinful. Some weeks later he was unable to remember anything about a film he had recently watched, even though he normally had an excellent memory. The reason was that the film included a story of a young couple having sexual relations for the first time, and this aroused unpalatable memories; his own recent sexual encounter, and the associated memory of the film, had been found to be repugnant to him (at a conscious level) and were therefore repressed from consciousness.

Other defence mechanisms include:

- *Denial.* The subject acts as if consciously unaware of a wish or reality.
- *Reaction formation.* The subject holds a psychological attitude diametrically opposed to an oppressed wish. For example, a man having a strong unconscious desire to look at pornographic images, who finds such a wish repugnant and distasteful at a conscious level, may become an ardent opponent of all pornography.
- *Isolation* is a way of breaking the links between certain thoughts and other thoughts held by the person. This is seen in obsessional neurosis.
- *Introjection* and *identification* are related defence mechanisms whereby the attitudes and behaviour of another are transposed into oneself, thereby helping one cope with separation from that person.
- *Undoing.* A person construes previous thoughts or actions as not having occurred.
- *Projection.* The person attributes repressed thoughts and wishes to other people or objects. In other words, *splitting* off of internal repressed thoughts and wishes takes place, which are then projected onto external objects.
- *Projective identification.* The subject not only sees another person as possessing repressed aspects of the self, but also actually constrains the other person to take on those aspects.
- In *displacement* the subject transfers thoughts and feelings about one person or object onto another.
- *Rationalization.* An attempt is made to explain in a rational way affects, ideas and wishes whose true motives are not consciously apparent.
- *Sublimation* is the way in which the pleasure principle is satisfied by means of socially acceptable gratifications. For example, someone who enjoys fires and has an unconscious wish to be a fire-setter might become a fire-fighter. Similarly, aggressive thoughts may be sublimated into competitive sporting activities.
- *Regression.* The person returns to an earlier stage of development, particularly at times of stress.

Transference

Transference (Figure 4.5) is a term derived from psychoanalysis, originating with Freud. The breadth of its meaning has varied over the years and also according to who is using it. In *The patient and the analyst* (1973), Sandler, Dare and Holder define transference as:

> . . . a specific illusion which develops in regard to the other person, one which, unbeknown to the subject, represents, in some of its features, a repetition of a relationship towards an important figure in the person's past. It should be emphasized that this is felt by the subject not as a repetition of the past, but as strictly appropriate to the present and to the particular person involved.

They also stated:

> Transference need not be restricted to the illusory apperception of another person . . . but can be taken to include the unconscious (and often subtle) attempts to manipulate or to provoke situations with others which are a concealed repetition of earlier experiences and relationships.

Such repetition can, of course, occur in everyday life (e.g. repeated failed relationships with the same sort of partner).

In getting to know people we initially 'project' on to them attributes from our experiences of others, and then gradually correct any misconceptions – this is called 'reality testing'. In the doctor–patient relationship there is a 'professional' distance that to some extent limits this reality testing. In psychoanalysis transference is fostered by reducing reality testing and by the exploration of fantasy. As an authority figure privy to intimate details of a patient's life, the doctor has a high likelihood of being unconsciously imbued with the attributes of previous authority figures known to the patient, most notably parents.

Transference may be positive, loving, even erotic. Such *positive transference* can be helpful to the patient in addressing upsetting experiences, but can also hinder, for example, the development of patient autonomy, which is usually the aim of

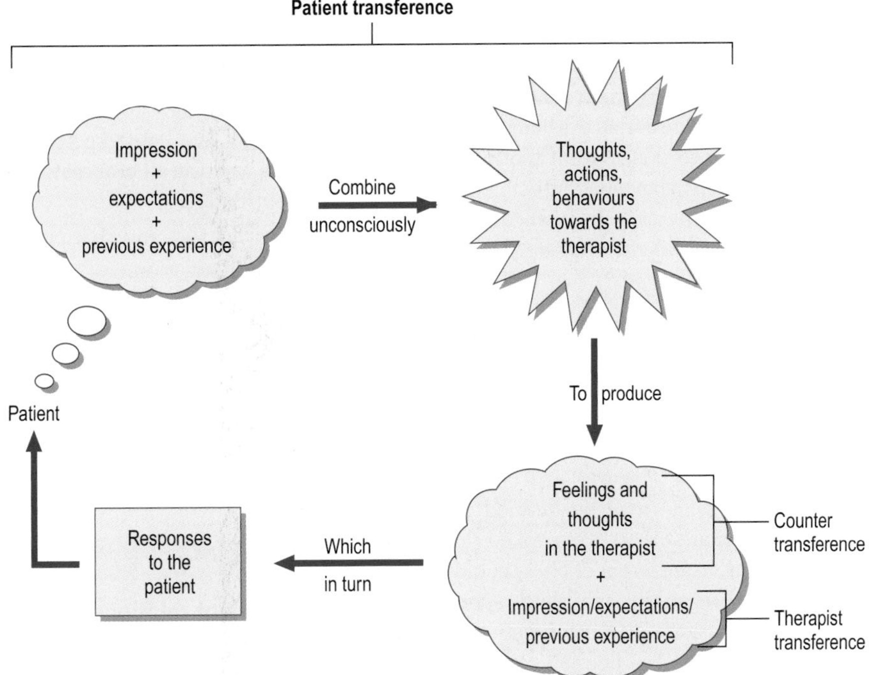

Figure 4.5 • Transference and countertransference.

treatment. *Negative transference* is the transfer of hostile or negative attributes, which are not reality-based. In extreme form this is paranoia (although the psychoanalysis of psychosis is an area that requires considerably more detailed examination than is possible here).

A more restrictive definition of transference reserves its use for the psychoanalytic setting, to phenomena that were not there before and develop in the context of the patient–analyst relationship (Figure 4.5). Even Freud, however, acknowledged that equivalent phenomena occur in other contexts and can have similar beneficial or detrimental influences. In group analysis, transferences occur to other members of the group as well as to the group facilitator.

Acting out is also known as 'acting in the transference' and refers to the second part of the definition above, i.e. actions based on previous experience. In lay terms, 'acting out' usually has negative connotations, and is used for antisocial or self-destructive behaviours. Other less obvious activities outside the relationship may also be encompassed. (For example, a young woman who acted in a flirtatious way towards the young male facilitator of a therapeutic group, described a new passionate relationship with someone outside the group who was soft, sympathetic and listened to all her woes. Although not interpreted, in supervision this relationship was pointed out as an example of 'acting out' of positive transference towards the therapist. The outside relationship was not sustained as it was found to be unfulfilling.)

There is a risk in relationships between doctor and patient of sexual acting out, particularly where intimate details are discussed, as in individual psychotherapy. The doctor must be aware of this, and maintain neutrality and distance while acknowledging any sexual feelings that may be felt. Awareness should include acknowledgement of the considerable power imbalance in such circumstances, and the strict ethical and disciplinary implications of acting on sexual feelings.

Dependency and regression

Dependency and regression are further features of the doctor–patient relationship that occur as a consequence of a person adopting the patient role. It is a familiar experience of surgical patients admitted to hospital for a minor procedure, even if they are quite well, to find it hard to resist donning night clothes and taking to bed. Also with the regression comes passivity, so that the patient will meekly agree to activities that would never be considered outside the patient role. A 'difficult' patient may simply not be fitting the required role model. Although the above is understandable, and to some extent soothing, in psychiatry in particular such behaviour conflicts with the aim of encouraging autonomy and self-reliance. The change from 'patient' to 'non-patient' may be abrupt and it may be difficult to adjust.

Countertransference

Countertransference is a term often used loosely to describe the whole of a therapist's feelings and attitudes towards the patient (Figure 4.5). More specifically, countertransference may be defined as those feelings and behaviours that are evoked in the therapist by the patient's transference. These could be (and were initially) regarded as 'blind spot' nuisances. More recently, countertransference has become regarded as a useful tool in helping patients, so long as it is used wisely and not too explicitly. Self-analysis or training analysis is advocated for analysts to identify such 'blind spots'. Most doctors and other health professionals are not so fortunate as to have the opportunity for such detailed investigation of their own psyche, but good clinical *supervision* can go some way towards filling this gap.

Conclusion

It is important to be aware of the nature and vagaries of the doctor–patient relationship in order to make best use of its therapeutic potential. Eric Cassell has described the 'art of medicine' as being composed of four areas:

- the ability to acquire and integrate both subjective and objective information to make decisions in the best interests of the patient
- the ability to use the doctor–patient relationship for therapeutic ends
- knowing how doctors and sick persons behave
- effective communication.

Whether medicine is art or science is for discussion elsewhere; however, it must be noted that doctors were earning a living well before the current technological revolution, which itself testifies to the power of the 'bedside manner'.

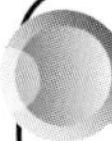

The doctor–patient relationship

- Communication between doctor and patient can be viewed at different levels, from the minutiae of non-verbal interactions to the sociocultural significance of the encounter. It is best not to make assumptions if the maximum is to be gained for both parties.
- Doctors should pay attention to their appearance, to the setting, to their own behaviour and to the function of contact with the patient.
- The structure of the relationship is modulated by boundaries, confidentiality and individual responsibility. These may be matters of negotiation.
- Transference and countertransference are important concepts that refer to those illusory feelings, behaviours and attitudes evoked in a relationship as a result of the unconscious interaction of current perception and previous experience.

Further reading

Balint, M., 1964. The doctor, his patient and the illness, second ed. Pitman, London.

Hughes, P., 1999. Dynamic psychotherapy explained. Radcliffe Medical Press, Oxford.

Silverman, J., Kurtz, S., Draper, J., 1998. Skills for communicating with patients. Radcliffe Medical Press, Oxford.

History taking and clinical examination

5

Introduction

As with other branches of medicine, a systematic approach to interviewing, history taking, clinical examination and investigations is necessary in order to make an appropriate differential diagnosis.

Psychiatric interviewing

The most important aims of psychiatric interviewing are (Institute of Psychiatry 1973):

- to obtain information
- to assess the emotions and attitudes of the patient
- to supply a supportive role and allow an understanding of the patient. This is the basis of the subsequent working relationship with the patient.

It is important to allow the patient to feel as relaxed and uninhibited about talking as possible by fostering a trusting relationship. At the same time, if the patient has troubling thoughts, he should feel that the interviewer can cope with these. The interviewer should provide a containing environment in the context of which the patient can believe that the interviewer can hold these burdens.

In general, and particularly at the beginning of the interview, open questions (e.g. 'How are you in your spirits?') should be used in preference to closed questions (e.g. 'Are you feeling low?'); it is important not to close off possible responses too soon. Indeed, it is often helpful to allow the patient to talk about his presenting problem for the first five minutes of the interview without being interrupted. In due course, when certain details in the history and mental state examination need to be established, the interviewer must set the agenda and can home in on the required details (see also Chapter 4).

When first taking a psychiatric history or carrying out a mental state examination, medical students and psychiatric trainees sometimes feel uncomfortable about certain aspects, such as asking about the psychosexual history. However, most patients, at least at an unconscious level, expect to be asked about such matters. Indeed, not being asked may feel rather like not having the abdomen palpated during a physical examination by a surgeon. Similarly, it is important to ask patients about any suicidal thoughts they may have: there is no particular evidence that one might thereby in some way put the idea into the patient's mind. Rather, the patient may again unconsciously expect to have this question asked.

For deaf patients who understand sign language, the services of a professional signer who has experience of psychiatry should be employed. Similarly, if the patient does not speak the same language as the interviewer, the services of a professional translator should be engaged.

Potentially violent patients

Patients who are hostile and angry cannot always be talked down, especially if they are very paranoid, psychotic or have an organic mental disorder. However, the risk of patients being violent to psychiatrists is less than that of patients being violent to general practitioners, or to those who work in casualty departments.

Always tell other members of staff which patient you will be interviewing and where. Be aware of relevant ward policies on violence, as well as alarm systems and bells. Training in simple breakaway techniques is always helpful.

Rapport is increased and the risk of violence reduced if you sit about a metre away from the patient, at the same level and in a position where you can always look at him but he can look away. This is usually achieved by sitting at approximately right angles (see Figure 4.1). Both you and the patient should have free access to the door, so that he does not feel trapped and you can make an easy exit.

Should a patient become acutely angry or threatening, you should adopt a calm manner, talk in a quiet voice, avoid eye contact and sit rather than stand to avoid making the patient feel overwhelmed. You may need to be prepared to talk him down for a prolonged period before relaxation can be achieved.

Psychiatric history

The psychiatric history should ideally be brought together from both the patient and sources of further information (see below).

Reason for referral

How and why the patient was referred are briefly stated.

Complaints

These are the complaints as described by the patient. The length of time each complaint has lasted should also be given.

History of presenting illness

A chronological account of the development of each symptom should be given, together with any precipitating factors. Note any associated impairments. For example, for a depressive episode, biological and cognitive symptoms of depression (see Chapter 9) should be included. Note the effects of the patient's condition on social functioning.

Family history

The patient should be asked details of parents and siblings, including their current age or age at death, occupation, health and relationship with the patient. The timing of parental separation and/or divorce, if relevant, should also be stated.

Family psychiatric history

Any family history of psychiatric or neurological disorder (e.g. epilepsy) should be detailed, including the nature of the disorder and any treatment. The patient should be asked about any history of suicide in the family.

Personal history

Childhood

This should include details of:

- date of birth
- place of birth
- abnormalities prior to or at birth, and whether the birth was premature
- early developmental milestones
- childhood health, including any history of 'nervous problems'
- any early emotional stresses, including separation (e.g. because of death) from close relatives such as siblings or parents.

Education

This requires details of:

- age on beginning schooling
- types of school attended
- relationship with peers and teachers
- any history of truancy or other trouble or difficulties at school
- qualifications achieved
- age on leaving school
- higher education.

Occupational history

Summarize the occupational history, giving details of promotion/demotion. Reasons for being sacked repeatedly (e.g. problem drinking) should be explored. Any other difficulties at work should be given.

Psychosexual history

For women, ask about the age of menarche, any menstrual abnormalities, history of pregnancies and the age of menopause, if relevant. The sexual orientation should also be given. Any history of sexual or physical abuse should be detailed, together with sexual and marital history (including any history of infidelity) and any sexual difficulties.

Children

Details of any children should be given, including any disturbances from which they suffer.

Current social situation

Give the patient's current:

- social situation, stating with whom they live
- marital status
- occupation and financial status
- nature and suitability of accommodation
- hobbies and social interests.

Past medical history

This is a chronological account of the past medical history, including the nature of physical disorders and injuries, where they were treated and the types of treatment administered. Any medication, and its side-effects, should also be enquired about, as should any history of hypersensitivity to drugs.

Past psychiatric history

This involves details of:

- the nature of any illness(es)
- their duration
- hospital(s) and outpatient department(s) attended
- treatment(s) received
- any current psychotropic medication being taken, and any side-effects from this.

Psychoactive substance use

Alcohol

Details should be obtained about the amount of alcohol the patient is currently drinking and the amount drunk in the past, including a history of any withdrawal symptoms (see Chapter 8). Also obtain any history of physical illnesses, injuries (e.g. road traffic accidents), legal problems (e.g. driving offences) or employment difficulties (e.g. being late regularly for work resulting in being sacked), as a result of alcohol intake. The CAGE Questionnaire (Chapter 7) should be routinely administered to patients to screen for alcohol problems; positive answers to two or more of the following four CAGE questions is indicative of problem drinking:

C Have you ever felt you should **C**ut down on your drinking?

A Have people **A**nnoyed you by criticizing your drinking?

G Have you ever felt **G**uilty about your drinking?

E Have you ever had a drink first thing in the morning (an **E**ye-opener) to steady your nerves or get rid of a hangover?

Tobacco

If the patient smokes, the type and number of nicotine-containing products smoked and any previous history of smoking should be obtained.

Illicit drug abuse

Detail the use of illicit drugs currently and in the past, including the types of drugs, the quantities taken, the methods of administration and the consequences.

Forensic history

Describe details of any history of delinquency and criminal offences, including a history of the punishments received (e.g. fines and custodial sentences).

Premorbid personality

The patient's personality consists of lifelong persistent and enduring characteristics and attitudes, including ways of thinking (cognition), feeling (affectivity) and behaving (impulse control and ways of relating to others and handling interpersonal situations). If the patient's personality has changed after the onset of psychiatric disorder, then details of personality prior to the disorder should be obtained by interviewing both the patient and other informants. This is summarized under the following headings:

- attitudes to others in social, family and sexual relationships

- attitude to self and character
- moral and religious beliefs and standards
- predominant mood
- leisure activities and interests
- fantasy life – daydreams and nightmares
- reaction pattern to stress, including defence mechanisms.

Psychiatric interviewing and history

- The most important aims of psychiatric interviewing are:
  - to obtain information
  - to assess the emotions and attitudes
  - a supportive role.
- Begin by using open questions.
- The psychiatric history:
  - reason for referral
  - complaints
  - history of presenting illness
  - family history
  - family psychiatric history
  - personal history: childhood, education, occupational history, psychosexual history, children, current social situation
  - past medical history
  - past psychiatric history
  - psychoactive substance use: alcohol, tobacco, illicit drug abuse
  - forensic history
  - premorbid personality.

Mental state examination and descriptive psychopathology

The mental state examination is an extremely important part of the psychiatric examination that should be practised repeatedly after carefully observing how trained psychiatrists carry it out. It covers the psychiatric symptomatology ('signs' of illness) exhibited at the time of the interview. In addition to recording information obtained from the interview itself, the mental state examination should also use information obtained by others, such as the observations of nursing staff in the case of an inpatient. This is important because the patient may not always be forthcoming about symptomatology. Thus, for example, a patient who is observed by the nursing staff to be responding to auditory hallucinations, may deny experiencing perceptual abnormalities during a formal interview.

The main areas that must be covered during the mental state examination are detailed in this section. Some of these need to be expanded according to the diagnosis. For example:

- in depression: expand on *mood*
- in schizophrenia: expand on *mood, abnormal beliefs* and *abnormal experiences*
- in obsessive–compulsive disorder: expand on *mood* and *thought abnormalities*
- in dementia: expand on *mood* and *cognitive state*.

Each heading of the mental state examination also makes reference to the corresponding abnormalities that can occur; this is known as descriptive psychopathology and corresponds to the physical examination of medical and surgical cases. Rather than trying to learn lists of signs and symptoms, it is usually easier and more useful to see how they fit in with individual disorders. The psychiatric signs and symptoms described here are referred to in the rest of this book under individual psychiatric disorders; it will therefore be useful to keep referring back to this chapter. The best way of understanding descriptive psychopathology, however, is by clerking patients who have different psychiatric disorders and eliciting their signs and symptoms.

Appearance and behaviour

General appearance

The patient's general appearance should be described, with particular reference to any features that may be consistent with a psychiatric disorder.

Self-neglect, as evidenced by a lack of personal cleanliness, with hair and clothes that have not been looked after, may be consistent with dementia, psychoactive substance use disorder (of both alcohol and illicit drugs), schizophrenia or a mood disorder. Poorly fitting clothes that appear too loose may be evidence of recent weight loss, as occurs in certain organic disorders such as carcinoma, and in depression. A patient suffering from mania may be dressed in a colourful, flamboyant way.

The presence of calluses on the dorsum of the hands may be consistent with a diagnosis of bulimia nervosa, the patient using the fingers to stimulate the gag reflex in self-induced vomiting. (In such cases the calluses are referred to as Russell's sign.)

Facial appearance

The facial appearance can also give clues to the diagnosis, particularly with respect to organic disorders, for example the typical facial appearances seen in endocrinopathies such as Cushing's syndrome, hyperthyroidism and hypothyroidism.

Depressed patients often have downcast eyes, a vertical furrow in the forehead and downturning of the corners of the mouth. Manic patients, on the other hand, may look euphoric and/or irritable. Anxiety in general may be associated with raised eyebrows, widening of the palpebral fissures, mydriasis and the presence of horizontal furrows in the forehead.

Relatively fixed unchanging facies may be caused by the parkinsonian side-effects of antidopaminergic neuroleptic treatment (used in the pharmacotherapy of schizophrenia and mania, for example) or by Parkinson's disease itself.

The presence of fine, downy 'lanugo' hair on the sides of the face (as well as on other parts of the body, which may not be visible until a physical examination is carried out, such as the arms and back) may occur in anorexia nervosa. In bulimia nervosa the face may have a chubby appearance owing to parotid gland enlargement; facial oedema may also occur as a result of purgative abuse.

Posture and movements

In schizophrenia, and sometimes also in other disorders, the following abnormal movements may occur: ambitendency, echopraxia, mannerisms, negativism, posturing and stereotypies. In *ambitendency* the patient makes a series of tentative incomplete movements when expected to carry out a voluntary action (Figure 5.1). *Echopraxia* is the automatic imitation by the patient of another person's movements, which occurs even when the patient is asked to refrain. *Mannerisms* are repeated involuntary movements that appear to be goal directed. *Negativism* is a motiveless resistance to commands and to attempts to be moved. In *posturing*, the patient adopts an inappropriate or bizarre bodily posture continuously for a long time. *Stereotypies* are repeated regular fixed patterns of movement (or speech), which are not goal directed. In *waxy flexibility* (also called *cerea flexibilitas*), there is a feeling of plastic resistance as the examiner moves part of the patient's body (resembling the bending of a soft wax rod) and that part then remains 'moulded' in the new position (Figure 5.2).

Tics are repeated irregular movements involving a muscle group and may be seen following encephalitis, in Huntington's disease and in Gilles de la Tourette's syndrome (see Chapter 16), for example.

Parkinsonism is associated with a festinant gait.

Depressed mood may be associated with poor eye contact – the eyes often being downcast – and hunched shoulders. Increased movements and an inability to sit still may be seen in mania. Restlessness is also often a feature of anxiety (which may be associated with depression).

Underactivity

Stupor in psychiatry refers to a patient who is mute and immobile (akinetic mutism) but who is also fully conscious. It is known that the patient is fully conscious because the eyes, which are often open, may follow objects. Moreover, following the episode of stupor the patient may be able to remember events that took place during it. The condition is sometimes

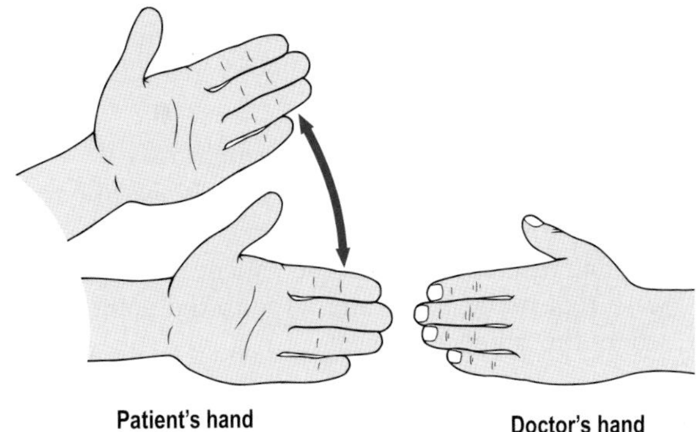

Figure 5.1 • An example of ambitendency. • The doctor proffers a handshake, the patient repeatedly alternates between extending and withdrawing the hand without ever reaching the point of actually shaking the doctor's hand.

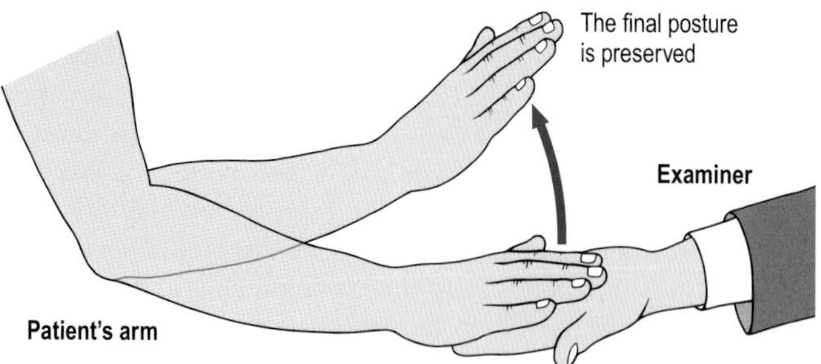

Figure 5.2 • Demonstrating waxy flexibility in a patient.

disturbed by periods of excitement and overactivity. It is seen in catatonic, depressive and manic stupor, and may also occur in epilepsy and hysteria. (In neurology stupor has a different meaning. A stuporose patient responds to pain and loud sounds, brief monosyllabic utterances may occur and some spontaneous motor activity takes place.)

Depressive retardation is a lesser form of psychomotor retardation occurring in depression, which, in its extreme form, merges with depressive stupor.

Obsessional slowness may be secondary to repeated doubts and compulsive rituals.

Overactivity

In *psychomotor agitation* there is overactivity, which is usually unproductive, and restlessness.

Overactivity, distractibility, impulsivity and excitability occur in *hyperkinesis*, which may be seen in children and adolescents, and is increasingly identified in adults.

In *somnambulism* (sleep walking) a complex sequence of behaviours is carried out by a person who rises from sleep and is not fully aware of the surroundings.

A *compulsion* is a repetitive and stereotyped seemingly purposeful behaviour. It is also referred to as a compulsive ritual, and is the motor component of an obsessional thought. Examples of compulsions include:

- checking rituals – in which the patient may repeatedly check that the front door is closed or that electrical switches are in the 'off' position
- cleaning rituals – in which the patient may hand wash repeatedly, sometimes even to the point where the skin is damaged
- counting rituals
- dressing rituals
- dipsomania – a compulsion to drink alcohol
- polydipsia – a compulsion to drink water
- kleptomania – a compulsion to steal
- trichotillomania – a compulsion to pull out one's hair
- nymphomania – a compulsive need in the female to engage in sexual intercourse
- satyriasis – a compulsive need in the male to engage in sexual intercourse.

Psychodynamic aspects

The psychodynamic aspects of movements should not be overlooked. For example, a married or engaged woman may play with her wedding or engagement ring during the interview because she has anxieties about her relationship; if she takes the ring off completely this may be indicative of an unconscious desire to end the relationship.

Social behaviour

Social behaviour may be altered in dementia, the patient not acting according to accepted conventions (e.g. the interviewer may be ignored). Schizophrenia may cause a patient to act bizarrely, aggressively or suspiciously. In mania, the patient may flirt with the interviewer and be sexually or otherwise disinhibited. In autistic spectrum disorders (pervasive developmental disorders), a person may act without seeming to have any concept of another's possible response.

Rapport

It is useful to record the nature of the rapport established with the patient. A positive rapport aids the formation of a constructive therapeutic relationship (see Chapter 4). A negative rapport may occur, for example, in the case of patients admitted to hospital against their will, and in some personality disorders (see Chapter 15). The rapport can be indicative of both the transference and the countertransference (see Chapter 4), and should be borne in mind when considering the underlying psychodynamics of the doctor's relationship with the patient and the latter's response to various types of treatment (such as individual psychotherapy). It is important that the doctor tries to establish a positive rapport.

Speech

Rate, quantity and articulation

The rate at which the patient speaks should be noted first. It may be increased in mania and reduced in dementia and depression. The quantity of speech may be increased in mania and anxiety but reduced in dementia, schizophrenia and depression.

There is an increase in both the quantity and rate of speech in *pressure of speech*, seen for example in mania; it is difficult to interrupt such speech. In *logorrhoea*, also called *volubility*, the speech is fluent and rambling, with the use of many words.

In *poverty of speech* there is a restricted amount of speech and any replies to questions may be monosyllabic. *Mutism* is the complete loss of speech.

The patient's *accent* may cause words to be pronounced in such a way as to be mistaken for neologisms by the interviewer. It should also be borne in mind that some people may normally speak in a way that could cause an incorrect psychiatric diagnosis to be made. For example, it is perfectly normal for some people from New York to speak in a rapid, pressured and loud manner; this should be taken into consideration before it is suggested that such a person is hypomanic.

Dysarthria is difficulty in the articulation of speech, *dysprosody* is the loss of its normal melody. In *stammering*, the flow of speech is broken by pauses and the repetition of parts of words.

Form of speech

The form of the patient's speech (i.e. the way in which he or she speaks) is noted (the content of the speech is considered later). If a disorder in the form of speech is suspected or found, it is useful to record a sample of the patient's speech that shows this.

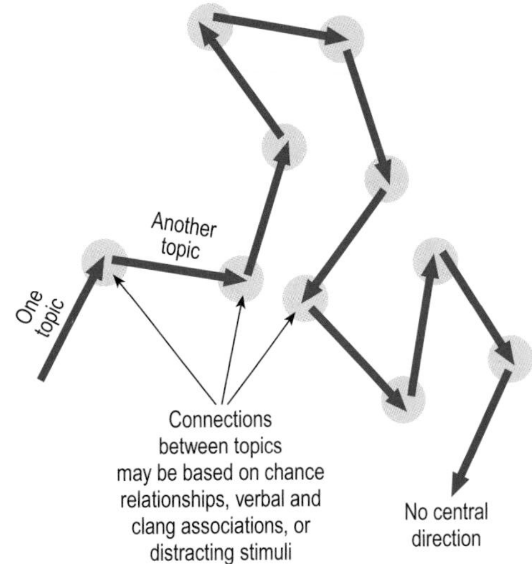

Figure 5.3 • Diagrammatic representation of flight of ideas.

In *flight of ideas*, the speech consists of a stream of accelerated thoughts, with abrupt changes from topic to topic and no central direction (Figure 5.3). The connections between the thoughts may be based on:

- chance relationships
- verbal associations, e.g. alliteration and assonance
- clang associations, e.g. 'The cat sat on the mat and that's that'
- distracting stimuli, e.g. a manic patient with flight of ideas is talking about why he has not been taking his prophylactic lithium carbonate medication, when he sees another patient with a long beard and abruptly changes the topic to that of beards in general.

In *circumstantiality*, thinking appears slow, with the incorporation of unnecessary trivial details, but the goal of thought is finally reached (Figure 5.4).

In *passing by the point* (also called *vorbeigehen*) the answers to questions, although clearly incorrect, demonstrate that the patient understands the question. For example, when asked 'How many legs does a cow have?' the patient may answer 'Five'. It is seen in the Ganser syndrome (first described in criminals awaiting trial).

A *neologism* is a new word constructed by the patient or an everyday word used in a special way. For instance, a woman suffering from schizophrenia who believed that electricity workers were interfering with her home said that they were doing this by means of instruments she termed 'electroenergators', which affected her electrical sockets.

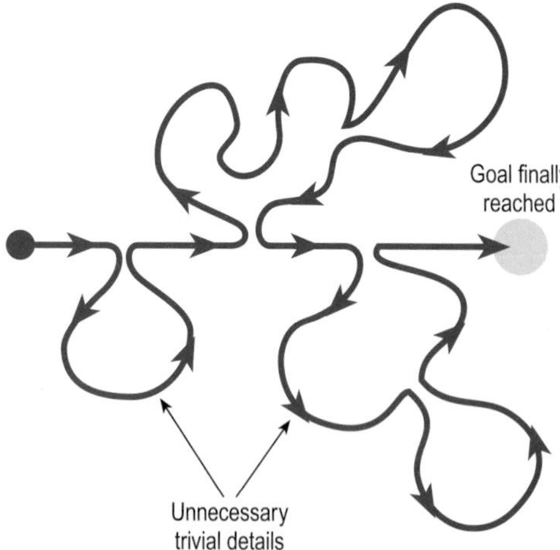

Figure 5.4 • Diagrammatic representation of circumstantiality, showing how the goal of thought is finally reached.

In *perseveration* (of both speech and movement), mental operations are continued beyond the point at which they are relevant. In *palilalia*, the patient repeats a word with increasing frequency; for example, a 79-year-old woman with Alzheimer's disease said 'Knife..knife..knife, knife, knife, . . .', faster and faster. In *logoclonia*, the patient repeats the last syllable of the last word. For example, a woman with Alzheimer's disease enquired 'What's the matter-er-er-er-er-er?'.

Echolalia is the automatic imitation by the patient of another person's speech, even when they do not understand it (e.g. another language).

In *thought blocking*, there is a sudden interruption in the train of thought, before it is completed, leaving a 'blank'. After a period of silence, the patient cannot recall what he or she had been saying or had been thinking of saying.

Disorders (loosening) of association occur particularly in schizophrenia and may be considered to be a schizophrenic language disorder. They are also sometimes called *formal thought disorder*. An example is *knight's move thinking*, in which there are odd tangential associations between ideas, leading to disruptions in the smooth continuity of speech. (This is like the knight's moves in a game of chess, which appear to jump abruptly from one square to another with which it is not directly connected.) In *schizophasia* – also called *word salad* or *speech confusion* – the speech is an incoherent and incomprehensible mixture of words and phrases.

The following five features of formal thought disorder were described by the psychiatrist Schneider:

- *Fusion*, in which heterogeneous elements of thought are interwoven with each other.
- *Omission*, in which a thought or part of a thought is senselessly omitted.
- *Derailment*, in which the thought derails onto a subsidiary thought.
- *Drivelling*, in which there is a disordered intermixture of the constituent parts of one complex thought.
- *Substitution*, in which a major thought is substituted by a subsidiary thought.

Schneider considered normal thinking to contain the features of *constancy*, in which a completed thought persists, *organization*, in which the contents of thought are separated from each other in an organized manner, and *continuity*, in which there is a continuity of the sense of the whole. In schizophrenia, the following three disorders of the form of thought were described by Schneider as corresponding to these three features of normal thinking:

- *Transitory thinking* (instead of constancy), in which omissions, derailments and substitutions occur.
- *Drivelling thinking* (instead of organization), in which the patient loses the preliminary organization of the thought, resulting in drivelling.
- *Desultory thinking* (instead of continuity), in which sudden ideas emerge but are not arranged in order in the whole content of consciousness.

Mood

DSM-IV-TR defines mood as 'A pervasive and sustained emotion that colors the perception of the world. Common examples of mood include depression, elation, anger, and anxiety.' An *objective assessment* should be made of the quality of the mood, based on the history, appearance, behaviour and posture of the patient. A *subjective assessment* of the quality of the mood as described by the patient can be obtained by asking a question such as 'How do you feel in yourself?', or 'How do you feel in your spirits?'

A *dysphoric mood* is an unpleasant mood. In *depression*, the patient has a low or depressed mood. This may be accompanied by *anhedonia*, in which the patient loses the ability to enjoy regular and pleasurable activities and no longer has any interest in them. In normal *grief* or mourning, the sadness is appropriate to the loss. If depression is apparent, the presence of depressive thoughts should be probed further, including asking about any *suicidal thoughts* the patient may have. If these are present, they should be recorded under 'Thought content' (see below).

Euphoria is a personal and subjective feeling of unconcern and contentment, usually seen after taking opiates or as a late sequel to head injury. *Elation* is an elevated mood or exaggerated feeling of well-being, which is pathological, and is seen in mania.

A patient with an *irritable mood* is easily annoyed and provoked to anger. A patient with *alexithymia* has difficulty in being aware of or describing emotions. In *apathy*, there is a loss of emotional tone and the ability to feel pleasure, associated with detachment or indifference.

Anxiety

When assessing mood it is important to remember that, in addition to depression and hypomania (or mania), anxiety can also be considered to be a mood disorder. Anxiety is a feeling of apprehension, tension or uneasiness owing to the anticipation of an external or internal danger. Types of anxiety include:

- *Phobic anxiety* – in which the focus of the anxiety is avoided (phobias are disorders of thought content).
- *Free-floating anxiety* – the anxiety is pervasive and unfocused.
- *Panic attacks* – anxiety is experienced in acute intense episodic attacks, and may be accompanied by physiological symptoms.

In the case of a patient who appears subjectively to be suffering from anxiety, the types of anxious thoughts should be enquired about; for example, 'When you're feeling anxious, what sort of thoughts do you have?'. The existence of situations that precipitate anxiety should be ascertained, as should the occurrence of somatic symptoms arising from the autonomic nervous system and from muscle tension, such as a dry mouth, palpitations, atypical chest pain, tremor, sweating and tension headaches.

Fear is anxiety caused by a realistic danger that is recognized at a conscious level. In *agitation*, there is excessive motor activity associated with a feeling of inner tension. In *tension*, there is an unpleasant increase in psychomotor activity.

Affect

According to DSM-III-R, affect is 'a pattern of observable behaviors that is the expression of a subjectively experienced feeling state (emotion) ... Affect is variable over time, in response to changing emotional states, whereas mood refers to a pervasive and sustained emotion.' The difference between affect and mood can be likened to that between the weather and the climate, with the first (affect/weather) being more short term and variable, and the second (mood/climate) more sustained. The appropriateness, constancy and reactivity of the patient's affect should be assessed.

Inappropriate affect is an affect that is inappropriate to the thought or speech it accompanies. For example, it is usually inappropriate to appear cheerful while talking about a recent bereavement. The externalized feeling tone is severely reduced in a patient with a *blunted affect*. A *flat affect* consists of a total or almost total absence of signs of expression of affect. A patient with a *labile affect* has a labile externalized feeling tone that is not related to environmental stimuli.

Thought content

Preoccupations

Any morbid thoughts, preoccupations and worries the patient has are noted. Suitable screening questions include 'What are your main worries and preoccupations?' and 'Do these interfere with your concentration and activities, such as sleep?'.

Hypochondriasis is a preoccupation with the fear of having a serious illness. This is not based on real organic pathology, but on an unrealistic interpretation of physical signs or sensations as being abnormal.

A pathological preoccupation with a single object is called *monomania*. *Egomania* is a pathological preoccupation with oneself.

Obsessions

Obsessions are repetitive senseless thoughts that are recognized as irrational by the patient and are unsuccessfully resisted. Themes include:

- fear of causing harm
- dirt and contamination
- aggression
- sexual
- religious, e.g. a religious person may have distressing recurrent blasphemous thoughts.

To check for their occurrence, the patient may be asked 'Do you keep having certain thoughts that don't make sense in spite of trying to avoid them?'. They may be accompanied by compulsions (compulsive rituals), described above, in which, for example, a patient may have to check repeatedly whether electric switches are off last thing at night.

Phobias

A phobia is a persistent irrational fear of an activity, object or situation, leading to avoidance. The fear is out of proportion to the real danger and cannot be reasoned away, being out of voluntary control. Some types are shown in Table 5.1. *Agoraphobia* is literally a fear of the market-place, and is a syndrome with a generalized high anxiety level and multiple phobic symptoms. It may include fears of crowds, open or closed spaces, shopping, social situations and travelling by bus or train. Phobias of *internal stimuli* include obsessive phobias and illness phobias, which overlap with hypochondriasis.

Suicidal and homicidal thoughts

Suicidal thoughts should be recorded. It is not only depressed patients who may have suicidal thoughts; but also they are common in schizophrenia, for example. Such thoughts may be accompanied by homicidal thoughts (see Chapter 9), which the patient should also therefore be asked about (e.g. 'Have you ever felt the wish to harm others?').

Table 5.1 Types of phobia

Phobia	Object of fear
Acrophobia	Heights
Agoraphobia	Crowds, open and closed spaces, shopping, social situations, travelling by public transport
Algophobia	Pain
Claustrophobia	Closed spaces
Simple phobia	Discrete objects (e.g. snakes and spiders) or situations
Social phobia	Personal interactions in a public setting, such as public speaking, eating in public, meeting people
Xenophobia	Strangers
Zoophobia	Animals

Abnormal beliefs and interpretations of events

Details of abnormal beliefs, including their content, onset and degree of intensity and rigidity, should be recorded. They may be referred to the environment. Persecutory delusions may occur in schizophrenia. Delusions of reference may occur in schizophrenia and can be enquired about: 'Do you ever feel that strangers or the radio, television or newspapers are referring to you in particular?' When similar thoughts are held but with less than delusional intensity (i.e. they are not unshakeable), they are referred to as *ideas of reference*.

Abnormal beliefs and interpretations of events may occur in relation to the patient's body, as in ideas or delusions of a hypochondriacal or nihilistic nature (as in depression). They may also occur with respect to the self in a more general way, in passivity phenomena such as thought insertion, thought withdrawal, thought broadcasting and made actions (see below). These may occur in schizophrenia. Similarly, delusions of poverty may occur in depression.

Overvalued ideas

An overvalued idea is an unreasonable and sustained intense preoccupation maintained with less than delusional intensity. The idea or belief held is demonstrably false and is not one that is normally held by others of the patient's subculture. There is a marked associated emotional investment.

Delusions

According to DSM-IV-TR, 'A delusion is a false belief based on incorrect inference about external reality that is firmly sustained despite what almost everyone else believes and despite what constitutes incontrovertible and obvious proof or evidence to the contrary. The belief is not one ordinarily accepted by other members of the person's culture or subculture (e.g., it is not an article of religious faith). When a false belief involves a value judgment, it is regarded as a delusion only when the judgment is so extreme as to defy credibility.' Some important types of delusion appear in Table 5.2. In a *mood congruent* delusion, the content of the delusion is appropriate to the mood of the patient, whereas the opposite is true in *mood incongruent* delusions. *Paranoid* delusions are not just persecutory delusions, but can also

Table 5.2 Types of delusion

Type of delusion	Delusional belief
Persecutory (querulant delusion)	One is being persecuted
Of poverty	One is in poverty
Of reference	The behaviour of others, and objects and events such as television and radio broadcasts and newspaper reports, refer to oneself in particular; when similar thoughts are held with less than delusional intensity they are called *ideas of reference*
Of self-accusation	One's guilt
Erotomania (de Clérambault's syndrome)	Another person is deeply in love with one (usually occurs in women, with the object often being a man of much higher social status)
Of infidelity (pathological jealousy, delusional jealousy, Othello syndrome)	One's spouse or lover is being unfaithful
Of grandeur	Exaggerated belief of one's own power and importance
Of doubles (l'illusion de sosies, seen in Capgras' syndrome)	A person known to the patient has been replaced by a double
Fregoli syndrome	A familiar person has taken on different appearances and is recognized in other people
Nihilistic	Others, oneself, or the world do not exist or are about to cease to exist
Somatic	Delusional belief pertaining to the functioning of one's body
Bizarre	Belief is totally implausible and bizarre
Systematized	A group of delusions united by a single theme or a delusion with multiple elaborations

include other types, such as delusions of grandeur and delusions of reference, as well as thought alienation (see below).

A *primary* delusion is one that arises fully formed without any discernible connection with previous events.

Passivity phenomena consist of the belief that an external agency is controlling aspects of the self that are normally entirely under one's own control. They include thought alienation (thought insertion, thought withdrawal and thought broadcasting), made feelings, made impulses, made actions and somatic passivity.

In *thought alienation*, the patient believes that his or her thoughts are under the control of an outside agency, or that others are participating in this thinking:

- *thought insertion* – belief that thoughts are being put into the mind by an external agency (Figure 5.5(a))
- *thought withdrawal* – belief that thoughts are being removed from the mind by an external agency (Figure 5.5(b))
- *thought broadcasting* – belief that thoughts are being 'read' by others, as if they were being broadcast (Figure 5.5(c))

The patient may feel that his own free will has been removed and that an external agency is controlling his feelings (*made feelings*), impulses (*made impulses*) or actions (*made actions* or *made acts*). He may feel under a form of hypnotic control.

In *somatic passivity*, the patient has the feeling of being a passive recipient of somatic or bodily sensations from an external agency.

Delusional perception

In a delusional perception, the patient attaches a new and delusional significance to a familiar real perception, without any logical reason. For example, when a patient with schizophrenia saw that a cupboard door was ajar, he immediately realized that this was a sign that meant that he was the King of Spain.

Abnormal experiences

Abnormal experiences may be referred to the environment (e.g. hallucinations, illusions and derealization), the body (e.g. alterations of somatic sensation and somatic hallucinations) or the self (e.g. depersonalization).

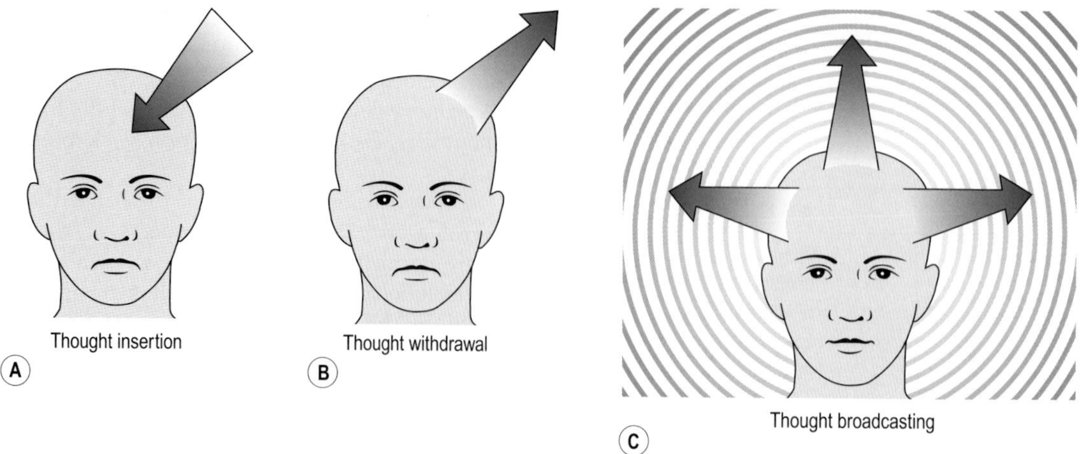

Figure 5.5 • Thought alienation.

Sensory distortions

Changes in intensity of sensations may occur, being either increased (*hyperaesthesia*) or decreased (*hypoaesthesia*).

Changes in quality of sensations occur particularly with visual stimuli, giving rise to *visual distortions*. When visual perceptions are coloured, for example because of toxins or retinal damage, they are named after the colours, such as:

- chloropsia – green
- erythropsia – red
- xanthopsia – yellow.

Changes in spatial form include *macropsia*, in which objects are seen as being larger or nearer than is actually the case, and *micropsia*, in which they are seen as being smaller or further away. (These changes are also called dysmegalopsia.)

Sensory deceptions

An *illusion* is a false perception of a real external stimulus. A *hallucination* is a false sensory perception in the absence of a real external stimulus. A hallucination is perceived as being located in objective space and as having the same realistic qualities as normal perceptions. It is not subject to conscious manipulation and only indicates a psychotic disturbance when there is also impaired reality testing. Hallucinations may occur in the auditory, visual, olfactory, gustatory or somatic modalities. Auditory hallucinations may occur in depression (particularly second-person hallucinations of a derogatory nature) and in schizophrenia (particularly third-person hallucinations and running commentaries). Somatic hallucinations can be divided into:

- *tactile hallucinations* (also called haptic hallucinations) which are superficial and usually involve sensations on or just under the skin in the absence of a real stimulus, including the sensation of insects crawling under the skin (called *formication*)
- *visceral hallucinations of deep sensations*.

Other special types of hallucination include:

- *Hallucinosis*. Hallucinations (usually auditory) occur in clear consciousness, usually as a result of chronic alcohol abuse.
- *Reflex*. A stimulus in one sensory field leads to a hallucination in another; for example, a man with schizophrenia would feel a sharp pain in his legs every time a certain patient called his name, and believed that this voice was the cause of the pain.
- *Functional*. The stimulus causing the hallucination is experienced in addition to the hallucination itself; for example, a woman with schizophrenia would hear voices commenting about her every time she flushed the lavatory.
- *Autoscopy* (also called the *phantom mirror image*). The patient sees himself and knows that it is he.
- *Extracampine*. The hallucination occurs outside the patient's sensory field; for example, a young man with schizophrenia believed he could just see Adolf Hitler standing behind him out of the corner of his eye, but every time he turned around Hitler disappeared.

- *Trailing phenomenon*. Moving objects are seen as a series of discrete discontinuous images, usually as a result of taking hallucinogens.
- *Hypnopompic*. The hallucination (usually visual or auditory) occurs while waking from sleep; it can occur in normal people.
- *Hypnagogic*. The hallucination (usually visual or auditory) occurs while falling asleep; it can occur in normal people.

As with delusions, hallucinations can be mood congruent or mood incongruent.

A *pseudohallucination* is a form of imagery arising in the subjective inner space of the mind. It lacks the substantiality of normal perceptions and occupies subjective rather than objective space. It is not subject to conscious manipulation.

An *eidetic image* is a vivid and detailed reproduction of a previous perception, as in a 'photographic memory'. In *pareidolia*, vivid imagery occurs without conscious effort while looking at a poorly structured background, such as a fire or plain wallpaper (Figure 5.6).

Disorders of self-awareness

These are also called *ego disorders* and include disturbances of:

- awareness of self-activity, including *depersonalization*, in which the patient feels that he is altered or not real in some way, and *derealization*, in which the surroundings do not seem real; both depersonalization and derealization may occur in normal people (e.g. during tiredness)
- the immediate awareness of self-unity
- the continuity of self
- the boundaries of the self.

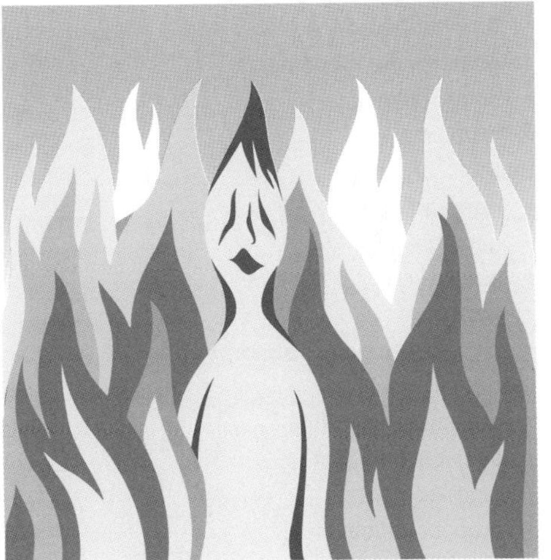

Figure 5.6 • Pareidolia. • Vivid imagery is seen without conscious effort while looking at a poorly structured background (in this case a fire).

Cognitive state

Orientation, attention and concentration, memory, general knowledge and intelligence should be checked. Further tests of the cognitive state that need to be carried out in those suspected of having an organic cerebral disorder, such as dementia, are detailed later.

Orientation

If disorientation is suspected, orientation in time, place and person should be assessed by asking the patient to give the time (day of the week, time of day, month, year), current location (name of the building if in hospital or outpatient department, and full address including the name of the town, county and country), and name, age and date of birth.

Attention and concentration

Attention and concentration can be checked by the 'serial sevens' test, in which the patient is asked to subtract seven from 100 and repeatedly subtract seven from the remainder as fast as possible, giving the answer at each stage. The time taken to reach a remainder less than seven is noted (the correct answers are 93, 86, 79, 72, 65 …). If this proves too difficult, perhaps because of poor arithmetical skills, a similar test using three instead of seven (serial threes) can be given. If this also proves too difficult, he can be asked to recite the days of the week or the months of the year backwards. As concentration is sustained attention, the serial sevens can be administered first and if the patient copes adequately there is no need to check attention separately. Disorders of attention include *distractibility*, in which the attention is drawn too frequently to unimportant or irrelevant external stimuli. If the patient is unable to attend to the task at hand, this should be noted, together with arousal level. In *selective inattention*, anxiety-provoking stimuli are blocked out.

Memory

There are a number of components to memory that should be assessed. Asking the patient to repeat immediately a sequence of digits can assess *immediate recall*. A normal person can immediately recall between five and nine digits, with a mean of seven. *Registration* can be assessed by saying a name and address and asking the patient to repeat them. Any mistakes should be recorded. The patient is asked to repeat this name and address five minutes later, and mistakes are again recorded; this is a test of *short-term memory*. *Memory for recent events* can be assessed by asking the patient to recall important news items from the previous two days. *Long-term memory* is assessed more formally by asking for the patient's date and place of birth.

Amnesia is the inability to recall past experiences, whereas in *hypermnesia* the degree of retention and recall is exaggerated.

Paramnesia is a distorted recall leading to falsification of memory, for example:

- *Confabulation*: gaps in the memory are unconsciously filled with false memories, as occurs in the amnesic (or Korsakov's) syndrome.
- *Déjà vu*: the subject feels that the current situation has been seen or experienced before.
- *Déjà entendu*: the illusion of auditory recognition.
- *Déjà pensé*: the illusion of recognition of a new thought.
- *Jamais vu*: the illusion of failure to recognize a familiar situation.
- *Retrospective falsification*: false details are added to the recollection of an otherwise real memory.

General knowledge and intelligence

General knowledge can be assessed by asking the patient to name the President of the USA, the colours of the national flag, five capital cities in a given continent or five state capitals. Whether the patient's intelligence lies within the normal range, clinically, can be judged from the answers to the general knowledge questions, from the responses to questions regarding the history and mental state examination thus far, and from the level of education achieved (from the history).

Learning disability or *mental retardation* is classified by DSM-IV-TR and ICD-10 according to the intelligence quotient (IQ) of the patient, as shown in Figure 5.7.

Dementia is a global organic impairment of intellectual functioning without impairment of consciousness. *Pseudodementia* resembles dementia clinically, but is not organic in origin; it may be caused by depression.

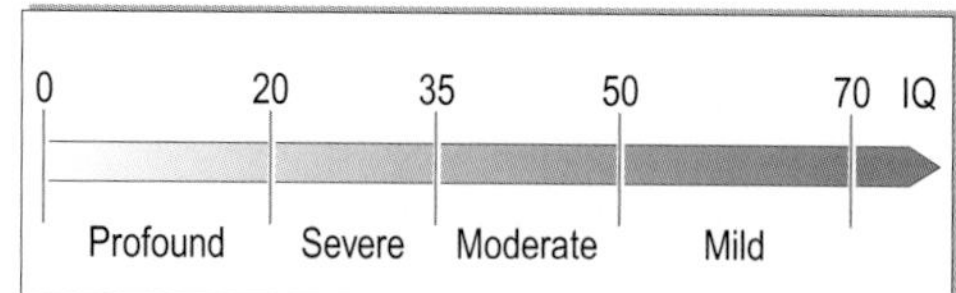

Figure 5.7 • The classification of mental retardation (learning disability) according to IQ.

Insight

If the patient has a psychiatric disorder, the degree of insight can be assessed by enquiring:

- 'Do you recognize that you are ill?'
- 'Do you accept that you have a psychiatric illness?'
- 'Do you accept that psychiatric treatment is necessary?'

The insight should not be recorded simply as being absent or present. Rather, reference should be made to the above three questions. For example: 'Mrs A had partial insight into her condition in that she recognized that she was ill but did not accept that it was psychiatric in nature and did not accept that she needed treatment.'

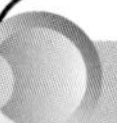

The mental state examination

- Appearance and behaviour:
  - general appearance
  - facial appearance
  - posture and movements
  - social behaviour
  - rapport.
- Speech:
  - rate and quantity
  - neologisms
  - accent
  - form
  - record a sample if abnormal.
- Mood:
  - objective– anxiety
  - subjective– affect.
- Thought content:
  - preoccupations
  - obsessions
  - phobias
  - suicidal and homicidal thoughts.

The mental state examination—cont'd

- Abnormal beliefs and interpretation of events:
  - referred to the environment – persecutory delusions, delusions of reference, ideas of reference
  - referred to the body – hypochondriacal and nihilistic delusions
  - referred to the self – passivity phenomena, delusions of poverty.
- Abnormal experiences:
  - referred to the environment – hallucinations, illusions, derealization, *déjà vu*
  - referred to the body – alterations in somatic sensations, somatic hallucinations
  - referred to the self – depersonalization.
- Cognitive state:
  - orientation in time, place and person
  - attention and concentration
  - memory – immediate recall, registration, short-term memory, memory for recent events, long-term memory
  - general knowledge and intelligence.
- Insight.

Physical examination

A full physical examination should routinely be carried out at the time of admission of a psychiatric inpatient. Organic disorders that can present with psychiatric symptomatology are described in Chapter 6.

Candidates for clinical examinations often do not have sufficient time when assessing a psychiatric case to carry out a full physical examination. In such cases it is usually possible to check the patient's blood pressure, fundi, neck (for a goitre) and so on. For example, the patient's pulse may be 'irregularly irregular' because of atrial fibrillation resulting from hyperthyroidism.

Organic cerebral disorder

Further tests of the cognitive state need to be carried out in those suspected of having an organic disorder affecting the brain, such as dementia and delirium (see Chapter 6). Further details are to be found in the excellent text by Hodges (1994).

Level of consciousness

The level of consciousness can vary, as shown in Figure 5.8, and the neurological terms somnolence (abnormal drowsiness), stupor and coma are described here.

A *drowsy* or *somnolent* patient can be awoken by mild stimuli and will be able to speak comprehensibly, albeit perhaps for only a little while before falling asleep again. A *stuporose* patient responds to pain and loud sounds and may make brief monosyllabic utterances, with some spontaneous motor activity. Note that the term stupor is used here in a neurological sense. In psychiatry, it means a patient who appears to be fully conscious (often with open eyes that follow objects) but who is mute and immobile and shows a lack of reaction to their surroundings; it is seen in catatonic, depressive and manic stupor. A *semicomatose* patient will withdraw from the source of pain but spontaneous motor activity does not take place. No response can be elicited in *deep coma*, there is no response to deep pain nor is there any spontaneous movement. Tendon, pupillary and corneal reflexes are usually absent.

Disorders of consciousness encountered in psychiatric practice include clouding of consciousness, delirium and fugue.

In *clouding of consciousness* the patient is drowsy and does not react completely to stimuli. There is disturbance of attention, concentration, memory, orientation and thinking. A patient suffering from *delirium* is bewildered, disoriented and restless. There may be associated fear and hallucinations. Variations include:

- *Oneiroid state* – a dreamlike state in a patient who is not asleep.
- *Twilight state* – a prolonged oneiroid state of disturbed consciousness, with hallucinations.
- *Torpor* – the patient is drowsy and falls asleep easily.

A *fugue* state is a state of wandering from the usual surroundings in which there is also loss of memory.

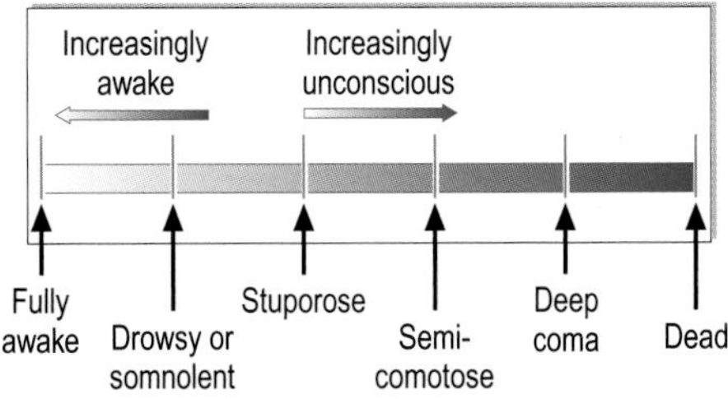

Figure 5.8 • The spectrum of conscious level.

Any change in the level of consciousness, including diurnal variation, should be asked about from nursing staff or other carers.

Language ability

Dysarthria, in which there is difficulty in the articulation of speech, can be tested by asking the patient to repeat a phrase such as 'West Register Street' or 'The Leith police dismisseth us'. Other defects of the motor aspects of speech that should be checked for include *paraphasias*, in which words are almost but not precisely correct, *neologisms* (see above), and *telegraphic speech*, in which sentences are abridged with words being missed out. In *jargon aphasia* the patient utters incoherent meaningless neologistic speech. *Expressive* or *motor aphasia*, also known as *Broca's non-fluent aphasia*, is a difficulty in expressing thoughts in words, while understanding remains and can be tested by asking the patient to:

- talk about his or her hobbies
- write to dictation
- write a passage spontaneously.

The types of *intermediate aphasia* include *central* or *syntactical aphasia*, in which there is difficulty in arranging words in their proper sequence, and *nominal aphasia*, in which there is difficulty in naming objects. The latter can be tested by carrying out a word-finding task, such as asking the patient to name objects or colours.

Receptive or *sensory aphasia*, also known as *Wernicke's fluent aphasia*, is difficulty in comprehending word meanings and includes the following types:

- *Agnosic alexia* – words can be seen but not read.
- *Pure word deafness* – words that are heard cannot be comprehended.
- *Visual asymbolia* – the patient can transcribe but has difficulty in reading.

Receptive or sensory aphasia can be tested for by asking the patient to read a passage, explain it, and respond to commands.

Global aphasia refers to the situation in which both receptive and expressive aphasia are present at the same time.

Handedness

If dysfunction in language ability is found, the handedness of the patient should be determined. The cerebral hemisphere associated with the expression of language is known as the *dominant hemisphere*, and in almost all right-handed people this is the left hemisphere. In left-handers, the left hemisphere is dominant in about 60%, the rest having either a right dominant hemisphere or a bilateral representation of language functions. The main functions of the cerebral cortex of each hemisphere are shown in Figure 5.9.

In determining handedness, it is not sufficient simply to ask which hand is used for writing: some left-handers may have been forced to learn to write with the right hand during childhood, for example. A more accurate picture is obtained by asking questions from a formal instrument such as the Annett Handedness Questionnaire (Table 5.3).

Memory

In addition to the tests of verbal memory (a dominant hemisphere function) carried out routinely in the mental state examination, tests of non-verbal memory (non-dominant hemisphere functions) should also be performed. A given design, such as that shown in Figure 5.10, should be drawn and the patient asked to redraw it immediately (registration and immediate recall) and then again after five minutes (short-term non-verbal memory).

Apraxia

Apraxia is an inability to perform purposive volitional acts, which does not result from paresis, incoordination, sensory loss or involuntary movements.

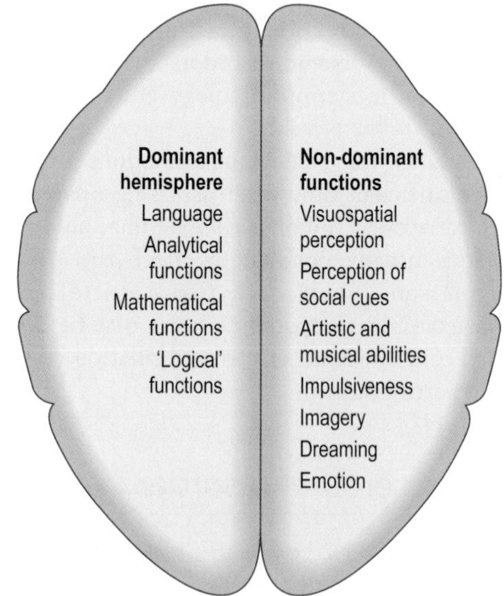

Figure 5.9 • Diagrammatic representation of the cerebral hemispheres, showing the typical lateralization of functions of the cerebral cortex.

Table 5.3 Modified version of the Annett Handedness Questionnaire

Which hand do you use:

1. To write a letter legibly?
2. To throw a ball to hit a target?
3. To hold a racket in tennis, squash or badminton?
4. To hold a match while striking it?
5. To cut with scissors?
6. To guide a thread through the eye of a needle (or guide needle on to thread)?
7. At the top of a broom while sweeping?
8. At the top of a shovel when moving sand?
9. To deal playing cards?
10. To hammer a nail into wood?
11. To hold a toothbrush while cleaning your teeth?
12. To unscrew the lid of a jar?

If you use the right hand for all these actions, are there any one-handed actions for which you use the left hand?

13. With which eye would you look through a telescope? (If you are not sure, roll a paper into a tube and look down it.)
14. Which foot would you use to kick a ball?

After Annett 1970; see Further reading.

Figure 5.10 • A typical geometric design that can be used in testing non-verbal memory.

Constructional apraxia is closely associated with *visuospatial agnosia*, with some authorities treating the two as being essentially the same. They are tested by asking the patient to construct a star or some other figure (such as a house) out of matchsticks, or else to draw them (Figure 5.11). The patient can also be asked to copy, at once and from immediate recall, a set of line drawings of progressive difficulty, as shown in Figure 5.12.

Dressing apraxia is tested by asking the patient to put on items of clothing.

Ideomotor apraxia is tested by asking the patient to carry out progressively more difficult tasks, for example touching parts of the face with specified fingers.

Ideational apraxia is tested by asking for a co-ordinated sequence of actions to be carried out, such as cutting a piece of paper in two using a pair of

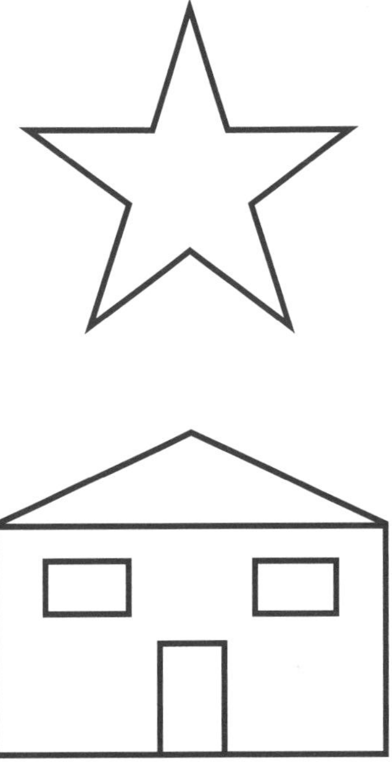

Figure 5.11 • Two typical figures that a patient can be asked to construct out of matchsticks, or else draw, when testing for constructional apraxia and visuospatial agnosia.

scissors and then folding one of the resulting pieces and placing it in an envelope. (If there is any evidence of dangerousness from the history and mental state examination, e.g. the presence of homicidal thoughts, then a potentially dangerous weapon such as a pair of scissors should not be made available to the patient.)

Agnosias and disorders of body image

Agnosia is an inability to interpret and recognize the significance of sensory information, which does not result from impairment of the sensory pathways, mental deterioration, and disorders of consciousness and attention or, in the case of an object, a lack of familiarity with the object.

Visuospatial agnosia has been considered above with constructional apraxia.

In *visual (object) agnosia*, a familiar object that can be seen, although not recognized by sight, can be recognized through another modality such as touch or hearing.

Prosopagnosia is an inability to recognize faces. In extreme cases this may involve an inability to recognize the reflection of one's own face in the mirror.

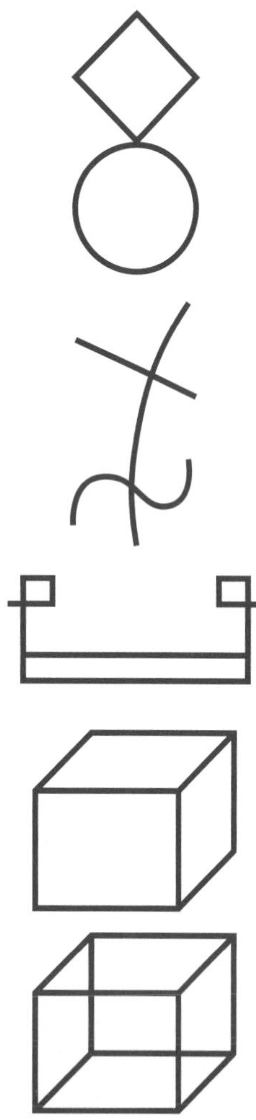

Figure 5.12 • A set of figures of progressive intricacy that a patient can be asked to copy, at once and from immediate recall, in order to test for constructional apraxia and visuospatial agnosia.

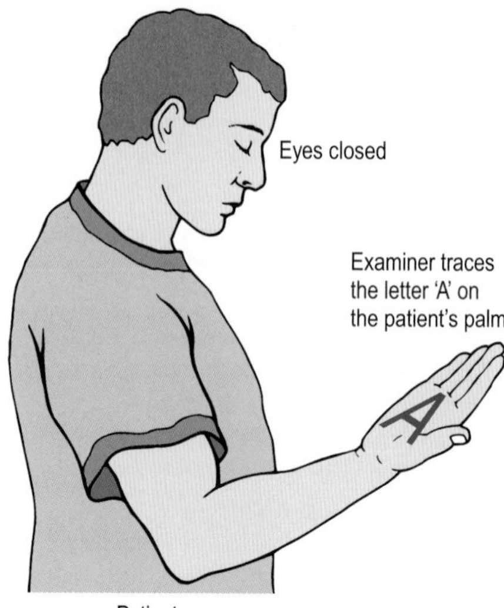

Figure 5.13 • Testing a patient for agraphognosia or agraphaesthesia.

For example, in advanced Alzheimer's disease a patient may misidentify their own mirrored reflection, a phenomenon known as the *mirror sign* (see Chapter 6).

In *agnosia for colours*, the patient is unable to name colours correctly even though colour sense is still present (e.g. coloured cards can be correctly sorted according to colour).

In *simultanagnosia*, the patient is unable to recognize the overall meaning of a picture, whereas its individual details are understood.

Agraphognosia or *agraphaesthesia* is present if the patient is unable to identify, with closed eyes, numbers or letters traced on the palm (Figure 5.13).

In *anosognosia* there is a lack of awareness of disease, particularly of hemiplegia (most often following a right parietal lesion). A localized distortion of body awareness is sometimes called a *coenestopathic state*.

Autotopagnosia is the inability to name, recognize or point on command to parts of the body. It can be tested by asking the patient to move certain parts of the body and to point to those parts both on him and on the examiner. The patient can also be asked the names of body parts.

In *astereognosia*, objects cannot be recognized by palpation. It is tested by placing an object in the patient's hand and asking for it to be identified with closed eyes (Figure 5.14).

Finger agnosia is the inability to recognize individual fingers, either the patient's own or another person's. This is tested by asking the patient to identify, with eyes closed, which finger has been touched.

Topographical disorientation can be tested using a locomotor map-reading task in which the patient is asked to trace out a given route on foot.

A patient may suffer from a *distorted awareness of size and shape* in which, for example, a limb may be felt to be growing larger. In *hemisomatognosis* or *hemidepersonalization*, the patient feels that a limb (which, in fact, is present) is missing, whereas in a patient whose limb *has* been removed the continued awareness of the presence of that limb is referred to as *phantom limb*. In the *reduplication phenomenon*, the patient feels that part or all of the body has been duplicated.

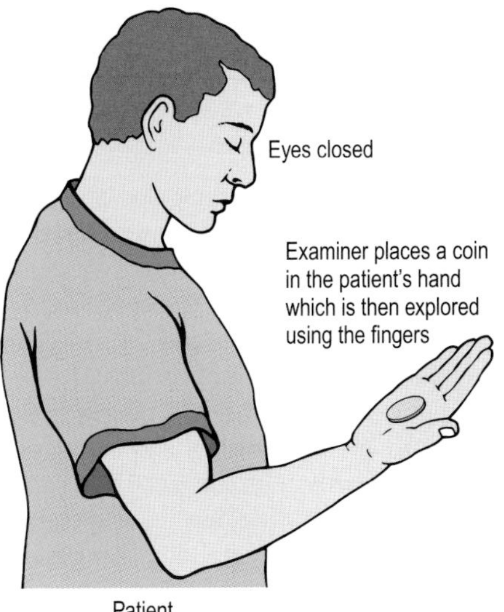

Figure 5.14 • Testing a patient for astereognosia.

Other cortical functions

Number functions (part of a test for Gerstmann's syndrome, also known as the *angular gyrus syndrome*) can be assessed by asking the patient to read aloud or write down numbers greater than 100, to count objects and to carry out arithmetical calculations (addition, subtraction, multiplication and division).

Right–left disorientation (part of a test for Gerstmann's syndrome) is tested by asking the patient to move his right and/or left hands, arms and feet, and by asking him to point to various objects on his right and left sides. He can be asked to carry out a command such as: 'Of the two pens in front of you, pick up the one on your right with your left hand and put it in my left hand.'

Verbal fluency (a test of frontal executive function) can be tested by asking the patient to recall as many words as possible, as quickly as possible, which begin with the letter F, in two minutes. He is instructed that proper nouns (e.g. France, Franco) are excluded as are variations in number, tense, etc. of the same word (e.g. flower *and* flowers, flower *and* flowered). The number of words is recorded and the test can be repeated using a different letter (often A and then S). In a further test of verbal fluency, he is asked to name as many (four-legged) animals as possible in one minute.

Abstraction (a test of frontal executive function) can be tested by asking the patient to interpret a proverb such as 'A rolling stone gathers no moss' or 'One swallow does not a summer make.'

Similarities (a test of frontal executive function) can be tested by asking the patient to state in what way the following are the same (Hodges 1994):

- an apple and a banana
- a coat and a dress
- a table and a chair
- a poem and a statue
- praise and punishment.

Alternating sequences (a test of frontal executive function) are tested by asking the patient to copy the simple alternating sequence shown in Figure 5.15 and to continue this alternating pattern.

Motor sequencing (a test of frontal executive function) may be tested by carrying out the Luria test. Here, the alternating hand sequence shown in Figure 5.16 (consisting of fist, side/edge, flat/palm, in this order and repeated) is demonstrated to the patient without verbal cueing four to five times and he is asked to repeat this sequence, without verbal cueing. Normal subjects can carry out this whole sequence at least four times in 10 seconds. If he cannot perform it, then verbal cueing ('fist, side, flat' or 'fist, edge, palm') is offered (but without a physical demonstration this time).

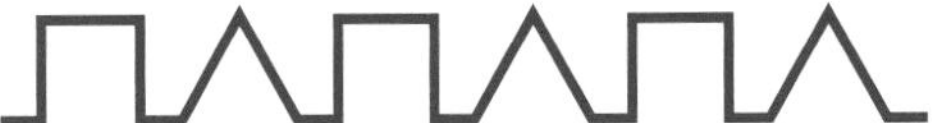

Figure 5.15 • Alternating sequences pattern to be copied and continued by the patient.

Physical examination

- A physical examination may allow organic causes of psychiatric symptomatology to be found.
- If an organic cerebral disorder is suspected, a fuller neurological examination should be carried out, including tests of:
  - level of consciousness
  - language ability
  - handedness
  - memory
  - apraxia
  - agnosia
  - number functions
  - right–left disorientation
  - verbal fluency.

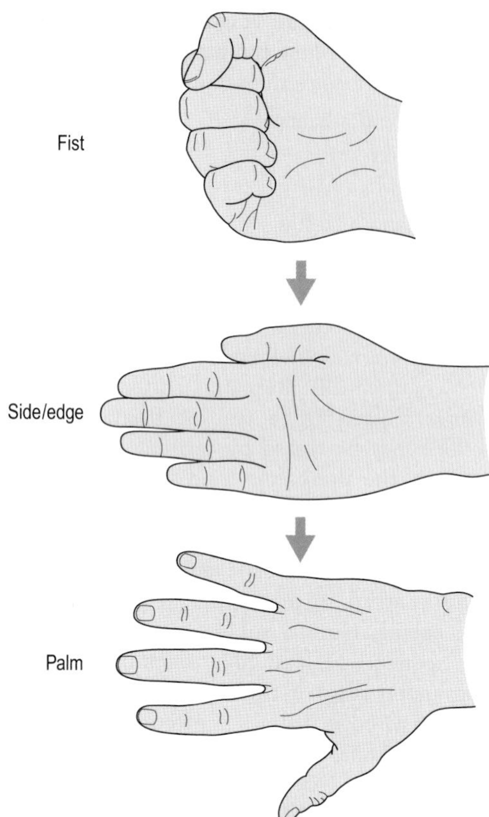

Figure 5.16 • The Luria test. • The subject gently slaps his or her thigh with their hand in the shape of a fist, and then with the side or edge of the same hand, and finally with the palm of the hand. This sequence is then repeated as rapidly as possible, and the number of complete sequences managed, without cueing, in 10 seconds is noted.

Investigations

Further information

When someone is admitted as a psychiatric inpatient, further information should be obtained from:

- relatives
- the GP (family doctor)
- other professionals involved in the case, such as social workers, community psychiatric nurses, psychologists and hostel nursing staff.

Further information should also be obtained from past psychiatric and medical case notes. If a patient has previously been admitted to other hospitals, time can be saved by requesting that the most important documents, such as discharge summaries, be faxed to the admitting unit.

Blood tests

An important reason for carrying out laboratory tests is to check for the presence of organic disorders, such as endocrinopathies and psychoactive substance-use disorders, that can present with psychiatric symptomatology (see Chapters 6 and 7). A second aim is to check for physical complications of psychiatric disorder. For example, self-neglect (as in schizophrenia and bipolar mood disorder) and eating disorders can lead to anaemia, electrolyte disturbances and the effects of vitamin deficiencies. Psychotic behaviour can also result in metabolic disturbances, for example as a result of compulsive water-drinking. A third aim of such tests is to detect metabolic disorders, such as hepatic disorders, which may influence pharmacotherapy.

Haematological, biochemical, endocrine and serological blood tests that should be carried out include:

- full blood count
- urea and electrolytes
- thyroid function tests
- liver function tests
- vitamin B_{12} and folate levels
- syphilis serology.

Second-line blood investigations, such as the calcium level, a cortisol assay and human immunodeficiency virus (HIV) serology, should be carried out only if indicated by the history or examination. In some countries, full informed consent must usually be obtained from the patient before a blood test for HIV can be carried out.

Urinary tests

A urinary drug screen should be carried out to check for covert psychoactive substance abuse. As with blood tests, second-line urinary investigations, such as levels of urinary porphyrins, should be carried out only if indicated by the history or examination.

Electroencephalography

Epilepsy can lead to psychiatric symptomatology. For example, complex partial seizures of the temporal lobe (temporal lobe epilepsy or temporolimbic epilepsy) can cause the symptomatology of schizophrenia and mood disorders. In first-episode admissions of such patients, electroencephalography (EEG) should therefore be carried out, as well as in other patients in whom epilepsy is suspected. In patients with learning disabilities (mental retardation) epilepsy is common, and this investigation may be required at the time of changing or stopping antiepileptic medication.

Neuropsychological tests

Psychometric testing by a clinical psychologist can be helpful in many cases, such as suspected dementia or pseudodementia, in child psychiatry and in the assessment of people with learning disabilities.

Neuroimaging

Structural neuroimaging is a second-line investigation, which is useful when an organic cerebral disorder is suspected. Thus, a magnetic resonance imaging (MRI) or computed tomography (CT) scan should be carried out if brain malignancy or the cortical atrophy of dementia is suspected, for example. MRI is also helpful as a second-line investigation if, for example, multiple sclerosis is suspected.

Functional neuroimaging with functional MRI (fMRI), positron emission tomography (PET) and single photon emission computer tomography (SPECT) are not currently routinely used as second-line investigations.

Human leucocyte antigen (HLA) typing

An example of a disorder for which HLA typing can be useful is narcolepsy. This sleep disorder is strongly linked with certain antigens. HLA typing, together with sleep laboratory testing (see below), is helpful because it helps corroborate the diagnosis and identifies those who are feigning the symptoms of narcolepsy in order to obtain stimulant drugs (including amphetamines).

Genetic tests

Karyotyping is a second-line investigation, which can confirm the presence of disorders caused by chromosomal abnormalities. This is particularly useful in the investigation of people with learning disabilities. For example, approximately 95% of cases of Down's syndrome are the result of trisomy 21 (47, +21) following non-disjunction during meiosis, giving rise to the abnormal karyotype shown in Figure 5.17. Figure 5.18 shows a pedigree in Down's syndrome resulting from a translocation involving chromosomes 13 and 21.

Genes associated with neuropsychiatric disorders will increasingly be characterized. In 1993 the gene mutation responsible for Huntington's disease, known since 1983 to be located on the distal short arm of chromosome 4, was identified. Such findings allow specific diagnostic genetic tests to be undertaken. It is also possible to carry out presymptomatic testing in the relatives (e.g. children and grandchildren) of affected patients; this raises ethical issues that are outside the scope of this chapter.

Sleep laboratory studies

These are used in the investigation of sleep disorders. Thus in narcolepsy, for example, the most striking physiological abnormality is the occurrence of rapid eye movement (REM) sleep at the onset of sleep or within 10 minutes thereafter. Although patients with excessive sleepiness and definite cataplexy can often be diagnosed on the basis of the history alone, laboratory investigations are helpful because of the reasons given above, and also, in the case of

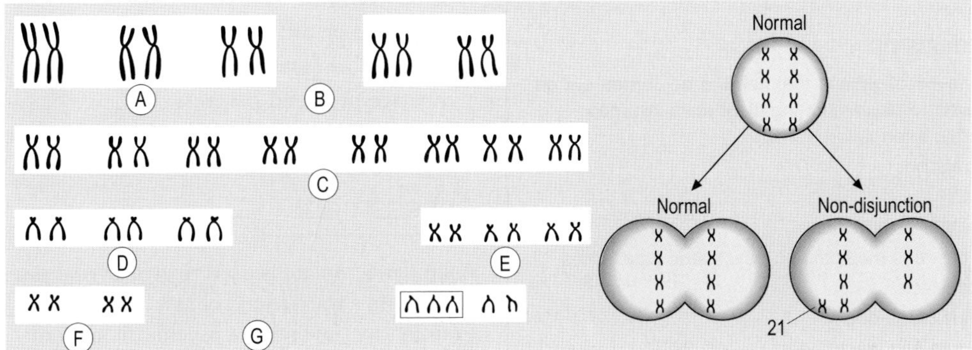

Figure 5.17 • Karyotype of Down's syndrome resulting from trisomy 21 following non-disjunction during meiosis.

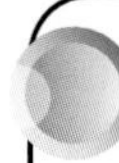

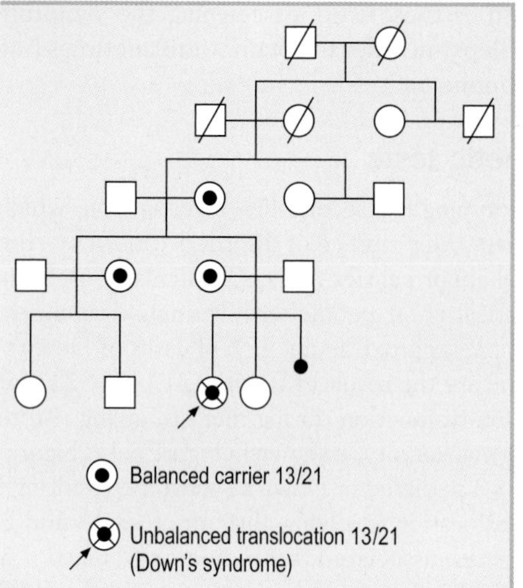

Figure 5.18 • Down's syndrome: 13/21 translocation pedigree.

sleep laboratory studies, they may disclose the presence of other disorders characterized by excessive sleepiness, such as sleep apnoea. The multiple sleep latency test is clinically the most useful technique for assessing sleepiness. The patient is asked to try to sleep at two-hourly intervals throughout the day. The length of time to the onset of sleep latency and the types of sleep that occur are monitored. More than 80% of patients with narcolepsy have a mean sleep latency of less than five minutes and at least two REM periods at the onset of sleep during this procedure. An EEG alone is inadequate for diagnosis, as REM sleep is recorded in less than 50% of patients with narcolepsy.

Investigations

First-line investigations that need to be carried out on admission to psychiatric inpatient units include:

- Further information from:
  - relatives
  - GP
  - other professionals
  - previous medical and psychiatric case notes.
- Blood tests:
  - full blood count
  - urea and electrolytes
  - thyroid function tests

Investigations—cont'd

  - liver function tests
  - vitamin B_{12} and folate levels
  - syphilis serology.
- Urinary drug screening.

Second-line investigations that can be carried out, as indicated by the history and/or mental state examination and/or physical examination, include:

- special blood and urine tests (e.g. HIV serology)
- EEG
- psychometric testing
- neuroimaging
- HLA typing
- genetic tests
- sleep laboratory studies.

The psychiatric report

The template given here is appropriate for most psychiatric patients, including children, adolescents and those with learning disabilities. A more specialized template is required in reporting on forensic psychiatry patients (see Chapter 21).

Components

The basic structure of a written psychiatric report (as detailed in this chapter and Chapter 3) is as follows:

- history
- mental state examination
- physical examination
- investigations
- diagnosis or differential diagnosis
- aetiological factors
- management and progress
- prognostic factors and further management.

Assessment

A similar template is used to give an oral assessment of a case in a ward round or as a candidate in a clinical examination involving a psychiatric patient:

- history
- mental state examination

- physical examination
- investigations to be performed (or already carried out)
- diagnosis or differential diagnosis
- aetiological factors
- management
- prognostic factors.

After the history, mental state examination and physical examination, a *brief* statement should be given that summarizes the main problems and the relevant positive and negative findings. After listing the investigations to be carried out, the diagnosis or differential diagnosis should be given. The main points in favour of and against each diagnosis should be indicated. Aetiological factors, the proposed management and the prognostic factors should then be given.

Letters to general practitioners

Since GPs are usually very busy, and already know most of the background information about their patients, it is usually appropriate to send them a short discharge letter in which the main points about the diagnosis, management and future management are outlined when the patient is discharged from hospital. This can then be filed with the GP's other notes on the patient.

Case history: sample case report

This case report is as an example of the application of the above template.

Mr A.B.
Date of birth: 12 June 1991
Address ...
Date of admission: 15 April 2011
Date of discharge: 16 May 2011
Consultant (Psychiatrist): Dr X

Reason for referral. Mr B. was admitted to Ward 3S by Dr X as an informal (voluntary) patient from the outpatient clinic with a three-week history of increasingly depressed mood and a three-day history of suicidal thoughts. These had worsened in spite of pharmacotherapy with 10 mg escitalopram daily.

History of presenting illness. Over the three weeks prior to admission, Mr B. had suffered from increasingly low mood, initial insomnia, early morning wakening and poor appetite. During the three days before admission, he began to feel that life was not worth living, and on the morning of the day of admission he reported considering hanging himself. He had been treated with escitalopram 10 mg daily but had not responded to this.

Family history. Father is a 51-year-old university professor of medicine. His mother is a 48-year-old accountant. Mr B. has no siblings. Mother and maternal grandmother have a history of depressive illness, for which mother has been treated in the past with electroconvulsive therapy. There is no other family psychiatric history.

Personal history. Mr B. was born in Oxford, UK, and his birth and early developmental milestones were normal. His childhood health was good and he made friends easily at school. After leaving school at the age of 18 with excellent academic qualifications, Mr B. went to the London School of Economics to read economics, and gained a second-class degree. He began his current postgraduate degree at the age of 21. Mr B. lives alone in student accommodation. He is heterosexually orientated and has had one serious relationship with a woman lasting about a year. This ended four weeks prior to admission, after she left him for one of his male friends. He has no children and there is no history of physical or sexual abuse in his past.

Past medical history. Unremarkable.

Past psychiatric history. Nil.

Psychoactive substance use. Drinks socially and does not smoke. No history of illicit drug abuse.

Forensic history. Nil.

Premorbid personality. He is normally sociable, outgoing and makes friends easily.

Mental state examination

Appearance and behaviour. Unshaven and unkempt young man who was wearing unwashed clothes. He sat quietly on a chair, made poor eye contact and kept looking at the floor during most of the interview. He was tearful at times. There was a good rapport and his answers to questions were appropriate.

Speech. He spoke slowly and there were long gaps between questions and his responses.

Mood. He was both objectively and subjectively depressed. He was not anxious. His affect was congruent and stable.

Thought content. He was preoccupied with thoughts about his girlfriend having left him recently, and how the man she left him for could do this to him. He had no thoughts of harming anyone other than himself.

Abnormal beliefs and abnormal experiences. He denied having any.

Cognitive state. His attention and concentration were poor, but there were no other abnormalities in his cognitive state.

Continued

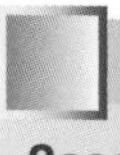

Case history: sample case report—cont'd

Insight. His insight was good in that he believed he was depressed and accepted that he needed inpatient psychiatric treatment for this.

Physical examination

Unremarkable.

Investigations

Routine haematological and biochemical tests were normal. His thyroid function tests, vitamin B_{12} and folate levels were also normal.

Diagnosis

Depressive episode.

Aetiological factors

The family history of depression on the maternal side indicates the possibility of a genetic loading for this disorder. This episode is likely to have been precipitated by the life event of his girlfriend leaving him for one of his friends.

Management and progress

In view of his suicidal thoughts, Mr B. was placed on continuous observations from the time of his admission until four days later, when he was no longer suicidal. The level of nursing observation was then gradually reduced to normal over the next three days. The escitalopram was increased to 15 and then 20 mg per day after admission. He was encouraged to vent his feelings about his ex-girlfriend and her new boyfriend in supportive psychotherapy sessions with his psychiatric nursing staff keyworker on the ward. Within two weeks his mood had improved, and his sleep and appetite were completely back to normal after another two weeks. After a successful weekend leave he was discharged on escitalopram 20 mg per day on 16 May to spend the following three weeks at his parents' home.

Prognosis and future management

Mr B. has come to terms with his separation from his girlfriend and he responded well to the increased dose of escitalopram. Therefore the prognosis for the present episode is likely to be very good. In view of the family psychiatric history he may be susceptible to further depressive episodes, and should continue to be followed up in the psychiatric outpatient department. It is planned that he will continue to take escitalopram 20 mg per day for the next six months.

Further reading

Annett, M., 1970. Classification of hand preference by association analysis. Br. J. Psychol. 61, 303–321.

Casey, P.R., Kelly, B., 2007. Fish's clinical psychopathology: signs and symptoms in psychiatry, third ed. Gaskell, London.

Hodges, J.R., 2007. Cognitive assessment for clinicians, second ed. Oxford University Press, Oxford.

Institute of Psychiatry, 1973. Notes on eliciting and recording clinical information. Oxford University Press, Oxford.

Leff, J.P., Isaacs, A.D., 1990. Psychiatric examination in clinical practice, third ed. Blackwell Scientific, Oxford.

Sims, A.C.P., 2003. Symptoms in the mind: an introduction to descriptive psychopathology, third ed. Saunders, London.

Organic psychiatry

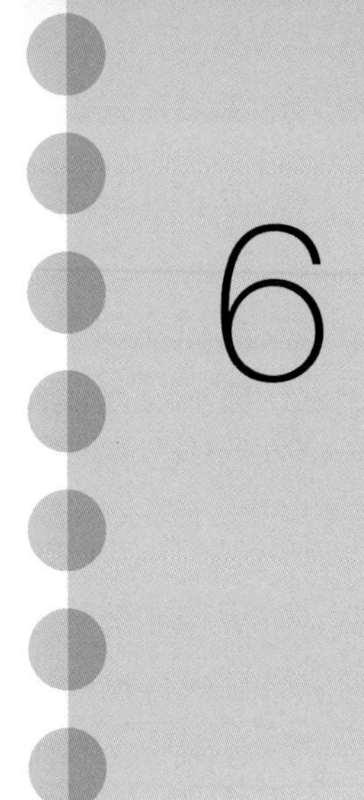

Introduction

In ICD-10 organic mental disorders are grouped on the basis of a common demonstrable aetiology being present in the form of cerebral disorder, injury to the brain or other insult leading to cerebral dysfunction (Table 6.1). The cerebral dysfunction may be:

- *primary* – disorders, injuries and insults affecting the brain directly or with predilection, e.g. Alzheimer's disease
- *secondary* – systemic disorders affecting the brain only in so far as it is one of the multiple organs or body systems involved, e.g. hypothyroidism.

Although, strictly speaking, they fall within the above definition, by convention the following disorders are excluded from the category of organic mental disorders and considered separately:

- *psychoactive substance-use disorders* (including brain disorder resulting from alcohol and other psychoactive drugs) – described in Chapter 7
- some *sleep disorders* – described in Chapter 6
- causes of learning *disability* – described in Chapter 17.

The use of the term 'organic' to describe the disorders discussed in this chapter does not mean that other disorders described in this book, such as schizophrenia and mania, are not organic (which they are in terms of genetics, biochemistry, pathology and so on), but simply that 'organic' disorders are attributable to independently diagnosable cerebral or systemic disorders.

Psychological dysfunction

The disorders described in this chapter result in psychological dysfunction in one or more of the following areas (see also Chapter 5):

- *cognitive functioning*, e.g. disorders of memory and intelligence
- the *sensorium*, e.g. disorders of consciousness and attention
- *thinking*, e.g. delusions
- *perception*, e.g. illusions and hallucinations
- *emotion/mood*, e.g. anxiety, depression and elation
- *behaviour and personality*, e.g. altered sexual behaviour.

Classification

In this chapter organic psychiatric disorders are classified according to whether they cause generalized psychological dysfunction or specific impairment in just one or two areas (e.g. thinking and mood) (Figure 6.1). Some disorders may cut across this classification. For example, at various stages in the course of its natural history, a brain tumour may cause psychological dysfunction that is acute and generalized (*delirium*), specific, and chronic and generalized (*dementia*).

Clinical aspects

Organic psychiatric disorders lie at the apex of the diagnostic hierarchy (see Figure 3.2). In other words, they should be excluded before a diagnosis of a

Table 6.1 ICD-10 classification: F00–F09 Organicorganic, including symptomatic, mental disorders

F00 Dementia in Alzheimer's disease
F01 Vascular dementia
Includes multi-infarct dementia and subcortical vascular dementia.
F02 Dementia in other diseases classified elsewhere
Includes dementia in Pick's disease, Creutzfeldt–Jakob disease, Huntington's disease, Parkinson's disease, and human immunodeficiency virus (HIV) disease.
F03 Unspecified dementia
F04 Organic amnesic syndrome, not induced by alcohol and other psychoactive substances
F05 Delirium, not induced by alcohol and other psychoactive substances
F06 Other mental disorders due to brain damage and dysfunction and to physical disease
Includes organic hallucinosis, organic catatonic disorder, organic delusional (schizophrenia-like) disorder, organic mood (affective) disorders, organic anxiety disorder, organic dissociative disorder, organic emotionally labile (asthenic) disorder, and mild cognitive disorder.
F07 Personality and behavioural disorders due to brain disease, damage and dysfunction
Includes organic personality disorder, postencephalitic syndrome and postconcussional syndrome.
F09 Unspecified organic or symptomatic mental disorder

'functional' psychosis, neurosis or personality disorder is entertained. For example, if a young man were to present for the first time with symptoms typically seen in schizophrenia, such as Schneiderian first-rank symptoms (see Chapter 8), it would be important to exclude the possibility that the symptoms resulted from an organic psychiatric disorder or psychoactive substance abuse, before treating the patient for schizophrenia. It could be that his symptoms were the result, for instance, of temporal lobe epilepsy or amphetamine abuse. Similarly, a middle-aged woman presenting with low mood may in fact be suffering from a brain tumour, hypothyroidism or Addison's disease, rather than a depressive illness. When such a primary organic cause is found, it should be the primary focus of treatment; in many cases it may be reversible.

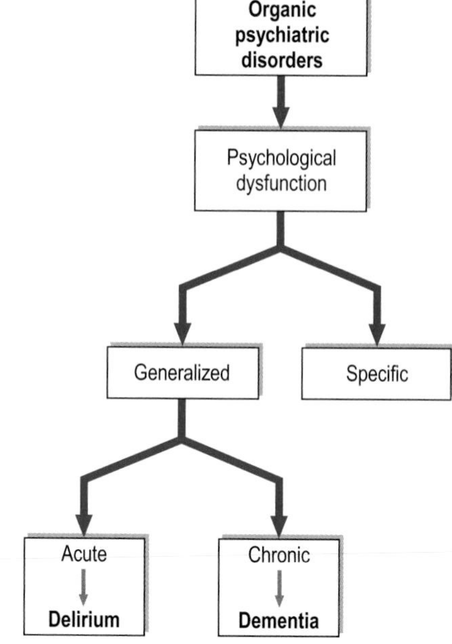

Figure 6.1 • Classification of organic psychiatric disorders.

To exclude an organic psychiatric disorder (including psychoactive substance abuse), it is necessary to take a detailed history, perform thorough mental state and physical examinations, and carry out appropriate investigations.

History

Aspects of the history that may indicate the presence of an organic psychiatric disorder (including psychoactive substance abuse) include:

- *History of presenting illness* – the patient may complain of psychological dysfunction (such as difficulties in cognitive functioning).
- *Family history* – of an organic disorder with a genetic component.
- *Personal history* – e.g. birth injury, childhood infections.
- *Past medical history* – physical disorders, operations and medication (interactions, side-effects and toxicity, e.g. steroid psychosis).
- *Drug history* – alcohol (e.g. Korsakov's syndrome), tobacco (e.g. carcinoma of the bronchus with cerebral metastases), illicit drugs (e.g. amphetamine psychosis).
- *Premorbid personality* – change in personality, e.g. in the frontal lobe syndrome.

Mental state examination

Pointers from the mental state examination that might indicate the presence of an organic psychiatric disorder (including psychoactive substance abuse) include:

- *Appearance* – e.g. the body build may suggest recent weight loss (as in malignancy and the AIDS-related complex); the facial appearance may suggest an endocrine disorder (such as hypothyroidism or Cushing's syndrome).
- *Behaviour* – e.g. bradykinesia, resting tremor, stooped flexed posture and festinant gait in Parkinson's disease; unsteady gait in normal-pressure hydrocephalus.
- *Speech* – e.g. aphasias (such as receptive or sensory aphasia resulting from a lesion in Wernicke's area).
- *Mood* – e.g. elevated mood in frontal lobe lesions.
- *Thoughts* – e.g. perseveration (common in both generalized and localized disorders of the brain), concrete thinking.
- *Perceptions* – visual hallucinations are usually caused by organic psychiatric disorders; hallucinations in other modalities may also occur (e.g. olfactory and auditory hallucinations in temporal lobe epilepsy, formication following cocaine use).
- *Orientation* – e.g. disorientation in time and place in delirium.
- *Attention* – e.g. impaired attention in dementia.
- *Memory* – e.g. loss of memory for recent events in dementia.
- *General information and intelligence* – e.g. there is impairment in these cognitive functions in dementia.

If an organic disorder is suspected it is important to carry out a detailed cognitive assessment including tests for apraxias, agnosias and language ability (see Chapter 5).

Physical examination

A detailed physical examination should be carried out if an organic psychiatric disorder is suspected. Together with the history and mental state examination, this may give a strong indication of the nature of the underlying pathology before any investigations are performed. For example, the presence of increased pigmentation in the mouth, skin creases and pressure points of a patient complaining of an insidious onset of low mood and lassitude points to Addison's disease. Similarly, in a young person presenting for the first time with auditory hallucinations, the presence of venepuncture marks points to the possibility that illicit drug abuse may be the underlying cause, although the relationship between drug use and psychiatric illness is not straightforward (see Chapter 7).

Investigations

The routine investigations detailed in Chapter 5 should be carried out: i.e. further information should be obtained from the GP, relatives and the case notes from any previous hospital treatment; routine haematological and biochemical tests, such as thyroid function tests; other blood tests as cited in Chapter 5 (such as syphilitic serology). In addition, other investigations should be carried out as appropriate: for example, cortisol assay in suspected Addison's disease, electroencephalography (EEG) in suspected epilepsy, magnetic resonance imaging (MRI) or computed tomography (CT) in suspected brain malignancy, and neuropsychological testing in suspected dementia or pseudodementia.

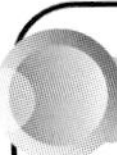

Introduction

- Organic psychiatric disorders cause psychological dysfunction in cognitive functioning, the sensorium, thinking, perception and/or emotion/mood.
- In order to exclude an organic psychiatric disorder, a detailed history, mental state examination, physical examination and appropriate investigations should be carried out.

Delirium

Delirium is characterized by acute generalized psychological dysfunction that usually fluctuates in degree. There is impairment of consciousness, often accompanied by abnormal perceptions (illusions and/or hallucinations) and mood changes (anxiety, lability or depressed mood). This is probably the most common psychiatric disorder encountered by medical students when first 'on the wards'.

Clinical features

The clinical features of delirium are summarized in Figure 6.2. Prodromal symptoms include:

- perplexion
- agitation
- hypersensitivity to light and sound.

Features of delirium itself include the following:

- *Impairment of consciousness*. The level of consciousness fluctuates, often being worse at night.
- *Mood changes*. The patient may be anxious, perplexed, agitated or depressed, with a labile affect.
- *Abnormal perceptions*. Transient illusions and visual, auditory and tactile hallucinations may occur.
- *Cognitive impairment*. Disorientation in time and place, poor concentration and impaired new learning, registration, retention and recall may all occur. Language disturbance may also occur.
- *Temporal course*. The disturbance develops over a short period (usually hours to days) and tends to fluctuate.

Epidemiology

Delirium can occur in patients suffering from physical illnesses, particularly hospital inpatients:

- general medical and surgical wards: delirium occurs in approximately 10%
- surgical intensive care units: 20–30%
- severely burned patients: approximately 20%.

Aetiology

Delirium can result from poisoning, psychoactive substance-use withdrawal, intracranial causes, endocrinopathies, metabolic disorders, systemic infections and postoperatively. Details of these causes, including psychoactive substance use (see Chapter 7), are summarized in Table 6.2. This is an appropriate place to consider briefly the more important clinical features of some of these endocrinopathies, particularly those that often present with psychiatric symptoms other than delirium.

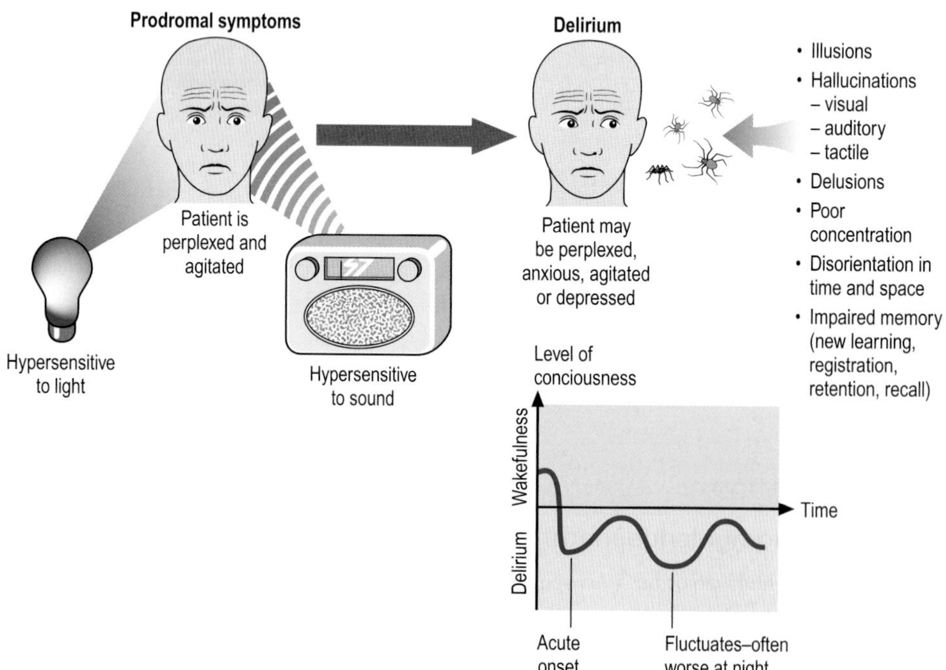

Figure 6.2 • Clinical features of delirium.

Table 6.2 Causes of delirium

Drugs and alcohol	Drug toxicity – antimuscarinic (anticholinergic) drugs, anticonvulsants, antihypertensives, anxiolytic-hypnotics, cardiac glycosides, cimetidine, insulin, levodopa, opiates, salicylate compounds, steroids; industrial poisons (e.g. organic solvents and heavy metals); carbon monoxide poisoning
Intracranial causes	Infections – encephalitis, meningitis Head injury Subarachnoid haemorrhage and space-occupying lesions – e.g. brain tumours, abscesses, subdural haematomas Epilepsy and postictal states Drug and alcohol withdrawal – withdrawal of anxiolytic-sedative drugs, amphetamine
Metabolic and endocrine disorders	Endocrinopathies – Addison's disease, Cushing's syndrome, hyperinsulinism, hypothyroidism, hyperthyroidism, hypopituitarism, hypoparathyroidism, hyperparathyroidism
Systemic infections	Hepatic failure, renal failure, respiratory failure, cardiac failure, pancreatic failure
Postoperative states	Hypoxia Hypoglycaemia Fluid and electrolyte imbalance Errors of metabolism – carcinoid syndrome, porphyria Vitamin deficiency – thiamine, nicotinic acid, folate, vitamin B_{12}

Primary hypoadrenalism (Addison's disease)

There is destruction of the adrenal cortex in this relatively uncommon endocrine disorder, leading to reduced production of glucocorticoids, mineralocorticoids and sex steroids. This condition often presents with symptoms similar to those that occur in depression, including weakness, tiredness, weight loss, depressed mood and anorexia. Important clinical features are shown in Figure 6.3(a) and (b).

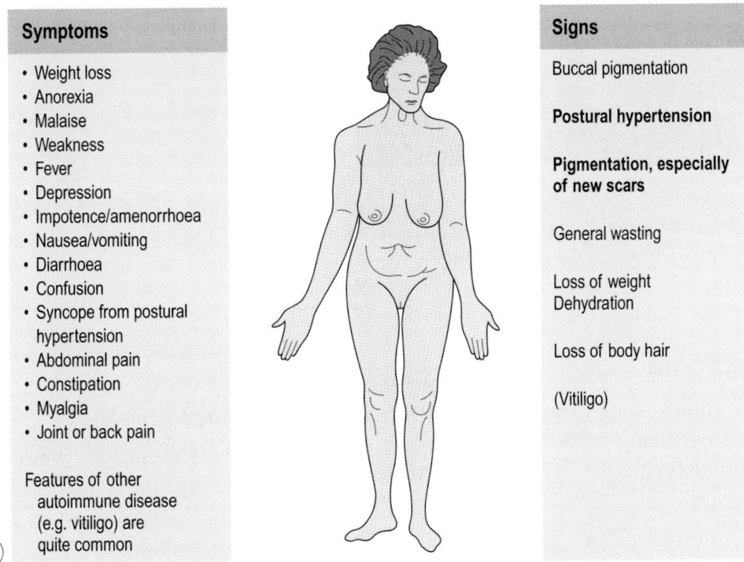

Figure 6.3 • Clinical features of primary hypoadrenalism (Addison's disease). (A) Bold type indicates signs of greater discriminant value. (Reproduced with permission from Kumar P, Clark M (eds) 1998 Clinical medicine. WB Saunders, Edinburgh.)

(continued)

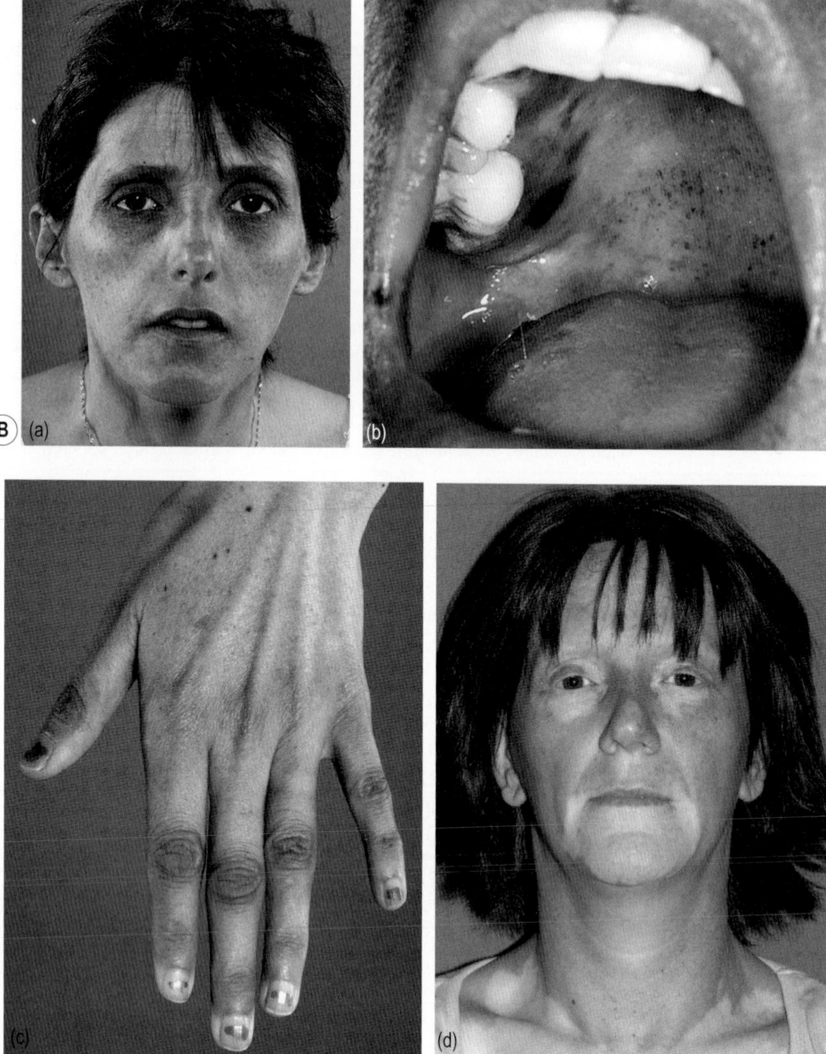

Figure 6.3—Cont'd (B) (a) Facial pigmentation. (b) Buccal pigmentation. (c) Skin crease pigmentation. (d) Vitiligo, which is particularly striking owing to Addisonian pigmentation of the 'normal' skin. (Reproduced with permission from Douglas G, Nicol F, Robertson C (eds) 2009 Macleod's clinical examination, 12th edn. Churchill Livingstone, Edinburgh.)

Cushing's syndrome

This describes the clinical state of increased free circulating glucocorticoid and occurs most commonly following the administration of synthetic steroids. Causes include:

- glucocorticoid administration
- pituitary-dependent (Cushing's disease)
- ectopic ACTH-producing tumours
- ACTH administration
- adrenal adenomas
- adrenal carcinomas
- alcohol-induced pseudo-Cushing's syndrome.

Cushing's syndrome may present with symptoms similar to those seen in depression, mania and schizophrenia (including mood changes, delusions, hallucinations and thought disorder). Important clinical features are shown in Figure 6.4(a) and (b).

Symptoms

- Weight gain (central)
- Change of appearance
- Depression
- Psychosis
- Insomnia
- Amenorrhoea/ oligomenorrhoea
- Poor libido
- Thin skin/easy bruising
- Hair growth/acne
- Muscular weakness
- Growth arrest in children
- Back pain
- Polyuria/polydipsia

Old photographs may be useful
Symptoms of hypopituitarism are rare

(A)

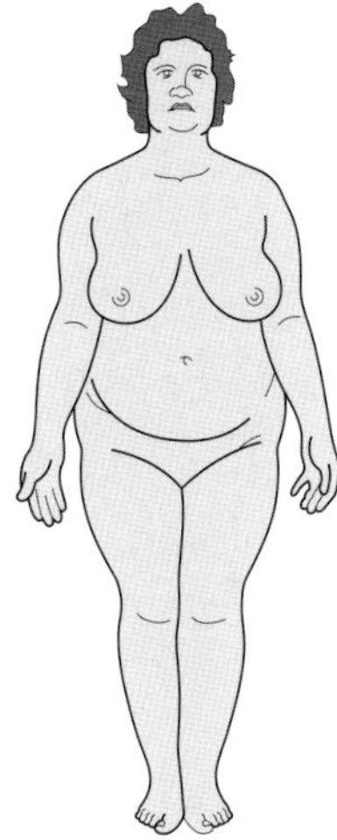

Signs

Depression/psychosis
Acne, hirsuties
Thin skin
Bruising
Hypertension
Rib fractures
Osteoporosis
Pathological fractures
Poor wound healing
Proximal muscle wasting
Proximal myopathy
Oedema

Frontal balding (female)
Moon face
Plethora
'Buffalo-hump'
Kyphosis
Centripetal obesity
Pigmentation
Striae (purple)
Skin infections
Glycosuria

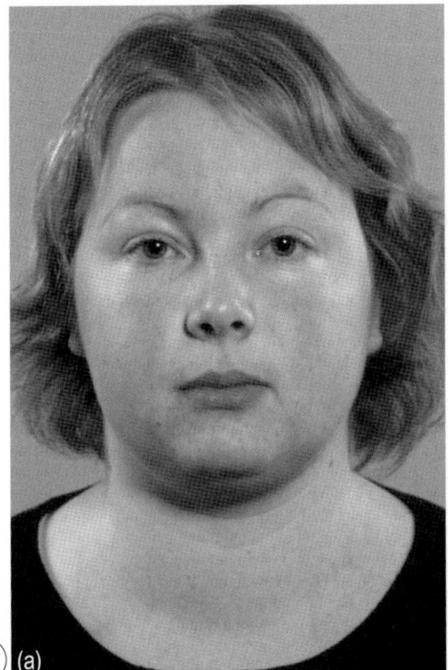

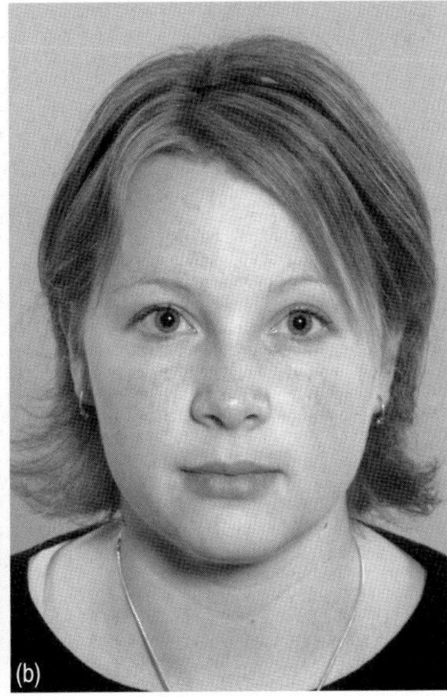

Figure 6.4 • Clinical features of Cushing's syndrome. (A) Bold type indicates signs of most value in discriminating Cushing's syndrome from simple obesity and hirsuties. (Reproduced with permission from Kumar P, Clark M (eds) 1998 Clinical medicine. WB Saunders, Edinburgh.) **(B)** (a) Cushingoid facies. (b) After curative pituitary surgery.

(continued)

Hypothyroidism

This is one of the most common endocrine disorders (particularly in women). Causes include:

- congenital causes – agenesis, ectopic thyroid remnants
- atrophic thyroiditis
- Hashimoto's thyroiditis
- iodine deficiency
- dyshormonogenesis
- antithyroid drugs
- other drugs – lithium, amiodarone, interferon
- postinfective thyroiditis
- postsurgery
- postirradiation

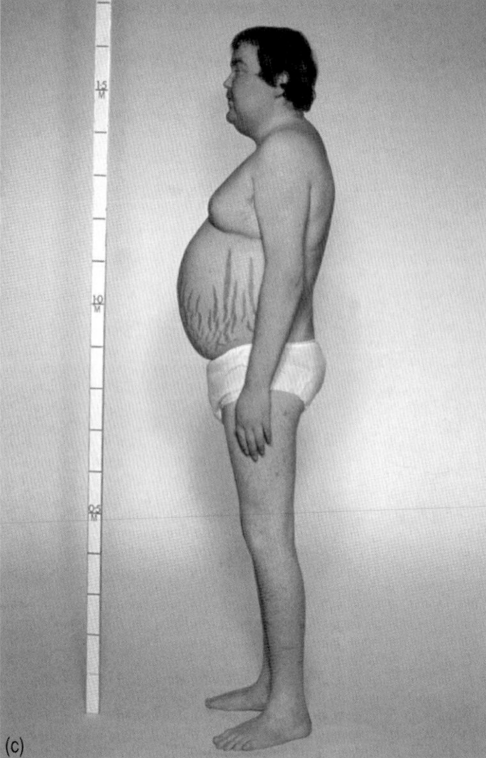

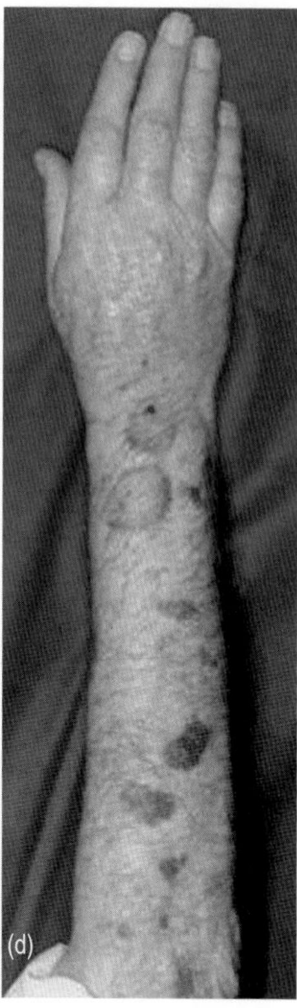

Figure 6.4—Cont'd (c) Typical features: facial rounding, central obesity, proximal muscle wasting and skin striae. (d) Skin thinning: purpura caused by wristwatch pressure. (Reproduced with permission from Douglas G, Nicol F, Robertson C (eds) 2009 Macleod's clinical examination, 12th edn. Churchill Livingstone, Edinburgh.)

- radioiodine therapy
- tumour infiltration
- peripheral resistance to thyroid hormone
- secondary hypopituitarism.

Hypothyroidism may present with symptoms similar to those seen in depression, mania and schizophrenia (myxoedema madness). Important clinical features are shown in Figure 6.5(a) and (b). Note that these features may not be seen in children and young women. The former often have slowed growth and perform poorly at school; pubertal development may be arrested. This condition should be excluded in any young non-pregnant, non-postpartum woman presenting with:

- oligomenorrhoea
- amenorrhoea
- menorrhagia
- infertility
- hyperprolactinaemia (e.g. manifesting with lactation).

Note also that the clinical features of hypothyroidism may be difficult to recognize in the elderly as some of them are similar to those that occur with normal ageing.

Hyperthyroidism

This is one of the most common endocrine disorders (particularly in women). Causes include:

- Graves' disease
- toxic solitary adenoma/nodule (Plummer's disease)
- toxic multinodular goitre
- de Quervain's thyroiditis
- postpartum thyroiditis
- thyrotoxicosis factitia
- exogenous iodine

Symptoms

- Tiredness/malaise
- Weight gain
- Anorexia
- Cold intolerance
- Poor memory
- Change in appearance
- Depression
- Psychosis
- Coma
- Poor libido
- Goitre
- Puffy eyes
- Dry, brittle unmanageable hair
- Dry coarse skin
- Arthralgia
- Myalgia
- Constipation
- Menorrhoea or oligomenorrhoea in women

A history from a relative is often revealing

Symptoms of other autoimmune disease may be present

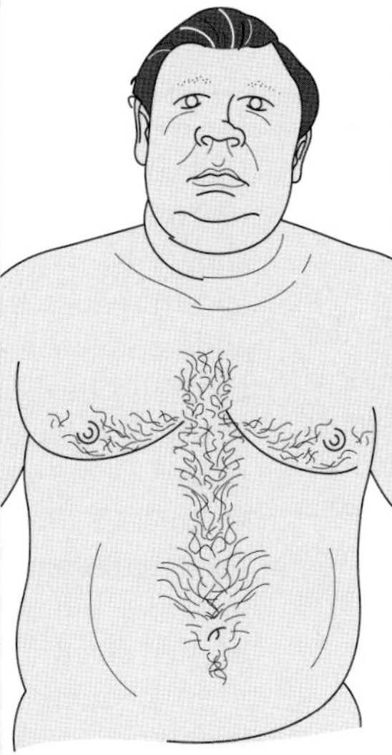

Signs

Mental slowness	Large tongue
Psychosis/dementia	
Ataxia	Periorbital oedema
Poverty of movement	Deep voice
Deafness	(Goitre)
'Peaches and cream' complexion	Dry skin Mild obesity
Dry thin hair	
Loss of eyebrows	Myotonia Muscular hypertrophy
Hypertension	Proximal myopathy
Hypothermia	Slow-relaxing reflexes
Heart failure	
Bradycardia	Anaemia
Pericardial effusion	
Cold peripheries	
Carpal tunnel syndrome	
Oedema	

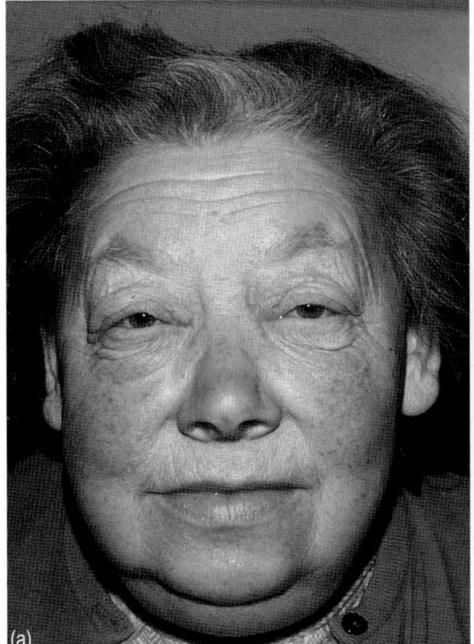

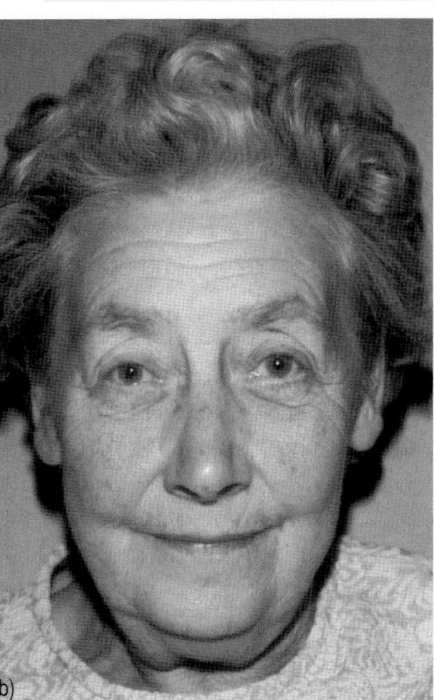

Figure 6.5 • Clinical features of hypothyroidism. **(A)** Bold type indicates signs of greater discriminant value. (Reproduced with permission from Kumar P, Clark M (eds) 1998 Clinical medicine. WB Saunders, Edinburgh.) **(B)** (a) Before treatment. Note the marked periorbital myxoedema, which may be particularly evident in older patients, and loss of eyebrow hairs. (b) After levothyroxine replacement. (Reproduced with permission from Douglas G, Nicol F, Robertson C (eds) 2009 Macleod's clinical examination, 12th edn. Churchill Livingstone, Edinburgh.)

- drugs – amiodarone
- metastatic differentiated thyroid carcinoma
- thyroid stimulating hormone (TSH)-secreting tumours
- human chorionic gonadotropin (HCG)-secreting tumours
- ovarian teratoma.

Hyperthyroidism may present with symptoms similar to those seen in mood disorders, panic disorder, generalized anxiety disorder and, in children, attention-deficit hyperactivity disorder (behavioural problems such as hyperactivity). Important clinical features are shown in Figure 6.6(a) and (b). Note that these features may not be seen in children, in whom hyperthyroidism may instead manifest as excessive growth or behavioural problems.

Management and prognosis

Appropriate investigations are carried out in order to determine the underlying cause of the delirium, which is then treated. In such cases, the episode of delirium usually lasts about a week, although it may sometimes last as long as a month. The prognosis is that of the underlying cause.

Good, calming nursing care is essential, preferably in a quiet single room. In general, it should be ensured that the delirious patient has an adequate fluid and electrolyte balance. The nature of the condition should be explained to the patient for reassurance and to reduce the effects of illusions, hallucinations and/or delusions (which may be persecutory in nature). The effects of disorientation can be reduced by, for example, allowing the patient to know the time, placing a television in the room and allowing visitors. A low level of lighting should be used at night, sufficient to reassure the patient of orientation in place, but not enough to interfere with much-needed sleep.

In patients who are very agitated, anxious or frightened, oral or intramuscular haloperidol can be used; if there is hepatic failure then benzodiazepines can be given. Benzodiazepines can also be given for their hypnotic effect at night. The treatment of alcohol withdrawal is described in Chapter 7.

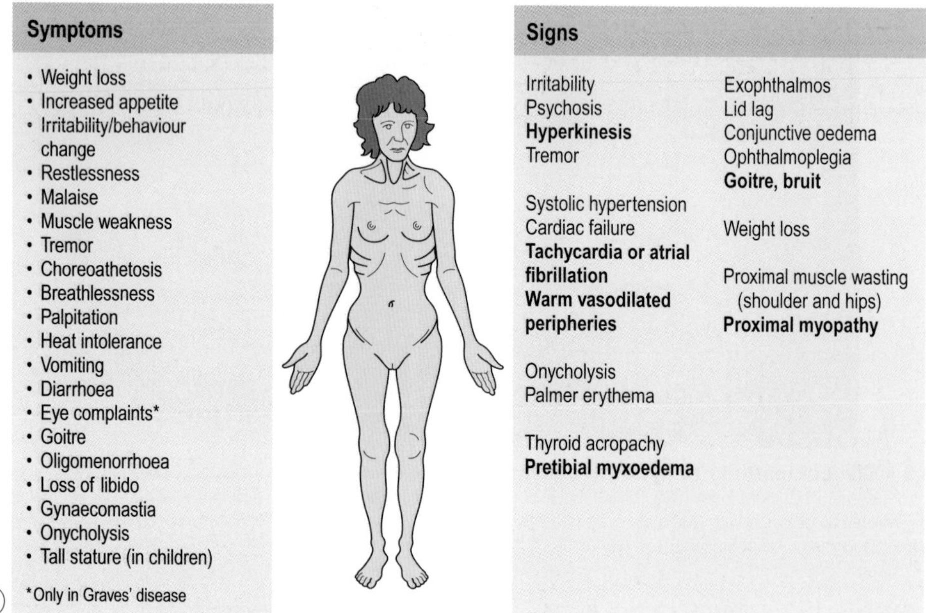

Figure 6.6 • Clinical features of hyperthyroidism. (A) Bold type indicates signs of greater discriminant value. (Reproduced with permission from Kumar P, Clark M (eds) 1998 Clinical medicine. WB Saunders, Edinburgh.)

(continued)

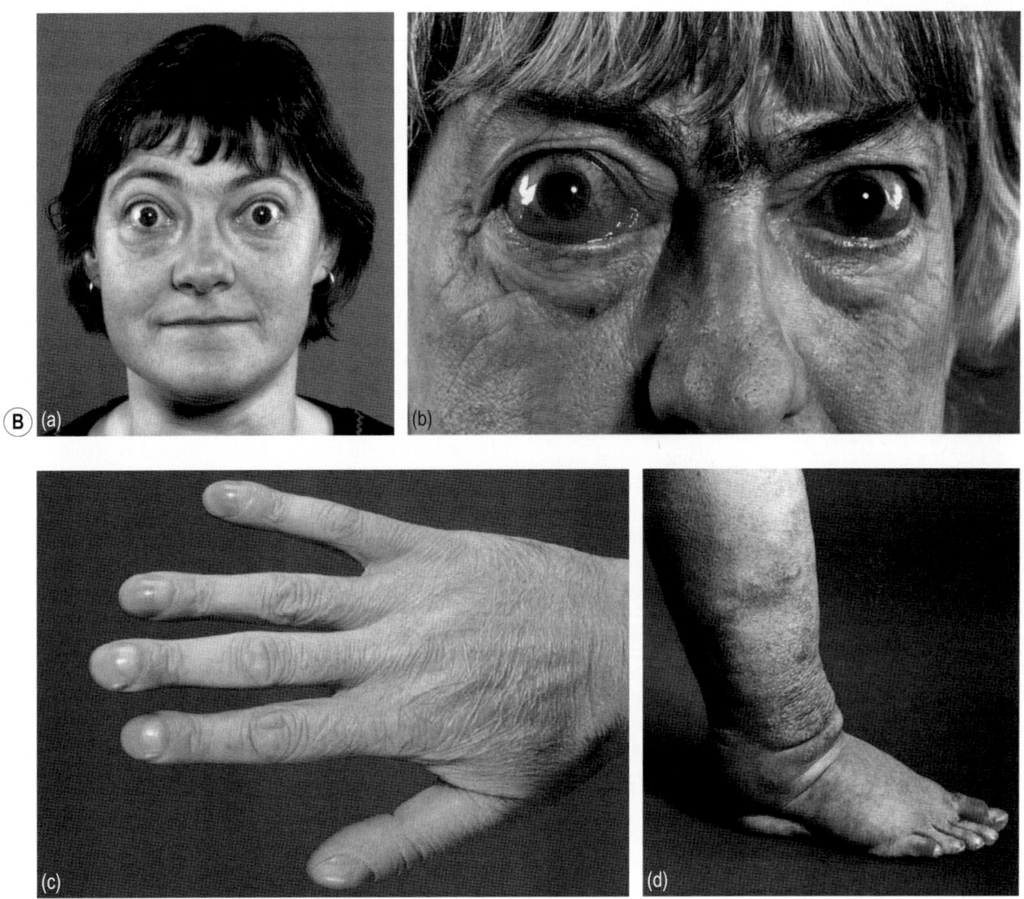

Figure 6.6—Cont'd (B) Clinical features of Graves' hyperthyroidism. (a) Typical facies. (b) Severe inflammatory thyroid eye disease. (c) Thyroid acropachy. (d) Pretibial myxoedema. (Reproduced with permission from Douglas G, Nicol F, Robertson C (eds) 2009 Macleod's clinical examination, 12th edn. Churchill Livingstone, Edinburgh.)

Dementia

Dementia is characterized by generalized psychological dysfunction of higher cortical functions without impairment of consciousness. In fully developed dementia the higher cortical functions affected include memory, thinking, orientation, comprehension, calculation, learning capacity, language and judgement. Dementia is an acquired and usually chronic or progressive disorder, although sometimes it may be reversible. In most sufferers the cause (e.g. Alzheimer's disease) is currently incurable; management strategies are discussed in Chapter 20.

Clinical features

The impairment of higher cortical functions mentioned above, which together form the cardinal feature of dementia, may be preceded, or more commonly accompanied, by impairment of:

- *emotional control* – anxiety, lability of mood, depression
- *social behaviour* – restlessness, inappropriate behaviour, e.g. shoplifting, sexual disinhibition
- *motivation* – the patient sinks into a set of rigid routines, with a loss of interest in new activities and reduced motivation; under stress the patient

is unable to cope and becomes markedly agitated, angry or upset (this is known as a *catastrophic reaction*).

Case history: postoperative delirium

Following a cardiac bypass operation, a 57-year-old man, while recovering in an intensive care unit, suddenly became very agitated and started shouting at the staff. He complained that the leads and tubes attached to his body were moving like snakes and he believed the nurses and doctors were trying to kill him. He was diagnosed as suffering from postoperative delirium. His fluid and electrolyte balance was normal. He was calmed by the nursing staff, who explained what was happening, and he agreed to take oral haloperidol (this was in order to prevent an accident, such as the intravenous tubing being pulled out and the monitoring equipment being disconnected). The haloperidol was given in syrup form to ensure compliance, as the patient was still somewhat suspicious and might have hidden tablets under his tongue, believing them to be poisonous. A night-time sleeping regime was instituted using benzodiazepines. At night, the lighting in the room was dimmed. By the fourth day the patient had made a full recovery from the episode of delirium, and had little memory of what had taken place.

Higher cortical functions

Higher functions that may become impaired in dementia include:

- *Memory*. Registration, storage and retrieval of new information are typically affected. Forgetfulness is a typical presenting feature. As the dementia advances, remote memory tends to be better than recent memory, which can result in confabulation. In advanced severe dementia even remote memory is affected, with the patient no longer remembering the names of spouse and children, for example.
- *Thinking and judgement*. Thinking becomes slower, with a reduced flow of ideas and impaired concentration. Judgement is impaired from early on and leads to poor insight. Paranoid thoughts and ideas of reference are common and may develop into delusions.
- *Orientation*. Disorientation for time, which may be present in early dementia, occurs in almost all cases of advanced dementia and precedes disorientation for place and person.
- *Comprehension and learning capacity*. The brain's ability to process incoming information is impaired.
- *Calculation*. This cognitive skill is usually impaired from early on in dementia.
- *Language*. Impairment in language manifests as difficulty in word finding and a reduced functional vocabulary in speech; a much greater use of clichés and set phrases; concretization; increasingly poor sentence construction and perseveration (e.g. echolalia). Careful examination may be needed to elicit nominal aphasia (e.g. by asking the patient to name objects), which may not otherwise be obvious.

In order to elicit the above clinical features it is particularly important to carry out a detailed mental state examination, including a full cognitive assessment (see Chapter 5), and to obtain further information from informants. Table 6.3 compares the features of delirium with those of dementia.

Table 6.3 Comparison of features of delirium and dementia

Delirium	Dementia
Acute onset	Insidious onset
Disorientation, bewilderment, anxiety, poor attention	
Clouding of/impaired consciousness, e.g. drowsy	Clear consciousness
Perceptual abnormalities (illusions, hallucinations)	Global impairment of cerebral functions (e.g. recent memory, intellectual impairment and personality deterioration with secondary behaviour abnormalities)
Paranoid ideas/delusions (term delirium sometimes only used if delusions and/or hallucinations present)	
Fluctuating course with lucid intervals	Progressive course (static course in head injury and brain damage)
Reversible	Irreversible

Epidemiology

The prevalence of dementia increases with age. In Western countries dementia afflicts at least 5% of the population aged over 65 and 10% of those aged over 80.

Aetiology

The causes of dementia are summarized in Table 6.4. Alzheimer's disease and vascular (including multi-infarct) dementia together account for approximately three-quarters of all cases of dementia. They are described in more detail in this section, with other specific causes of dementia: Lewy body dementia, frontotemporal dementia, Pick's disease, Huntington's disease (chorea), Creutzfeldt–Jakob disease and normal-pressure hydrocephalus. Other disorders that can result in dementia, for example Parkinson's disease, are described in the next section of this chapter and in Chapter 7.

Table 6.4 Causes of dementia

Degenerative diseases of the CNS	Alzheimer's disease Pick's disease Huntington's disease (or chorea) Creutzfeldt–Jakob disease Normal-pressure hydrocephalus Parkinson's disease Multiple sclerosis Lewy body disease
Intracranial causes	Space-occupying lesions – tumours, chronic subdural haematomas, chronic abscesses, aneurysms Infections – encephalitis, meningitis, neurosyphilis, AIDS and AIDS-related complex (ARC), cerebral sarcoidosis Trauma – head injury, punch-drunk syndrome
Metabolic and endocrine disorders	Endocrinopathies – Addison's disease, Cushing's syndrome, hyperinsulinism, hypothyroidism, hypopituitarism, hypoparathyroidism, hyperparathyroidism Hepatic failure, renal failure, respiratory failure Hypoxia Renal dialysis Chronic uraemia Chronic electrolyte imbalance – hypocalcaemia, hypercalcaemia, hypokalaemia, hyponatraemia, hypernatraemia Porphyria Hepatolenticular degeneration (Wilson's disease) Vitamin deficiency – thiamine, nicotinic acid, folate, vitamin B_{12} Vitamin intoxication – vitamin A, vitamin D Paget's disease Remote effects of carcinoma or lymphomas
Vascular causes	Multi-infarct dementia Cerebral artery occlusion Cranial arteritis Arteriovenous malformation Binswanger's disease
Intoxication	Alcohol Heavy metals – lead, arsenic, mercury, thallium Carbon monoxide Drug and alcohol withdrawal – withdrawal of anxiolytic-sedative drugs, amphetamine

Alzheimer's disease

Alzheimer's disease is the most common cause of dementia in people over the age of 65. The same pathological changes take place in both the senile (onset over the age of 65) and the presenile forms (onset under the age of 65). A 39–43 amino acid fragment of β-amyloid precursor protein (APP), Aβ, accumulates in the brain parenchyma to form the typical lesions associated with Alzheimer's disease.

Pathological features

Macroscopically there is global atrophy of the brain, which is shrunken with widened sulci and ventricular enlargement. The atrophy is usually most marked in the frontal and temporal lobes, as shown in Figure 6.7. The structural neuroimaging appearances seen are shown in Figure 6.8.

Histologically there is neuronal loss, shrinkage of dendritic branching and a reactive astrocytosis in the cerebral cortex. Other neuropathological features include the abundant presence, particularly in the cerebral cortex, of neurofibrillary tangles; the presence, mainly in the cortex, of silver-staining neuritic plaques (senile plaques) (Figure 6.9); granulovacuolar degeneration, particularly in the middle pyramidal layer of the hippocampus; and

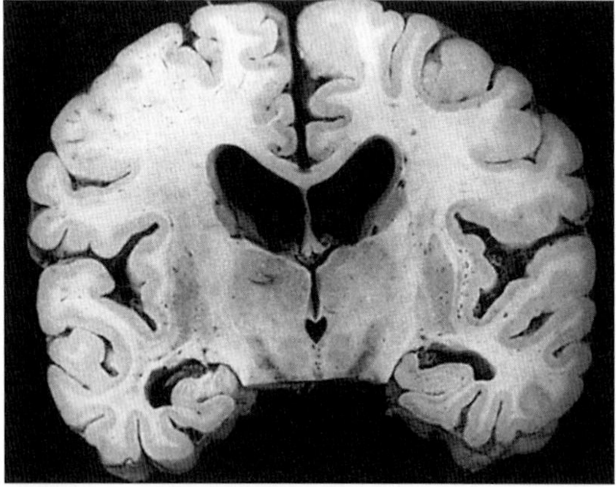

Figure 6.7 • Alzheimer's disease. • The coronal section shows gross atrophy, affecting in particular the temporal lobes, and associated lateral ventricular enlargement. (Reproduced with permission from Graham DI, Nicoll JAR, Bone I (eds) 2006; see Further reading.)

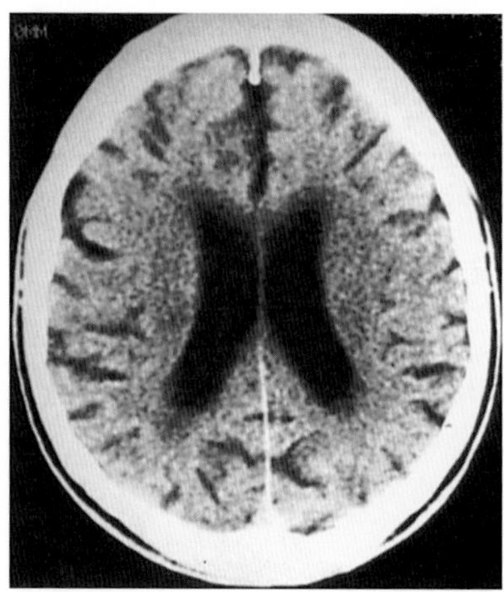

Figure 6.8 • Alzheimer's disease seen on CT scan. (Reproduced with permission from Suohami RL, Moxhum J (eds) 1994 Textbook of medicine, 2nd edn. Churchill Livingstone, Edinburgh.)

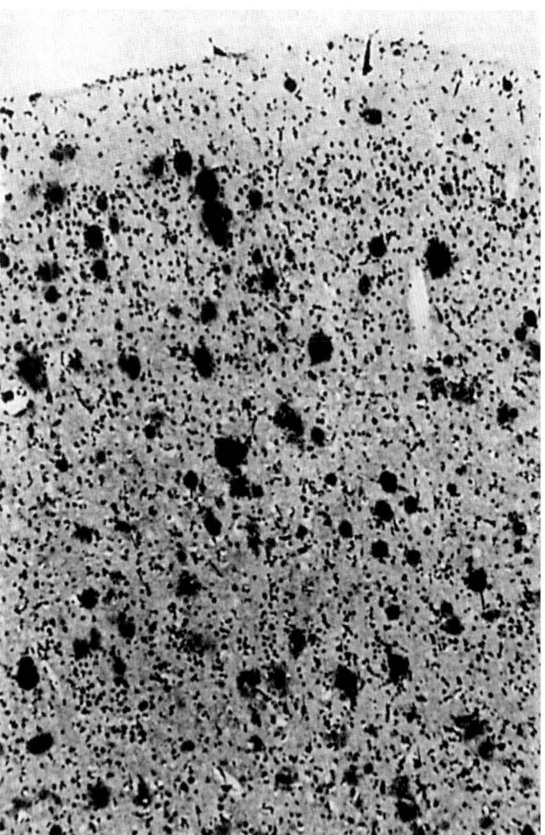

Figure 6.9 • Alzheimer's disease. • There are many silver-staining neuritic plaques in the cerebral cortex which can be seen to be granular and filamentous. Some of the plaques have dense cores. (Reproduced with permission from Graham DI, Nicoll JAR, Bone I (eds) 2006; see Further reading.)

eosinophilic rod-shaped filamentous intracytoplasmic neuronal inclusion bodies known as Hirano bodies. Neurofibrillary tangles are silver-staining highly insoluble neuropathological structures of the neuronal perikaryon, made up of thick bundles of neurofibrils. The numbers of neurofibrillary tangles and neuritic plaques correlate with the degree of cognitive impairment.

Electron microscopy reveals that each neuritic plaque contains an amyloid core made of Aβ. Abnormal neurites surround the amyloid. The gene coding for Aβ has been localized to the long arm of chromosome 21.

Biochemically, in the post-mortem brain there is reduced activity of both acetylcholinesterase and choline acetyltransferase. These enzymes are involved in the metabolism and biosynthesis, respectively, of the neurotransmitter acetylcholine. Other neurotransmitters, for example γ-aminobutyric acid (GABA), may also play a role.

Clinical features

Alzheimer's disease is more common in women and in those with a family history of:

- Alzheimer's disease
- Down's syndrome
- lymphoma.

It usually presents with memory loss. Other clinical features may include: apathy or lability of mood; progressive impairment of intellectual function; progressive deterioration of personality; features typical of parietal lobe dysfunction (see below); paranoid features; parkinsonism; the mirror sign, in which individuals may fail to recognize their own reflection; disorders of speech such as logoclonia and echolalia; epilepsy; and aspects of the Klüver–Bucy syndrome, which includes hyperorality, hypersexuality, hyperphagia and placidity.

Patients with Down's syndrome are very likely to develop the neuropathology and clinical features of Alzheimer's disease by the time they reach the fourth decade (see Chapter 17). This is probably related to the fact that Down's syndrome results from trisomy 21.

Lewy body dementia

The generic term 'dementia with Lewy bodies' was proposed at the first International Workshop on Lewy Body Dementia in 1995. (It was described in 1923 by Frederick H. Lewy in a large proportion of his patients with paralysis agitans who had coincident plaques and neurofibrillary tangles.) It includes various types of dementia such as:

- diffuse Lewy body disease
- senile dementia of Lewy body type
- Lewy body variant of Alzheimer's disease.

Lewy body dementia is the second most common neurodegenerative cause of dementia.

Pathological features

The histological appearance of a typical Lewy body is shown in Figure 6.10. A Lewy body is an intracytoplasmic concentrically laminated round to elongated eosinophilic inclusion, which often has a dense central core surrounded by a paler peripheral rim.

Each Lewy body consists of protein neurofilaments intermingled with granular material and dense core vesicles. The neurofilaments are packed densely in the core and radially oriented in the paler rim, hence the histological appearance. In addition to the presence of neurofilament antigens, immunohistochemical studies have detected the presence of microtubule assembly protein, ubiquitin and tau

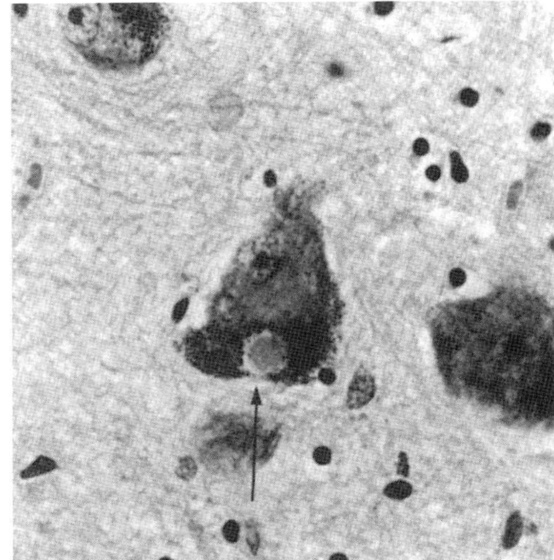

Figure 6.10 • Lewy body in Parkinson's disease. • There is a rounded concentric hyaline inclusion (arrow) in the perikaryon of a pigmented neurone of the substantia nigra. (Stained with H & E.) (Reproduced with permission from Graham DI, Nicoll JAR, Bone I (eds) 2006; see Further reading.)

protein. It has therefore been argued that Lewy bodies may have a cytoprotective function, being formed by a neurone in response to stress. (For example, in stress, ubiquitin facilitates the degradation of proteins denatured beyond repair, thereby protecting the cell from further injury.)

Classically, Lewy bodies are found in idiopathic Parkinson's disease. In this condition there is substantial (>70% at the time of motor symptoms and signs) loss of pigmented catecholaminergic neurones in the substantia nigra and locus coeruleus, with Lewy bodies being found in remaining neurones. Parkinson's disease patients may also have Lewy bodies in other subcortical nuclei, such as the cholinergic cells of the basal nucleus of Meynert, and in cortical areas, particularly the cingulate and parahippocampal gyri.

In Lewy body dementia, the occurrence of Lewy bodies is widespread. For example, their density in the cingulate and parahippocampal gyri and temporal cortex is much greater than is the case in Parkinson's disease.

Clinical features

Characteristic clinical features of Lewy body dementia include:

- marked fluctuating cognitive impairment over weeks or months affecting memory and higher cortical functions (language, visuospatial ability, praxis or reasoning), with intervening episodic lucid intervals
- mild spontaneous extrapyramidal symptoms
- recurrent visual hallucinations
- neuroleptic sensitivity syndrome (in which marked extrapyramidal symptoms, particularly parkinsonism, occur in response to standard doses of antipsychotic drugs).

Antipsychotics should be avoided (or used only with extreme caution) in such patients, owing to a high incidence of adverse and life-threatening reactions.

Frontotemporal dementia

Frontotemporal dementia is a clinical dementia syndrome characterized by behavioural changes, including character changes such as altered personal and social conduct, arising from frontotemporal involvement and distinct from Alzheimer's disease. Such changes may include:

- disinhibition
- inattention
- stereotypic behaviours
- antisocial acts
- reduced speech.

Mood disorder and psychiatric symptoms of a transient nature may occur and may mark the beginning of cognitive and behavioural deterioration. Spatial skills are preserved. Recognized features of the late stages include:

- apathy
- withdrawal
- akinesia
- mutism
- rigidity
- frontal release sign.

The term frontotemporal dementia covers both the temporal and frontal presentations of this condition. (The frontal variant presents with insidious changes in personality and behaviour, with neuropsychological evidence of disproportionate frontal dysfunction.) Many pedigrees have been described in which this disorder is inherited as an autosomal dominant trait. It is genetically heterogeneous with loci defined on chromosomes 17 and 3. At least three histological entities are recognized:

- Pick's disease
- non-specific frontotemporal degeneration
- frontal lobe abnormalities associated with motor neurone disease.

Pick's disease

Pick's disease is slightly more common in women, with a peak age of onset between 50 and 60. Clinical features include: personality deterioration, with features of frontal lobe dysfunction (see below); nominal aphasia; memory impairment; perseveration; and aspects of the Klüver–Bucy syndrome. Table 6.5 compares Pick's disease with Alzheimer's disease.

In terms of neuropathological changes, macroscopically there is selective asymmetrical atrophy of the frontal and temporal lobes, which, because of its severity, causes the gyri to become very thin – this is known as knife-blade atrophy of the gyri (Figure 6.11).

Table 6.5 Comparison of Pick's and Alzheimer's disease

	Pick's	Alzheimer's
Concept of space and time	Retained until late	Early disorientation, dressing and handling difficulties
Memory loss	Late	Early
Dysphasia	Nominal – mute	Expressive and receptive – impoverished or garrulousness
Personality and mood	Egocentric	Not characteristic
	Rigid (stereotype)	Eager for emotional rapport
	Obstinant	
Psychotic manifestations	Never	Auditory and visual hallucinations
		Paranoid ideas
Physical	Rare	Epilepsy
		Emaciation – late
Extrapyramidal symptoms	+	–
Apraxia of gait	–	+
Hyperalgesia	+	–
EEG	Normal	Reduced α–θ

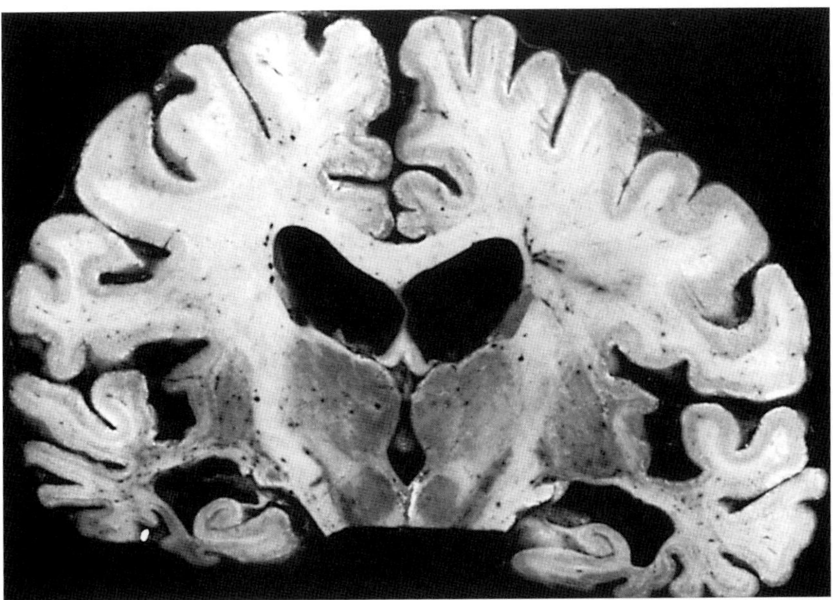

Figure 6.11 • Pick's disease. • The coronal section shows gross atrophy of the temporal lobes (with sparing of the superior temporal gyri) and, in addition, associated ventricular enlargement. (Reproduced with permission from Graham DI, Nicoll JAR, Bone I (eds) 2006; see Further reading.)

A characteristic histological feature of Pick's disease is the presence of argyrophilic intracytoplasmic neuronal inclusion bodies (Pick's bodies). They consist of neurofilaments, paired helical filaments and endoplasmic reticulum. Other histological changes include loss of neurones, most marked in the outer layers of the cerebral cortex, and a reactive astrocytosis. These changes may also occur in the basal ganglia, locus coeruleus and substantia nigra.

Vascular (multi-infarct) dementia

Multi-infarct dementia is also known as arteriosclerotic dementia and is an ischaemic disorder caused by multiple cerebral infarcts, with the extent of cerebral infarction being related to the degree of cognitive impairment. It is associated with chronic hypertension and arteriosclerosis.

ICD-10 classes multi-infarct dementia under vascular dementia. In practice, the term vascular dementia usually applies to multi-infarct dementia.

Pathological features

Macroscopically there are multiple cerebral infarcts, local or general atrophy of the brain with secondary ventricular dilatation and evidence of arteriosclerotic changes in major arteries (Figure 6.12). In most cases in which cognitive impairment is detectable the volume of the infarcts is greater than 50 mL, whereas a volume of greater than 100 mL is particularly likely to be associated with dementia. The histological changes of infarction and ischaemia are seen.

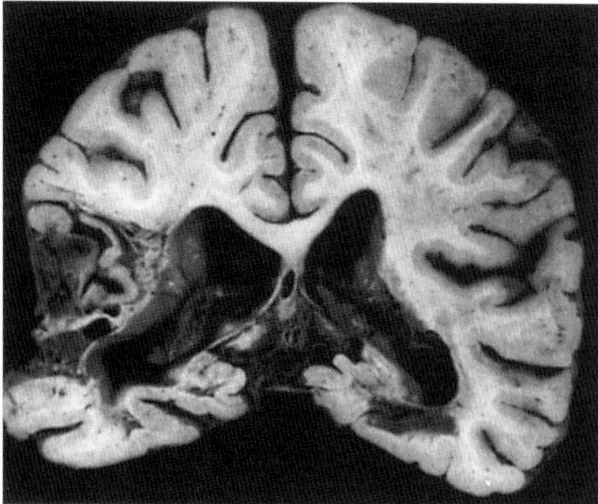

Figure 6.12 • Vascular (multi-infarct) dementia. (Reproduced with permission from Graham DI, Nicoll JAR, Bone I (eds) 2006; see Further reading.)

Clinical features

It is more common in men, and a history and clinical features of hypertension are usually present. The onset is usually acute, peaks in the 60s and 70s, and may be associated with a cerebrovascular accident. Other clinical features include: stepwise deterioration; focal neurological features; nocturnal confusion; fits; fluctuating cognitive impairment; and emotional incontinence and low mood. Death tends to occur on average between four and five years after diagnosis. The commonest causes of death are ischaemic heart disease (in around 50%), cerebral infarction and renal complications.

Table 6.6 compares the clinical features of Alzheimer's disease with those of vascular dementia.

Huntington's disease (chorea)

Huntington's disease is an autosomal dominant disorder caused by a gene on 4p16.3, containing an abnormal sequence of repeated CAG repeats (encoding a polyglutamine). Therefore, on average, 50% of the children of one affected parent can develop this disorder. Spontaneous mutations can also give rise to sporadic cases in which there is no known family history.

Pathological features

Macroscopically the brain is usually small, with reduced mass, and there is marked atrophy of the corpus striatum of the basal ganglia, particularly the caudate nucleus, and of the cerebral cortex, particularly the gyri of the frontal lobes (Figure 6.13). Histological changes include: neuronal loss in the cerebral cortex, particularly affecting the frontal lobes, and in the corpus striatum, particularly affecting GABA neurones with relative sparing of large neurones; and astrocytosis in the affected regions.

Clinical features

Males and females are affected equally and the average age of onset is 35–44 years; some cases occur in childhood. It causes an insidious onset of involuntary choreiform movements, which, early in the course of the disorder, typically affect the face, hands and shoulders or the gait (ataxia). These motor abnormalities usually begin before the onset of progressive dementia, which, in turn, usually involves impairment of frontal lobe functions (see below) relatively early on; memory is usually not affected to any

Table 6.6 A comparison of the features of Alzheimer's disease and vascular dementia

	Alzheimer's disease (previously senile dementia)	Vascular dementia (previously arteriosclerotic dementia)
Age of onset	Usually after 65	Usually after 40
Sex	More common in women	More common in men
Course	Progressive	'Step ladder'
Impairment of insight, intelligence and personality	Early	Late
Somatic symptoms	Absent	Present
Physical signs	Few and late	Often present, e.g. focal neurological signs

One-half of elderly depressives have cognitive impairments. One-quarter of Alzheimer's patients have depressive symptoms.

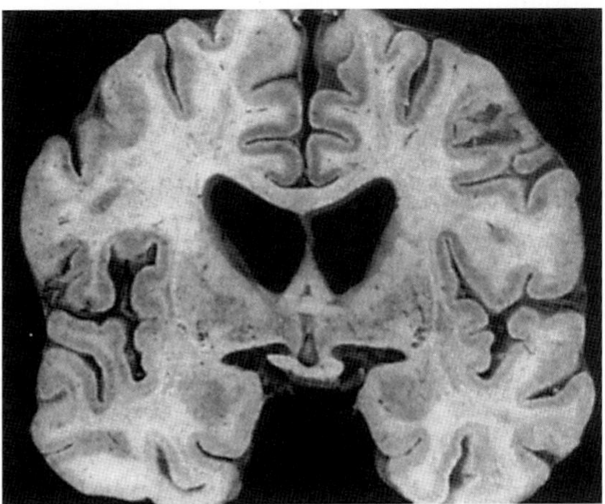

Figure 6.13 • Huntington's disease. • The coronal section shows atrophy of the caudate nucleus. (Reproduced with permission from Graham DI, Nicoll JAR, Bone I (eds) 2006; see Further reading.)

major degree until later. Other features include slurring of speech, extrapyramidal rigidity and epilepsy. Psychiatric features include depression, increased risk of suicide and schizophreniform and delusional disorders. Insight tends to be retained until a late stage. Death usually occurs within 15 years of the onset of symptoms.

Phenothiazine antipsychotics in low doses may be given to help with emotional disturbance, whereas depression may be treated with antidepressants. Involuntary movements may be decreased by giving tetrabenazine. This may act by causing dopamine depletion at nerve endings, but may cause depression to develop, thereby limiting its use. Huntington's disease may respond to treatment with eicosapentaenoic acid.

Creutzfeldt–Jakob disease (CJD)

Aetiology

CJD is a rare progressive dementia, which is believed to be transmitted by infection with a prion – a glycoprotein viral subparticle lacking ribonucleic acid. Infection may be transmitted from infected humans through procedures such as corneal transplantation, human pituitary glands (used as a source of human somatotropin for clinical use), depth EEG with contaminated electrodes and neurosurgery using contaminated instruments. In 1995, in Britain, a new variant of CJD (nvCJD) was reported, which is thought to be linked to transmission, via the food chain, of the neuropathologically related bovine disorder bovine spongiform encephalopathy (BSE). It is believed that the preceding increased incidence of BSE in Britain in the late 1980s may have been the result of including bone-meal derived from scrapie-infected sheep in cattle feed. An alternative theory suggests that BSE and/or nvCJD is/are associated with the combination of the use of organophosphate pesticides and exposure to excess manganese (and reduced copper).

Pathological features

There may be little or no gross atrophy of the cerebral cortex evident in rapidly developing cases. In those who survive longest, gross neuropathological changes seen may include selective cerebellar atrophy, generalized cerebral atrophy and ventricular dilatation.

Histologically there is evidence of neuronal degeneration without inflammation. Astrocytic proliferation occurs particularly in the cerebral cortex, basal ganglia, brainstem motor nuclei and spinal cord anterior horn cells. A characteristic feature of the grey matter of the cerebral cortex is the presence of multiple vacuoles. This gives the cerebral cortex a spongy appearance and is known as status spongiosus (Figure 6.14). Degeneration also occurs in spinal cord long descending tracts.

Clinical features

CJD is a rare form of presenile dementia with an equal incidence in men and women. Its clinical features depend on the parts of the brain most affected, the most important being a rapidly progressing devastating dementia (leading to memory impairment and personality change with slowing, fatigue and depressed mood) and motor abnormalities that usually follow the onset of the dementia (consisting of a progressive spastic paralysis of the limbs, accompanied by extrapyramidal signs with tremor, rigidity and choreoathetoid movements). Other clinical features may include: features typical of parietal lobe dysfunction, such as Gerstmann's syndrome (see below); epileptic fits; myoclonic jerks; psychotic symptomatology; cerebellar ataxia; visual failure; muscle fibrillation; dysarthria; and dysphagia. Owing to the mental manifestations, and particularly in cases of temporary remission of early neurological features, the presentation may be mistaken for a functional psychiatric disorder. ICD-10 therefore recommends that CJD should be suspected in all cases of a dementia that progresses fairly rapidly over months to one to two years, and is accompanied or followed by multiple neurological symptoms. In some cases the neurological signs may precede the onset of dementia. A useful investigation is the EEG, which shows a characteristic triphasic pattern. Death usually occurs within two years.

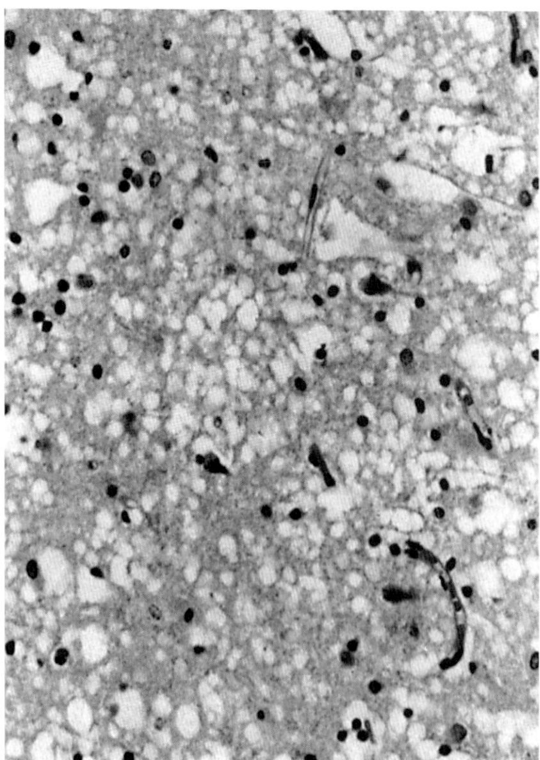

Figure 6.14 • Creutzfeldt–Jakob disease. • The section shows status spongiosus in the cerebral cortex. (Reproduced with permission from Graham DI, Nicoll JAR, Bone I (eds) 2006; see Further reading.)

Normal-pressure hydrocephalus

Hydrocephalus is an increase in the intracranial cerebrospinal fluid (CSF) volume associated with dilatation of the ventricular system. The normal production and flow of CSF is shown in Figure 6.15. In the case of primary hydrocephalus, an increased volume of CSF within the cranial cavity can result from increased formation of CSF, an obstruction to its circulation or decreased absorption. This, in turn, leads to raised CSF pressure. Normal-pressure hydrocephalus is a special type of primary hydrocephalus in which the CSF pressure is normal most of the time.

Aetiology

Normal-pressure hydrocephalus is both obstructive and communicating. It is caused by an obstruction in the subarachnoid space that prevents CSF from being reabsorbed, but allows it to flow into the subarachnoid space from the ventricular system (see Figure 6.15). Monitoring studies have demonstrated that there may be episodes of raised CSF pressure during sleep, and it has therefore been suggested that a better term for this syndrome might be intermittent hydrocephalus.

Pathological features

There is dilatation of the ventricular system (Figure 6.16). Cortical atrophy is usually absent.

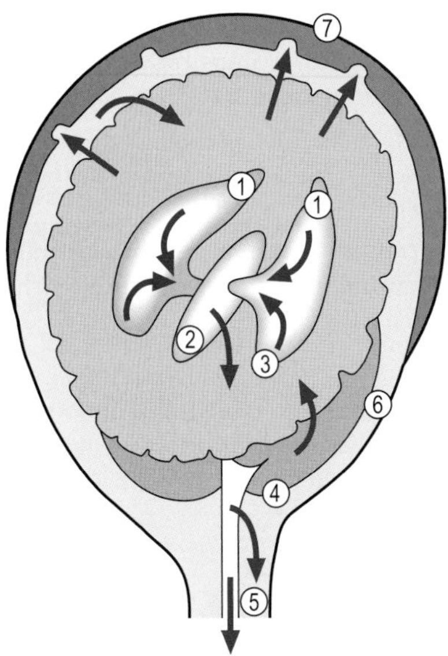

Figure 6.15 • The normal production and flow of CSF. • CSF is secreted by the choroid plexuses in the lateral, IIIrd and IVth ventricles. It flows from the lateral ventricles (1), into the IIIrd ventricle (2), through the cerebral aqueduct (3), into the IVth ventricle (4). From the IVth ventricle, CSF passes downwards into the central canal of the spinal cord, and through the foramina of Magendi and Lushka out into the subarachnoid space (5). CSF flows over the whole surface of the brain in the subarachnoid space (6) and is reabsorbed into the dural sinuses (7) via the arachnoid granulations. (Reproduced with permission from Souham RL, Moxhum J (eds) 1990 Textbook of medicine. Churchill Livingstone, Edinburgh.)

Clinical features

In normal-pressure hydrocephalus the features of raised intracranial pressure are generally absent. The syndrome mainly occurs in the seventh and eighth decades of life. Varying degrees of cognitive impairment and physical slowness occur. Other features include unsteadiness of gait, urinary incontinence and nystagmus. When it causes presenile dementia, particularly if physical features are absent, it may prove difficult to differentiate normal-pressure hydrocephalus from Alzheimer's disease.

Treatment is usually by means of ventriculoperitoneal shunting (Figure 6.16).

Case history: normal-pressure hydrocephalus

A 58-year-old man was noticed by his wife to have begun gradually to suffer from forgetfulness over the past few months. He would typically forget recently learnt addresses and telephone numbers, even though in the past he had had a good memory, and he was no longer always able to follow conversations. Occasionally he was rather moody. His wife asked for a medical opinion when her husband began to suffer from urinary incontinence.

On entering the consulting room the patient was noticed to walk with an unsteady, somewhat broad-based, gait. A mental state examination revealed no evidence of a mood disorder. A CT scan of the brain revealed the presence of enlarged ventricles without any cortical atrophy. This result, together with the finding that on lumbar puncture the CSF pressure was normal, strongly confirmed the clinical diagnosis of normal-pressure hydrocephalus. The patient was treated with ventriculoperitoneal shunting and two months later improvement was continuing to occur in both the cognitive and physical deficits.

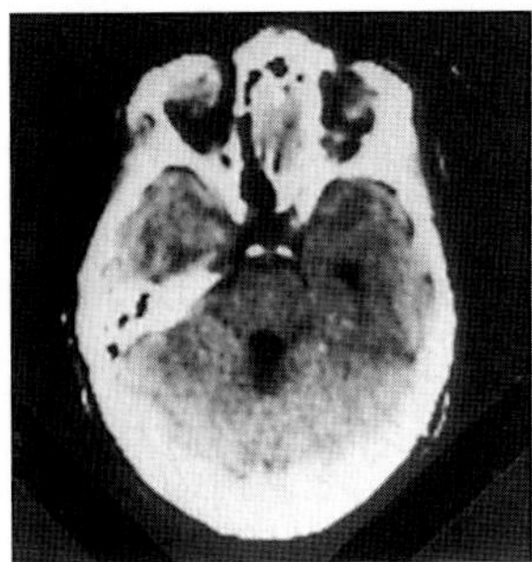
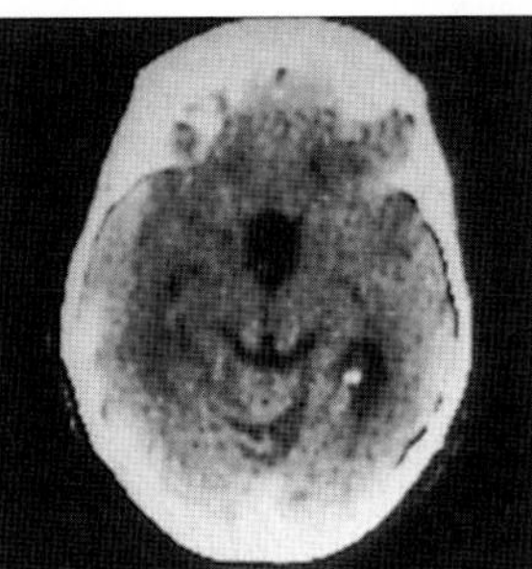
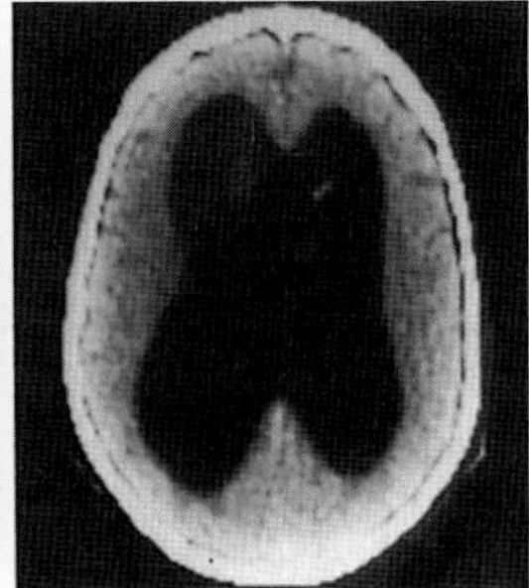

Figure 6.16 • Normal-pressure hydrocephalus treated by ventriculoperitoneal shunt (tube seen in right lateral ventricle). (Reproduced with permission from Suohami RL, Moxhum J (eds) 1994 Textbook of medicine, 2nd edn. Churchill Livingstone, Edinburgh.)

Delirium and dementia

- Delirium is characterized by acute generalized fluctuating impairment of consciousness, abnormal perceptions and mood changes.
- The management of delirium includes appropriate investigations, good calming nursing care in a quiet room with a low level of lighting, reassurance, reorientation, haloperidol or benzodiazepines (as a hypnotic or in hepatic failure).
- Dementia is characterized by generalized psychological dysfunction of higher cortical functions without impairment of consciousness.
- Alzheimer's disease, the most common cause of dementia in those aged over 65 years, is more common in females and usually presents with memory loss.
- Vascular/multi-infarct/arteriosclerotic dementia, an ischaemic disorder caused by multiple cerebral infarcts, is associated with chronic hypertension and arteriosclerosis; it is more common in males and usually has an acute onset followed by stepwise deterioration.
- Pick's disease, associated with asymmetrical atrophy of the frontal and temporal lobes, is more common in females.
- Huntington's disease, an autosomal dominant disorder, affects males and females equally, presenting with an insidious onset of involuntary choreiform movements.
- CJD, a rare rapidly progressing dementia known to be transmissible, affects males and females equally with death usually occurring within two years.
- Normal-pressure hydrocephalus occurs mainly in the seventh and eighth decades and may present with dementia, unsteadiness of gait, urinary incontinence and nystagmus.
- Lewy body disease may cause fluctuating cognitive impairment, mild/variable short-term memory loss, hallucinations, delusions, depressed mood, spontaneous extrapyramidal symptoms and neuroleptic sensitivity syndrome.

Causes of specific psychological dysfunction

Amnesic syndrome

The amnesic (or amnestic, dysmnesic, dysmnestic or Korsakov's) syndrome is characterized by prominent impairment of recent and remote memory with preservation of immediate recall in the absence of generalized cognitive impairment. The following two types of amnesia occur:

- *retrograde amnesia* – pathological inability to recall events that occurred prior to the onset of the illness
- *anterograde amnesia* – pathological inability to lay down new memories after the onset of the illness.

Aetiology

This is summarized in Table 6.7. The most common cause in the Western world is thiamine deficiency secondary to alcohol abuse (see Chapter 7).

Pathology

The causes listed in Table 6.7 typically affect either or both of the hypothalamic–diencephalic system and the bilateral hippocampal region of the brain. For example, if the cause is cerebral neoplasia, the tumour is usually found to involve the third ventricle (and thereby the hypothalamic–diencephalic system) or both hippocampal regions. Figure 6.17

Table 6.7 Causes of the amnesic syndrome

Thiamine (vitamin B_1) deficiency	Chronic alcohol abuse Malabsorption – lesions of the stomach (e.g. gastric carcinoma), duodenum or jejunum Hyperemesis Starvation
Intoxication	Heavy metals – lead, arsenic Carbon monoxide
Intracranial causes	Head injury Brain tumours affecting the third ventricle or hippocampal formations Bilateral hippocampal damage – e.g. following neurosurgery or vascular lesions Subarachnoid haemorrhage Infections – herpes simplex encephalitis, tuberculous meningitis Epilepsy
Hypoxia	Anaesthetic accidents Asphyxiation – e.g. non-fatal strangulation or hanging
Alzheimer's disease	

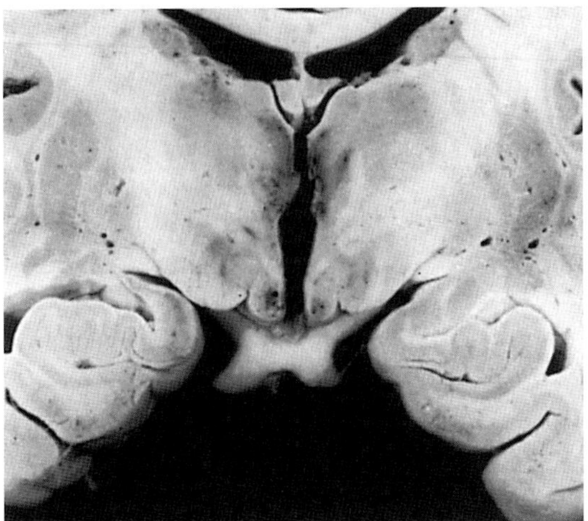

Figure 6.17 • Amnesic syndrome. • There are multiple petechial haemorrhages in the mammillary bodies and in the walls of the third ventricle. (Reproduced with permission from Graham DI, Nicoll JAR, Bone I (eds) 2006; see Further reading.)

shows a brain section from a patient who suffered from thiamine deficiency during life.

Clinical features

Anterograde amnesia is associated with an impaired ability to learn and disorientation for time. If the underlying pathology improves, this can result in a lessening of the extent of the retrograde amnesia. Confabulation, whereby gaps in memory are unconsciously filled with false memories, is often a feature. Other cognitive functions are usually normal, as is perception.

The course and prognosis are those of the primary pathology; if the latter is treatable, then complete recovery of the memory impairment is possible.

Focal cerebral disorder: clinical features

Figure 6.18 illustrates the normal localization of function in the cerebral cortex, whereas Figure 6.19 illustrates the regional localization of cognitive function and dysfunction. It is convenient to describe the clinical features of focal cerebral disorders before describing neuropathological conditions (e.g. tumours) that can give rise to them; some causes of dementia that can lead to focal cerebral disorder have already been described in the previous section. Clinical features give an indication of the location of the pathology, but usually do not imply the nature of the pathology itself. For example, the frontal lobe syndrome can be caused by a number of different disorders, such as a tumour, trauma, Pick's disease and neurosyphilis.

Frontal lobe

Personality changes occurring in association with frontal lobe lesions may include disinhibition, reduced social and ethical control, sexual indiscretion, financial and personal errors of judgement, elevated mood, lack of concern for the feelings of other people and irritability. These are primarily related to prefrontal impairment, and in frontal lobe damage are associated with perseveration, utilization behaviour (e.g. putting on a pair of spectacles when seen, writing when a pen comes within grasp, and eating and drinking whenever food and water are seen) and palilalia (repetition of sentences or phrases). These features demonstrate rigidity of thinking and stereotyped repetition. Other characteristic features include impairment of attention, concentration and initiative. Aspontaneity, slowed psychomotor activity, motor Jacksonian fits and urinary incontinence may also occur as part of the frontal lobe syndrome. Frontal lobe lesions can also give rise to a recrudescence of primitive reflexes, especially rooting, grasp, pout and palmomental reflexes. If frontal lobe syndrome is suspected, these reflexes should be tested for clinically.

If the motor cortex or deep projections are affected, this may result in a contralateral spastic paresis or aphasia. Posterior dominant frontal lobe lesions may cause apraxia of the face and tongue, primary motor aphasia or motor agraphia. Anosmia and ipsilateral optic atrophy may result from orbital lesions.

Temporal lobe

Dominant temporal lobe lesions may cause sensory aphasia, alexia and agraphia. Posterior dominant temporal lobe lesions may cause features of the parietal lobe syndrome mentioned below. Non-dominant temporal lobe lesions may cause hemisomatognosia, prosopagnosia, visuospatial difficulties and impaired retention and learning of non-verbal patterned stimuli such as music. Bilateral medial temporal lobe lesions may cause the amnesic syndrome described above. The personality changes that may occur are similar to those seen in frontal lobe syndrome. Other features include psychotic symptomatology, epilepsy and a contralateral homonymous upper quadrantic visual field defect.

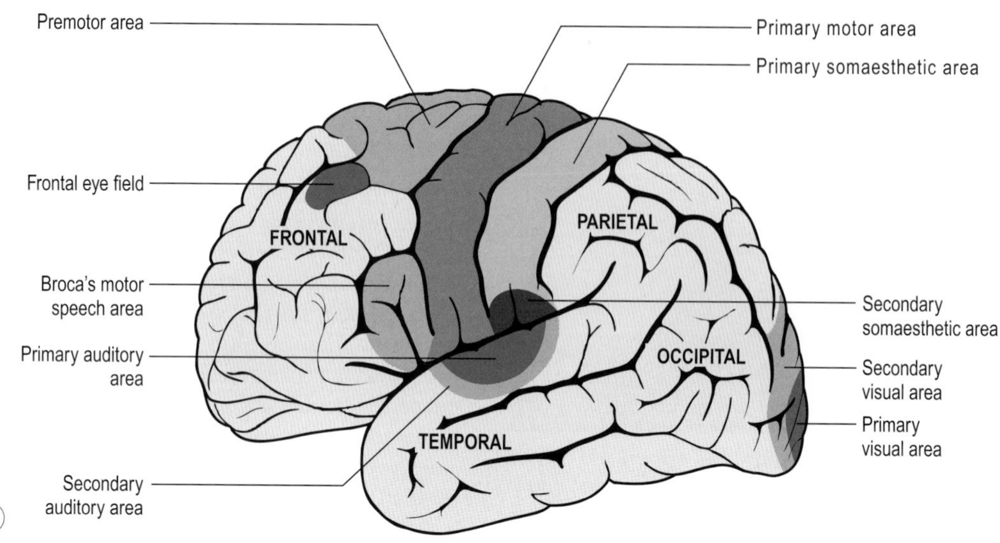

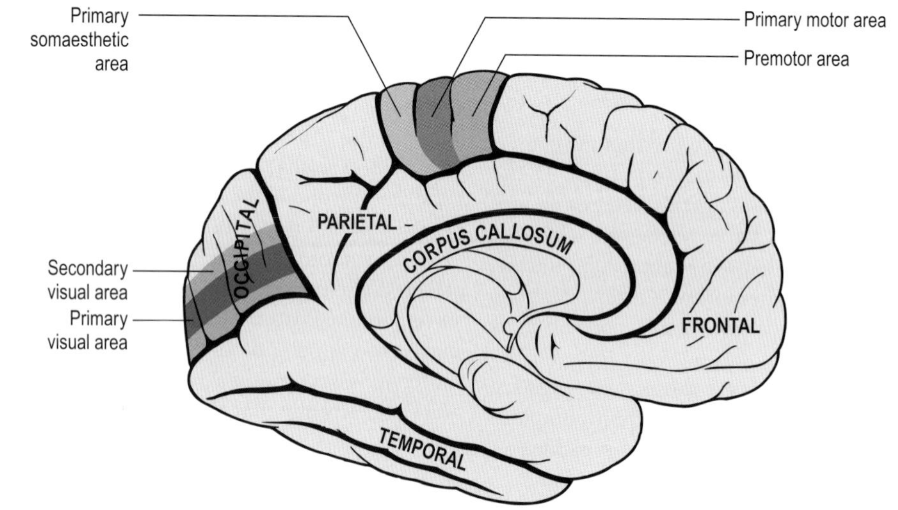

Figure 6.18 • Localization of function in the cerebral cortex. • (A) Lateral aspect. (B) Medial aspect.

Parietal lobe

Features of the parietal lobe syndrome include visuospatial difficulties such as constructional apraxia (e.g. difficulty in buttoning one's coat) and visuospatial agnosia, topographical disorientation, visual inattention, sensory Jacksonian fits and cortical sensory loss. Cortical sensory loss results in agraphaesthesia, asterognosis, impaired two-point discrimination and sensory extinction.

Dominant parietal lobe lesions may cause primary motor aphasia (caused by anterior lesions), primary sensory aphasia (caused by posterior lesions and leading to agraphia and alexia), motor apraxia, Gerstmann's syndrome (dyscalculia, agraphia, finger agnosia and right–left disorientation), bilateral tactile agnosia and visual agnosia (caused by parieto-occipital lesions).

Non-dominant parietal lobe lesions may cause anosognosia, hemisomatognosia, dressing apraxia and prosopagnosia.

Occipital lobe

Features of the occipital lobe syndrome include a contralateral homonymous hemianopia, scotomata and simultanagnosia. Bilateral lesions may result in

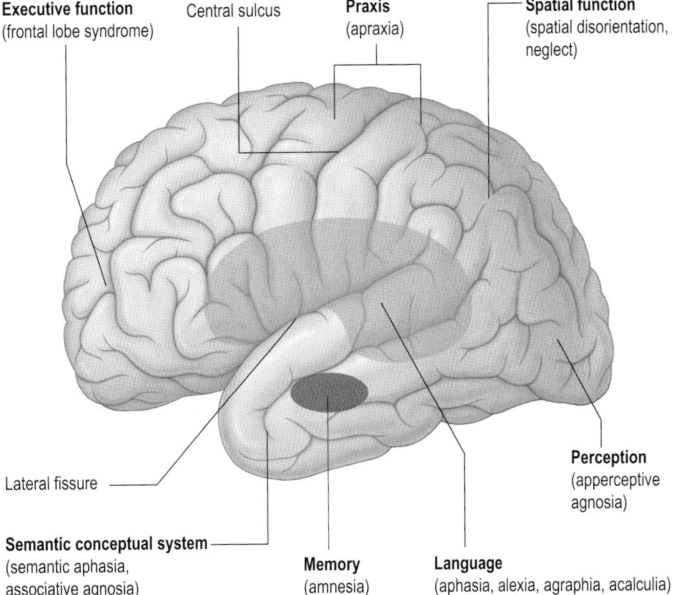

Figure 6.19 • Localization of cognitive function (dysfunction) in the cerebral hemisphere. (Reproduced with permission from Standring S (ed) 2008 Gray's anatomy, 40th edn. Churchill Livingstone, Edinburgh.)

cortical blindness. Dominant occipital lobe lesions may cause alexia without agraphia, colour agnosia and visual object agnosia. Visuospatial agnosia, prosopagnosia, metamorphopsia (image distortion) and complex visual hallucinations are more common with non-dominant lesions.

Corpus callosum

Acute severe intellectual impairment may occur. With extension into other parts of the central nervous system, neurological signs of involvement of the frontal lobe, parietal lobe or diencephalon may result. For a patient in whom the left hemisphere is dominant, loss of contact between the dominant hemisphere speech centres and the non-dominant hemisphere can lead to left-sided apraxia to verbal commands and asterognosis in the left hand.

Diencephalon and brainstem

Characteristic features of midline lesions include the amnesic syndrome, hypersomnia and akinetic mutism. Intellectual impairment, or occasionally a rapidly progressive dementia, may also be seen. Personality changes resemble those caused by frontal lobe lesions, except that loss of insight is less likely. Features of raised intracranial pressure may occur. Pressure on the optic chiasma may lead to visual field defects. Thalamic lesions may cause hypalgesia to painful stimuli and sensory disorders similar to those seen in the parietal lobe syndrome. Hypothalamic lesions may cause polydipsia, polyuria, increased body temperature, obesity, amenorrhoea or impotence and an altered rate of sexual development in children. Pituitary lesions may cause various endocrine disorders. Brainstem lesions may cause palsies of the cranial nerves and disorders of long-tract motor and sensory functions.

Other organic mental disorders

For the following organic mental disorders the treatment, course and prognosis are essentially those of the underlying pathology.

Organic hallucinosis

In ICD-10, organic hallucinosis is defined as being a disorder of persistent or recurrent hallucinations, in any modality but usually visual or auditory, which occurs in clear consciousness without any significant intellectual decline and which may or may not be recognized by the subject as such. Delusional elaboration of the hallucinations may occur, but often insight is preserved. The causes of organic hallucinosis are summarized in Table 6.8. Psychoactive substance abuse is described in Chapter 7.

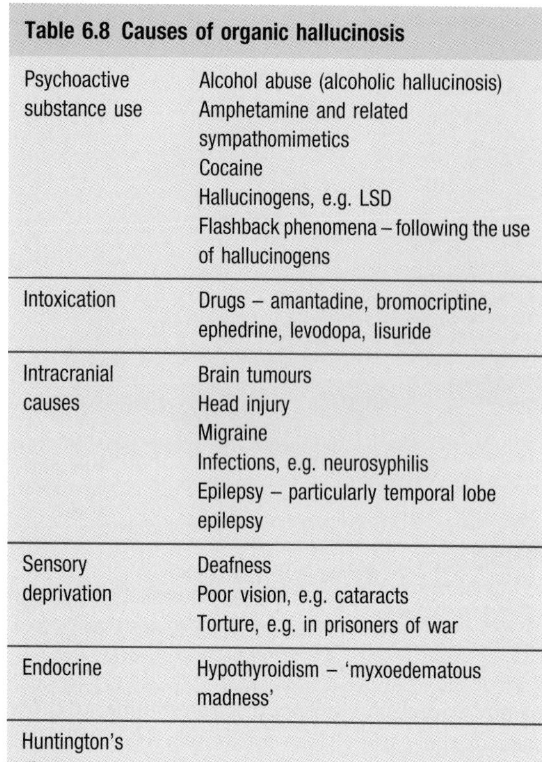

Table 6.8 Causes of organic hallucinosis

Psychoactive substance use	Alcohol abuse (alcoholic hallucinosis) Amphetamine and related sympathomimetics Cocaine Hallucinogens, e.g. LSD Flashback phenomena – following the use of hallucinogens
Intoxication	Drugs – amantadine, bromocriptine, ephedrine, levodopa, lisuride
Intracranial causes	Brain tumours Head injury Migraine Infections, e.g. neurosyphilis Epilepsy – particularly temporal lobe epilepsy
Sensory deprivation	Deafness Poor vision, e.g. cataracts Torture, e.g. in prisoners of war
Endocrine	Hypothyroidism – 'myxoedematous madness'
Huntington's disease	

Organic catatonic disorder

ICD-10 defines organic catatonic disorder as a disorder of diminished (stupor) or increased (excitement) psychomotor activity associated with catatonic symptoms; the extremes of psychomotor disturbance may alternate. The stuporose symptoms may include complete mutism, negativism and rigid posturing. Excitement manifests as gross hypermotility. Other catatonic symptoms that may occur include stereotypies and waxy flexibility. The most important causes are encephalitis and carbon monoxide poisoning.

Organic delusional or schizophrenia-like disorder

In ICD-10, organic delusional or schizophrenia-like disorder is defined as being a disorder in which the clinical picture is dominated by persistent or recurrent delusions, with or without hallucinations. The delusions are most often persecutory, but grandiose delusions or delusions of bodily change, jealousy, disease or death may occur. Memory and consciousness are not affected.

The most common cause is psychoactive substance use, particularly amphetamine and related substances, cocaine and hallucinogens. Intracranial causes, such as tumours and epilepsy, are particularly important if they affect the temporal lobe of the brain, for example temporal lobe epilepsy. Huntington's disease can also be a cause.

Organic mood disorder

Organic mood disorder is characterized by a change in mood (depressive or (hypo)manic), usually accompanied by a change in the overall level of activity, which is caused by organic pathology. Its causes are summarized in Table 6.9.

Organic anxiety disorder

Organic anxiety disorder is characterized by the features of generalized anxiety disorder and/or panic

Table 6.9 Causes of organic mood disorder

Psychoactive substance use	Amphetamine and related sympathomimetics Hallucinogens, e.g. LSD
Medication	Corticosteroids Levodopa Centrally acting antihypertensives – clonidine, methyldopa, reserpine and rauwolfia alkaloids Cycloserine Oestrogens – hormone replacement therapy, oral contraceptives Clomifene
Endocrine disorders	Hypothyroidism, hyperthyroidism Addison's disease Cushing's syndrome Hypoglycaemia, diabetes mellitus Hyperparathyroidism Hypopituitarism
Other systemic disorders	Pernicious anaemia Hepatic failure Renal failure Rheumatoid arthritis Systemic lupus erythematosus Neoplasia – particularly carcinoma of the pancreas, carcinoid syndrome Viral infections – e.g. influenza, pneumonia, infectious mononucleosis (glandular fever), hepatitis
Intracranial causes	Brain tumours Head injury Parkinson's disease Infections, e.g. neurosyphilis

disorder (see Chapter 10) caused by organic pathology. The symptoms include tremor, paraesthesia, choking, palpitations, chest pain, dry mouth, nausea, abdominal pain ('butterflies'), loose motions and increased frequency of micturition. Some of these symptoms, such as paraesthesia, are related to associated hyperventilation. There may be secondary cognitive impairment, for example poor concentration.

The causes of this condition are manifold (see Table 6.10). The most important conditions to exclude in clinical practice are hyperthyroidism, phaeochromocytoma and hypoglycaemia.

Organic personality disorder

ICD-10 defines organic personality disorder as being characterized by a significant alteration in the habitual patterns of behaviour displayed by the subject premorbidly. Such alteration always involves more profoundly the expression of emotions, needs and impulses. Cognition may be defective, mostly or exclusively in the areas of planning actions and anticipating their likely consequences.

The most common cause is head injury. Other intracranial causes include brain tumours, brain abscesses, subarachnoid haemorrhage, neurosyphilis and epilepsy, particularly when the frontal or temporal lobes are involved. For example, temporal lobe epilepsy may result in aggressive behaviour, hyposexuality or hypersexuality. Other causes of organic personality disorder include Huntington's disease, hepatolenticular degeneration (Wilson's disease), medication such as corticosteroids, psychoactive substance use and endocrinopathies.

Other neuropsychiatric disorders

Systemic lupus erythematosus

Systemic lupus erythematosus (SLE) affecting the central nervous system can cause cranial and peripheral nerve lesions, depression, phobias and epilepsy. Disorientation and hallucinations may also occur, but usually secondary to pharmacotherapy with corticosteroids.

Cerebral arterial syndromes

Figure 6.20 shows the circle of Willis and the arteries of the brainstem, whereas Figure 6.21 depicts the regions of the cerebral cortex supplied by the anterior, middle and posterior cerebral arteries. The clinical features resulting from the occlusion of different cerebral arteries are briefly outlined.

Table 6.10 Causes of organic anxiety disorder

Psychoactive substance use	Alcohol and drug withdrawal Amphetamine and related sympathomimetics Cannabis
Intoxication	Drugs – penicillin, sulphonamides Caffeine and caffeine withdrawal Poisons – arsenic, mercury, organophosphates, phosphorus, benzene Aspirin intolerance
Intracranial causes	Brain tumours Head injury Migraine Cerebrovascular disease Subarachnoid haemorrhage Infections – encephalitis, neurosyphilis Multiple sclerosis Hepatolenticular degeneration (Wilson's disease) Huntington's disease Epilepsy
Endocrine	Pituitary dysfunction Thyroid dysfunction Parathyroid dysfunction Adrenal dysfunction Phaeochromocytoma Hypoglycaemia Virilization disorders of females
Inflammatory disorders	Systemic lupus erythematosus Rheumatoid arthritis Polyarteritis nodosa Temporal arteritis
Vitamin deficiency	Vitamin B_{12} deficiency Pellagra (nicotinic acid deficiency)
Other systemic disorders	Hypoxia Cardiovascular disease Cardiac arrhythmias Pulmonary insufficiency Anaemia Carcinoid syndrome Systemic neoplasia Febrile illnesses and chronic infections Porphyria Infectious mononucleosis (glandular fever) Posthepatic syndrome Uraemia Premenstrual syndrome

Based on Cummings J 1985 Clinical neuropsychiatry. Grune & Stratton, Orlando.

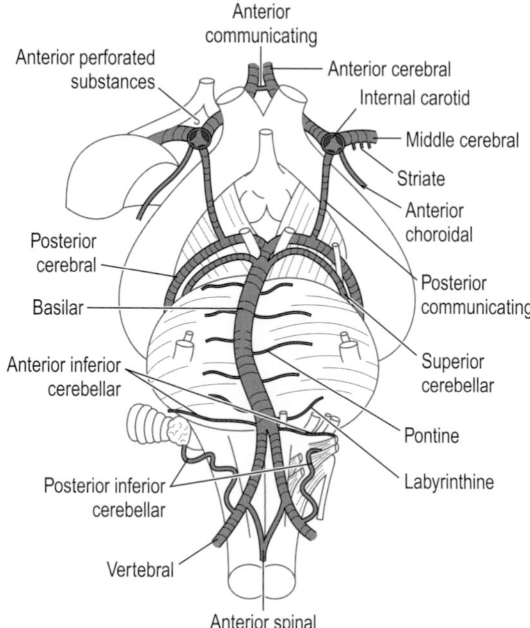

Figure 6.20 • The circle of Willis and the arteries of the brainstem. • The arterial circle (horizontal) lies at right angles to the basilar artery (vertical). (Reproduced with permission from Last RJ 1978 Last's anatomy, 6th edn. Churchill Livingstone, Edinburgh.)

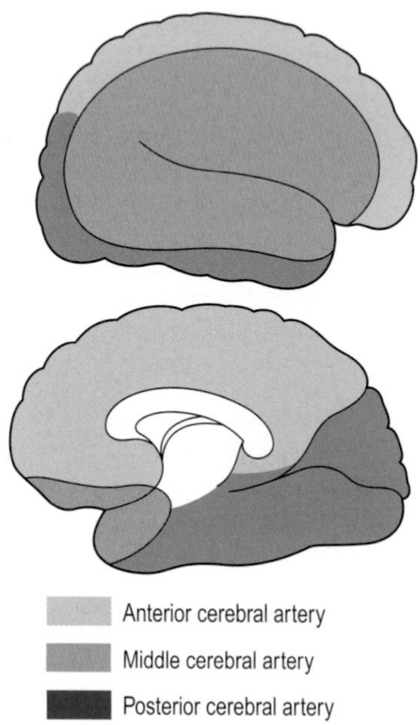

Figure 6.21 • Diagram of (a) the lateral areas and (b) the medial areas of the cerebral cortex supplied by the cerebral arteries. (Reproduced with permission from Aitken JT, Sholl DA, Webster KE, Young JZ 1971 A manual of human anatomy, vol V: central nervous system, 2nd edn. Churchill Livingstone, Edinburgh.)

Middle cerebral artery occlusion can result in:

- contralateral hemiparesis
- cortical sensory loss
- contralateral hemianopia
- aphasia, if the dominant hemisphere is affected
- agnosic syndromes and body image disturbances if the non-dominant hemisphere is affected
- clouding of consciousness.

Anterior cerebral artery occlusion can result in:

- contralateral hemiparesis, with the leg being affected more severely than the arm
- grasp reflex
- cortical sensory loss
- motor aphasia
- clouding of consciousness.
- personality change of the frontal lobe dysfunction type
- changes in mental functioning similar to those seen in dementia
- incontinence.

Occlusion of the *internal carotid artery* may be asymptomatic if the circle of Willis is patent. Otherwise it may cause a middle cerebral infarction-type picture, together with monocular blindness, unilateral loss of the carotid pulse and an ipsilateral Horner's syndrome.

Posterior cerebral artery occlusion can result in:

- contralateral hemianopia
- visual hallucinations
- visual agnosia
- spatial disorientation
- visual perseveration
- alexia without agraphia, if the dominant occipital lobe and the splenium of the corpus callosum are affected
- a contralateral thalamic syndrome
- cerebellar ataxia
- cortical blindness, in the case of bilateral occipital lobe infarction.

So far as the *vertebrobasilar system* is concerned, total occlusion of the basilar artery is rapidly fatal. Partial occlusion of the basilar artery may cause:

- features of brainstem, pyramidal and ipsilateral cerebellar lesions
- ipsilateral cranial nerve palsies
- peduncular hallucinosis (vivid well-formed hallucinations, sometimes confined to a half-field

of vision, which the patient recognizes as being unreal in spite of their dramatic nature)
- the locked-in syndrome
- states of bizarre disorientation
- excessive dreaming.

Cerebrovascular accidents

The psychiatric sequelae of cerebrovascular accidents include:

- dementia
- organic personality change, such as irritability and apathy, which may be more the result of widespread atherosclerosis than of focal changes following cerebrovascular accidents
- depressed mood
- paranoid–hallucinatory syndromes occur rarely.

Subarachnoid haemorrhage

Psychiatric sequelae have been found to be relatively common in individuals who survive. They include:

- cognitive impairment
- personality impairment, including 'organic moodiness' and frontal lobe syndrome-like changes
- occasional improvement in personality following anterior bleeds
- symptoms of anxiety and depression
- the amnesic syndrome.

Neurosyphilis

The CSF changes in neurosyphilis include increased cells and protein, in addition to positive results to the appropriate antibody tests. The most important manifestations of neurosyphilis are meningovascular syphilis, tabes dorsalis and general paralysis of the insane.

Syphilitic *gummata* are granulomatous lesions that occur in the meninges attached to the dura mater alone or also to the underlying part of the brain. Central necrosis and lymphocytic and plasma cell invasion of the lesions occur. Gummata typically occur over the cerebral hemispheres and cerebellum. They can give rise to convulsions and, depending on their location, focal neurological features such as aphasia and hemiplegia.

Meningovascular syphilis typically occurs within a decade or so of the time of the initial infection. A characteristic granulomatous meningitis occurs in which fibrosis of the meninges may affect the cranial nerves. Cranial nerve palsy may also be the result of endarteritis obliterans, leading to ischaemic necrosis and arterial thrombosis. Other pathological features include hypertrophic pachymeningitis, causing thickening of the cervical dura mater, and myelitis. Clinically, meningovascular syphilis may present with headache, lethargy, irritability and malaise. Neck stiffness, convulsions, delirium and psychotic symptomatology may also occur. An alternative presentation is the occurrence of focal neurological features such as cranial nerve palsy, particularly affecting the second, third, fourth or eighth cranial nerves, and features of cerebrovascular accidents. Meningeal anterior and posterior spinal root thickening may cause muscle wasting and pain respectively.

Tabes dorsalis develops some 10–35 years after the primary infection, and sometimes occurs with general paralysis of the insane. Initially there is spinal cord posterior root sensory neuronal degeneration, usually in the lower thoracic and lumbar nerve roots. The rarer cases, in which the cervical nerve roots are mainly affected, are known as cervical tabes. This is followed by posterior white column atrophy (Figure 6.22). The spinal cord posterior root involvement leads to the characteristic clinical feature of lightning pains, which are severe stabbing pains lasting a few seconds and most often affecting the legs, although other regions of the body may also be affected. Another characteristic feature is the occurrence of sudden severe episodes of abdominal pain and vomiting that may last for days, which are known as tabetic crises. Posterior white column involvement leads to loss of proprioception, which, in turn, causes an ataxia with a characteristic gait that is wide-based and stamping; Romberg's sign is positive.

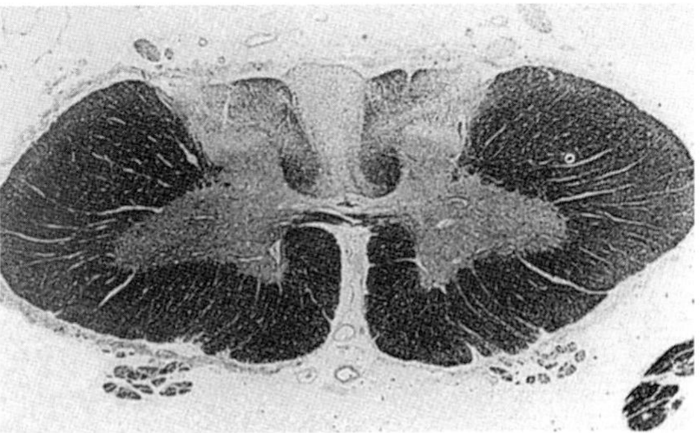

Figure 6.22 • Tabes dorsalis. • There is shrinkage and loss of myelin in the posterior columns. (Stained with Luxol fast blue/cresyl violet.) (Reproduced with permission from Graham DI, Nicoll JAR, Bone I (eds) 2006; see Further reading.)

Loss of vibration sense in the lower limbs can be demonstrated clinically. There may be loss of deep pain sensation, leading to neuropathic or Charcot's joints. Severe foot ulceration can result from loss of cutaneous sensation. Areflexia occurs in the legs, but in pure tabes dorsalis the plantar reflexes are flexor. A neurogenic bladder is also sometimes present. Argyll Robertson pupils are seen mainly in tabes dorsalis and general paralysis of the insane. The pupils are small and irregular; there is no light reflex but the pupils do constrict with accommodation.

General paralysis of the insane (or general paresis) usually develops 10–20 years after the initial infection. There is atrophy of the cerebral cortex, which is usually most severe in the frontal and temporal lobes. Histologically, a subacute encephalitis is present in the regions of cortical atrophy, with neuronal degeneration, astrocytosis and the presence of siderophages, lymphocytes, plasma cells and spirochaetes. A chronic ventriculitis is present and there is meningeal thickening with lymphocytic infiltration. Presenting clinical features include impairment of memory and concentration, frontal lobe dysfunction-type personality changes and minor emotional symptoms. Depression, mania, dementia and schizophreniform presentations may be seen, hence the usefulness of carrying out syphilitic serological tests. Other clinical features include: epilepsy; Argyll Robertson pupils; tremor, either cerebellar or extrapyramidal, affecting the tongue, limbs and trunk; dysarthria; and focal neurological features such as aphasia and hemiplegia.

Virus encephalitis

Generalized clinical features include headache, nausea and vomiting, drowsiness and fits. Focal neurological features may also occur. Features of raised intracranial pressure may also be present, as may neck stiffness if there is meningeal involvement. Pyrexia, if present, is usually low grade. Impaired consciousness, delirium and, more rarely, psychiatric disorders may also be part of the presentation. For example, cases have been reported in which such patients were admitted as psychiatric inpatients with a provisional diagnosis of schizophrenia.

With resolution of the acute episode a number of complications may emerge. These include personality changes, depression, chronic anxiety and dementia. Episodes of virus encephalitis may also contribute to childhood behaviour disorders.

Cases of encephalitis lethargica are now very rare. This is also known as epidemic encephalitis and postencephalitic parkinsonism, owing to the occurrence of the features of Parkinson's disease as a complication. Postencephalitic personality change and psychosis have also been reported.

Chronic fatigue syndrome is also known as myalgic encephalomyelitis (ME) or postviral syndrome. Prolonged periods of lethargy occur, often accompanied by headache, myalgia and features of depression. The disorder often affects young people and may occur in epidemics (such as the outbreak at the Royal Free Hospital in London in 1955) and may follow an illness. Some cases may be associated with viral infections, but others are associated with either other infective agents or no known infective cause.

Cerebral abscess

Cerebral abscesses are caused by bacteria such as streptococci, staphylococci, pneumococci and the enterobacteriaceae. The primary infection is usually in the middle ear, the sinuses or the lungs. Although the diagnosis is often clear, with a presentation of the primary infection and features caused by an intracranial expanding lesion, cerebral abscesses may form insidiously and be wrongly diagnosed as psychiatric disorders because of the development of depressive symptoms and changes in personality.

Acquired immunodeficiency syndrome (AIDS)

A case of AIDS is a reliably diagnosed disease indicative of a defect in cell-mediated immunity occurring in a person who has serum antibodies to the human immunodeficiency virus (HIV) and no other known cause. Diseases indicative of diminished cell-mediated immunity include opportunistic viral, bacterial, fungal, protozoal and helminthic infections, for example pneumonia caused by *Pneumocystis carinii*, and secondary neoplasia such as Kaposi's sarcoma occurring in individuals aged less than 60 years.

Encephalitis, usually subacute, affects approximately one-third of patients overall, and almost all survive for a relatively long time. It is usually caused by HIV but may also result from opportunistic infections, such as cytomegalovirus, herpes simplex, herpes zoster and mycobacteria. *Meningitis* may be caused not only by the more common pathogens responsible for meningitis in non-AIDS cases, but also by less common pathogens such as *Cryptococcus neoformans*, fungi and amoebae. Another common neuropathological feature of AIDS is the occurrence of *cerebral abscesses*, usually multiple and caused by

Toxoplasma gondii. Other neuropathological features include primary cerebral lymphoma, myelopathy associated with subacute encephalitis, retinitis and peripheral neuropathy.

The clinical development of AIDS in infected individuals is the basis of the classification system of the Centers for Disease Control, Atlanta, Georgia. The first group is the development of an *acute seroconversion illness* soon after infection in some individuals. The second group refers to the *asymptomatic infection* that occurs in most infected individuals, who are seropositive, for a few months to several years. During this stage, HIV can be transmitted to others. The next stage that usually follows (Group III) is *persistent generalized lymphadenopathy*. Approximately one-third of this group goes on to develop AIDS itself within the next five years. The fourth group includes:

- *AIDS-related complex* (ARC) – generalized features such as decreased body mass, chronic fatigue, night sweats, pyrexia, myalgia, diarrhoea and cutaneous infections.
- HIV-related *neurological disease* – a wide range of neurological and neuropsychiatric complications can occur, including *AIDS dementia*, with loss of cognitive functioning. Initially the progressive loss of cognitive function may be mistaken for a depressive illness. If it occurs, *primary cerebral lymphoma* may present with headache, seizures and focal neurological deficits, or with a progressive dementia. When present, clinical features of other neuropathological changes, such as peripheral neuropathy, are also seen.
- Diseases resulting from *opportunistic infections*, such as *P. carinii* pneumonia. *Meningitis* may be caused most often by C. *neoformans* and *encephalitis* by cytomegalovirus, JC virus and SV40. Cytomegalovirus infections are more likely to cause *retinitis*, and therefore blindness.
- *Secondary neoplasia*, the most common being Kaposi's sarcoma.
- Other conditions, such as thrombocytopenia.

Head injury

The acute effects of head injury include: impairment of consciousness, or concussion; acute post-traumatic psychosis; and memory disorders evident following recovery of consciousness. Clinically, an important measure of memory impairment is the length of the *post-traumatic amnesia*, i.e. the interval of time between the moment of head injury and the resumption of normal continuous memory. It has been found that the duration of the post-traumatic amnesia is a good indicator of the degree of psychiatric disablement, post-traumatic personality change and neurological and cognitive impairment.

The chronic psychological sequelae of head injury comprise: cognitive impairment, which may be focal or generalized; personality change, which is related to the site of damage, being particularly common following frontal lobe lesions; psychoses, including schizophrenia, delusional disorders and mood disorder; suicide; and neuroses. Post-traumatic epilepsy commonly takes the form of temporal lobe epilepsy (complex partial seizures), which is, in turn, associated with psychological sequelae.

Punch-drunk syndrome

This is also known as dementia pugilistica, post-traumatic dementia and boxing encephalopathy. It develops in individuals such as boxers who have received repeated blows to the head. A characteristic gross neuropathological feature is cerebral atrophy. Particularly affected regions are the cerebral cortex and the hippocampal–limbic region, and enlargement of the lateral ventricles is common. Other changes that commonly occur include perforation of the septum pellucidum and thinning of the corpus callosum. Histological changes include cortical neuronal loss and neurofibrillary degeneration, with the presence of a type of neurofibrillary tangle in the cortex and brainstem similar to that seen in Alzheimer's disease; neuritic plaques, however, are not present.

Clinical features include: progressive impairment of memory and intellect, without any confabulation; personality deterioration, with irritability and reduced drive; features of cerebellar dysfunction; extrapyramidal signs; and pyramidal signs. In addition to dementia, pathological (delusional) jealousy (see Chapter 8) and rage reactions may also occur.

Multiple sclerosis

As plaques of demyelination may occur in any place in the white matter of the CNS (see Figures 6.23 and 6.24), the clinical presentation of multiple sclerosis (MS) can vary. The most common presentations are cervical spinal cord involvement leading variously to motor, sensory, bladder, bowel and erectile dysfunction; retrobulbar neuritis secondary to involvement of the optic nerve; cerebellar signs; diplopia secondary to an ocular nerve palsy or an internuclear ophthalmoplegia; and vertigo secondary to vestibular nuclear complex involvement.

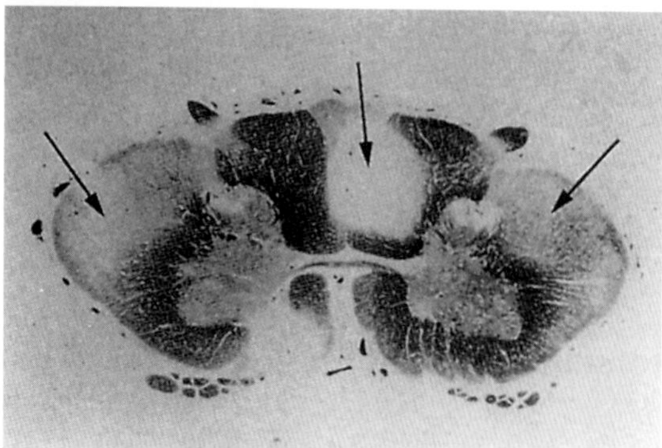

Figure 6.23 • Multiple sclerosis. • Cross-section of the spinal cord showing demyelination (arrows) in the posterior column and lateral corticospinal tracts. (Reproduced with permission from Kumar P, Clark M (eds) 1998 Clinical medicine. WB Saunders, Edinburgh.)

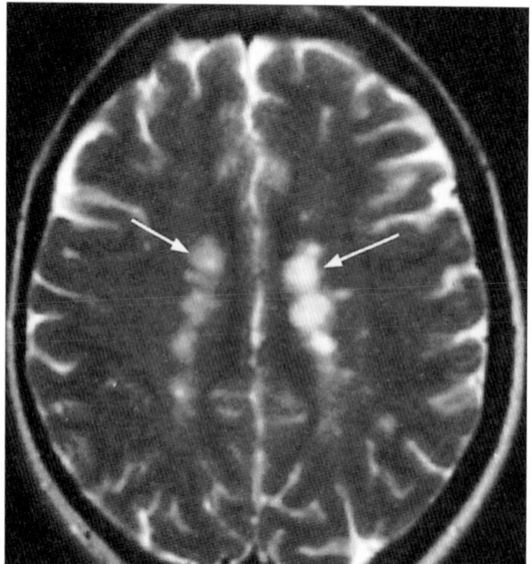

Figure 6.24 • Transverse T_2-weighted MRI scan of the brain in a patient with multiple sclerosis, showing multiple areas of high signal (arrows) in the periventricular white matter. (Reproduced with permission from Kumar P, Clark M (eds) 1998 Clinical medicine. WB Saunders, Edinburgh.)

The course of MS may be one of progressive deterioration or, particularly in those with a younger age of onset, there may be spontaneous partial remissions interwoven with periods of relapse. In most affected individuals there is eventually an accumulation of multiple neurological handicaps, with the development of dementia, quadriplegia and blindness.

Psychiatric complications include: intellectual impairment, usually leading eventually to dementia; abnormalities of mood and associated personality changes, with episodes of depression and – particularly as the condition progresses – inappropriate euphoria; and psychotic symptomatology including, rarely, a psychotic presentation. There are also reports of conversion reactions (see Chapter 11) occurring in chronic MS.

Hepatolenticular degeneration

Hepatolenticular degeneration (or Wilson's disease) is an autosomal recessive disorder of copper metabolism. There is a decrease in the plasma copper-binding protein ceruloplasmin, an increase in the albumin-bound copper and an increased urinary excretion of copper. The pathological features are principally the result of abnormal deposition of copper in hepatocytes, leading to cirrhosis; in the limbus of the cornea, leading to a zone of golden-brown, yellow or green corneal pigmentation known as a Kayser–Fleischer ring (Figure 6.25); and in the CNS.

The neurological features are principally those of an extrapyramidal disorder, and include choreiform movements of the face and hands, athetoid movements of the limbs, tremor, rigidity and bradykinesia. The mask-like facies of parkinsonism may also occur. Occasionally, dysarthria is the presenting feature. Mental manifestations include loss of emotional control and dementia. Alterations in personality and

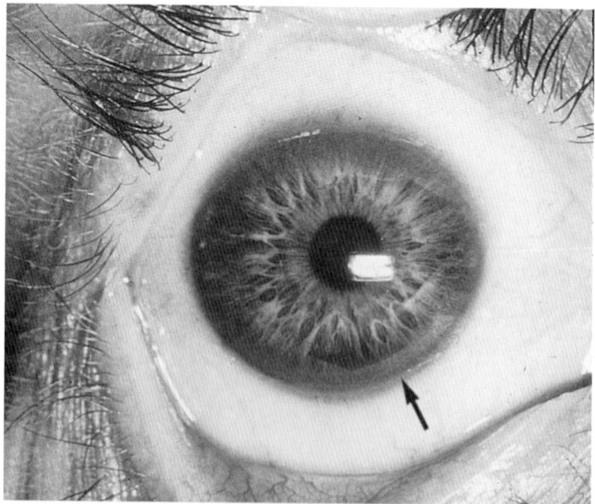

Figure 6.25 • Kayser–Fleischer rings at the junction of the cornea and sclera (arrow) in a patient with hepatolenticular degeneration (Wilson's disease). (Reproduced with permission from Edwards CRW, Bouchier IAD, Haslett C, Chilvers ER (eds) 1998; see Further reading.)

behaviour occur, which are related to neurological disease. Depressive symptomatology is associated with hepatic and biochemical abnormalities.

Acute porphyrias

The porphyrias can be classified into acute (including acute intermittent porphyria, variegate porphyria and hereditary coproporphyria) and non-acute. The non-acute porphyrias are not associated with neuropsychiatric complications.

In a reaction occurring mainly in the liver and bone marrow and catalyzed by the mitochondrial enzyme δ-ALA synthetase, δ-ALA (δ-aminolaevulinic acid) is formed from glycine and succinyl CoA (Figure 6.26). Two molecules of δ-ALA then react to form a molecule of porphobilinogen. These are the precursors of porphyrins, pigments found in haemoglobin, myoglobin and cytochromes.

The porphyrias, acute and non-acute, are associated with increased activity of δ-ALA synthetase. The acute porphyrias are autosomal dominant disorders in which the increased δ-ALA synthetase activity leads to an abnormal accumulation of δ-ALA and porphobilinogen. Neuropsychiatric complications are believed to result partly from the binding of δ-ALA to central GABA receptors.

Neuropathological features include those of cerebrovascular accidents and retinal ischaemia, as a result of cerebral arterial spasm, and chromatolysis of spinal cord neurones (as a result of peripheral neuropathy) and motor nuclear neurones.

Acute episodes occur with gastrointestinal features such as abdominal pain, vomiting and constipation; cardiovascular features such as tachycardia, hypertension and left ventricular failure; neurological and psychiatric features such as peripheral neuropathy, seizures, emotional disturbance, depression, delusional and schizophreniform psychoses; and delirium, which may progress to coma. In acute intermittent porphyria and variegate porphyria, acute episodes may be precipitated by drugs such as barbiturates, sulphonamides and the oral contraceptive pill; by acute infections; and by fasting or alcohol. Often the diagnosis is missed and in the past many such patients were diagnosed as suffering from hysteria.

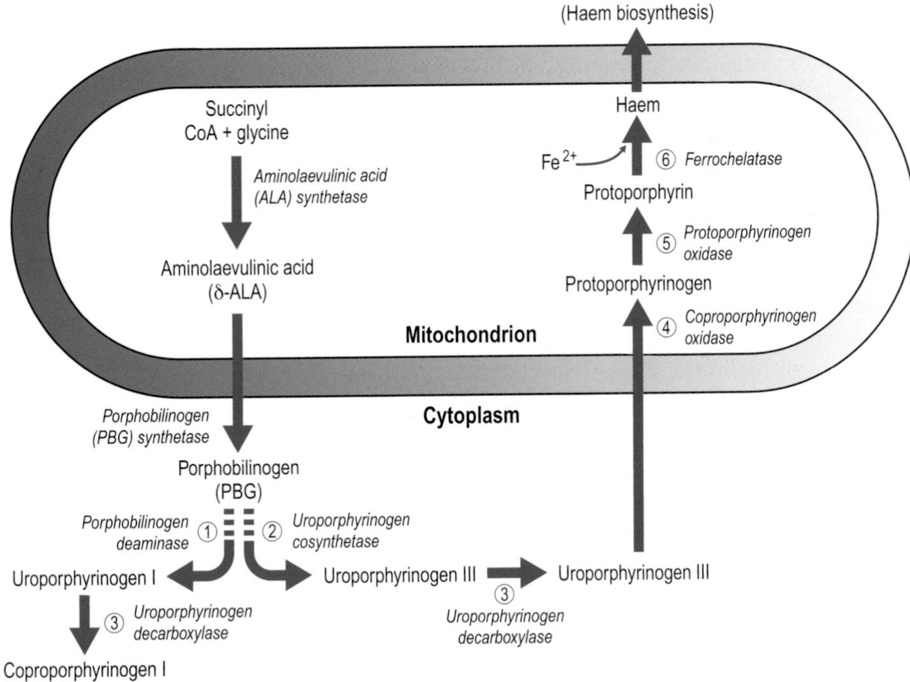

Figure 6.26 • Metabolic pathways for haem biosynthesis. • A block in porphyrin metabolism at the following sites results in a particular form of porphyria: (1) PBG deaminase – acute intermittent porphyria; (2) uroporphyrinogen cosynthetase – congenital (erythropoietic) porphyria; (3) uroporphyrinogen decarboxylase – porphyria cutanea tarda; (4) coproporphyrinogen oxidase – hereditary coproporphyria; (5) protoproporphyrinogen oxidase – variegate porphyria; (6) ferrochelatase – erythropoietic protoporphyria. (Reproduced with permission from Edwards CRW, Bouchier IAD, Haslett C, Chilvers ER (eds) 1998; see Further reading.)

Parkinson's disease

In addition to idiopathic Parkinson's disease or paralysis agitans, parkinsonism can result from drugs such as neuroleptics, methyldopa and reserpine; intoxication with poisons such as carbon monoxide, carbon disulphide, manganese, mercury and MPTP, a synthetic opiate analogue that was a contaminant of illicitly synthesized heroin in the USA in the 1980s; head injury; infection, with parkinsonism having commonly developed in survivors of the 1919–1924 pandemic of encephalitis lethargica – known as postencephalitic parkinsonism; and the parkinsonism–dementia complex of Guam, which occurs in the population of Guam and is of uncertain origin. Cerebral arteriosclerosis is a controversial cause. Other diseases that may give rise to parkinsonism include cerebral palsy, Huntington's disease, progressive supranuclear palsy and hepatolenticular degeneration (Wilson's disease).

Idiopathic Parkinson's disease is considered here, but many of the features outlined also apply to parkinsonism resulting from other causes. The characteristic site of neuropathological change is the substantia nigra of the brainstem, leading to a reduction in the dopaminergic neurones of this part of the extrapyramidal motor system. Parkinsonism can also result from a functional deficiency of dopamine in this system, caused, for example, by antipsychotic medication (see Chapter 3).

The most important neurological features of Parkinson's disease are bradykinesia, a resting tremor, cogwheel rigidity and postural abnormalities. Other features include hypersalivation, seborrhoea, oculomotor abnormalities, fatigue, poor balance, micrographia, dysarthria and urinary disturbance. Psychiatric features include cognitive impairment, personality changes, mood disorder (primarily depressive illness) and, very rarely, schizophreniform psychoses.

Cerebral tumours

The general neurological effects of cerebral tumours include the effects of intracranial expanding lesions, including raised intracranial pressure and cerebral oedema. Epilepsy occurs in approximately one-third of cases and may be focal or generalized. It is particularly common with tumours in the frontal and temporal lobes. Depending on their location, cerebral tumours may cause varying focal neurological features. The clinical features of focal cerebral disorder were described earlier. Invasion of the meninges may give rise to signs of meningism.

Certain cerebral tumours give rise to particular manifestations that are not generally seen with other types of cerebral tumour. For example, pituitary adenomas may cause endocrinological effects, whereas neurilemmomas affecting the eighth cranial nerve (acoustic neuromas) cause progressive deafness and occasionally vertigo and tinnitus.

General psychological and psychiatric effects of cerebral tumours include: impairment of consciousness and other cognitive changes, both focal and generalized; mood changes, such as emotional dullness, apathy and irritability; hallucinations in any modality and also in association with epilepsy; and neurotic and other psychotic phenomena.

Case history: cerebral tumour

A 68-year-old woman was compulsorily admitted to a psychiatric ward after being found to be deteriorating in the community. She was living on tins of custard and was therefore very poorly nourished, her home was in a very disorganized state, and she claimed to be following the commands of the (deceased) actor Cary Grant, whom she believed to be alive and in his 90s. She said she had been able to hear him clearly for at least the past six years. The mental state examination revealed a complex delusional system involving Cary Grant.

A CT brain scan revealed the presence of a frontal meningioma. As this type of cerebral tumour is slow growing, it is possible that it had been causing psychiatric symptoms for the past six years. The patient was referred for neurosurgery, and six weeks postoperatively she was no longer experiencing auditory hallucinations and it was clear that the systematized delusions were diminishing in intensity.

Epilepsy

Epilepsy is a symptom, which may not necessarily be complained of, rather than a disease. It may give rise to psychiatric symptoms.

Classification

Table 6.11 summarizes the 1981 International Classification of Seizures, excluding infantile and childhood epilepsies, which is based on clinical features rather than aetiology.

In simple partial seizures, consciousness is not impaired. Its manifestations are a function of the cerebral region giving rise to the seizure. With impairment of consciousness the seizure is a complex partial one and may include automatisms.

Table 6.11 Summary of the International Classification of Seizures (excluding infantile and childhood epilepsies)

Partial seizures (beginning locally)	Simple partial seizures (consciousness is not impaired): — with motor symptoms — with somatosensory or special sensory symptoms — with autonomic symptoms — with psychic symptoms Complex partial seizures (consciousness is impaired): — starting as a simple partial seizure — impaired consciousness at onset with or without automatism Partial seizures becoming generalized
Generalized seizures (convulsive or non-convulsive)	Absence: — simple (petit mal) — complex Myoclonic Clonic Tonic Tonic–clonic (grand mal) Atonic
Adolescent epilepsies	Early morning myoclonus associated with tonic–clonic seizures Myoclonus and simple absence
Progressive myoclonic epilepsies	
Unclassified epilepsy seizures (because of incomplete data)	

Generalized seizures include the simple absence (petit mal) and tonic–clonic (grand mal) forms. Generalized seizures can be convulsive or non-convulsive. Simple absences (petit mal) begin in childhood or adolescence. During an episode, the affected person suddenly stops whatever he or she is doing and adopts a frozen vacant appearance; 5–20 seconds later the person returns to what he or she was doing, as if nothing had happened. Generalized tonic–clonic seizures cause a loss of consciousness, falling, a tonic phase with rigidity and cyanosis, followed by generalized rhythmic jerking of all limbs. The attack usually lasts one to ten minutes and is followed by postictal drowsiness. Tongue biting and single or double incontinence may occur during a seizure. Some children and adolescents experience generalized seizures (absence, tonic–clonic or myoclonic) as a result of being exposed to certain stimuli such as the flicker of a television screen or computer monitor.

Psychiatric disorders causing fits

Seizures can result from organic psychiatric disorders, for example Alzheimer's disease and vascular (multi-infarct) dementia. Focal cerebral lesions also cause fits.

Seizures can also result from withdrawal from psychoactive substances and as a side-effect of those psychotropic medications that reduce the seizure threshold (e.g. antipsychotic drugs and tricyclic antidepressants). In these cases, however, the fits tend to be isolated single occurrences.

Many patients with a learning disability suffer from epilepsy. The prevalence of seizures has been found to be positively related to the severity of the mental retardation.

Infantile autism is associated with the development of seizures in adolescence.

Psychiatric disorders resulting from epilepsy

In the preictal phase, epilepsy can give rise to prodromal symptoms such as dysphoria and irritability.

Complex partial seizures affecting the temporal lobe and limbic system (temporolimbic epilepsy) can cause a wide variety of psychiatric symptoms, including disorders of perception, such as illusions and hallucinations, mood disorder, cognitive changes and abnormal experiences such as *déjà vu* and *jamais vu*. This form of epilepsy may be clinically indistinguishable from schizophrenia. It can also give rise to automatic behaviour. Simple partial seizures arising in the temporal lobe can also give rise to similar manifestations. In the postictal phase there may be clouding of consciousness.

A high frequency of simple absences in childhood and adolescence can lead to learning disabilities owing to frequent interruptions of attention.

Other disorders associated with epilepsy include personality changes, neuroses and psychosexual disorders. The suicide rate in epilepsy is five times that in the general adult population.

Finally, it is important to bear in mind that non-convulsive generalized seizures can be misdiagnosed as psychiatric disorders by the unwary.

Causes of specific psychological dysfunction

- The amnesic/amnestic/Korsakov's syndrome is characterized by prominent impairment of recent and remote memory with preservation of immediate recall in the absence of generalized cognitive impairment; it is most commonly caused in the West by alcohol abuse (leading to thiamine deficiency).
- Frontal lobe lesions may cause personality change (e.g. disinhibition, reduced social and ethical control), perseveration, utilization behaviour and impaired attention.
- Temporal lobe lesions may cause sensory aphasia, alexia, agraphia, psychotic symptoms, epilepsy and a contralateral homonymous upper quadrantic visual field defect.
- Parietal lobe lesions may cause visuospatial difficulties, topographical disorientation, sensory Jacksonian fits and cortical sensory loss.
- Occipital lobe lesions may cause a contralateral homonymous hemianopia, scotomata, simultanagnosia and cortical blindness; complex visual hallucinations are more common in non-dominant lesions.
- Acute severe intellectual impairment may occur in corpus callosum lesions.
- For organic mental disorders the treatment, course and prognosis are essentially those of the underlying pathology.
- SLE affecting the CNS can cause depression, phobias and epilepsy; corticosteroid treatment can lead to disorientation and hallucinations.
- CVAs can cause dementia, organic personality change and depression.
- Subarachnoid haemorrhage can cause cognitive impairment, personality impairment, anxiety, depression and the amnesic syndrome.
- Virus encephalitis may present with impaired consciousness, delirium or as a psychiatric disorder (e.g. a schizophreniform picture); complications following resolution of the acute episode may include personality changes, depression, anxiety and dementia.
- ME/chronic fatigue syndrome is associated with prolonged periods of lethargy, often with headache and myalgia.
- Cerebral abscesses may cause depression and personality change.
- AIDS may cause dementia, depression and symptoms from associated infections.
- Head injury may, acutely, cause concussion, acute post-traumatic psychosis and memory disorders; the length of the post-traumatic amnesia is a good indicator of the degree of psychological disability.
- Psychiatric complications of MS include dementia, depression with episodes of inappropriate euphoria, psychotic symptoms and conversion reactions.
- Psychiatric complications of hepatolenticular degeneration/Wilson's disease include loss of emotional control, dementia, personality and behavioural changes and depression.
- Psychiatric complications of acute porphyrias include depression, delusional and schizophreniform psychoses and delirium.
- Psychiatric complications of Parkinson's disease include cognitive impairment, personality change, depression and, rarely, schizophreniform psychoses.

Further reading

Douglas, G., Nicol, F., Robertson, C. (Eds.), 2009. Macleod's clinical examination. twelfth ed. Churchill Livingstone, Edinburgh.

Edwards, C.R.W., Bouchier, I.A.D., Haslett, C., Chilvers, E.R. (Eds.), 1998. Davidson's principles and practice of medicine. seventeenth ed. Churchill Livingstone, Edinburgh.

Graham, D.I., Nicoll, J.A.R., Bone, I. (Eds.), 2006. Adam's and Graham's introduction to neuropathology. third ed. Hodder Arnold, London.

Moore, D.P., 2008. Textbook of clinical neuropsychiatry, second ed. Hodder Arnold, London.

Yudofsky, S.C., Hales, R.E. (Eds.), 2008. The American Psychiatric Publishing textbook of neuropsychiatry and behavioral neurosciences. fifth ed. American Psychiatric Publishing, Arlington, VA.

Psychoactive substance use disorders

Introduction

The administration of a *psychoactive substance* can lead to relatively rapid central nervous system (CNS) effects, including a change in the level of consciousness or the state of mind. This chapter considers the effects of alcohol and other psychoactive drugs, both illicit (such as cocaine and heroin) and licit (such as caffeine). Table 7.1 gives the ICD-10 classification of these disorders. First, however, it is necessary to define some of the terms used.

Definitions

The following definitions are based mainly on recommendations published by the World Health Organization (WHO) in 1965 and on ICD-10.

Acute intoxication. This is a transient condition following the administration of a psychoactive substance resulting in disturbances or changes in the patterns of physiological, psychological or behavioural functions and responses.

Harmful use. This is defined as a pattern of psychoactive substance use that is causing damage to health. The damage may be physical (as in cases of hepatitis from the self-administration of injected drugs) or mental (such as episodes of depression secondary to heavy drinking).

Tolerance. This is said to take place when the desired CNS effects of a psychoactive substance diminish with repeated use, so that increasing doses need to be administered to achieve the same effects.

Dependence syndrome. This is defined as a cluster of physiological, behavioural and cognitive phenomena in which the use of psychoactive substances takes on a much higher priority for the individual than other behaviours that once had higher value. There is a desire, which is often strong and sometimes overpowering, to take the psychoactive substance(s) on a continuous or periodic basis. Tolerance may or may not be present. Dependence may be psychological, physical or both:

- *Psychological dependence*: a condition in which a psychoactive substance produces a feeling of satisfaction and a psychological drive that requires periodic or continuous administration of the substance in order to produce pleasure or to avoid the psychological discomfort (such as anxiety and depression) of its absence.
- *Physical dependence*: an adaptive state that manifests itself by intense physical disturbance when the administration of a psychoactive substance is suspended. There is a desire to take the substance in order to avoid the physical symptoms of a withdrawal state (see below) occurring (e.g. tremor, myalgia and insomnia).

Withdrawal state. This is a group of physical and psychological symptoms occurring on absolute or relative withdrawal of a psychoactive substance after repeated, and usually prolonged and/or high-dose, use of that substance. The onset and course of the withdrawal state are time-limited and are related to the type of substance and the dose being administered immediately prior to abstinence. The withdrawal state may be complicated by delirium (see Chapter 6) and/or convulsions.

Table 7.1 ICD-10 classification: F10–F19 mental and behavioural disorders due to psychoactive substance use

F10 Mental and behavioural disorders due to use of alcohol
F11 Mental and behavioural disorders due to use of opioids
F12 Mental and behavioural disorders due to use of cannabinoids
F13 Mental and behavioural disorders due to use of sedatives or hypnotics
F14 Mental and behavioural disorders due to use of cocaine
F15 Mental and behavioural disorders due to use of other stimulants, including caffeine
F16 Mental and behavioural disorders due to use of hallucinogens
F17 Mental and behavioural disorders due to use of tobacco
F18 Mental and behavioural disorders due to use of volatile solvents
F19 Mental and behavioural disorders due to multiple drug use and use of other psychoactive substances

Four- and five-character codes may be used to specify the clinical conditions:

F1x.0 Acute intoxication
.00 Uncomplicated
.01 With trauma or other bodily injury
.02 With other medical complications
.03 With delirium
.04 With perceptual distortions
.05 With coma
.06 With convulsions
.07 Pathological intoxication

F1x.1 Harmful use

F1x.2 Dependence syndrome

F1x.3 Withdrawal state
.30 Uncomplicated
.31 With convulsions

F1x.4 Withdrawal state with delirium
.40 Without convulsions
.41 With convulsions

F1x.5 Psychotic disorder
.50 Schizophrenia-like
.51 Predominantly delusional
.52 Predominantly hallucinatory
.53 Predominantly polymorphic
.54 Predominantly depressive symptoms
.55 Predominantly manic symptoms
.56 Mixed

F1x.6 Amnesic syndrome

F1x.7 Residual and late-onset psychotic disorder
.70 Flashbacks
.71 Personality or behaviour disorder
.72 Residual affective disorder
.73 Dementia
.74 Other persisting cognitive impairment
.75 Late-onset psychotic disorder

F1x.8 Other mental and behavioural disorders

F1x.9 Unspecified mental and behavioural disorder

Alcohol problems

Of all the alcohols known to chemistry, ethanol (C_2H_5OH) is to all intents and purposes the only one that is self-administered to any extent by humans; most of the others would be far too toxic to be ingested. Thus, when we refer to alcohol in this book we mean ethanol unless otherwise stated.

The concentration of alcohol in alcoholic beverages is often stated by manufacturers in terms of 'proof' scales. In the USA, one degree (1°) proof is equal to a concentration of 0.5% by volume (v/v). In the UK, however, 1° proof is equal to 0.5715% by volume.

There are four major types of alcohol problem: excessive consumption, alcohol-related disabilities, problem drinking and alcohol dependence.

A description of each of these is followed by a consideration of the epidemiology, aetiology, assessment and treatment of alcohol problems.

Excessive consumption

Units of alcohol

In the assessment of alcohol consumption it is useful to have a standardized measure of alcohol. It has been found that the amount (mass) of alcohol contained in a standard measure of spirits, in a standard glass of sherry or fortified wine, a standard glass of table wine, and in one half-pint of beer or lager of standard strength (3–3.5% by volume) is approximately the same, at 8–10 g. This amount is known as a *unit of alcohol* (Figure 7.1). Note that some (European continental) lagers can be as strong as 5–6% by volume, and some wines can be as strong as 17% (or even higher) by volume; the figures given in Figure 7.1 have to be adjusted accordingly in such cases. Also, although Figure 7.1 considers 25 mL to be a standard measure for spirits, some public houses and bars now use larger 'standard' measures for spirits, so that the number of units of alcohol is correspondingly higher.

Levels of consumption

The Royal College of Physicians has defined *low-risk levels* of alcohol consumption as being up to 21 units per week for men and up to 14 units per week for women (Figure 7.2). This amount of alcohol should not be consumed in one go, and alcohol should not be consumed every day, for these levels to apply.

Alcohol consumption in greater amounts constitutes *excessive consumption* and carries a much greater risk of developing alcohol-related disabilities and alcohol dependence. The definitions of *increasing hazard* and *dangerous levels* of alcohol consumption are also shown in Figure 7.2.

=
=
=
= 1 unit of alcohol
1 single measure of spirit (whisky, brandy, gin, rum, vodka)
1 glass of sherry or fortified wine (e.g. port)
1 glass of table wine
½ pint of beer or cider (or ¼ pint of strong lager)
1 bottle of spirits
= 30 units of alcohol

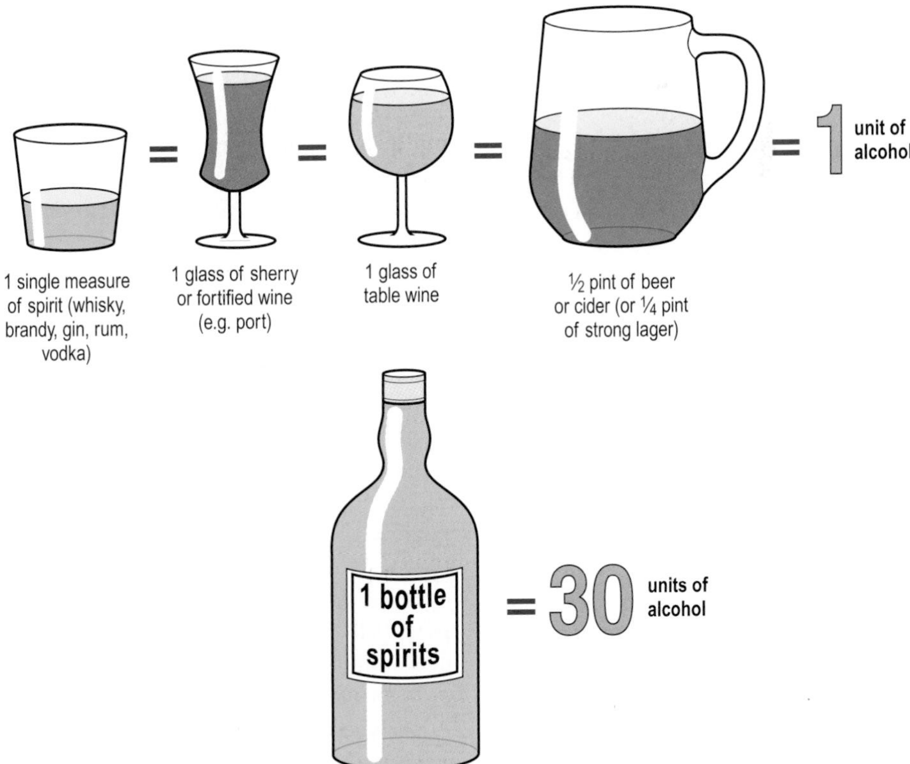

Figure 7.1 • Alcoholic beverages and units of alcohol.

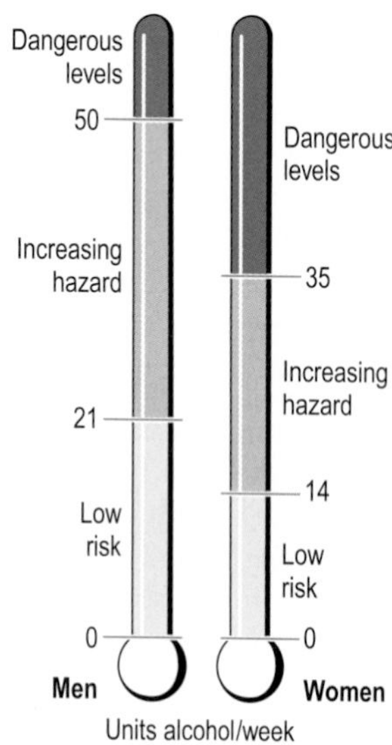

Figure 7.2 • Levels of alcohol consumption.

Abstinence or minimal alcohol consumption is recommended in pregnancy, as otherwise there is a risk of the development of fetal alcohol syndrome (see below).

Alcohol-related disabilities

Excessive alcohol consumption can lead to physical, psychiatric and social morbidity.

Physical (medical) morbidity

Excessive alcohol consumption is associated with an increased mortality, with approximately one-fifth of men admitted to general medical wards having been found to suffer from problem drinking (defined below). *Gastrointestinal disorders* are a common consequence of excessive alcohol consumption and include:

- nausea and vomiting, particularly in the morning, which can be prevented by drinking more alcohol
- gastritis, peptic ulcers, Mallory–Weiss tears and oesophageal varices.

Malnutrition occurs mainly as a result of poor food intake, particularly of protein and the B vitamins. Other causes include the gastrointestinal disorders just mentioned.

Hepatic damage takes place chronologically in the following order:

1. Fatty infiltration of the liver, leading to an acute increase in the size of the liver, takes place within a few days of excessive alcohol consumption; this change is reversible if alcohol consumption is stopped.
2. Alcoholic hepatitis.
3. Cirrhosis.

Both *acute pancreatitis* and, following years of excessive alcohol consumption, *chronic pancreatitis* can occur.

Cardiovascular system changes include hypertension and cardiac arrhythmias, particularly after binge drinking.

Haematological complications include:

- "idxB978-7020-1.00007-2,3))"]>iron deficiency anaemia, often as a result of haemorrhage from the gastrointestinal pathology mentioned above
- macrocytosis
- folate deficiency
- impaired clotting because of vitamin K deficiency and/or reduced platelet functioning.

Cancer of the oropharynx, oesophagus, pancreas, liver and lungs is increased in incidence.

Excessive alcohol consumption in pregnancy can lead to permanent fetal damage. The clinical features of the consequent presentation of the *fetal alcohol syndrome* following birth are shown in Figure 7.3.

Accidents and trauma may result from alcohol consumption. These include:

- road accidents
- assaults (including head injuries)
- falls (including head injuries)
- drowning
- burns and death by fire.

There is an increased risk of *infections* such as tuberculosis, particularly in homeless people who drink heavily.

Nerve and muscle disorders, some of which are potentially reversible in the early stages if alcohol consumption is stopped, include:

- myopathy
- peripheral neuropathy
- cerebellar degeneration
- epilepsy

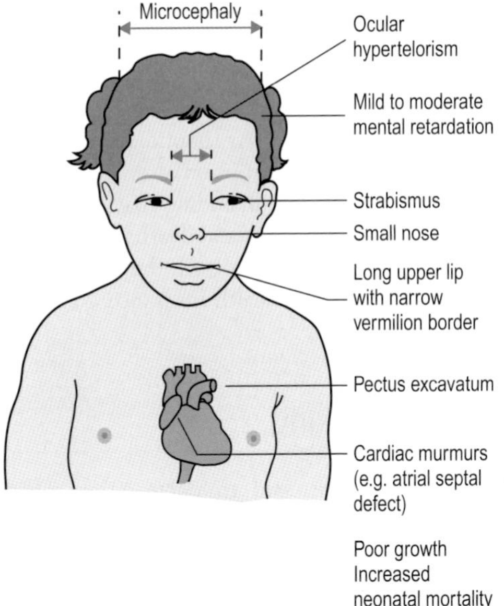

Figure 7.3 • Fetal alcohol syndrome in a child whose mother consumed excess alcohol during pregnancy.

- optic atrophy
- central pontine myelinolysis
- Marchiafava–Bignami disease, which is a rare fatal demyelinating disease characterized neuropathologically by widespread demyelination affecting the central corpus callosum, and often also the middle cerebellar peduncles, the white matter of the cerebral hemispheres and the optic tracts. There is usually a clinical presentation of emotional disturbance and cognitive impairment, followed by epilepsy, delirium, paralysis and coma.

Psychiatric morbidity

Alcohol affects the *mood* of the drinker. Excessive alcohol consumption may initially take place because the drinker wishes to relieve disagreeable mood states, such as anxiety and low mood. However, chronic heavy drinking can itself produce such unpleasant states. Indeed, the rate of *suicide* is at least 50 times greater in such drinkers than in the general population.

Alcohol also affects the *personality* of the drinker, who may initially drink to achieve such superficial effects as appearing more sociable and sexually desirable. However, the effects of chronic heavy drinking on personality are often negative, causing boastfulness, embarrassing speech and actions and offensiveness. With persistent heavy drinking personality deterioration occurs, which may simulate a personality disorder (see Chapter 15).

Intoxication frequently leads to episodes of short-term amnesia or *blackouts*. For example, the events that occurred during heavy drinking the night before, while the subject was still conscious, are no longer recalled the following morning. This phenomenon does not necessarily imply chronic alcohol use; it may occur after just one bout of heavy drinking, and indeed is estimated to have been experienced by 15–20% of those who drink.

In chronic heavy drinkers, a fall in the blood alcohol concentration leads to withdrawal symptoms (see below). These include *delirium tremens* or *DTs*. The features of delirium have been described in Chapter 6. Another important withdrawal symptom is *withdrawal fits*, which may occur within 48 hours of stopping drinking.

A rarer psychiatric disorder caused by chronic alcohol intake is *alcoholic hallucinosis*, which is characterized by the occurrence of auditory hallucinations in clear consciousness. These may be in the form of noises or voices uttering derogatory remarks and threats; they may sometimes be in the third person and describe the patient's actions. Alcoholic hallucinosis should therefore be considered in the differential diagnosis of schizophrenia when there is a history of chronic alcohol consumption.

A number of *psychosexual disorders* can result from taking alcohol. Although it reduces inhibitions and may increase the desire for sexual intercourse, in men intoxication leads to erectile impotence and delayed ejaculation. Chronic heavy drinking in men can cause loss of libido, reduction in the size of the testes and penis, loss of body hair and gynaecomastia, whereas in women it can lead to menstrual cycle abnormalities, loss of breast tissue and vaginal dryness.

Chronic heavy drinking is one cause of *pathological (delusional) jealousy* (see Chapter 8). Alcohol is also a cause of *fugue states* (see Chapter 11).

Heavy drinking is often associated with gambling and the use of other psychoactive substances. It can also be a cause of *dementia* (see Chapter 6).

The most common cause in the Western world of the *amnesic* or *Korsakov's syndrome* is thiamine (vitamin B_1) deficiency secondary to alcohol abuse. Alcohol-induced amnesic syndrome is frequently preceded by *Wernicke's encephalopathy*. This is also caused by severe thiamine deficiency, which, in turn, is usually caused by alcohol abuse in Western countries, when the term *alcoholic encephalopathy* may also be used. Other causes include: lesions of the stomach (e.g. gastric carcinoma), duodenum or jejunum, causing malabsorption; hyperemesis; and starvation. The most important clinical features of Wernicke's encephalopathy are:

- ophthalmoplegia
- nystagmus
- ataxia
- clouding of consciousness
- peripheral neuropathy.

In its early stages, Wernicke's encephalopathy may be reversible through abstinence and the administration of high doses of thiamine; the amnesic syndrome is irreversible. As the latter may emerge from Wernicke's encephalopathy in chronic alcohol abuse, the term Wernicke–Korsakov syndrome is sometimes used.

Social morbidity

The social costs of excessive alcohol consumption are very high, and include the following:

- *Breakdown of relationships, marriages and families*. This may be a result of mood changes, personality deterioration, verbal abuse, physical violence, psychosexual disorders, pathological jealousy, and associated gambling and other psychoactive substance use. Such breakdowns, particularly when children are involved, can lead to an increased financial burden on the taxpayer in those countries with a well-developed social security/support system. Furthermore, the children of such broken families may suffer emotionally in years to come from the trauma of having lived with a parent or parents who drank heavily.
- *Poor performance at work*. This may result, for example, from morning hangovers leading to lateness, particularly on the first day of the working week. This can clearly lead to a financial cost to companies and to the overall economy. In the case of certain professionals, for example doctors and airline pilots, there is also the direct risk to others.
- *Crime*. Alcohol often plays a part in crimes, such as arson, sexual offences (e.g. rape) and crimes of violence (such as homicide) (see Chapter 21). There are clearly associated financial costs to individuals and the country resulting from such crimes.
- *Accidents and trauma*. As mentioned above, excessive alcohol consumption often plays a part in accidents and trauma, including road accidents, falls, drowning and burns and death by fire. As well as the emotional costs involved, the economic cost to health services or health insurance companies can be very high.

Problem drinking

Problem drinking is said to occur when chronic heavy drinking leads to alcohol-related disabilities (described above). Problem drinking does not necessarily imply the concurrent existence of alcohol dependence (described below), although the two can and do occur together.

Alcohol dependence

Chronic heavy drinkers exhibit a cluster of common symptoms that form the alcohol dependence syndrome:

- *Primacy of drinking over other activities*, such as family, career and social position.
- *Subjective awareness of a compulsion to drink and difficulty in controlling the amount drunk.* Attempted abstinence leads to tension and increasing craving for alcohol.
- *A narrowing of the drinking repertoire*, in which the drinker no longer has control of when to drink and when to abstain or drink moderately.
- *Increased tolerance to alcohol.*
- *Repeated withdrawal symptoms*. A fall in the blood alcohol concentration leads to tremor, insomnia, nausea, increasing sweating, anorexia and anxiety symptoms. These early symptoms occur within 12 hours after the last intake of alcohol, and may take place on waking because of the nocturnal fall in the alcohol concentration. They are relieved by drinking more alcohol. Continued abstinence can lead to the development of generalized *withdrawal fits* between 10 and 60 hours after the last intake of alcohol. Persisting withdrawal symptoms may

lead, after 72 hours, to the development of *delirium tremens*. Alcohol withdrawal should be borne in mind as a possible cause of fits in medical and surgical cases, for example postoperatively.
- *Relief or avoidance of withdrawal symptoms by further drinking.*
- *Reinstatement after abstinence.* After a period of abstinence of, say, two weeks, the drinker may no longer have a subjective craving for alcohol and may believe that it is now possible to drink in moderation. However, such an attempt is highly likely to lead to a reinstatement of the previous undesirable drinking pattern and the other features of the alcohol dependence syndrome.

Epidemiology

Figure 7.4, which shows data for European countries in the mid-1970s, demonstrates a close association between *liver cirrhosis* mortality and the consumption of alcohol. Such figures are a useful index of alcohol consumption. Other indices that can be used include the number of *drunkenness offences*, including drink-driving offences, the number of *psychiatric hospital admissions* for alcohol abuse, and *surveys* of the general population.

Gender

Although the prevalence and lifetime expectancy among heavy drinkers is generally much higher in men than in women, recently there has been a relative increase in the rates in women in some Western countries, such as England and Wales.

Age

In Western countries the highest rates of heavy drinking occur in adolescence and the early 20s.

Occupation

Those occupations at higher risk than normal of problem drinking can be deduced by studying the statistics for higher than normal mortality rates from alcoholic cirrhosis of the liver (Figure 7.5).

Aetiology

The main aetiological factors involved in problem drinking can be divided into individual and social causes.

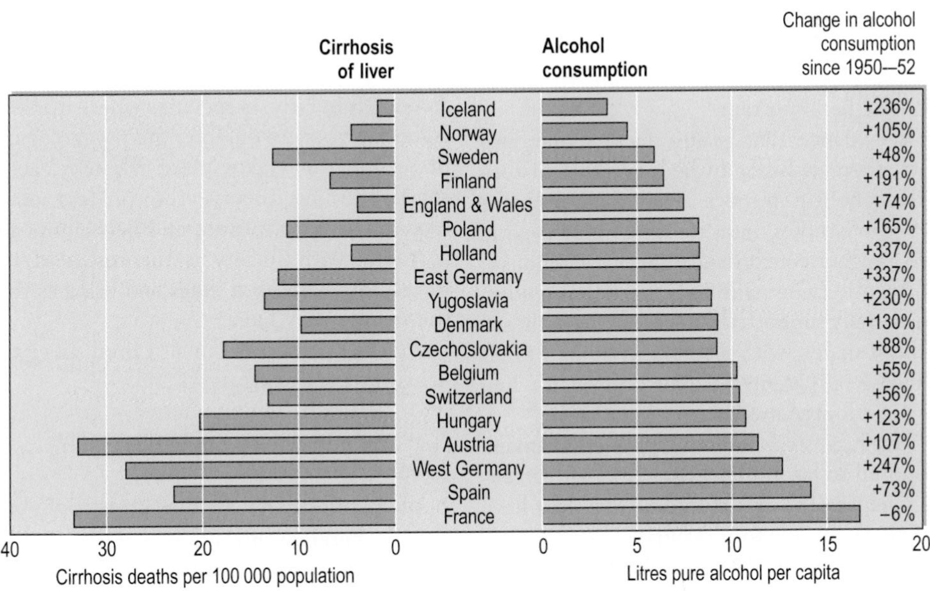

Figure 7.4 • The relationship between liver cirrhosis mortality and alcohol consumption in selected European countries in the mid-1970s. • Czechoslovakia = Czech Republic and Slovakia. (Reproduced with modifications from the Office of Health Economics 1981 *Alcohol, reducing the harm.*)

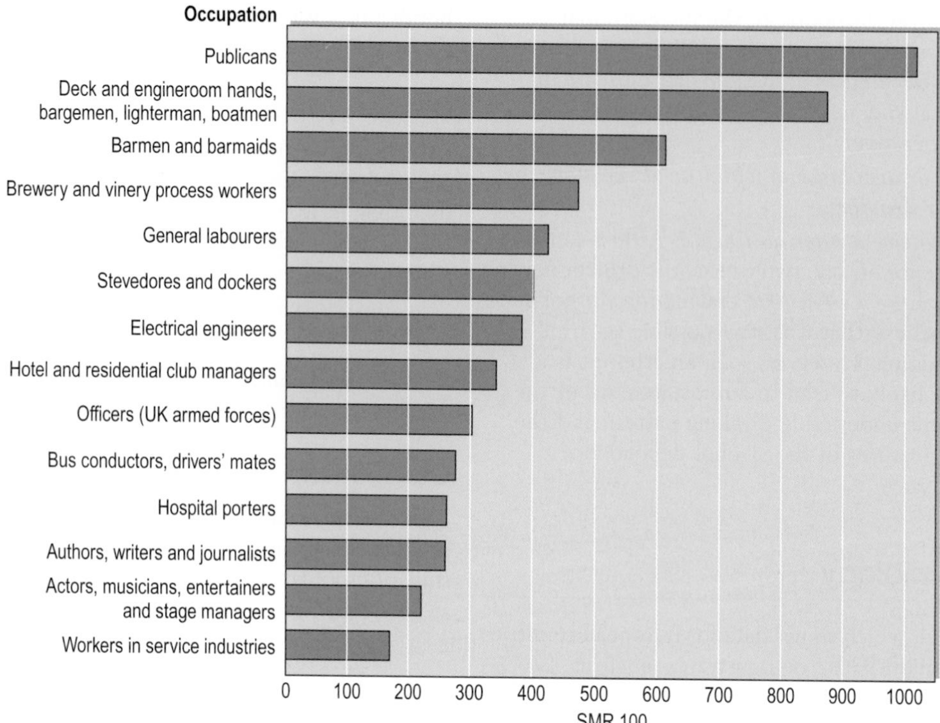

Figure 7.5 • Occupations with higher than normal mortality rates from alcoholic cirrhosis of the liver.

Individual causes

In some of the occupational groups at high risk of problem drinking enumerated below, such as publicans and brewery workers, the ready *availability* of alcohol is highly likely to be an important aetiological factor. In others, such as medicine, the *stress* of the job may be important.

There is evidence that *genetic* factors may also play a part: there is likely to be a positive history of familial alcoholism in more severe male problem drinkers. Twin studies indicate that monozygotic twins have a higher concordance rate for alcoholism than do dizygotic twins. Similarly, adoption studies have also generally supported this genetic hypothesis, particularly in males, with alcoholism being passed on from biological parents to their sons even when the latter are adopted away.

It has been suggested that some problem drinkers are predisposed to harmful drinking by their *personality* (see Chapter 15), but studies in this area have tended to give contradictory results.

Advertising pressures predispose to drinking, particularly in adolescents and young people. Such advertisements often associate drinking with physical attraction and being socially at ease with the opposite sex, possibly gaining their influence through the psychological process of observational learning.

Similarly, *peer group pressures* can also cause drinking. For example, in some universities and colleges new students take part in 'tribal initiation' rites, which frequently involve drinking large quantities of alcohol. Similarly, in societies where drinking alcohol is looked upon favourably, the psychological process of *socialization* takes place whereby, according to social learning theory, the process of acquiring characteristics, attitudes and behaviours that are in harmony with society is the result of individuals interacting with each other and using as role models the people they like.

Psychiatric illness can also predispose to harmful drinking, particularly:

- depressive illness and bereavement
- anxiety disorders
- phobic disorders, such as claustrophobia
- more rarely, schizophrenia, particularly in withdrawn patients with affective flattening and possibly experiencing auditory hallucinations; such a patient may also be homeless

- patients suffering from bipolar mood disorder may also drink heavily while in the elated mood of (hypo)mania.

Social causes

Religion can affect the overall consumption of alcohol in a society. For example, excessive alcohol consumption is relatively rare in some Islamic countries because the sale and drinking of alcoholic beverages is strictly limited in public.

Similarly, *tradition* and *cultural factors* can influence the amount of alcohol consumed. In France, for example, wine is drunk regularly from an early age in many families.

Economic factors have been found to play a major role in the overall consumption of alcohol. There is a close relationship between consumption and the price of alcoholic beverages.

Assessment

History

Important pointers to look for in the history include: *difficulties at work*, including repeatedly losing one's job and absenteeism, particularly on the first day of the working week; *psychosexual and relationship difficulties*, such as a deterioration in the patient's marriage as a direct or indirect result of alcohol; *repeated accidents*; a *family history of alcohol problems*; an *occupational history* that includes working in high-risk jobs such as those mentioned earlier; and a positive *forensic history*, particularly for drink-related offences such as drink-driving.

In the *alcohol history*, the pattern of drinking should be noted as well as the number of units of alcohol drunk on average each week.

The *CAGE questionnaire* (Table 7.2) can be routinely administered to patients to screen for alcohol problems; positive answers to two or more of the four CAGE questions is indicative of problem drinking.

Withdrawal symptoms should also be asked about if there is a suspicion of problem drinking.

Table 7.2 The CAGE questionnaire
C Have you ever felt you should **C**ut down on your drinking?
A Have people **A**nnoyed you by criticizing your drinking?
G Have you ever felt **G**uilty about your drinking?
E Have you ever had a drink first thing in the morning (an **E**ye-opener) to steady your nerves or get rid of a hangover?

Mental state examination

Evidence of the psychopathology associated with chronic heavy alcohol consumption should be looked for, such as low mood, delusional jealousy and confabulation.

Physical examination

Evidence of the following should be looked for in particular when problem drinking is suspected:

- *withdrawal symptoms*, such as tremor and flushing
- *hepatic disease*, such as spider naevi, liver palms and hepatomegaly
- *accidents* or *fighting*, such as haematomas, cuts and broken ribs
- *concomitant illicit drug abuse*, such as venepuncture marks.

Investigations

Further information should be sought from relatives, other doctors and the case notes of previous hospital admissions. The following should also be checked:

- Mean corpuscular volume (MCV) may be raised.
- γ-Glutamyl-transpeptidase (γGT or GGT) may be raised.
- Aspartate aminotransferase (AST) may be raised.
- Blood alcohol concentration, determined by analysing the alcohol level in expired air using an Alcometer, or by means of a direct blood test, gives an index of alcohol consumption in the previous 24 hours.
- Plasma uric acid concentration may be raised.

Treatment

When treating a patient with a drinking problem as an inpatient, it is useful to form a signed *contract* whereby the patient agrees not to drink alcoholic beverages or other substances containing alcohol (e.g. aftershave lotion, perfume) during the time spent as an inpatient.

Reinstatement after abstinence is likely to occur. That is, after a period of abstinence the drinker may no longer have a subjective craving for alcohol and may believe that it is now possible to drink in moderation. However, such an attempt is highly likely to lead to a reinstatement of the previous undesirable drinking pattern and the other features of the alcohol dependence syndrome. Therefore, in general it is probably better to aim for *total abstinence*.

Withdrawal symptoms

The treatment of withdrawal symptoms, also known as *detoxification*, is aimed not only at attending to early symptoms (see above), but also at preventing *withdrawal fits* and *delirium tremens*. Not all alcohol withdrawal needs to be conducted on an inpatient basis, and indeed most is not. The treatment consists of the following:

- *Support and explanation* from the nursing staff, with care preferably taking place in a single quiet side room.
- *Rehydration* and *correction of electrolyte imbalance*, as required. If the patient is hypoglycaemic, oral or parenteral glucose replacement should be given slowly with great care, together with *thiamine*, as there is a risk of precipitating Wernicke's encephalopathy if the patient is thiamine-deficient.
- *Oral thiamine*.
- *Pharmacotherapy* with a *reducing regimen* of *benzodiazepines* (e.g. diazepam or chlordiazepoxide) or *clomethiazole*. The initial starting dosage should be reduced gradually to zero over five to seven days.

Withdrawal fits should be treated with intravenous or rectal *diazepam*. The treatment of *delirium tremens* is that of delirium (see Chapter 6).

Wernicke's encephalopathy

In its early stages, Wernicke's encephalopathy may respond to abstention from alcohol and treatment with *thiamine*. (Note that parenteral administration of B vitamins may be associated with anaphylaxis.)

Alcoholic hallucinosis

As with the drug treatment of acute schizophrenia (see Chapter 8), alcoholic hallucinosis usually responds to pharmacotherapy with *phenothiazines*, although these antipsychotics lower the threshold for seizures and so may increase the risk of withdrawal fits.

Long-term prevention of problem drinking

The following are useful approaches:

- Encourage the patient to keep a *drinking diary*, such as the one shown in Figure 7.6. This can enable an objective measure of the number of units of alcohol drunk each week to be noted by both the patient and the doctor.
- *Psychological treatments* include *individual* or *supportive psychotherapy*, *group psychotherapy* and *behaviour therapy*.
- *Prophylactic adjunctive pharmacotherapy* with *disulfiram (Antabuse)*, which is taken regularly. The ingestion of even small amounts of alcohol leads to very unpleasant systemic reactions, including facial flushing, headache, palpitations, tachycardia, nausea and vomiting. Large amounts of alcohol can lead to air hunger, arrhythmias and severe hypotension.
- *Acamprosate* (taken regularly), used in combination with *counselling*, may be helpful in maintaining abstinence. This treatment should be initiated as soon as possible after the alcohol withdrawal period (i.e. after abstinence has been achieved) and maintained if the patient relapses. Its therapeutic benefit is negated if there is continued alcohol abuse. The recommended treatment period is one year.
- *Agencies and resources* that may be of help include *Alcoholics Anonymous (AA)* for patients, *Al-Anon* for their spouses, and *Al-Ateen* for their teenage children. *Hostels and group homes* may also be helpful in the rehabilitation of problem drinkers.

Prognosis

Good prognostic factors include:

- good insight
- strong motivation
- good social support, including somewhere to live
- good family support.

Factors that can precipitate relapse include:

- emotional states
- interpersonal conflicts
- social pressures.

		Name	A. N. Other				
		Week starting Sunday	17th October			201 0	

Day	Beer in pints	Spirits (no. of measures)	Wine and other drinks (no. of glasses)	Where drunk	With whom	When	Circumstance
Sun	4	6	1	pub	alone	afternoon	Following argument with children
Mon	4	4	nil	home	alone	evening	Following argument with wife
Tue	2	nil	nil	pub	friend	evening	Colleague from work
Wed	nil	nil	nil				
Thu	nil	8	nil	hotel	colleagues	evening	Conference
Fri	nil	8	4	hotel	colleagues	evening	Conference
Sat	2	4	4	hotel	colleagues	evening	Conference

Figure 7.6 • A typical drinking diary.

Case history: chronic alcoholism

A 46-year-old separated man is admitted to a psychiatric hospital complaining of hearing voices. He gives a history of having worked in the hospital canteen for the past two months and says he does not know why his wife left him recently. He refuses to answer questions from the CAGE questionnaire. In the mental state examination it is found that the auditory hallucinations, which occur in clear consciousness, are derogatory in content, frequently telling the patient that he is a bad person. There is prominent impairment of recent memory, with preservation of immediate recall in the absence of generalized cognitive impairment. Physical examination reveals spider naevi, hepatic palms, fetor hepaticus and hepatomegaly.

Further information from his wife and family doctor reveals that some of the history given by the patient, particularly concerning the previous two months, is incorrect. For example, he has never worked in the hospital, but has in fact worked as a chef in five different hotels over the past 18 months, having been sacked each time for persistently turning up late. He has been unemployed for the last two months. According to his wife, the patient had drunk heavily for years, had suffered from erectile dysfunction and had become increasingly verbally and physically abusive towards her. Two years ago he received hospital treatment for Wernicke's encephalopathy. His blood tests show a raised MCV, γGT and AST.

A diagnosis of alcoholic hallucinosis and Korsakov's syndrome was made, accounting respectively for the auditory hallucinations in clear consciousness and the confabulation. The former responded rapidly to pharmacotherapy with oral chlorpromazine; no treatment could be offered for the Korsakov's syndrome.

Alcohol problems

- One unit of alcohol = 8–10 g pure alcohol = one standard measure of spirits = one glass of standard table wine = $\frac{1}{2}$ pint beer = $\frac{1}{2}$ pint standard-strength lager.
- Low-risk level of alcohol consumption is up to 21 units in men and up to 14 units in women.
- Physical consequences of excessive alcohol consumption include gastrointestinal disorders, malnutrition, hepatic damage, pancreatitis, hypertension, cardiac arrhythmias, haematological complications, cancer, fetal alcohol syndrome, accidents and trauma, and neuromuscular disorders.
- Psychiatric consequences include low mood, suicide, personality deterioration, blackouts, delirium tremens, withdrawal fits, alcoholic hallucinosis, psychosexual disorders, delusional (pathological) jealousy, fugue states, gambling, illicit drug abuse, dementia, alcoholic encephalopathy, Wernicke's encephalopathy and the amnesic (Korsakov's) syndrome.
- Social consequences include the breakdown of relationships and families, poor performance at work, criminal behaviour and accidents and trauma.
- Problem drinking is said to occur when chronic heavy drinking leads to alcohol-related disabilities.
- In the alcohol dependence syndrome there is:
  - primacy of drinking over other activities
  - subjective awareness of a compulsion to drink and difficulty controlling the amount drunk
  - a narrowing of the drinking repertoire
  - increased tolerance to alcohol
  - repeated withdrawal symptoms
  - relief or avoidance of withdrawal symptoms by further drinking
  - reinstatement after abstinence.

Other psychoactive substances

Table 7.3 gives colloquial names often used for some of the illicit drugs described in this section.

Table 7.3 Colloquial names for some abused drugs

Drug	Colloquial name
Heroin	Smack
Cannabinoids	Grass, hash, ganja, pot
Temazepam capsules	Jellies
Barbiturates	Downers
Cocaine	Snow, coke, girl, lady
Amphetamines	Speed, whizz
LSD	Acid
PCP	Angel dust, Peace Pill
MDMA	Ecstasy, XTC, Adam, E

Opioids

Opioids are used clinically as analgesics and antitussives. They also produce euphoria. Other side-effects include nausea and vomiting, constipation, drowsiness, anorexia, lowered libido and, in large doses, hypotension and respiratory depression. Although regular use leads to tolerance and both physical and psychological dependence, this is not a contraindication for the administration of the more powerful analgesic opioids for the management of pain in terminal illness.

The opioids can be divided into:

- *natural*, such as morphine and heroin (diamorphine), which can be derived from the opium poppy
- *synthetic*, such as methadone and oxycodone
- *synthetic compounds that have both opioid agonist and antagonist properties*, such as buprenorphine and pentazocine.

The most widely abused of the opioids in Western countries are heroin and morphine. Although they can be administered by most routes, the most common method of taking heroin is intravenously, as this leads to a very intense transient 'rush' of pleasurable feelings. The clinical features of chronic opioid dependence are shown in Figure 7.7.

Withdrawal symptoms

These include: an intense craving for the opioid drug; nausea and vomiting; muscle aches and joint pains; lacrimation and rhinorrhoea; dilated pupils; piloerection; sweating; diarrhoea; yawning; changes in body temperature, such as the development of pyrexia; restlessness and insomnia; increased cardiac rate; and cramp-like abdominal pains. This syndrome is sometimes referred to colloquially as 'cold turkey'.

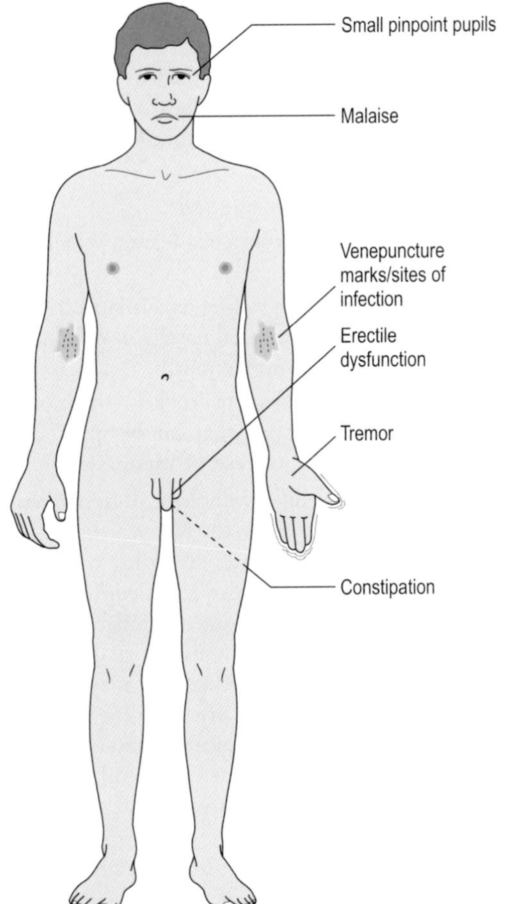

Figure 7.7 • Clinical features seen in chronic opioid dependence.

Treatment

Detoxification can be carried out over a mutually agreed timescale using another drug, such as clomethiazole or a benzodiazepine, to help with the effects of reducing the dose of opioid administered. In the case of dependency on high doses of heroin, the less potent opioid methadone is often used.

A patient presenting with apparent opioid withdrawal symptoms or with great pain (such as abdominal cramps) may be exaggerating the intensity of the symptoms to try to obtain further drugs such as the opioids pethidine and methadone.

Cannabinoids (cannabis)

The major psychoactive substance found in this group is *Δ-9-tetrahydrocannabinol*. The group includes substances derived from the cannabis plant, such as marijuana ('grass') and hashish, and synthetic substances that are similar to tetrahydrocannabinol. The most common route of administration is by smoking as a cigarette ('joints'), but the oral route may also be used with the substance being mixed with food. Cannabinoids do not cause physical dependence, but can give rise to marked psychological dependence. Occasionally, cannabinoids may be used clinically, for example in MS.

Physical symptoms of cannabinoid administration are shown in Figure 7.8. Psychological effects include: euphoria; anxiety; suspiciousness; the feeling that time is slowed down; impairment of judgement (so that it can be dangerous for the user to drive a car); and social withdrawal. The suspiciousness may occasionally develop into persecutory delusions. Depersonalization, derealization and hallucinations have been reported in cases of very high blood cannabinoid levels.

Sedatives and hypnotics

The main groups of psychoactive substances used clinically as sedatives and hypnotics are:

- *Benzodiazepines*, such as diazepam, temazepam and chlordiazepoxide.
- *Barbiturates* with an intermediate half-life, such as amobarbital and butobarbital. Barbiturates with

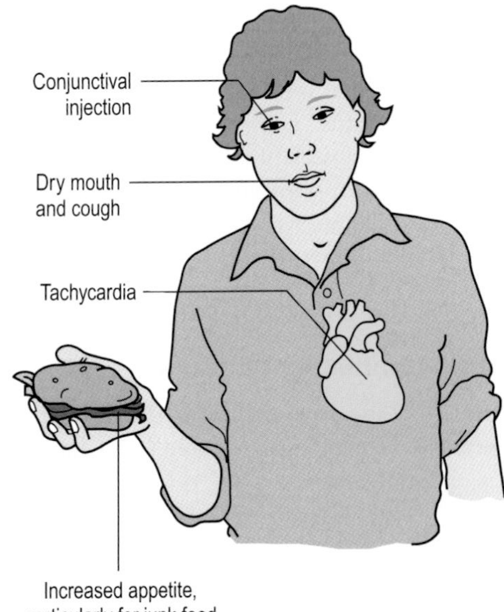

Figure 7.8 • Physical symptoms of cannabinoid administration.

a very short half-life, such as thiopental, are used as anaesthetics, whereas those with a long half-life, such as phenobarbital and methylphenobarbital, can be used in the prophylaxis of epilepsy.
- *Chloral hydrate derivatives.*

The most common route of administration is orally. However, some individuals attempt intravenous injection of the contents of capsules (which may be heated first), for example temazepam, or a solution of ground-down tablets. This gives a 'rush'-like experience, but carries a very high risk of damage to the veins. Physical dependence on sedatives and hypnotics can occur very quickly.

Neurological symptoms of intoxication include slurred speech, incoordination, unsteady gait and impaired attention or memory. Behavioural and psychological symptoms of intoxication include: a paradoxical increase in aggressive, hostile or sexual impulses, caused by disinhibition; mood lability; impaired judgement; and impaired social or occupational functioning.

Withdrawal symptoms

These are similar to those caused by withdrawal from alcohol, and occur after several weeks or more of moderate use of the drug. They may not occur for up to three weeks following drug use and include: nausea and vomiting; malaise or weakness; autonomic hyperactivity, such as tachycardia and sweating; anxiety or irritability; orthostatic hypotension; a coarse tremor of the hands, tongue and eyelids; insomnia; *grand mal* fits; loss of appetite and body weight; and tinnitus. Delirium may also develop, usually within one week of sudden cessation of drug use. It is associated with visual, auditory or tactile hallucinations. Delusions, agitation, tremor, pyrexia and autonomic hyperactivity are also commonly occurring features.

Amnesic (amnestic) disorder

Chronic use of the drug can lead to the development of an amnesic (amnestic) syndrome (see Chapter 6).

Treatment

Owing to the withdrawal syndrome and the possibility of delirium, it is important that detoxification takes place gradually, over a period of from four weeks to, say, one year.

Cocaine

Cocaine is derived mainly from the leaves of the coca plant and is used clinically as a local anaesthetic, for example in eye-drops. The main types of cocaine that are abused are:

- *coca leaves*, which are chewed
- *coca paste*, derived from coca leaves, which is usually smoked
- *cocaine hydrochloride*, which is available as a powder that can be inhaled nasally or dissolved in water and injected intravenously
- *crack cocaine* ('freebase' or 'rock'), which is an alkaloid form of cocaine that can be smoked (which leads to the release of vapours).

Cocaine causes strong psychological dependence. Cocaine intoxication leads to: tachycardia; dilated pupils; raised blood pressure; sweating; nausea and vomiting; behavioural changes such as euphoria, grandiosity, agitation, impairment of judgement and social or occupational functioning; visual or tactile hallucinations. Tactile hallucinations may take the form of feeling that insects are crawling under the skin, known clinically as formication and colloquially as the 'cocaine bug'. High doses may lead to ideas of reference, increased sexual interest and a delusional disorder.

Withdrawal symptoms

When the 'rush' of well-being and confidence produced by crack and intravenous cocaine abates, there follows a rebound 'crash' typified by a dysphoric mood, a craving for more cocaine, anxiety and irritability, and fatigue. Stopping or reducing the amount administered after chronic use leads to similar symptoms, together with insomnia or hypersomnia, and paranoid and suicidal thoughts. Sudden cessation of use can also lead to the development of delirium within 24 hours.

Other stimulants

Amphetamine and related substances

The amphetamines, such as dexamfetamine, are used clinically in the treatment of narcolepsy and ADHD. Illicit users tend to administer these substances orally or, for a more intense 'rush', intravenously; methamphetamine ('speed') is also sometimes inhaled nasally.

Their effects include euphoria, excitement, a feeling of well-being and increased confidence, increased energy and drive, and a reduced need for sleep. Physical effects include tachycardia, dilated pupils and raised blood pressure. Increased doses, particularly with chronic use, lead additionally to sweating, nausea and vomiting, and behavioural and psychological changes, which include: grandiosity; hypervigilance; agitation; impairment of judgement and social or occupational functioning; illusions; tactile, auditory and visual hallucinations; and a delusional disorder. In the acute stages the psychosis produced by amphetamines can be indistinguishable clinically from schizophrenia. However, the psychosis usually abates with drug cessation, although sometimes it may precipitate a schizophrenic illness.

Within 24 hours of taking the drug delirium may develop (substance intoxication delirium). Withdrawal symptoms occur following cessation of chronic use and include: dysphoric mood (including depression, irritability and anxiety); fatigue; insomnia or hypersomnia; and agitation. These withdrawal symptoms last for more than 24 hours after stopping the drug.

Case history: amphetamine addiction

A 21-year-old man was admitted to hospital in an agitated state with a two-day history of third-person auditory hallucinations and delusions of persecution. There was no family psychiatric history and no previous psychiatric history. The patient denied abusing alcohol or illicit drugs.

Physical examination revealed an area of sepsis in the left antecubital fossa; the patient was right-handed. The possibility of illicit intravenous drug abuse was suspected and a urine sample was sent to the laboratory for a drug screen. Meanwhile, the patient was given oral chlorpromazine to settle his agitation and symptomatology. The screen proved positive for amphetamine and a diagnosis of an amphetamine-induced psychotic disorder was made. After a further three days the patient was symptom-free and no longer on psychotropic medication. He now admitted a long history of amphetamine abuse and, as he had shared needles in the past, he was referred for counselling with a view to considering being tested for HIV. He was also put in contact with a drug-dependency unit.

Caffeine

Caffeine is a drug legally available and widely consumed in beverages such as coffee, tea, cola and hot chocolate, and in the form of chocolate. It is also included by manufacturers in many analgesic preparations and 'cold' remedies. It is not known to have a clinically useful analgesic or anti-inflammatory action. Caffeine tablets are also available legally as stimulants. The doses contained in various legal preparations are shown in Figure 7.9. Note that a can of diet cola may contain 40–50 mg caffeine. Caffeine can lead to psychological but not physical dependence.

Caffeine intoxication, with doses as small as 250 mg, can lead to clinical features similar to those seen in panic disorder, generalized anxiety disorder and hypomania. However, the effects are usually transient and temporally related to the intake of caffeine. They include: restlessness, agitation and

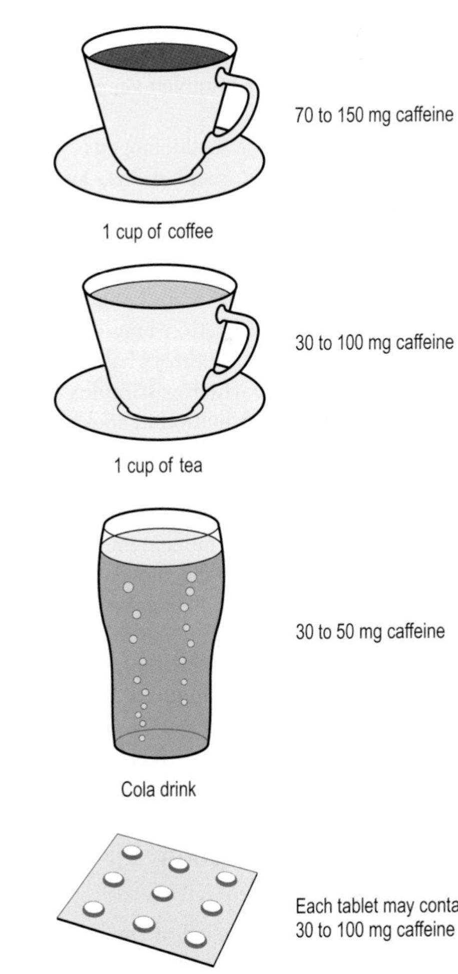

Figure 7.9 • Doses of caffeine in legally available preparations.

anxiety; excitement; insomnia; facial flushing; diuresis; gastrointestinal changes; muscle twitching; tachycardia and, sometimes, cardiac arrhythmias; a rambling flow of thought and speech; and periods of inexhaustibility.

Hallucinogens

The main types of hallucinogen are:

- substances *related to serotonin* (*5-HT*), such as lysergic acid diethylamine (LSD), dimethyltryptamine (DMT), mescaline and psilocybin (from 'magic mushrooms')
- *phencyclidine (PCP) and related arylcyclohexylamines* such as ketamine
- *3, 4-methylenedioxymethamphetamine (MDMA)*, also known as 'Ecstasy', 'XTC', 'Adam' and 'E'.

These substances are usually taken orally and do not usually cause dependence, a notable exception being MDMA (Ecstasy).

The physical effects of hallucinogens include dilated pupils, tachycardia, palpitations, sweating, blurred vision, incoordination and tremor. The psychological effects involve perceptual abnormalities, sometimes (but not always) including hallucinations. Perceptions in all modalities may be intensified, depersonalization and derealization may occur, and illusions may also be present. Auditory hallucinations are rare. Synaesthesias, in which a stimulus in one sensory field leads to a hallucination in another, may also occur. Other psychological symptoms include: anxiety; depression, which may lead to suicide; ideas of reference; a fear that one is going mad; paranoid thoughts; and impairment of judgement and social or occupational functioning. Hallucinogens may give rise to a delusional disorder, which may be life-threatening. For example, cases have occurred of people jumping out of tall buildings under the LSD-induced delusion that they have the ability to fly. MDMA (Ecstasy) also makes the user have 'loving feelings' towards others, so that they may feel the need to engage in bodily contact with others.

Posthallucinogen perception disorders (flashbacks)

This refers to the re-experiencing of the perceptual changes that occurred while intoxicated with a hallucinogen after regular use of that hallucinogen has ceased. These flashback phenomena may occur many years after regular use has stopped, and lead to great distress for the patient; panic disorder, depression and suicide may result.

Tobacco

The widespread legal availability of tobacco products, with consumption encouraged by means of expensive advertising, allows the psychoactive substance nicotine to be self-administered in a variety of forms, including the smoking of cigarettes, pipes and cigars, the chewing of tobacco and the nasal inhalation of snuff. The cerebral effects of nicotine take place most quickly with cigarette smoking. The short-term physical effects are sympathomimetic in nature, whereas psychologically nicotine acts as a central stimulant. Both psychological and physical dependence occur.

Withdrawal symptoms

These include: craving for nicotine; irritability, frustration or anger; anxiety symptoms; poor concentration and restlessness; and increased appetite.

Volatile solvents

Substances giving off psychoactive vapours include solvents, adhesives, petrol, butane gas, paint, paint thinners, typewriter correction fluid and some cleaning agents. They may be inhaled directly or from plastic bags or other containers (which runs the risk of suffocation). Death can also result from direct toxicity and from inhalation of gastric contents. This form of abuse is also known as 'glue sniffing'. As these substances are usually freely available, this type of psychoactive substance use is particularly prevalent in children. Psychological dependence can occur with prolonged use. As these substances are highly flammable, burns may be caused.

The physical effects of intoxication include: dizziness; nystagmus; blurred vision; incoordination; slurred speech; unsteady gait; lethargy; decreased reflexes; tremor; muscle weakness; and, in high doses, stupor, leading to coma. Behavioural and psychological effects include: apathy and psychomotor retardation; belligerence; impairment of judgement and social or occupational functioning; and euphoria.

Assessment

In the *history*, the patient may reveal the use of a psychoactive substance, particularly if it is legally available. It is important to ask about this and to take a detailed history of the pattern of use. The symptoms, including their temporal relationship to substance use, may suggest a suitable line of enquiry. For example, in someone who suffers from regular headaches on weekday afternoons it may be useful to determine the amount of coffee drunk on weekday mornings, as they may be suffering from caffeine withdrawal. A past history of psychoactive substance use is also suggestive of present use of such substances.

In the *mental state examination*, the presence of the behavioural and psychological effects of the substances given above should suggest the possibility of their use.

In the *physical examination*, it is important to look for evidence such as venepuncture marks or the complications of venepuncture (such as local infection). The patient may smell of cannabis or solvents, for example, and there may be traces of the solvent on clothes or skin.

Investigations

Further information should be obtained from other sources. Laboratory investigation methods are available for detecting the presence of many psychoactive substances in the blood or urine, including opioids, cannabinoids, many sedatives and hypnotics, amphetamines and cocaine. Therefore, a drug screen should be carried out if psychoactive substance use is suspected.

Other psychoactive substances

- The natural opioids heroin and morphine are often taken intravenously to give an intense 'rush'; withdrawal leads to 'cold turkey'.
- Cannabinoids contain tetrahydrocannabinol and are commonly taken by smoking; they can cause euphoria, anxiety, suspiciousness, persecutory delusions and social withdrawal.
- The contents of temazepam capsules may be abused by being injected intravenously to give a 'rush'.
- Cocaine hydrochloride is abused by being inhaled nasally or injected intravenously, whereas crack cocaine is smoked, leading to the release of vapours; cocaine can cause euphoria, grandiosity, formication and, in high doses, increased sexual interest and a delusional disorder.
- Amphetamines are usually abused by being taken orally or intravenously (for a more intense 'rush'); they can cause a transient acute psychotic picture clinically indistinguishable from schizophrenia.
- Caffeine is legally available; intoxication can cause a transient picture clinically similar to that seen in panic disorder, generalized anxiety disorder and hypomania.
- Hallucinogens (e.g. LSD, PCP, Ecstasy) are usually taken orally; they can cause hallucinations, depersonalization, derealization, synaesthesia, depression, ideas of reference, delusional disorders and flashbacks.
- Volatile solvents are usually abused by inhalation, either directly or from containers ('glue sniffing'); they can cause apathy, psychomotor retardation and impaired social functioning.

Further reading

Edwards, G., 2003. Alcohol: the world's favourite drug. St. Martin's Press, London.

Heather, N., Robertson, I., 1997. Problem drinking, third ed. Oxford University Press, Oxford.

Royal College of Psychiatrists, 2000. Drugs: dilemmas and choices. Gaskell, London.

Schizophrenia and delusional (paranoid) disorders

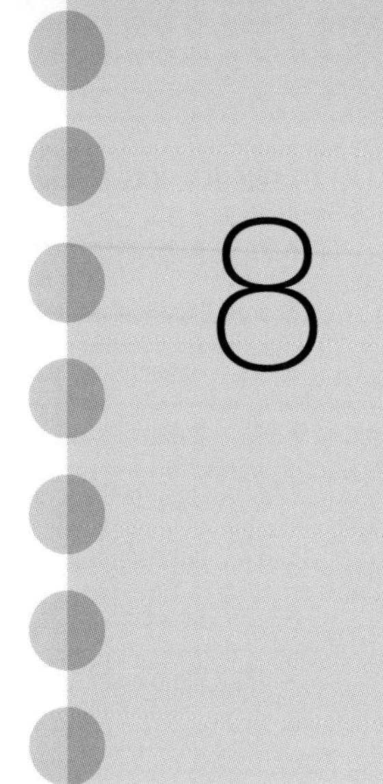

Introduction

Schizophrenia is one of the most debilitating psychiatric disorders. It is a major psychosis that can manifest itself in a variety of ways, described below. This is followed by a discussion of less severe related psychotic disorders known as delusional or paranoid disorders. The chapter ends with a consideration of schizoaffective disorders, which combine elements of both schizophrenia and mood disorders (see Chapter 9). Table 8.1 gives the ICD-10 classification of these disorders.

Schizophrenia

Clinical features

The clinical features of schizophrenia characteristically include one or more of the following:

- changes in *thinking*
- changes in *perception*
- blunted or inappropriate *affect*
- a reduced level of *social functioning*.

Cognitive functions are usually intact in the early stages.

Schneiderian first-rank symptoms

One important set of features that can be used in diagnosing schizophrenia is the presence of any of a number of symptoms brought together by Kurt Schneider and known as *Schneider's first-rank symptoms* (Table 8.2). In the absence of organic cerebral pathology, the presence of any of these is indicative of, though not pathognomonic of, schizophrenia.

The first-rank symptoms include three types of *auditory hallucination*: the voices heard by the patient (through the ears) may repeat his thoughts out loud as they are being thought (*Gedankenlautwerden*), just after they have been thought (*écho de la pensée*), or in anticipation just before they have been thought; voices may talk about the patient in the third person; or the voices may give a running commentary about the patient.

Three types of *thought alienation* (see Figure 5.5; p. 68), in which the patient believes his thoughts are under the control of an external agency or that others are participating in this thinking, are included as first-rank symptoms. He may believe that external (alien) thoughts are being inserted into his mind by an external agency (*thought insertion*), or that his own thoughts are being withdrawn from his mind by an external agency (*thought withdrawal*). The third type of thought alienation is *thought broadcasting*, in which the patient believes that his thoughts are being 'read' by others, as if they were being broadcast.

The patient may experience the feeling that his free will has been removed and that an external agency is controlling his feelings (*made feelings*), impulses (*made impulses*) or actions (*made actions* or *made acts*). He may feel under a form of hypnosis.

A related symptom is feeling that one is a passive recipient of somatic or bodily sensations from an external agency (*somatic passivity*).

A *delusional perception* involves a real perception (such as seeing a real object or hearing a real sound), which is followed by a delusional misinterpretation of

Table 8.1 ICD-10 classification of schizophrenia and delusional disorders

F20 Schizophrenia	
F20.0	Paranoid schizophrenia
F20.1	Hebephrenic schizophrenia
F20.2	Catatonic schizophrenia
F20.3	Undifferentiated schizophrenia
F20.4	Post-schizophrenic depression
F20.5	Residual schizophrenia
F20.6	Simple schizophrenia
F20.8	Other schizophrenia
F20.9	Schizophrenia, unspecified
F22 Persistent delusional disorders	
F22.0	Delusional disorder
F22.8	Other persistent delusional disorders
F22.9	Persistent delusional disorder, unspecified
F23 Acute and transient psychotic disorders	
F23.0	Acute polymorphic psychotic disorder without symptoms of schizophrenia
F23.1	Acute polymorphic psychotic disorder with symptoms of schizophrenia
F23.2	Acute schizophrenia-like psychotic disorder
F23.3	Other acute predominantly delusional psychotic disorders
F23.8	Other acute and transient psychotic disorders
F23.9	Acute and transient psychotic disorder, unspecified
F24 Induced delusional disorder	
F25 Schizoaffective disorders	
F25.0	Schizoaffective disorder, manic type
F25.1	Schizoaffective disorder, depressive type
F25.2	Schizoaffective disorder, mixed type
F25.8	Other schizoaffective disorders
F25.9	Schizoaffective disorder, unspecified
F28 Other non-organic psychotic disorders	
F29 Unspecified non-organic psychosis	

that perception. For example, a patient suffering from chronic schizophrenia once saw that a door had been left slightly open (a real visual perception) and realized as a result that he was the King of Spain (a delusional misinterpretation of that perception).

Other ICD-10 symptoms

Besides Schneider's first-rank symptoms, there are other symptoms of schizophrenia that are described by ICD-10 as having special importance for diagnosis. None of these is pathognomonic of schizophrenia. They include:

Table 8.2 Schneider's first-rank symptoms of schizophrenia
Auditory hallucinations: voices repeating thoughts out loud
Auditory hallucinations: discussing the subject in the third person
Auditory hallucinations: running commentary
Thought insertion
Thought withdrawal
Thought broadcasting
Made feelings
Made impulses
Made actions
Somatic passivity
Delusional perception

- *Other persistent delusions*. These include religious or political identity, or superhuman powers and abilities (e.g. being able to control the weather or being in communication with aliens from another planet).
- *Persistent hallucinations*. These are important in any modality, particularly when accompanied by fleeting or half-formed delusions without clear affective content, by persistent overvalued ideas or when occurring every day for weeks on end. An *overvalued idea* is an unreasonable and sustained intense preoccupation maintained with less than delusional intensity; the idea or belief is demonstrably false and is not normally held by others of the patient's subculture. There is a marked emotional investment associated with overvalued ideas.
- *Breaks or interpolations in the train of thought*. These can result in *incoherence* or *irrelevant speech*. They can also cause *neologisms* – new words constructed by the patient or everyday words used in a special way.
- *Catatonic behaviour*. The symptoms of catatonia include *stupor*, in which the patient is unresponsive, akinetic, mute and fully conscious, and *excitement*; the patient may change between these two states. Other symptoms include: *posturing*, in which the patient adopts an inappropriate or bizarre bodily posture continuously for a substantial period of time; *waxy flexibility* (also known as *cerea flexibilitas*), in which the patient's limbs can be 'moulded' into a position and remain fixed for long periods of time; and *negativism*, in which motiveless resistance occurs to instructions and to attempts to be moved.
- *Negative symptoms*. These typically occur in *chronic* schizophrenia. They include marked apathy, poverty of speech, lack of drive, slowness and blunting or incongruity of affect, and usually result in social withdrawal and lowered social performance. In identifying the presence of negative symptoms, other possible causes of such symptomatology (e.g. depression and antipsychotic medication) should first be excluded. The *positive symptoms* typically occur in *acute* schizophrenia, and have been discussed above; they include delusions, hallucinations and thought interference.
- *Change in personal behaviour*. This can be noted as a significant and consistent change in the overall quality of some aspects of personal behaviour, manifest as loss of interest, aimlessness, idleness, a self-absorbed attitude and social withdrawal.

Subtypes

ICD-10 distinguishes the following major types of schizophrenia.

Paranoid schizophrenia

The clinical picture is dominated by the presence of *paranoid symptoms*, such as:

- *delusions of persecution*, such as the patient believing that others are plotting against him
- *delusions of reference*, such as believing that strangers or the television, radio or news papers are referring to the patient in particular; when such thoughts do not reach delusional intensity they are known as *ideas of reference*
- *delusions of exalted birth*, or of having a special mission; for example, the belief that one has been born with a messianic role
- *delusions of bodily change*
- *delusions of jealousy* (described below)
- *hallucinatory voices* of a threatening nature or that issue commands to the patient
- *non-verbal auditory hallucinations*, such as laughing, whistling and humming
- *hallucinations in other modalities*, such as smell, taste, vision or of sexual or other somatic sensations.

Paranoid schizophrenia is the most common type and the patient may not look psychiatrically ill until the paranoid symptoms are exposed.

Hebephrenic schizophrenia

The following features are typical of this form of schizophrenia:

- *irresponsible and unpredictable behaviour*, with the patient often exhibiting mannerisms and playing pranks
- rambling and incoherent *speech*
- *affective changes*, including an incongruous affect and shallow mood, often with giggling and fatuousness
- poorly organized *delusions*
- fleeting and fragmentary *hallucinations*.

The age of onset of hebephrenic schizophrenia is usually between 15 and 25 and it generally has a poor prognosis, associated with the onset of 'negative' symptoms.

Catatonic schizophrenia

Here, catatonic symptoms, as described above, are prominent.

Simple schizophrenia

In this form there is an insidious onset of functional decline. Negative symptoms develop without the prior occurrence of 'positive' symptoms. For this reason the diagnosis is often made confidently only in retrospect.

Residual or chronic schizophrenia

This form of schizophrenia is preceded by one of the above types and is characterized by negative symptoms.

Other classifications

The above ICD-10 subtypes can be argued to be unsatisfactory because many patients show clinical features characteristic of more than one. Two alternative types of classification are considered here.

Syndromal classifications

From a research viewpoint, the heterogeneous nature of schizophrenia limits the value of studies that group patients under this global label. One method of addressing such heterogeneity is to adopt a syndromal approach. There are a number of such approaches, one example being that of Liddle, who has classified the symptoms of schizophrenia into three syndromes:

- *psychomotor poverty syndrome*, characterized by poverty of speech, flatness of affect and decreased spontaneous movement
- *disorganization syndrome*, characterized by disorders of the form of thought and inappropriate affect
- *reality distortion syndrome*, characterized by the occurrence of delusions and hallucinations.

These syndromes can coexist in the same individual. Positron emission tomography (PET) regional cerebral blood flow (rCBF) studies have shown that each of these is associated with a specific pattern of perfusion in paralimbic and associated cerebral cortex and in related subcortical nuclei (Figure 8.1).

A neurodevelopmental classification

On the basis of genetic, epidemiological, neuropathological, neuroimaging and gender difference studies, a neurodevelopmental classification has been put forward in which schizophrenia is subdivided into the following three groups:

- *Congenital schizophrenia*. The abnormality is present (although not necessarily recognizable) at birth, and may be caused by a genetic predisposition and/or an environmental insult such as maternal influenza, obstetric complications and early brain injury or infection. Patients are more likely to have minor physical abnormalities, to show abnormal personality or social impairment in childhood, to present to the psychiatric services early, to exhibit negative symptoms and to show morphological brain changes and cognitive impairment. They are also more likely to be male and to have a poor outcome.
- *Adult-onset schizophrenia*. These patients are more likely to exhibit positive symptoms, including Schneiderian first-rank symptoms, and mood (affective) symptoms. They may have a genetic predisposition to manifest symptomatology anywhere along a continuum from bipolar mood disorder (see Chapter 9), through schizoaffective disorder (see below) to acute schizophrenia (Figure 8.2).
- *Late-onset schizophrenia*. This is the group of late paraphrenia, discussed in Chapter 20, in which patients usually present after the age of 60 and

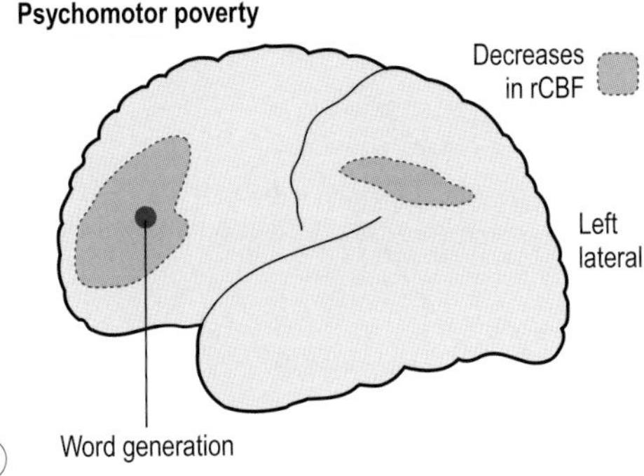

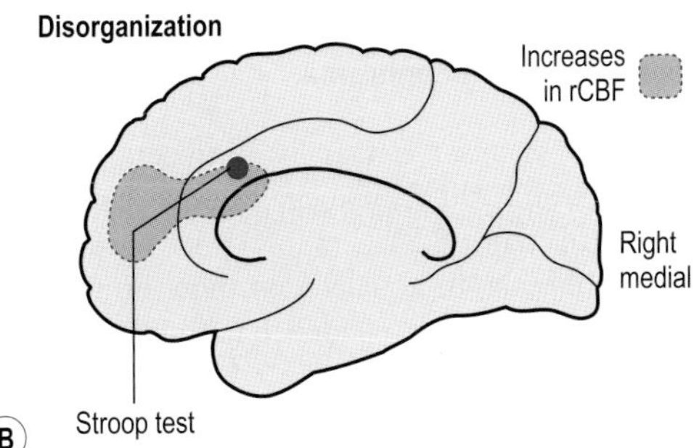

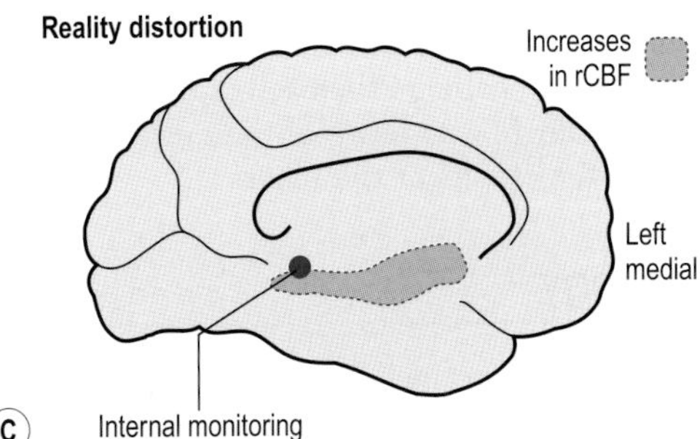

Figure 8.1 • Liddle's classification. • (a) Locus of maximal activation of the prefrontal cortex during the internal generation of words in normal subjects superimposed on the areas of decreased cortical blood flow associated with psychomotor poverty in schizophrenia. (b) Locus of maximal activity of the anterior cingulate cortex during performance of the Stroop test superimposed on the area of increased cortical blood flow associated with disorganization in schizophrenia. (c) Locus of maximal activation of the parahippocampal gyrus during the internal monitoring of eye movements superimposed on the area of increased medial temporal blood flow associated with reality distortion in schizophrenia.

have good premorbid functioning in the intellectual and occupational spheres. It is more common in females and is often associated with auditory and visual sensory deprivation, for example as a result of age-related hearing and visual impairment. It is sometimes related to a paranoid personality or to a mood disorder. Organic brain dysfunction is often found to be present.

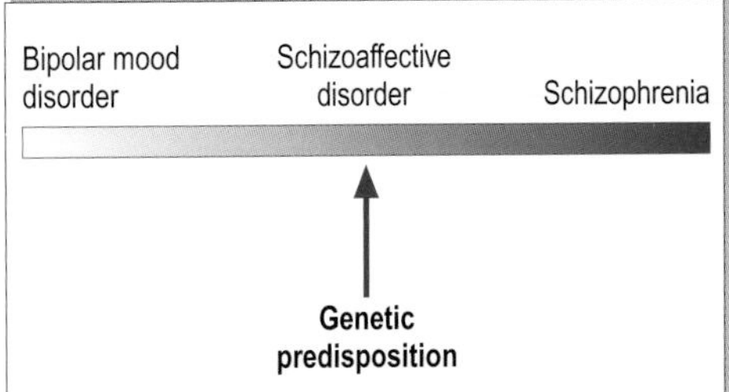

Figure 8.2 • The spectrum of 'adult-onset' psychotic disorders.

Clinical features and classification

- Schizophrenia can lead to changes in thinking, perception, affect and social functioning; cognitive functions are usually intact in the early stages.
- Schneider's first-rank symptoms of schizophrenia include: auditory hallucinations; thought insertion, withdrawal or broadcasting; made feelings, impulses or actions; somatic passivity and delusional perception.
- Other important symptoms include: other persistent delusions; persistent hallucinations in any modality; persistent overvalued ideas; formal thought disorder; catatonic behaviour; social withdrawal.
- Positive symptoms typically occur in acute schizophrenia and include delusions, hallucinations and thought disorder; negative symptoms typically occur in chronic schizophrenia and include poverty of speech, blunting/incongruity of affect and social withdrawal.
- ICD-10 subtypes of schizophrenia include paranoid, hebephrenic, catatonic, simple and residual/chronic schizophrenia.
- Liddle's three syndromes, which can coexist in the same individual, are psychomotor poverty, disorganization and reality distortion.
- A recent neurodevelopmental classification subdivides schizophrenia into the following three groups: congenital schizophrenia, adult-onset schizophrenia and late-onset schizophrenia.

Investigations

The investigations carried out in a patient presenting for the first time with schizophrenic symptomatology are those described in Chapter 5, and include:

- further information
- urea and electrolytes, full blood count, thyroid function tests, liver function tests
- a screen for illicit drugs, if psychoactive substance use is suspected as a cause
- vitamin B_{12} and folate levels
- syphilitic serology
- electroencephalography (EEG) (the symptoms may be caused by complex partial seizures of the temporal lobe)
- computed tomography (CT) or magnetic resonance imaging (MRI) scan (if clinically indicated).

In the case of first presentation in the elderly, i.e. when the diagnosis being considered is paraphrenia (see Chapter 20), tests of hearing and vision should be carried out at an early stage, as sensory deprivation is an important cause in this age group.

Differential diagnosis

Organic disorders and *psychoactive substance use disorders*, described in Chapters 6 and 7, should be excluded before making a diagnosis of schizophrenia. A full physical examination and appropriate further investigations (see below) should be carried out, particularly with a first presentation, in order to do this.

Mood disorders (see Chapter 9) may present with symptoms similar to schizophrenia. Negative symptoms and the early stages of simple schizophrenia may be difficult to distinguish from depression. In such cases care should be taken to look for other symptoms of depression. Moreover, depression may itself be a symptom of schizophrenia, both in the acute phase and following an episode of schizophrenic illness (*post-schizophrenic depression*). Schneider's first-rank symptoms can occur in mania. Therefore, one should look for other features of mania, particularly if there is no previous history of schizophrenia.

The onset of schizophrenia can lead to personality deterioration, which may simulate a *personality disorder* (see Chapter 15).

Epidemiology

The *incidence* of schizophrenia is between 15 and 30 new cases per 100 000 of the population per year. The *point prevalence* is less than 1%. There is a *lifetime risk* of developing schizophrenia of approximately 1% in the general population.

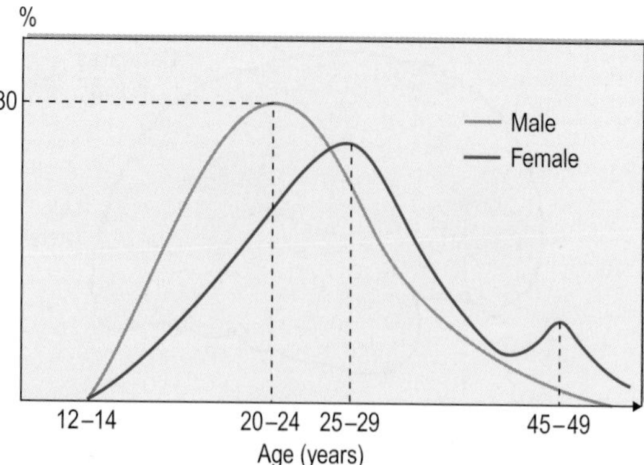

Figure 8.3 • Sex-specific age distribution of the index admission for schizophrenia.

The *age of onset* is usually between 15 and 45 years, with an earlier mean age of onset in men than in women (Figure 8.3).

Schizophrenia is equally common in males and females. It has a higher incidence in those who are not married.

Schizophrenia has also been found to be most common in social classes IV and V. This may be the result of *social drift*: the parents of patients with schizophrenia have a more normal social class distribution but the patients themselves may drift downwards socially (e.g. in terms of their occupation) as a result of the effects of the illness.

Aetiology

Predisposing factors include genetic, prenatal, perinatal and personality factors. *Precipitating factors* include psychosocial stresses. *Perpetuating factors* include the patient's family and social factors. *Mediating factors* may include neurotransmitters and neurodegeneration, and psychoneuroimmunological and psychoneuroendocrinological factors.

Genetics

Family studies have shown that the lifetime risks for developing schizophrenia are much greater in the biological relatives of patients than the approximately 1% for the general population. These are shown in Table 8.3, from which it can also be seen that the lifetime risk is generally greater in first-degree relatives (such as full siblings) than in second-degree relatives (such as grandchildren, uncles and aunts). Table 8.3 also shows that a greater genetic loading is associated with a greater risk. Thus,

Table 8.3 Approximate lifetime risks for the development of schizophrenia in the relatives of patients (probands) with schizophrenia

Relationship	Lifetime expectancy rate to the nearest percentage point
Parents	6
All siblings	10
Siblings (when one parent has schizophrenia)	17
Children	13
Children (when both parents have schizophrenia)	46
Grandchildren	4
Uncles, aunts, nephews and nieces	3

the risk in children is greater if both parents have schizophrenia, rather than just one.

Twin studies have reported a higher concordance rate for monozygotic (identical) twins (approximately 46%) than for dizygotic (fraternal) twins (approximately 14%).

Adoption studies have shown that when the children of schizophrenic mothers have been adopted soon after birth by non-schizophrenic families, they have a similar likelihood of developing schizophrenia (approximately 11%) as the rates suggested by family studies and shown in Table 8.3 (13% when one parent has schizophrenia). There is no such increased risk in the children of non-schizophrenic parents who are similarly adopted.

Taken together, family studies, twin studies and adoption studies support the hypothesis that there is an important genetic component to schizophrenia. It is hoped that studies in *molecular genetics* will characterize causative genes. However, the fact that the concordance rate for schizophrenia is not 100% in monozygotic twins indicates that there is also an important environmental component; it seems probable that a genetic–environmental interaction is important in the aetiology of this disorder.

Prenatal factors

Schizophrenia is more common in those born in the late winter and early spring months. It is particularly common in those exposed prenatally to influenza epidemics between the third and seventh months of gestation. It has been suggested that the cause may be *maternal viral infection*.

Perinatal factors

Some studies have shown that schizophrenia is more common in those who suffered from *obstetric complications* during birth. This may be related to trauma to the brain – for example during forceps delivery – and hypoxia.

Personality

Those with *schizotypal personality disorder* (see Chapter 15) have peculiarities and anomalies in ideation, appearance, speech and behaviour (which may be eccentric), as well as deficits in interpersonal relationships. This is more common in the first-degree relatives of patients and is considered to be part of a *genetic spectrum* of schizophrenia.

Psychosocial stressors

The notion of a triggering effect considers that *life events* (see Chapter 3) may act as precipitating factors in a person with a predisposition to schizophrenia. Overall, the current evidence is inconsistent and does not give strong support for this hypothesis.

The patient's family

There is an increased relapse rate of schizophrenia in those who live with families that display *high expressed emotion*, where the relatives are apt to make critical comments about the patient and tend to become over-involved emotionally. It may be that changes in physiological arousal account for this effect.

Figure 8.4 summarizes a model of the interaction of predisposing factors, psychosocial stressors, high expressed emotion and the modifying action of medication.

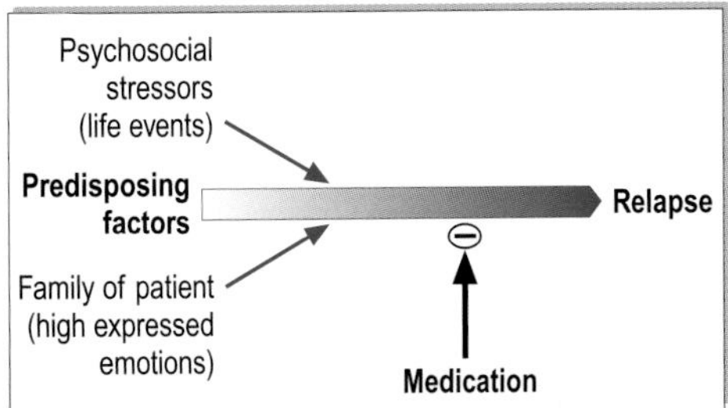

Figure 8.4 • The interaction of predisposing factors, psychosocial stressors, high expressed emotion and the modifying action of medication.

Social factors

It has been shown that understimulation in the social environment of patients with chronic schizophrenia is associated with increased negative symptoms, particularly social withdrawal, affecting blunting and poverty of speech. This has been termed *poverty of the social milieu*. Conversely, social overstimulation can act as a psychosocial stressor and possibly precipitate a relapse.

Neurotransmitters

The *mesolimbic–mesocortical system* is a *dopaminergic* system originating in the ventral tegmental area of the brain, which can be thought of as being made up of two subsystems. The mesolimbic system projects to the limbic system, whereas the mesocortical system innervates the cingulate, entorhinal and medial prefrontal cortices. According to the *dopamine hypothesis of schizophrenia*, the clinical features of this disorder are the result of central dopaminergic hyperactivity in the mesolimbic–mesocortical system.

Evidence *supporting* the dopamine hypothesis includes:

- Antipsychotic (neuroleptic) drugs (see Chapter 3 and below), such as chlorpromazine and haloperidol, which are effective in the treatment of schizophrenia, are dopamine blocking agents.
- There is a positive correlation between the ability of neuroleptic drugs to block dopamine receptors and their antipsychotic effectiveness.
- The administration of drugs such as amphetamine, which increase the functional central activity of catecholamines, including dopamine, by causing their release from catecholaminergic neurones, can cause the development of a psychotic clinical picture very similar to that seen in the 'positive symptoms' of acute schizophrenia.
- Similarly, amphetamine and related drugs can worsen the psychotic symptomatology in schizophrenia.
- Administration of levodopa (L-dopa), the precursor of dopamine, can have similar effects to those caused by amphetamine.
- In a study comparing the clinical actions of two structural isomers of the antipsychotic flupentixol (one with and one without dopamine receptor-blocking activity) and a placebo in a double-blind trial on patients with acute schizophrenia, only those receiving the dopamine antagonist improved.
- Post-mortem studies of neuroleptic binding (and therefore of dopamine binding) have shown increased binding in the brains of those with schizophrenia compared with controls.
- In animal models of dopamine function, the administration of dopamine agonists produces a behavioural picture said to be similar to human psychosis. This can be reversed by giving dopamine antagonists.

Evidence *against* the dopamine hypothesis includes:

- The CSF concentration of the dopamine metabolite homovanillic acid (HVA) in schizophrenia patients has generally not been found to be higher than in controls.
- Dopamine inhibits the release of prolactin from the adenohypophysis. Therefore, if increased central dopaminergic activity also occurred in this dopaminergic system (the tuberoinfundibular system), one might expect there to be a decrease in the baseline prolactin level. This has not generally been found to be the case.
- The proposed increased central dopaminergic activity might also be expected to occur in the nigrostriatal dopaminergic system. If this were the case, it should mean that Parkinson's disease, which is caused by reduced dopaminergic activity in this system, should not occur in a patient with schizophrenia. In practice, the two conditions can coexist.
- Pharmacotherapy with neuroleptics may take at least two weeks to cause antipsychotic effects in schizophrenia. This time interval is much greater than that required for its biochemical action, as outlined in Figure 8.5, which shows that the increase in plasma prolactin levels caused by the antidopaminergic action of neuroleptics in the tuberoinfundibular system takes place much more rapidly. Similarly, the extrapyramidal side-effects of neuroleptics may begin within two days of starting the drug.
- Not all cases of acute schizophrenia respond to dopamine antagonists.

There is some evidence that central *serotonergic* and *glutamate* dysfunction may be associated with schizophrenia. For example, the hallucinogenic drug lysergic acid diethylamide (LSD) acts at serotonin receptors.

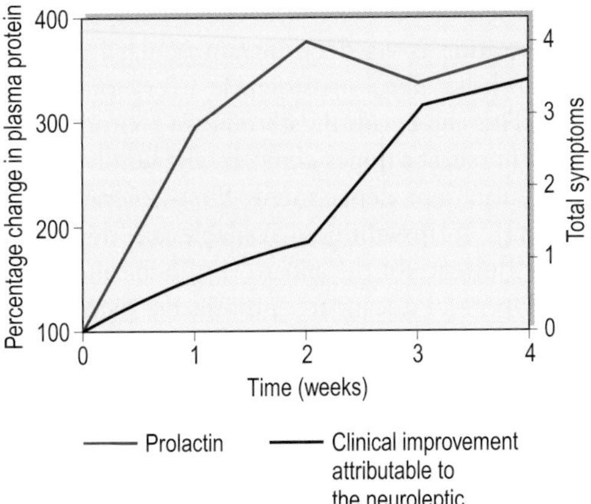

Figure 8.5 • Comparison of the time course of the change in plasma prolactin levels in patients treated with a neuroleptic with the time course of the clinical improvement attributable to the drug. (After Cotes *et al.* 1978 Psychological Medicine 8: 657.)

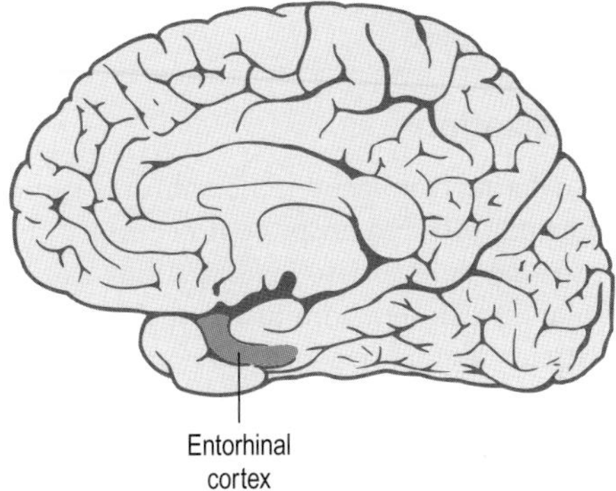

Figure 8.6 • Medial view of a normal brain, showing the location of the entorhinal cortex.

Neurodevelopmental pathology

Structural neuroimaging studies show that cerebral ventricular enlargement is present in a proportion of patients with schizophrenia.

It is generally believed that this is not caused by treatment and is present at the time of onset of the illness. It may be associated with poor premorbid adjustment. Similarly, a diffuse reduction in the volume of cortical grey matter has been found in schizophrenic patients by MRI; this has also been found to be associated with poor premorbid function. If these findings are correct, and in particular if it is the case that ventricular enlargement is non-progressive, then this would be consistent with neurodevelopmental changes having taken place in such patients.

Post-mortem neuropathological studies have revealed changes in the cytoarchitecture of the temporal lobes and limbic system in schizophrenia. Compared with control brains, the brains of patients with schizophrenia have been found to be a little lighter and to have a reduced hippocampal size and fewer neurones in the hippocampus, with these changes being particularly marked on the left side. Abnormalities have also been found in the entorhinal cortex, which forms the anterior part of the parahippocampal gyrus and lies superficial to the amygdala and to the uncal and most anterior parts of the body of the hippocampal formation (Figure 8.6). These abnormalities include invaginations of the cortical surface and heterotopic displacement of neurones. They are likely to be caused by abnormal neuronal migration. As neuronal migration is usually almost complete by the time of birth, such abnormalities probably represent neurodevelopmental pathology. The hippocampus and entorhinal cortex are interconnected and are involved jointly in the functions of memory and reality testing, so that abnormalities in their cytoarchitecture may be responsible for some of the symptoms of schizophrenia.

Investigations, differential diagnosis, epidemiology and aetiology

- Standard first-line investigations for a first presentation of a psychotic disorder in the elderly should include tests of hearing and vision to exclude sensory deprivation.
- The differential diagnosis of schizophrenia includes organic disorders and psychoactive substance use disorders, mood disorders and personality disorder.
- Incidence = 15–30 new cases per 100 000/year; point prevalence $<1\%$; lifetime risk $\simeq 1\%$; age of onset is earlier in men; sex ratio is equal; increased incidence in the unmarried; commonest in social classes IV and V.
- Predisposing factors include genetic factors, prenatal factors, perinatal factors and personality.
- Life events may act as a precipitating factor.
- Perpetuating factors include the family of the patient (high expressed emotion) and social factors (poverty of the social milieu).
- Mediating factors include neurotransmitters, neurodevelopmental pathology, psychoimmunological factors and psychoneuroendocrinological factors.

Management

Hospitalization

Those suffering from acute schizophrenic symptoms should be admitted to hospital, if necessary compulsorily, so that appropriate investigations can be carried out and treatment administered. After discharge such patients require regular follow-up appointments with a psychiatrist and, particularly in chronic schizophrenia, a community psychiatric nurse.

Patients with chronic schizophrenia should be admitted for relapses, but can otherwise often be maintained in the community or in sheltered accommodation.

Physical treatments

Pharmacotherapy. The mainstay of schizophrenia treatment is *antipsychotic drugs*, which are dealt with more fully in Chapter 3. Acute positive symptoms generally respond better than chronic negative symptoms.

In the Western world, second-generation antipsychotics are often used as first-line drug treatment. Examples are given in Chapter 3.

Clozapine may be used in those patients who either do not respond to or cannot tolerate other antipsychotics. As clozapine can cause agranulocytosis, such patients need to have regular checks (initially weekly) of their white blood count and neutrophil and platelet levels. They must also be monitored clinically for signs of infection, such as a sore throat or the development of influenza.

Patients admitted to hospital with acute positive symptoms should be treated with oral neuroleptics if they are willing to take medication by mouth. If there is any doubt at all about the compliance of such a patient (e.g. one suffering from paranoid schizophrenia and who fears being poisoned but nonetheless agrees to oral medication) then the medication should be given in the form of orodispersible tablets (many second-generation antipsychotics) or syrup (for some of the older first-generation antipsychotics). Otherwise, there is a risk that the patient may simply hide the tablets under the tongue and not swallow them. If a compulsorily detained patient refuses medication then intramuscular administration should be considered.

For patients with chronic schizophrenia living in the community, maintenance antipsychotic pharmacotherapy can help reduce the frequency of relapses. Although such patients can be asked to self-administer an oral neuroleptic, a more convenient method of administration is via deep intramuscular injection of a slow-release *depot* neuroleptic every one to four weeks. This can be administered by a community psychiatric nurse, at a depot clinic, by the family doctor or in the outpatient department. First-generation (conventional) antipsychotics available in depot form include flupentixol decanoate, fluphenazine decanoate, haloperidol decanoate, pipotiazine palmitate and zuclopenthixol decanoate. The first injection of such a conventional antipsychotic should be a small test dose to check for any unacceptable side-effects. The second-generation antipsychotic risperidone is also available in a long-acting depot injection form.

As mentioned in Chapter 3, the central antidopaminergic activity of neuroleptics gives rise to the following types of *extrapyramidal side-effects*:

- *parkinsonian symptoms* including a resting tremor, bradykinesia, cogwheel rigidity, postural abnormalities and a festinant gait
- *dystonias*, which are abnormal involuntary facial and bodily movements caused by slow and continuous muscle contraction or spasm, such as tongue protrusion, grimacing, opisthotons (involving most of the body), spasmodic torticollis (involving the neck) and oculogyric crisis (involving movement of the eyes superiorly and to one side)
- *akathisia*, in which a disagreeable inclination to move leads to restlessness
- *tardive dyskinesia*, which is abnormal involuntary movements of the face, limbs and respiratory muscles, including chewing and sucking movements, tongue protrusion, grimacing, finger movements, clenching and torticollis.

The parkinsonian symptoms can be treated with antimuscarinic (anticholinergic) drugs, such as:

- trihexyphenidyl (benzhexol)
- orphenadrine
- procyclidine.

These should be prescribed only to patients who are affected by parkinsonian symptoms. This is because some patients do not develop parkinsonism, and the antimuscarinic drugs have a number of unwanted actions, including the worsening of tardive dyskinesia.

Dystonias and akathisia usually respond to antimuscarinic drugs or improve when the antipsychotic dosage is reduced or the antipsychotic changed. If an oculogyric crisis or other drug-induced acute dystonic reaction develops, the antimuscarinic drug should be administered parenterally.

Tardive dyskinesia, on the other hand, may not be reversible even when antipsychotic medication is stopped. It usually only occurs following long-term antipsychotic therapy, although cases have been reported following short-term low-dose treatment.

The other major side-effects of antipsychotics are considered in Chapter 3.

Electroconvulsive therapy (ECT) (see Chapter 3) is used in the treatment of catatonic stupor, which occurs only rarely these days (possibly because of the ready availability and early use of antipsychotics).

Psychosocial treatments

Social milieu. Poverty of the social milieu, referred to above, should be reduced in order not to increase negative symptoms. This can involve *social skills training*, in which group psychotherapeutic methods are used to teach patients how to interact appropriately with other people. *Occupational therapy* is also very useful and can be used to teach patients useful skills for living outside hospital, such as cooking. It should be remembered that social overstimulation can also cause adverse effects by acting as a psychosocial stressor.

Expressed emotion. For those patients who are exposed to high expressed emotion, *group work* can be carried out. If it is not possible to reduce the level of expressed emotion, it may be better for the patient not to return to live with such a family but instead to be accommodated in a *staffed hostel*.

Behaviour therapy. In addition to social skills training, another type of behaviour therapy that may be used is the application of a *token economy*, whereby desired behaviour is rewarded with tokens that can be exchanged for privileges or goods.

Sheltered workshops. Attendance at such workshops, which are run especially for patients, can allow both inpatients and outpatients to gain a sense of achievement by carrying out some work each week and earning what is usually a relatively small wage. In addition, a useful skill, such as woodwork, can be mastered.

Prognosis

Approximately one-quarter of cases of schizophrenia show good clinical and social recovery, and most studies show that less than half have a poor long-term outcome. Factors associated with a good prognosis include:

- being female
- having a relative who suffers from bipolar mood disorder (in which case the patient is more likely to have affective or mood symptoms during the acute schizophrenic illness)
- older age of onset
- sudden onset
- rapid resolution
- good response to treatment
- affective loading
- good psychosexual adjustment
- not showing cognitive impairment
- not having ventricular enlargement (as demonstrated on CT or MRI).

Case history: chronic schizophrenia

A research psychiatrist carrying out a PET neuroimaging study of patients with schizophrenia interviewed a 39-year-old woman who lived in the community. She had first suffered from acute schizophrenia at the age of 19 and had been treated with antipsychotic medication ever since. For the past four years she had been receiving a depot neuroleptic, fluphenazine decanoate. Because of acute extrapyramidal side-effects, she also took oral procyclidine as required. At interview there was no evidence of positive symptoms. However, the negative symptoms of apathy, poverty of speech and low drive were noted. There was no evidence that the patient was clinically depressed. Her case notes recorded that almost five years ago, when she was not compliant with neuroleptic medication for several weeks, she had exhibited a similar clinical picture to the one she now presented. The researcher concluded that the patient was suffering from the negative symptoms of chronic schizophrenia.

Case history: paranoid schizophrenia

A 23-year-old man was referred to the psychiatric outpatient clinic by his GP with a possible low mood. In a careful interview during which the patient was encouraged to talk openly, he admitted that he had been upset for at least a year owing to the fact that he had been hearing voices when he was on his own and when there were no obvious causes. He would typically hear two male voices who would talk to each other about him and who would also sometimes comment on his

Continued

Case history: paranoid schizophrenia—cont'd

actions. He had put off going to see his doctor for over a year because he had 'realized' that the voices were the result of his being spied on by security agents, who were plotting to kill him. The patient had a positive family history in that both his sister and his mother were receiving treatment for schizophrenia. The mental state examination revealed no other important signs; in particular, there was no evidence that the patient was clinically depressed.

The patient agreed to hospital admission. Arrangements were made to interview his nearest relatives, and the positive family history of schizophrenia was confirmed. All the routine blood tests proved to be normal, as did his EEG and CT brain scan. He was diagnosed as suffering from paranoid schizophrenia and was commenced on treatment with aripiprazole. Within two weeks the persecutory delusions had disappeared and the auditory hallucinations had become very infrequent and much reduced in intensity. The patient was discharged from hospital shortly thereafter. As he was compliant with medication, he was given a prescription for oral aripiprazole. He was followed up in the psychiatric outpatient department.

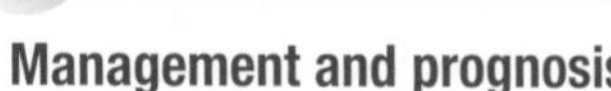

Management and prognosis

- Patients suffering from acute schizophrenic symptoms generally need to be treated as inpatients, whereas those with chronic schizophrenia can often be maintained in the community, needing admission only for relapses.
- The mainstay of treatment is with antipsychotic (neuroleptic) medication.
- Parkinsonian side-effects can be treated with antimuscarinic (anticholinergic) drugs.
- ECT is used in the treatment of catatonic stupor.
- Psychosocial treatments include reducing poverty of the social milieu (social skills training, occupational therapy), reducing expressed emotion (family therapy), behaviour therapy and sheltered workshops.
- The prognosis is good in one-quarter and poor in < one-half; a good prognosis is associated with female sex, having a relative with bipolar mood disorder, older age of onset, sudden onset, rapid resolution, good treatment response, affective loading, good psychosexual adjustment, no cognitive impairment and no ventricular enlargement.

Delusional (paranoid) disorders

The core feature of delusional (paranoid) disorders is the development of a delusion or delusional system, which is usually persistent, sometimes lifelong, and has no identifiable organic basis. The patient does not suffer from schizophrenia or a mood disorder, although depressive symptoms may be present intermittently. According to ICD-10, occasional or transitory auditory hallucinations, particularly in elderly patients, do not rule out this diagnosis, provided they are not typically schizophrenic and form only a small part of the overall clinical picture. According to ICD-10:

> The delusions are highly variable in content. Often they are persecutory, hypochondriacal, or grandiose, but they may be concerned with litigation or jealousy, or express a conviction that the individual's body is misshapen, or that others think that he or she smells or is homosexual. Other psychopathology is characteristically absent, but depressive symptoms may be present intermittently, and olfactory and tactile hallucinations may develop in some cases . . . Apart from actions and attitudes directly related to the delusion or delusional system, affect, speech, and behaviour are normal.

A number of special delusional disorders having specific features are described here. Paraphrenia is considered in Chapter 20.

Epidemiology

The *point prevalence* of delusional disorders is much lower than that of schizophrenia, being in the order of 0.03%, with a *lifetime risk* of 0.05 and 0.1%. The mean age of onset is between 40 and 55 years. Overall, delusional disorders are slightly more common in females.

Specific disorders

Pathological (delusional) jealousy

In this condition the patient holds the delusional belief that his or her spouse or sexual partner is being unfaithful, and will go to great lengths to find evidence of this. For example, the partner's underclothing may be examined for semen stains, other belongings may be searched regularly (e.g. for love letters) and the partner may be constantly interrogated or followed.

Also called the Othello syndrome, morbid jealousy, erotic jealousy, sexual jealousy, psychotic jealousy and conjugal paranoia, pathological or delusional jealousy is more common in men.

It should be noted that it may occasionally be true that the partner is being unfaithful, but it is not the truth or otherwise of the delusional belief that is its essential quality; rather it is the fact that it is based on an incorrect inference about external reality that is important.

Pathological jealousy may result from or be associated with the following conditions:

- *organic disorders* and *psychoactive substance use disorders* such as excessive alcohol consumption, cerebral tumours, punch-drunk syndrome, endocrinopathies, dementia, cerebral infection, and the use of amphetamines and cocaine
- *paranoid schizophrenia*
- *depression*
- *neurosis and personality disorder.*

If one of the above conditions is found, then treatment should be directed at the underlying or associated disorder, for example a drinking problem. If no primary cause can be identified, pharmacotherapy with a neuroleptic such as chlorpromazine and/or psychotherapy may be helpful. If there is a risk of violence (including a risk of murder) to the patient's partner, then it may be best to recommend that the couple separate.

Erotomania (de Clérambault's syndrome)

In this relatively rare delusional disorder the patient holds the delusional belief that someone else, usually of a higher social or professional status, or a famous personality or in some other way 'unattainable', is in love with them, and may make repeated attempts to contact that person. The patient may initially believe that because the other person is of a higher status it is not possible to tell the patient explicitly that he or she is loved, and rejections may be seen as actually representing coded messages of love. Eventually, the rejections may lead to animosity and bitterness on the part of the patient.

In hospital and outpatient clinical psychiatry, patients are more likely to be female than male, whereas in forensic psychiatry male patients are more common. Overall, females outnumber males.

Persecutory (querulant) delusions

Persecutory delusions are the most common of the delusional disorders. In these, patients believe they are being persecuted in various ways, for example by being defrauded or plotted against. They often lodge complaints and may engage in legal actions.

Cotard's syndrome

Cotard's syndrome, also called *délire de négation,* is a nihilistic delusional disorder in which the patient believes, for example, that all his wealth has gone, or that relatives or friends no longer exist. It may take a somatic form, with the patient believing that parts of his body do not exist. It can be secondary to very severe depression or to an organic disorder.

Capgras syndrome

Although Capgras syndrome is also called *illusion des sosies*, or illusion of doubles, it is actually not an illusion but a delusional disorder. The essential feature of this rare symptom (it is not strictly speaking a syndrome) is that a person who is familiar to the patient is believed to have been replaced by a double. This disorder is more common in females, with the apparently replaced person often being a relative, such as the husband. Common primary causes are schizophrenia, mood disorder and organic disorder. Derealization commonly occurs.

Case history: Capgras syndrome

A 46-year-old mother complained that her son, who was visiting home during his university holidays, was not actually her son, even though he looked as if he was, but was actually a 'photocopy' of her son. A psychiatrist and the family doctor visited the patient at home and found that her abnormal belief was unshakeable; this delusion was identified as being Capgras syndrome. They also elicited other clinical evidence consistent, in the absence of organic disorder, with a diagnosis of schizophrenia. The patient was admitted against her will to a psychiatric ward. Investigations for organic disorders proved negative and pharmacotherapy with quetiapine (modified release formulation) was commenced. After three weeks the patient no longer suffered from Capgras syndrome and recognized her son as being who he really was.

Fregoli syndrome

In this very rare delusional disorder, the patient believes that a familiar person, who is often believed to be the patient's persecutor, has taken on different appearances. The patient 'recognizes' this person in others who may look completely different from the actual other person. Primary causes include schizophrenia and organic disorder.

Induced psychosis (*folie à deux*)

This rare delusional disorder is shared by two – or, rarely, more than two – people who are closely related emotionally. One has a genuine psychotic disorder and his/her delusional system is induced in the other person, who may be dependent on or less intelligent than the first. When two people are involved this is also referred to as *folie à deux*; when three people are involved it is called *folie à trois*, and so on. Geographical separation of the people involved leads to the recovery of those who are originally psychiatrically well; psychotherapy is also often used in combination with separation.

Schizoaffective disorders

In ICD-10, the term schizoaffective disorders is used to refer to episodic disorders in which both symptoms of a mood (affective) disorder and schizophrenic symptoms are prominent within the same episode of illness, either simultaneously or within a few days of each other. The occurrence of mood-incongruent delusions or hallucinations in mood disorders does not change the diagnosis from that of a mood disorder to schizoaffective disorder.

When schizophrenic and manic symptoms are prominent in the same episode of illness, the disorder is termed *schizoaffective disorder, manic type*. The patient usually makes a full recovery.

In *schizoaffective disorder, depressive type*, schizophrenic and depressive symptoms are prominent in the same episode of illness. The prognosis of this subtype is not as good as that of the manic subtype, with there being a greater chance of patients going on to develop 'negative' symptoms of schizophrenia.

Differential diagnosis

This includes the differential diagnosis of schizophrenia (see above) and of mood disorders (see Chapter 9).

Management

The management of schizoaffective disorders is similar to that of schizophrenia described above, except that antipsychotic medication is used mainly for the treatment of acute schizophrenic symptoms and in the treatment of schizoaffective disorder (manic type), whereas in the case of schizoaffective disorder (depressive type) the treatments for depression described in Chapter 9 (usually starting with antidepressants but possibly requiring ECT in unresponsive cases) are given.

Case history: schizoaffective disorder

A 28-year-old man with no past psychiatric history had been admitted to a psychiatric hospital for the assessment and treatment of a probable depressive illness. Investigations for organic disorders proved negative. The nursing staff and doctors on the ward noticed that he suffered from early morning wakening, loss of appetite (he had lost 10 pounds in weight over the previous eight weeks), anhedonia, poor concentration, prominent guilt feelings, loss of energy and suicidal thoughts. These clinical features would ordinarily have allowed a diagnosis of a depressive episode to be made. However, the patient was also found to be suffering from the following symptoms of schizophrenia: he believed aliens from another planet were trying to control his actions and feelings; he also believed he was being spied on, not just by these aliens but also by agents of a foreign power; and he admitted to experiencing third-person auditory hallucinations, which he believed to originate from the aliens, who discussed him among themselves and commented on his actions. The patient held all these abnormal beliefs with delusional intensity.

He was diagnosed as suffering from schizoaffective disorder, depressive type. Initially he showed some improvement in his schizophrenic symptoms after several days' pharmacotherapy with amisulpride, but after this there was no further improvement in spite of further treatment. The patient was also treated with the tricyclic antidepressant amitriptyline. However, after four weeks there had been no real improvement in his depressive symptoms. In the fifth week of treatment the amitriptyline was stopped and a course of ECT commenced. Most of the depressive and schizophrenic symptoms resolved after a course of eight sessions.

Prognosis

Overall, the prognosis of schizoaffective disorders probably lies between that of mood disorders and schizophrenia.

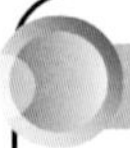

Delusional (paranoid) and schizoaffective disorders

- The core feature of delusional (paranoid) disorders is the development of a delusion or delusional system, which is usually persistent, has no identifiable organic basis and is not secondary to schizophrenia or a mood disorder.
- Point prevalence of delusional disorders
    - ~ 0.03%; lifetime risk
    - = 0.05–0.1%; mean age of onset

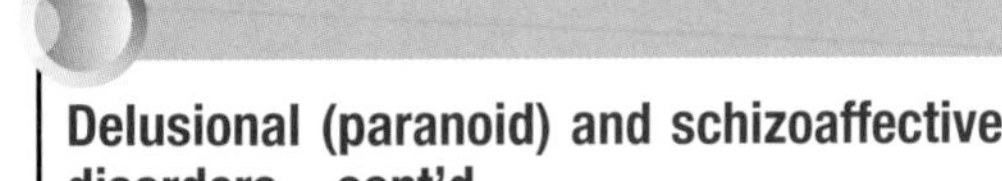

Delusional (paranoid) and schizoaffective disorders—cont'd

- = 40–55 years; f > m.
- Schizoaffective disorders are episodic disorders in which both symptoms of a mood disorder and schizophrenic symptoms are prominent within the same episode of illness either simultaneously or within a few days of each other (ICD-10).
- Antipsychotic drugs are used mainly in treating acute schizophrenic symptoms in schizoaffective disorders and in treating schizoaffective disorder, manic type; antidepressants and/or ECT are used mainly to treat schizoaffective disorder, depressive type.
- The prognosis of schizoaffective disorders probably lies between that of mood disorders and schizophrenia.

Further reading

Frangou, S., Murray, R.M., 2000. Schizophrenia, second ed. Martin Dunitz, London.

Frith, C., Johnstone, E.C., 2003. Schizophrenia: a very short introduction. Oxford University Press, Oxford.

Lawrie, S., Johnstone, E., Weinberger, D. (Eds.), 2004. Schizophrenia: from neuroimaging to neuroscience. Oxford University Press, Oxford.

Mortimer, A.M., McKenna, P., 2010. Therapeutic strategies in schizophrenia. Clinical publishing.

Mood disorders, suicide and parasuicide

Introduction

As discussed in Chapter 5, the terms *affect* and *mood* have different meanings, although both refer to emotional states. Definitions based on the DSM are:

- *Affect*. A pattern of observable behaviours that is the expression of a subjectively experienced feeling state (emotion). Common examples of affect are euphoria, anger and sadness. Affect is variable over time, in response to changing emotional states.
- *Mood*. A pervasive and sustained emotion that colours the person's perception of the world. Common examples of mood include depression, elation and anxiety.

The disorders of mood discussed in this chapter are depressive episodes, bipolar disorder and persistent mood disorders. Schizoaffective disorders are discussed in Chapter 8, whereas anxiety disorders, which can be considered to be disorders of emotion, are described in Chapter 10. Table 9.1 gives the ICD-10 classification of the mood disorders.

In the past, disorders of mood were often referred to as affective disorders; in this book the more correct term mood disorders is used. ICD-10 uses the term bipolar affective disorder, whereas a more correct term would be bipolar mood disorder; in order to avoid confusion, the term bipolar disorder is used here.

Suicide and parasuicide (deliberate self-harm) are also considered in this chapter. It should be remembered, however, that they can be associated with psychiatric disorders other than mood disorders, for example schizophrenia.

Depressive episode

Clinical features

In depressive episodes there is depression of mood and:

- loss of interest and enjoyment (known as anhedonia)
- reduced energy, which, in turn, causes tiredness and reduced activity
- reduced attention and concentration
- ideas of guilt and worthlessness
- lowered self-esteem.

These, in turn, can lead to hopelessness and a belief that life is not worth living. As a result, suicidal thoughts may occur.

Depressive episodes frequently cause somatic or physiological changes. These are known as *biological symptoms* of depression and are summarized in Table 9.2. *Reduced appetite* leads to *weight loss*, which is often taken as meaning a loss of at least 5% of body weight in a month. *Constipation* is also a common feature of depressive episodes. Compared with normal sleep (Figure 9.1), the following types of *insomnia* may occur:

- initial insomnia – difficulty getting off to sleep
- broken sleep
- waking in the morning at least two hours before the usual time, known as early morning wakening or terminal insomnia.

Patients often wake up feeling very depressed and possibly suicidal, with the mood gradually lifting

Table 9.1 ICD 10 classification of mood (affective) disorders
F30 Manic episode
F30.0 Hypomania F30.1 Mania without psychotic symptoms F30.2 Mania with psychotic symptoms F30.8 Other manic episodes F30.9 Manic episode, unspecified
F31 Bipolar affective disorder
F31.0 Bipolar affective disorder, current episode hypomanic F31.1 Bipolar affective disorder, current episode manic without psychotic symptoms F31.2 Bipolar affective disorder, current episode manic with psychotic symptoms F31.3 Bipolar affective disorder, current episode mild or moderate depression .30 Without somatic symptoms .31 With somatic symptoms F31.4 Bipolar affective disorder, current episode severe depression without psychotic symptoms F31.5 Bipolar affective disorder, current episode severe depression with psychotic symptoms F31.6 Bipolar affective disorder, current episode mixed F31.7 Bipolar affective disorder, currently in remission F31.8 Other bipolar affective disorders F31.9 Bipolar affective disorder, unspecified
F32 Depressive episode
F32.0 Mild depressive episode .00 Without somatic symptoms .01 With somatic symptoms F32.1 Moderate depressive episode .10 Without somatic symptoms .11 With somatic symptoms F32.2 Severe depressive episode without psychotic symptoms F32.3 Severe depressive episode with psychotic symptoms F32.8 Other depressive episodes F32.9 Depressive episode, unspecified
F33 Recurrent depressive disorder
F33.0 Recurrent depressive disorder, current episode mild .00 Without somatic symptoms .01 With somatic symptoms F33.1 Recurrent depressive disorder, current episode moderate .10 Without somatic symptoms .11 With somatic symptoms F33.2 Recurrent depressive disorder, current episode severe without psychotic symptoms F33.3 Recurrent depressive disorder, current episode severe with psychotic symptoms F33.4 Recurrent depressive disorder, currently in remission F33.8 Other recurrent depressive disorders F33.9 Recurrent depressive disorder, unspecified
F34 Persistent mood (affective) disorders
F34.0 Cyclothymia F34.1 Dysthymia F34.8 Other persistent mood (affective) disorders F34.9 Persistent mood (affective) disorder, unspecified

Continued

Table 9.1 ICD 10 classification of mood (affective) disorders—cont'd

F38 Other mood (affective) disorders
F38.0 Other single mood (affective) disorders .00 Mixed affective episode F38.1 Other recurrent mood (affective) disorders .10 Recurrent brief depressive disorder F38.8 Other specified mood (affective) disorders
F39 Unspecified mood (affective) disorder

Table 9.2 Biological symptoms of depression
Reduced appetite
Reduced weight
Constipation
Early morning wakening (terminal insomnia)
Diurnal variation of mood
Reduced libido
Amenorrhoea

during the day until it reaches its best in the evening; this diurnal cycle may repeat itself day after day and is called *diurnal variation of mood*. There is usually a markedly *reduced libido* and, in women who normally menstruate, *amenorrhoea* may occur.

Mental state examination

Appearance (Figure 9.2). Depressive facies typically include downturned eyes, sagging of the corners of the mouth and, often, the presence of a vertical furrow between the eyebrows. The patient usually makes poor eye contact with the interviewer. There may be direct

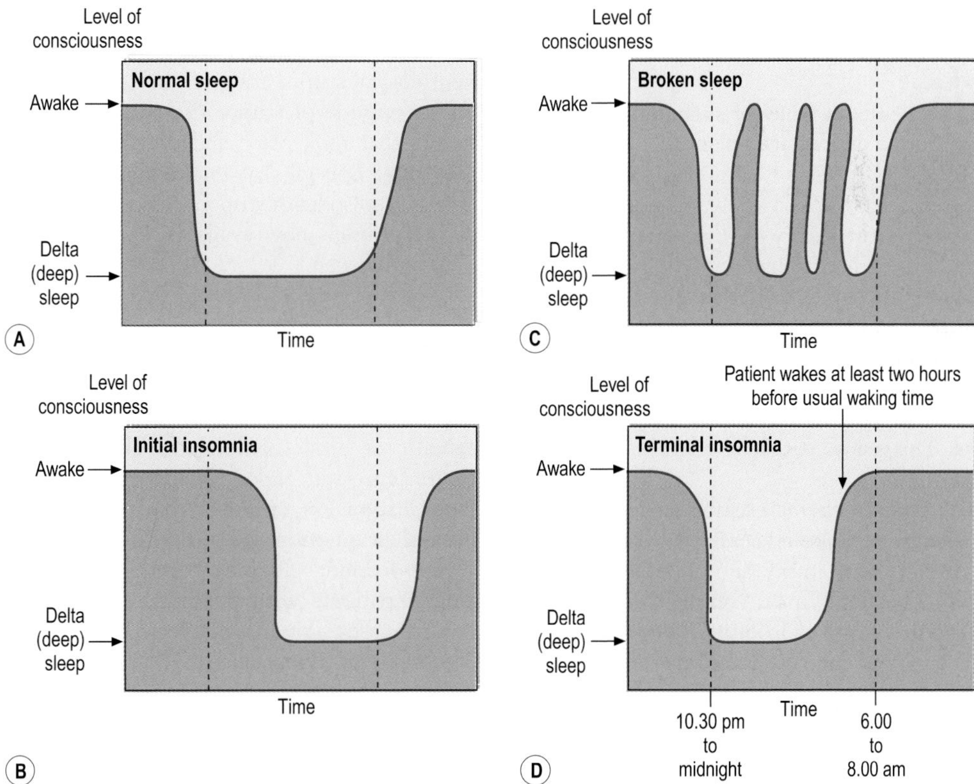

Figure 9.1 • Types of sleep disturbance in depressive episodes. • (a) Normal sleep. (b) Initial insomnia. (c) Broken sleep. (d) Early morning wakening or terminal insomnia.

• Downturned eyes
• Poor eye contact
• Expressionless, frown
• 'Knitted' brow
• Weight loss/emaciation (baggy clothes)
• Unkempt appearance
• Dirty clothes
• Poor personal hygiene
• Slow speech

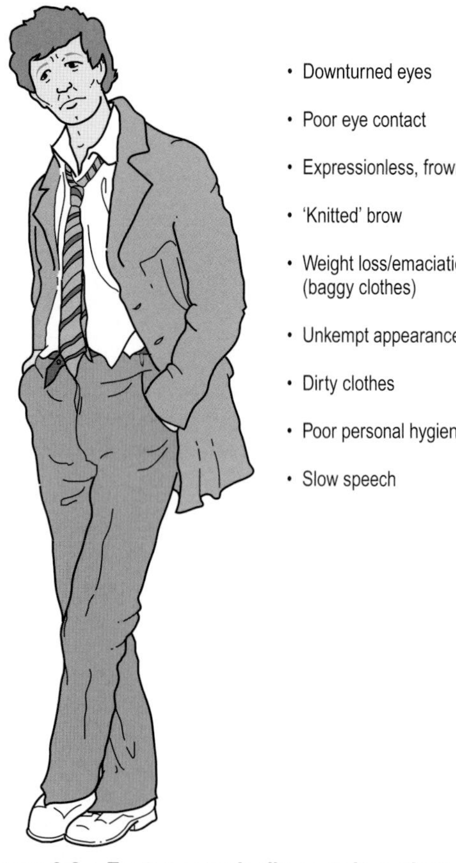

Figure 9.2 • Features typically seen in patients suffering from a depressive episode.

evidence of weight loss, with the patient appearing emaciated and perhaps dehydrated. Indirect evidence of recent weight loss may be clothes appearing to be too large. Evidence of poor self-care and general neglect may include an unkempt appearance, poor personal hygiene and dirty clothing.

Behaviour. Psychomotor retardation typically occurs.

Speech. This is slow, with long delays before answering questions.

Mood. This is characteristically low and sad, with feelings of hopelessness; the future seems bleak. Anxiety, irritability and agitation may also occur. The patient may complain of reduced energy and drive, and an inability to feel enjoyment. There is a loss of interest in normal activities and hobbies.

Thoughts. Pessimistic thoughts concerning the patient's past, present and future occur. For example, minor misdemeanours in the past, such as taking home an office pencil many years ago, may be exaggerated out of all proportion and used as 'proof' that the patient is evil and undeserving of current status in life. The patient may suffer from delusions of poverty or illness. Suicidal thoughts may occur and should be ascertained. Homicidal thoughts may also be present. For example, a depressed mother may decide the future is equally bleak for her children and plan to kill them before committing suicide. Similarly, an elderly depressed man may persuade his wife to enter into a suicide pact.

Perceptions. In severe depressive episodes mood-congruent auditory hallucinations may occur. They are typically second person and derogatory in content. For example, the depressed patient may hear sentences such as 'You are an evil, sinful man'; 'You should die'.

Cognition. Poor concentration may lead the patient to think (mistakenly) that memory is also impaired. In elderly patients the presentation of depression may be very similar to that of dementia; this is known as (depressive) pseudodementia (see Chapter 20).

Depressive stupor

The patient exhibits features of stupor, being unresponsive, akinetic, mute and fully conscious. (Details of the differences between depressive stupor and neurological stupor are given in Chapter 5.) Following an episode of stupor the patient can recall the events that took place and the depressed mood at the time. Episodes of excitement may take place between episodes of stupor. Owing to effective treatment regimens now available, depressive stupor is only rarely seen.

Masked depression

Depressed patients may not always present with a depressed mood, but may instead present with somatic or other complaints. They may somatize their depressed mood owing to cultural factors (see Chapter 19), or indeed may not be able to articulate their emotions, as in the case of patients with severe learning disability (see Chapter 17) and elderly patients with dementia (see Chapter 20). In such cases, the presence of biological symptoms of depression is particularly helpful in making the diagnosis. In the case of learning disability, diurnal variation in abnormal behaviour may be observed and mirror diurnal variation in mood. The effective treatment of masked depression usually leads to a resolution of the somatic or other presentations.

Seasonal affective disorder (SAD)

In SAD there is a regular temporal relationship between the onset of depressive episodes and a particular time or season of the year. This often takes the form of untreated depressive episodes, commencing in the autumn or winter months and ending in the spring or summer months as the hours of daylight increase in each 24-hour cycle. The onset of bipolar disorders may also be seasonal. During depressive episodes, patients with SAD often exhibit carbohydrate craving, hypersomnia and weight gain; in these they differ from symptoms more typical of depression.

Cases in which there is a clearly distinguished seasonal psychosocial stressor, such as becoming depressed each winter because of regular winter unemployment, are excluded from the category of SAD.

Other types of depression

Agitated depression can occur in the elderly and is considered in Chapter 20. Neurotic depression or dysthymia is considered below. Another neurotic disorder, known as mixed anxiety and depressive disorder or anxiety depression, in which both anxiety and depressed mood are present but neither is clearly prominent, is considered in Chapter 10.

Investigations

The investigations carried out in a patient presenting for the first time with depressive symptomatology are those described in Chapter 5, and include:

- further information
- urea and electrolytes, full blood count, thyroid function tests, liver function tests
- a screen for illicit drugs, if psychoactive substance use is suspected as a cause
- vitamin B_{12} and folate levels
- syphilitic serology
- electroencephalography (EEG) and/or computed tomography (CT)/magnetic resonance imaging (MRI) brain scan (if clinically justified).

In the case of first presentation with auditory hallucinations in the elderly, i.e. when a differential diagnosis being considered is paraphrenia (see Chapter 20), tests of hearing and vision should be carried out at an early stage, as sensory deprivation is an important cause in this age group.

The physical examination should include a careful inspection for any evidence of self-harm, such as scars on the wrists.

Differential diagnosis

Organic disorders and *psychoactive substance use disorders* should be excluded before making a diagnosis of a depressive episode. These are described in Chapters 6 and 7. A full physical examination and appropriate further investigations (see above) should be carried out, particularly in a case of first presentation, to exclude such disorders.

Negative symptoms and the early stages of simple *schizophrenia* may be difficult to distinguish from depression. In such cases other symptoms of depression, such as the biological symptoms, should be carefully investigated. Moreover, depression may itself be a symptom of schizophrenia, both in the acute phase and following an episode of schizophrenic illness (*post-schizophrenic depression*).

Epidemiology

Depressive episodes are more common in females. The *incidence* of depressive episodes is between 80 and 200 new cases per 100 000 of the population per year in men, and between 250 and 7800 new cases per 100 000 of the population per year in women. The *point prevalence* in Western countries is between 1.8 and 3.2% for men and between 2.0 and 9.3% for women. The point prevalence of depressive *symptoms* is much higher, at up to 20%. The *lifetime risk* in the general population of Western countries is 5–12% in men and 9–26% in women.

The average *age of onset* is around the late 30s, but it can start at any age from childhood onwards. It has a higher incidence in those who are not married, including those who are divorced or separated.

Depressive episodes have also been found to be more common in working-class women than in women from the middle classes. They may also be more common in women who:

- have three or more children under the age of 14 to look after
- do not work outside the home
- do not have somebody to confide in, i.e. there is a lack of intimacy
- lost their own mother before the age of 11, through death or separation.

Aetiology

The aetiology of depressive episodes is considered in the section on bipolar disorder.

The reasons for the increased prevalence of depressive episodes in women compared with men are not known, but the following possibilities have been suggested (see also Chapter 12):

- Women may be more likely to admit to feeling depressed.
- Depression may be underdiagnosed in men, who may be more likely to engage in excessive alcohol consumption as a result of depression and therefore be diagnosed as suffering from psychoactive substance use disorder instead.
- Women may suffer from greater stresses, such as childbirth and hormonal effects (menarche, premenstrual syndrome and menopause).

Management

Hospitalization

Less severe depressive episodes can be treated by GPs in the community or by psychiatrists in outpatient clinics. However, patients suffering from severe episodes should be admitted to hospital. This may need to be compulsory if severe life-threatening features are present, such as a risk of *suicide* or *poor intake of food and fluids*.

Physical treatments

Pharmacotherapy. The mainstay of physical treatment is *antidepressant medication*. As detailed in Chapter 3, there are now available many antidepressants which are relatively safe in overdose, such as those belonging to the selective serotonin reuptake inhibitor (SSRI), serotonin–noradrenaline reuptake inhibitor (SNRI), noradrenaline reuptake inhibitor (NARI), reversible inhibitor of monoamine oxidase A (RIMA) and noradrenergic and specific serotonergic antidepressant (NaSSA) groups. (There is some evidence that many antidepressants may actually be only marginally more effective than placebos in treating depression. The reader is referred to the excellent book by Professor Irving Kirsch (see Further reading). It may not be a good idea to mention this in psychiatry examinations though.) Certain antidepressants, particularly SSRIs, may actually *increase* the risk of suicide. The 58th edition (2009) of the British National Formulary (BNF) warns: 'The use of antidepressants has been linked with suicidal thoughts and behaviour; children, young adults, and patients with a history of suicidal behaviour are particularly at risk. Where necessary, patients should be monitored for suicidal behaviour, self-harm, or hostility, particularly at the beginning of treatment or if the dose is changed.'

Electroconvulsive therapy (ECT). In the following relatively uncommon circumstances, ECT may be considered as a first-line treatment:

- life-threatening illness resulting from refusal of food or fluids
- attempted suicide
- a dangerously high risk of suicide, with strong ideas/plans.

It may be considered in severe depression associated with:

- stupor
- severe psychomotor retardation
- depressive delusions/hallucinations

Psychosurgery. In extremely rare cases, when all other treatments have failed, the extreme option of psychosurgery may be considered in severe chronic handicapping depression.

Phototherapy. For those patients suffering from SAD in whom the onset of depression is in the autumn or winter months, treatment with high-intensity light is possible.

Psychosocial treatments

Cognitive behavioural therapy (CBT). CBT has been found to be effective for mild to moderate depression. Unlike antidepressants, it clearly does not have any drug-related side-effects. Therefore, where eadily available, CBT should be considered as a first choice treatment in non-severe cases of depression. If a practitioner is not available, then CBT can be delivered in a self-help format, such as:

- bibliotherapy – written books
- workbooks
- computerized CBT (CCBT) – free packages include www.livinglifetothefull.com and www.moodgym.anu.edu.au/welcome.

Other psychotherapies. A number of other different types of psychotherapy are available for mildly or moderately depressed patients or for patients who have recovered from severe depressive episodes. These include: group therapy; psychoanalytic psychotherapy; and, in the case of family or marital difficulties, family therapy and marital therapy. All can be used in combination with pharmacotherapy.

Increased activity and social contact. It is important not to allow depressed patients to withdraw totally from work and social activities. Instead, they should be encouraged gradually to increase such activities. Meeting other people and developing confiding relationships has a protective function in preventing relapse. *Occupational therapy* can be useful in enabling depressed inpatients to learn to cope with life skills such as cooking.

Prognosis

The outcome of depressive episodes varies, but, in general, is better the greater the length of follow-up. The risk of relapse is reduced if antidepressant medication is continued for six months after the end of the depressive episode. Overall, there is a suicide rate of around 9%.

Case history: depressive episode

A 39-year-old married ex-nurse was referred by her GP to a psychiatric outpatient clinic with a six-month history of depressed mood. She was a slim woman of medium height who had been suffering from tearfulness, lack of energy, anhedonia, reduced appetite and a moderate degree of weight loss. She was suffering from initial insomnia of one to two hours but there was no early morning wakening. During the past six months she had not had sexual intercourse with her husband owing to her very low libido. She had also noticed that her menstrual cycle, which was normally regular, had stopped three months ago. Prior to referral, her physical condition had been extensively investigated by an endocrinologist and all tests had proved negative. Although the patient was suffering from depressed mood, she denied having suicidal thoughts. Her husband confirmed that she had never seriously considered suicide.

A diagnosis of a depressive episode was made and it was decided to treat her as an outpatient with a course of an SSRI. The potential side-effects were carefully explained to her, and in particular it was emphasized that she should endeavour to continue with the medication even if she suffered from nausea and/or vomiting early in the treatment. Within eight weeks almost all the depressive symptoms had resolved and the patient was able to cope with everyday activities again. Her relationship with her husband, including their sex life, was also improving and her menstrual periods had returned. She continued to be followed up in the psychiatric outpatient department and was continued on the course of the SSRI for a further six months.

Depressive episode

- The biological symptoms of depression include reduced appetite, reduced weight, constipation, sleep disturbance (e.g. early morning wakening), diurnal variation of mood, reduced libido and amenorrhoea.
- Other symptoms include depressed mood, anhedonia, reduced energy, tiredness, reduced activity, low attention and concentration, ideas of guilt and worthlessness, low self-esteem and suicidal thoughts.
- Other types of depression include depressive stupor, masked depression, SAD, agitated depression and neurotic depression (dysthymia).
- The differential diagnosis of a depressive episode includes organic disorders and psychoactive substance use disorders, and schizophrenia (negative symptoms and post-schizophrenic depression).
- The mean age of onset is in the late 30s and the condition is more common in women than in men.
- Mild to moderate depression responds well to CBT. If a practitioner is not available, then a self-help format might be considered.
- Those suffering from severe episodes should be treated as inpatients, particularly if there is a risk to life (suicide risk and/or low food and fluid intake); less severe episodes can be treated by GPs or psychiatrists in the community.
- The mainstay of treatment for severe episodes is antidepressant medication.
- ECT can be used in resistant depression.
- The risk of relapse is reduced if antidepressants are continued for six months after the end of the episode.

Bipolar disorder

Terminology

In DSM-IV-TR, the essential feature of bipolar disorder is the occurrence of at least one episode of mania, usually, but not necessarily, accompanied by at least one depressive episode. Thus, by definition, any previously well person suffering from a first episode of mania (or hypomania) would be classed as suffering from bipolar disorder. On the other hand, if a previously well person suffered from one or more depressive episodes, a diagnosis of bipolar disorder would not be made unless and until the first episode of mania occurred.

In ICD-10, the definition of bipolar disorder is slightly different, in that there must be a history of at least two episodes of mood disturbance, at least one of which should have been mania (or hypomania). The similarities and differences between the two classification systems are illustrated in Figure 9.3.

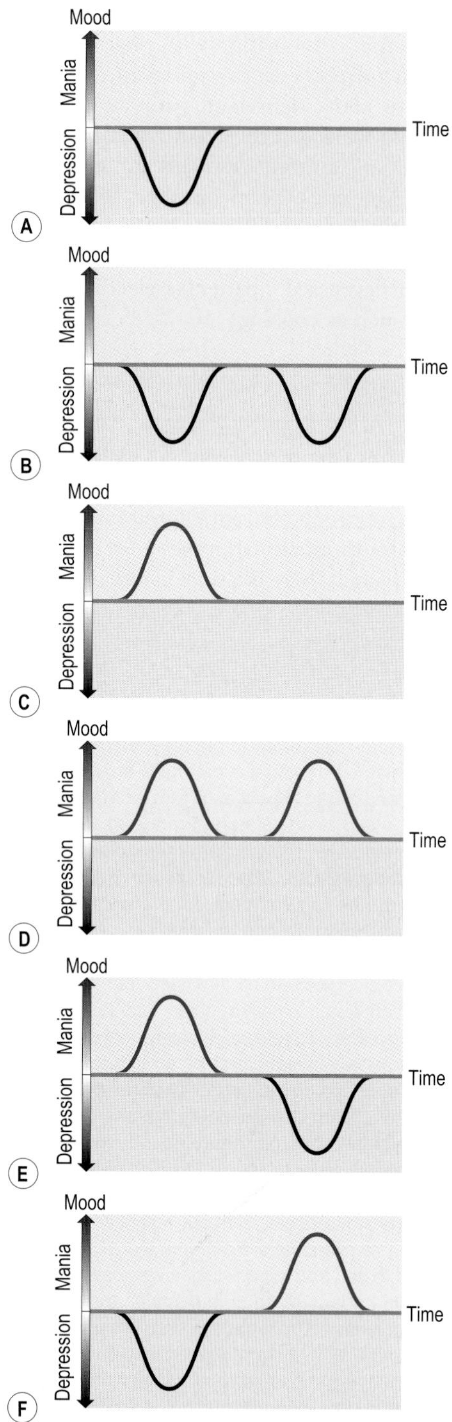

Figure 9.3 • Terminology. • (a) Depressive episode; (b) recurrent depressive episodes; (c) bipolar disorder in DSM-IV-TR, manic episode in ICD-10; (d) to (f) bipolar disorder in both DSM-IV-TR and ICD-10.

Clinical features

In mania there is elevation of mood, increased energy, overactivity, pressure of speech, reduced sleep, loss of normal social and sexual inhibitions, and poor attention and concentration. The elevated mood may manifest itself as elation, but sometimes patients can be irritable and angry instead.

During a manic episode a patient may overspend, start unrealistic projects, be sexually promiscuous and, if irritable or angry, be inappropriately aggressive.

In severe mania there may be severe and sustained physical activity and excitement that may result in aggression or violence. Neglect of eating, drinking and personal hygiene may result in dangerous states of dehydration and self-neglect.

Mental state examination

Appearance. The patient may be flamboyantly dressed in colours that are unusually bright for him or her. In severe cases the patient may show signs of self-neglect, such as appearing unkempt and dehydrated.

Behaviour. Overactivity is a characteristic feature, and it may prove difficult to persuade the patient to sit still and be interviewed for even a few minutes. (In less severe cases the patient is likely to eat and drink greedily whatever is desired.)

Speech. There is pressure of speech, in which the speech is increased in rate and amount and is difficult to interrupt.

Mood. The patient may be euphoric, or else irritable and angry.

Thoughts. The patient has an inflated view of his or her importance and there may be expansive and grandiose ideas about the significance of personal opinions and work. Flight of ideas is common in severe mania, with the stream of accelerated thoughts showing abrupt changes of topic and no central direction; the connections between thoughts may be based on:

- chance relationships
- verbal associations, such as alliteration (in which successive words start with the same letter, for example 'Crazy cool cat cannot catch cabbages…')

- clang associations (e.g. 'The cat sat on the mat and that's that')
- distracting stimuli.

In severe mania there may be additional delusions and hallucinations (see below); this is classified in ICD-10 as *mania with psychotic symptoms*:

> Inflated self-esteem and grandiose ideas may develop into delusions, and irritability and suspiciousness into delusions of persecution. In severe cases, grandiose or religious delusions of identity or role may be prominent, and flight of ideas and pressure of speech may result in the individual becoming incomprehensible.... If required, delusions ... can be specified as congruent or incongruent with the mood. 'Incongruent' should be taken as including affectively neutral delusions ... for example, delusions of reference with no guilty or accusatory content.

Perceptions. Perceptual abnormalities, according to ICD-10, include 'the appreciation of colours as especially vivid (and usually beautiful), a preoccupation with fine details of surfaces or textures, and subjective hyperacusis' (an increased sensitivity to sounds). In severe mania, hallucinations may occur, which may be auditory, for example confirming the patient's grandiose delusions ('You are the most important person in the world') or visual (seeing oneself seated on a throne, or in a scene laden with religious motifs). As with delusions, the hallucinations may be mood congruent or incongruent. Incongruent delusions include affectively neutral hallucinations, such as hearing voices speaking about events that have no special emotional significance.

Cognition. Attention and concentration are poor.

Insight. Insight is absent during the manic episode. Realization of this behaviour while 'high' can subsequently tip the patient into depression.

Subtypes of mania

Hypomania

According to ICD-10:

> Hypomania is a lesser degree of mania, in which abnormalities of mood and behaviour are too persistent and marked to be included under cyclothymia [see below] but are not accompanied by hallucinations or delusions. There is a persistent mild elevation of mood..., increased energy and activity, and usually marked feelings of wellbeing and both physical and mental efficiency. Increased sociability, talkativeness, overfamiliarity, increased sexual energy, and a decreased need for sleep are often present but (unlike mania) not to the extent that they lead to severe disruption of work or result in social rejection. Irritability, conceit, and boorish behaviour may take the place of the more usual euphoric sociability.

Attention and concentration may be reduced, although not to the same extent as in mania.

Mania without psychotic symptoms

In this ICD-10 subtype, the clinical features of mania, excluding delusions and hallucinations, occur.

Mania with psychotic symptoms

In this ICD-10 subtype, delusions and hallucinations occur in addition to the other clinical features of mania already described. As mentioned in Chapter 8, Schneider's first-rank symptoms can occur in mania: they have been reported in 8–23% of cases.

Manic stupor

In this condition the patient is unresponsive, akinetic, mute and fully conscious. The facies indicate elation, and on recovery the patient remembers experiencing the flight of ideas typical of mania. Owing to effective pharmacotherapy with neuroleptics (see below), manic stupor is only rarely seen where these drugs are available.

Investigations

The investigations carried out in a patient presenting for the first time with manic symptomatology are those described in Chapter 5.

Differential diagnosis

Organic disorders and *psychoactive substance use disorders* should be excluded before making a diagnosis of mania. These are described in Chapters 6 and 7. For example, increased activity and restlessness (and often loss of weight) may also occur in hyperthyroidism and anorexia nervosa. A full physical examination and appropriate further investigations should be carried out.

Schizophrenia may present with similar symptoms to mania (see Chapter 8). Diagnostic guidelines in ICD-10 note that:

> One of the commonest problems is differentiation (of mania with psychotic symptoms) from schizophrenia, particularly if the stages of development through hypomania have been missed and the patient is seen only

> at the height of the illness when widespread delusions, incomprehensible speech, and violent excitement may obscure the basic disturbance of (mood). Patients with mania that is responding to neuroleptic medication may present a similar diagnostic problem at the stage when they have returned to normal levels of physical and mental activity but still have delusions or hallucinations ... (If) hallucinations and delusions are prominent and persistent, the diagnosis of schizoaffective disorder (may be) appropriate.

In *agitated depression* in the elderly (see Chapter 20) the early stages may present in a similar way to the irritability of hypomania. In severe *obsessive–compulsive disorder* patients may stay up at night in order to perform household rituals. However, in this case the affect is not likely to be one of elation (see Chapter 10). Hypomania, with its associated increase in irritability, disinhibited behaviour and increased sexual drive, may present as *dyssocial personality disorder* (see Chapter 15), especially when mild and chronic.

Epidemiology

Males and females are affected equally. The *point prevalence* of bipolar disorder in Western countries (based mainly on US studies) is between 0.4 and 1% in the general population. The *lifetime risk* in the general population of Western countries is 0.6–1.1%.

The average *age of onset* is around the mid-20s. It should be noted, however, that this disorder can start for the first time in old age. When occurring in adolescence, it may be mistaken for schizophrenia (although recent research shows that the accuracy of diagnosis of the first-episode is as good in adolescence as in adulthood).

Bipolar disorders have been found to be more common in the upper social classes.

Aetiology

This subsection considers the aetiology of both bipolar disorders and depressive episodes together. Predisposing factors include genetic factors and personality. Precipitating factors include psychosocial stresses and physical illness. Perpetuating and mediating factors include:

- psychological factors
- social factors
- neurotransmitters
- psychoneuroendocrinological factors
- water and electrolyte changes
- sleep changes
- photic changes.

Genetics

Family studies have shown that the lifetime risks for developing a mood disorder are much greater in biological relatives of patients (probands) than in the general population. When mood disorders are divided into bipolar disorder (in which at least one episode of mania has occurred) and unipolar disorder (in which only depressive episodes have occurred) then, in general, family studies demonstrate increased lifetime risks of both bipolar and unipolar disorder for the first-degree relatives of patients with bipolar disorder, but an increased lifetime risk of only unipolar disorder in the first-degree relatives of patients with unipolar disorder. This is illustrated in Table 9.3.

Twin studies also provide support for the presence of an important genetic component in mood disorders. For depression, the monozygotic to dizygotic concordance rate ratio is around 40–50% to 20–25%. It is even higher for bipolar disorder. As with family study results, this supports the hypothesis that there may be a greater genetic contribution in bipolar disorder than in unipolar disorder.

Table 9.3 Approximate lifetime risks for the development of unipolar and bipolar mood disorder in first-degree relatives of patients (probands) with such disorders

	Lifetime expectancy rate to the nearest percentage point	
Proband type	Bipolar disorder	Unipolar disorder
Bipolar disorder	8	11
Unipolar disorder	1	9

Adoption studies in general also support the hypothesis of an important genetic component. In an adoption study published in 1977 on 29 adoptees with a history of bipolar disorder, it was found that 28% of the biological parents suffered from a mood disorder, compared with 12% of the adoptive parents. By comparison, 26% of the biological parents of 31 bipolar non-adoptees were also found to suffer from a mood disorder.

Studies in *molecular genetics* are being carried out in order to characterize causative genes.

Personality

Cyclothymic or *cycloid personality disorder* (see Chapter 15 and the section on persistent mood disorders below) is characterized by persistent instability of mood, with numerous periods of mild depression and mild elation. It may predispose to bipolar disorder.

Psychosocial stressors

The notion of a triggering effect in depression considers that recent *life events* (see Chapter 3) may act as precipitating factors. In support of this hypothesis, it has been shown that excess life events occur in the six months before a depressive episode starts. Predisposing life events have also been postulated as occurring. As mentioned above, depressive episodes are more common in working-class women. These have been termed *vulnerability factors*, and they have not been successfully replicated in all studies. It has been suggested that they operate by reducing self-esteem.

Physical illness

Many physical illnesses are accompanied or followed by depressed mood. The association of mood disorders with childbirth is considered in Chapter 12.

Psychological factors

In experiments involving mammals repeatedly subjected to unavoidable aversive stimuli, the animal learns that there is no behaviour that will allow it to avoid such stimuli and it may then move very little and look and act in a helpless manner, for example by curling up in a corner of its cage. Such *learned helplessness* may then become generalized to other circumstances, and it has been suggested that some of its features, such as reduced voluntary movement and a belief that one has no control over the environment, occur in cases of depression.

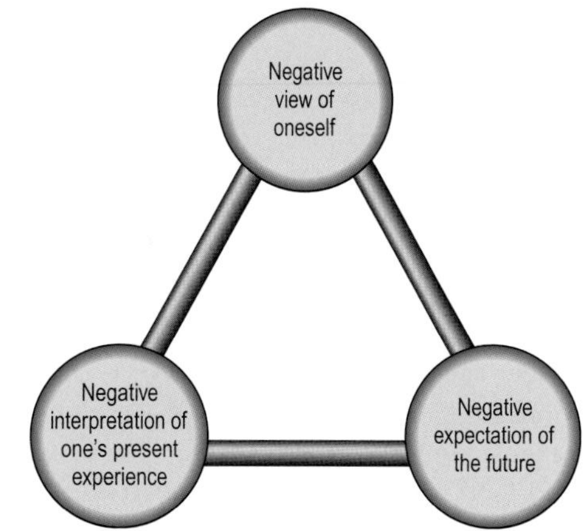

Figure 9.4 • Cognitive triad occurring in depressive episodes.

According to *cognitive theory*, in depression cognitive dysfunction takes place, manifested in the following ways (Figure 9.4):

- irrational automatic intrusive thoughts
- inflexible primary assumptions concerning the patient and his or her relationship with other people
- cognitive distortions, which include arbitrary inference, selective abstraction, overgeneralization, dichotomous thinking, magnification and minimization.

Social factors

As mentioned above, a lack of a *confiding relationship* is a vulnerability factor so far as depression in women is concerned.

As with schizophrenia (see Chapter 8), a high *expressed emotion* at home is associated with an increased risk of relapse of depression.

Neurotransmitters

The *monoamine hypothesis of mood disorders* has undergone a number of changes from the original, which stated that depression was associated with a depletion of central functional noradrenaline and that mania was associated with an excess. It is now emphasizes the role of serotonin, rather than just noradrenaline. Evidence in favour of this includes:

- Tricyclic antidepressants act as monoamine reuptake inhibitors. They inhibit the reuptake of noradrenaline and serotonin by presynaptic neurones, so leading to an increase in the availability of these monoamines in the synaptic cleft.

- MAOIs also increase the availability of monoamines by inhibiting their metabolic degradation by monoamine oxidase. They also act as antidepressants.
- SSRIs increase the availability of serotonin. They also act as antidepressants.
- The use of tricyclic antidepressants in bipolar disorder can precipitate mania.
- Amphetamine is structurally similar to the catecholamines and releases them from neurones. It is a CNS stimulant that lifts mood.
- Reserpine, an antihypertensive drug derived from the Indian plant *Rauwolfia*, depletes central monoaminergic neuronal stores of catecholamines and serotonin. In accordance with the monoamine hypothesis, its use can lead to severe depression and suicide.
- The CSF level of the serotonin metabolite 5-hydroxyindoleacetic acid (5-HIAA) is often reported as being reduced in depressed patients.

Evidence against the monoamine hypothesis includes:

- Pharmacotherapy with antidepressants takes at least two weeks to cause antidepressant effects clinically. This is much greater than the relatively rapid onset of biochemical action.
- Not all drugs that act as monoamine reuptake inhibitors have a therapeutic antidepressant action. One such example is cocaine.

Psychoneuroendocrinological factors

As mentioned in Chapter 6, mood disorders are associated with a number of endocrinopathies, such as Cushing's syndrome, Addison's disease and thyroid disorders. Disturbances of the hypothalamic–pituitary–adrenal axis have been reported in depression. The thyroid system may also be implicated, and the hypothalamic–growth hormone axis is also being considered by researchers.

Water and electrolyte changes

It has been reported that there are increases in the body's *residual sodium* (an index of intracellular sodium ion concentration) in both depression and mania. This may be related to the prophylactic action of lithium ions in bipolar disorder. Further studies have indicated that the erythrocyte sodium ion concentration decreases following recovery from depression or mania as a result of increased sodium–potassium ATPase activity.

Sleep changes

The interval between the onset of sleep and the onset of the first episode of rapid eye movement (REM) sleep is called the *REM latency*. In depressed patients this is shortened. The changes in the architecture of sleep may be related to the circadian rhythm changes mentioned above. One of the biological symptoms of depression is early morning wakening, which again is probably related to circadian rhythm changes.

Photic changes

Modulation of the rhythmic secretion of melatonin by the pineal gland is believed to be the means by which changes in the photoperiod lead to changes in circadian and seasonal physiological rhythms. The biosynthesis of melatonin from its precursor serotonin occurs via *N*-acetylation followed by O-methylation. The step involving serotonin *N*-acetyltransferase is probably rate-limiting and is stimulated at night. The suprachiasmatic nucleus of the hypothalamus acts as a biological clock and probably acts as the endogenous pacemaker for this nocturnal biosynthesis. Compared to normal subjects, patients with SAD have been found to have an increased sensitivity of melatonin biosynthesis to inhibition by phototherapy.

Management

Hospitalization

It is almost always best to admit a patient suffering from mania (or hypomania) as a psychiatric inpatient. Despite the patient protesting a willingness to take medication in the community, the lack of insight that occurs in this disorder, together with the feeling of well-being that often accompanies it, is very likely to lead to non-compliance and a risk of the mania worsening. As mentioned above, severe mania can lead to a dangerous level of self-neglect and dehydration. In the case of a first episode, the patient's relatives will need to have the nature of the condition and the need for admission carefully explained; relatives of previous sufferers are usually very pleased for admission to take place, having witnessed its social and medical effects.

Physical treatments

Pharmacotherapy. The mainstay of treatment is a *mood-stabilizing drug* (lithium or carbamazepine) plus an *antipsychotic (neuroleptic) drug* (see Chapter 3).

Lithium compounds (lithium carbonate and lithium citrate) are commonly used mood-stabilizing drugs. They are used in the prophylaxis of mania and, therefore, of bipolar disorder. Lithium salts can also be used in the treatment of acute mania, but patients generally take at least a week to respond, so that antipsychotic drugs are preferred. Lithium has a low therapeutic ratio and therefore regular plasma level monitoring is essential. By adjusting the dose, its plasma concentration is kept between 0.4 and 1.0 mmol l^{-1} (measured 12 hours after the preceding, usually bedtime, dose). Lithium and sodium cations compete for proximal tubular reabsorption and therefore lithium retention can be caused by sodium deficiency and sodium diuresis. Contraindications to the use of lithium include:

- renal insufficiency
- cardiovascular insufficiency
- Addison's disease
- untreated hypothyroidism.

The side-effects of lithium vary according to the plasma concentration and are shown in Figure 9.5. Other side-effects are mentioned in Chapter 3.

In addition to monitoring the plasma lithium level, other tests that should be carried out regularly include the urea and electrolytes and the thyroid function tests.

In cases of bipolar disorder resistant to lithium, alternative mood-stabilizing prophylactic treatment with *carbamazepine* can be tried. Again, the plasma level must be monitored regularly.

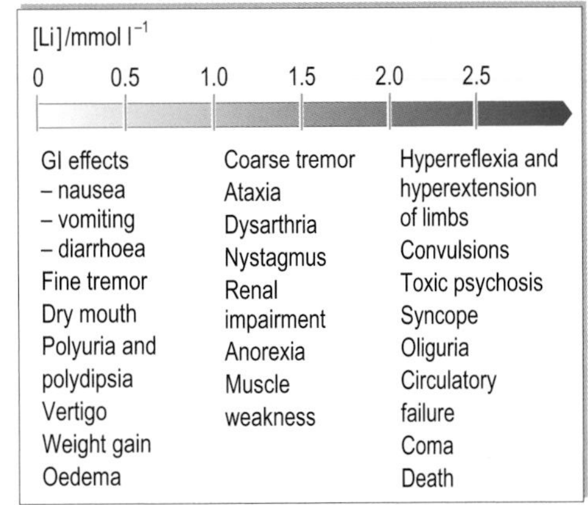

Figure 9.5 • Side-effects of lithium according to lithium level.

ECT. This is considered if the patient is suffering from severe mania coupled with physical exhaustion that is life-threatening or resistance to treatment with medication (antipsychotic plus lithium/carbamazepine).

Psychosocial treatments

If the patient is subjected to a high level of expressed emotion, then the relatives should be seen and educated about the need to reduce the degree of critical comment in order to reduce the chances of relapse. Family therapy may be offered. Marital problems may benefit from marital therapy. The nature of bipolar disorder should also be explained to the relatives, as well as to the patient when he or she is well, and the need to continue with prophylactic medication should be emphasized.

Prognosis

The prognosis of bipolar disorder is much better in those who regularly take prophylactic medication (lithium salts or carbamazepine).

Case history: bipolar disorder

A 23-year-old unmarried postgraduate student was assessed in the community by his GP, a psychiatrist and a social worker, after the police had been alerted by members of the public. He had been running up and down a street in the middle of the night, shouting out that he was going to save all humans. The GP noted that he had been treated for a depressive episode two years previously, and that his mother suffered from bipolar disorder. It was difficult to question the patient, but from his friends it emerged that over the past week he had become increasingly elated, though at times he

Continued

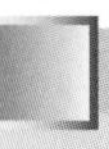

Case history: bipolar disorder—cont'd

would seem irritable. He was normally quiet, shy and studious, but over the past week he had been unable to sleep for more than two hours per night and had been sexually promiscuous. He had also been overspending and had gone into debt, something that again was very much out of character. A provisional diagnosis of mania was made and the patient was admitted to a psychiatric ward against his will under mental health legislation.

The patient was prescribed haloperidol, which he agreed to take orally. This was administered in syrup form to ensure compliance. Meanwhile, a full physical examination, blood tests and tests for illicit drugs proved negative. The patient's mood was brought down very quickly by the antipsychotic drug, and within two weeks he had recovered from this episode. When well, he mentioned that his mother was coping well on lithium prophylaxis and that he, too, felt he would benefit from such medication. The psychiatric team agreed and, as his renal and thyroid functions were normal, he was started on prophylactic treatment with lithium carbonate, the dose being adjusted to give a therapeutic plasma level of 0.6 mmol l^{-1}. After discharge the patient was followed up regularly in an outpatient clinic.

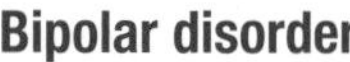

Bipolar disorder

- Clinical features of mania include elevation of mood (elation or irritability), low energy, overactivity, pressure of speech, grandiosity, lack of sleep, loss of normal social and sexual inhibitions, and low attention and concentration. Neglect of eating, drinking and personal hygiene may lead to dangerous states of dehydration and self-neglect.
- Mania may rarely cause stupor.
- The differential diagnosis of mania includes organic disorders and psychoactive substance use disorders, schizophrenia, agitated depression, severe obsessive–compulsive disorder and dyssocial personality disorder.
- The mean age of onset is around the mid-20s; it is more common in upper social classes.
- Predisposing factors of mood disorders (both depressive episodes and bipolar disorders) include genetic factors and personality (cyclothymic or cycloid personality) disorder.
- Precipitating factors of mood disorders include psychosocial stressors (recent life events, vulnerability factors) and physical illness (e.g. viral infections).
- Perpetuating and mediating factors of mood disorders include psychological factors (e.g. learned helplessness, depressive cognitive triad), social factors (lack of a confiding relationship, high expressed emotion), neurotransmitters (monoamine hypothesis of mood disorders), psychoneuroendocrinological factors, water and electrolyte changes, sleep changes (low REM latency in depression) and photic changes.
- Patients with mania should be treated as inpatients.
- The mainstay of the treatment of acute (hypo)mania is antipsychotic medication plus a mood-stabilizer (lithium or carbamazepine).
- Lithium is also used in the prophylaxis of bipolar disorder.
- ECT may be considered in severe mania that is accompanied by life-threatening exhaustion or treatment resistance.
- Compliance with prophylactic medication (lithium or carbamazepine) leads to a better prognosis in bipolar disorder.

Persistent mood disorders

In ICD-10, persistent mood disorders are defined as follows:

> These are persistent and usually fluctuating disorders of mood in which individual episodes are rarely if ever sufficiently severe to warrant being described as hypomanic or even mild depressive episodes. Because they last for years at a time, and sometimes for the greater part of the individual's adult life, they involve considerable subjective distress and disability.

The two most important persistent mood disorders are cyclothymia and dysthymia (depressive neurosis), which are described below. In ICD-10, the persistent mood disorders are classed with the mood disorders rather than with the personality disorders because of evidence from family studies, which suggests that they are genetically related to the other mood disorders.

Cyclothymia

Cyclothymia is defined in ICD-10 as 'A persistent instability of mood, involving numerous periods of mild depression and mild elation. This instability usually develops early in adult life and pursues a chronic course, although at times the mood may be normal and stable for months at a time'.

The lifetime risk of cyclothymia is reported to be between 0.4 and 3.5%, with the sex ratio being equal. The first-degree biological relatives of patients are more likely than the general population to suffer from depressive episodes and bipolar disorder. Many people with cyclothymia do not come to the attention of doctors, and are just treated by their friends as suffering from mild 'mood swings'. Some patients, however, are treated successfully with lithium and/or psychotherapy. Hospitalization is not usually indicated.

Dysthymia

Dysthymia, also called depressive neurosis, is defined in ICD-10 as:

> A chronic depression of mood which does not fulfil the criteria for recurrent depressive disorder ... The balance between individual phases of mild depression and intervening periods of comparative normality is very variable. Sufferers usually have periods of days or weeks when they describe themselves as well, but most of the time ... they feel tired and depressed; everything is an effort and nothing is enjoyed. They brood and complain, sleep badly and feel inadequate, but are usually able to cope with the basic demands of everyday life.

Dysthymia is probably more common in women than in men. It is also more common in the first-degree biological relatives of patients with a history of depressive episodes than it is in the general population.

In more severe cases, treatment with antidepressants, individual psychotherapy or cognitive therapy may be helpful. Hospitalization is not usually indicated unless the patient becomes suicidal.

Persistent mood disorders

- Cyclothymia, a persistent instability of mood involving numerous periods of mild depression and mild elation, has a lifetime risk of 0.4–3.5% and is equally common in males and females.
- Dysthymia (depressive neurosis), a chronic depression of mood that does not fulfil the criteria for recurrent depressive disorder, is more common in women.

Suicide and parasuicide (deliberate self-harm)

Suicide

Suicide is, unfortunately, a fundamental and sometimes unavoidable consequence of mental illness.

Epidemiology

Suicide is more common in men than in women and also in those aged over 45 (Figure 9.6). Recently, there has been a reported increase in suicides among young males. The highest rates are in those who are

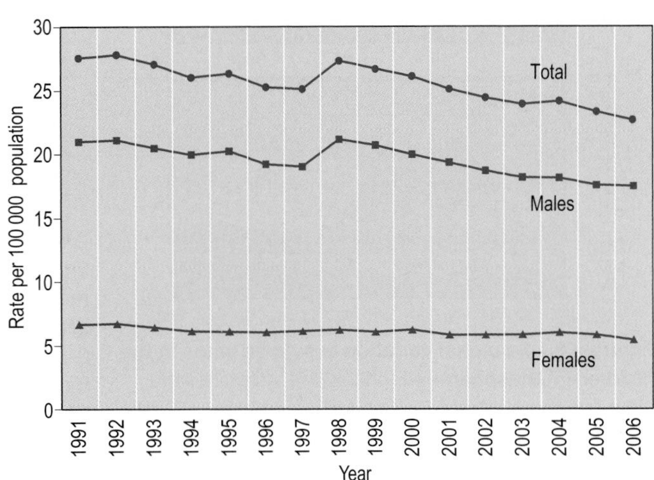

Figure 9.6 • UK age-standardized suicide rates per 100 000 population by age and gender for 1991–2006. (Reproduced with permission from Hawley C, St John Smith P, Padhi A 2010; see Further reading)

divorced, single or widowed, with those who are married having the lowest rate. The highest rates are in social classes I and V.

Suicide is associated with lack of employment, including both unemployment and retirement. As shown in Figure 9.7, suicide rates fell in England and Wales during the World Wars. There is also a seasonal variation in suicide, rates being highest during the spring and early summer (Figure 9.8) no matter whether in the northern or the southern hemisphere.

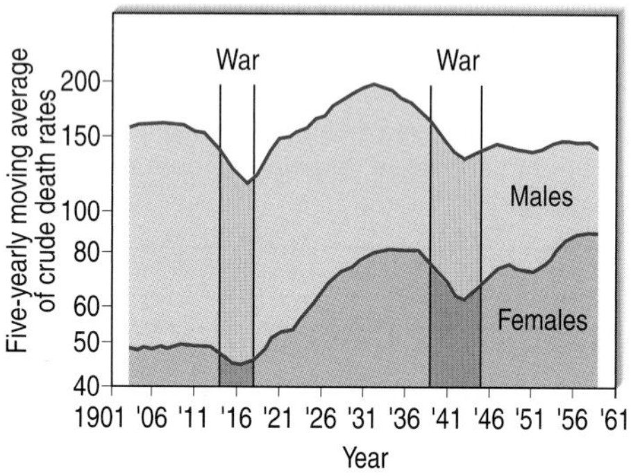

Figure 9.7 • Suicide rates for England and Wales, showing the drop during World Wars I and II. (Reproduced with permission from Kreitman N 1988; see Further reading)

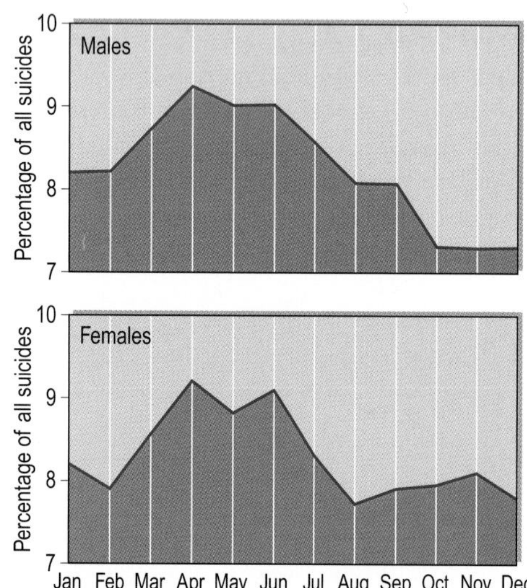

Figure 9.8 • Seasonal variation in suicide rates in the northern hemisphere. • In the southern hemisphere there is also an increase in the spring and early summer months. (Reproduced with permission from Kreitman N 1988; see Further reading)

Aetiology

Approximately 90% of people who commit suicide have been found to suffer from a psychiatric disorder. The most common include:

- depressive episodes – some of these patients actually use their antidepressant drugs to kill themselves; the newer SSRIs are much safer in this respect
- alcohol dependence
- other psychoactive substance use disorders, particularly illicit drugs
- personality disorders
- chronic neuroses
- schizophrenia, particularly in young men with low mood; such patients may commit suicide in unusual ways (Figure 9.9).

There is probably also an association with chronic painful illnesses and epilepsy.

It is important to note that following an act of parasuicide (deliberate self-harm) the risk of committing suicide in the following year is approximately 100 times that in the general population.

Assessment

It is important to ask patients about any suicidal thoughts they may have as there is no evidence that doing so might put the idea into the patient's mind.

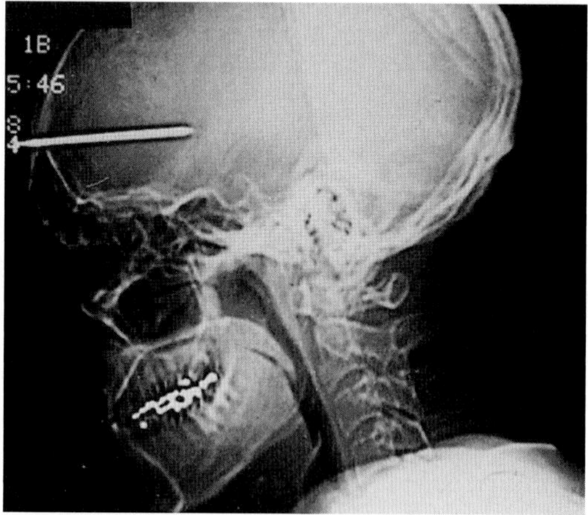

Figure 9.9 • Lateral skull radiograph of a 36-year-old man suffering from persecutory delusions who attempted to commit suicide by holding the head of a 3-inch masonry nail against a wall and head-butting its point until he had driven it fully into his forehead. The radiograph shows the nail *in situ*. (Reproduced with permission from Puri BK *et al.* 1994 British Journal of Psychiatry 164:841.)

Indeed, only 1% of individuals who have undertaken deliberate self-harm will successfully commit suicide in the following year. Rather, they may expect such questions to be asked. If there is any evidence of suicidal thoughts, the reasons for them and the methods being considered should be explored.

Any statement that the patient feels there is no future, that life is pointless or that suicide is being considered, should be taken very seriously indeed. It has been found that the majority of people who commit suicide have actually told somebody of their thoughts beforehand. Indeed, most may have seen their GP in the previous month and around half have seen a psychiatrist in the previous week.

It is important to look for any evidence of the psychiatric and physical illnesses mentioned above that have an association with an increased suicide risk. Relatives and friends should also be interviewed, and information obtained about any losses, such as:

- break-up of a relationship
- death of a relative or close friend
- loss of job
- financial loss
- loss of position or status in society, for example as a result of being arrested for shoplifting.

Evidence of loneliness and reduced or no social contacts should also be sought.

The predictive validity of the above factors is very poor, and consequently even experienced psychiatrists are frequently unable to predict suicide.

Management

If there is a serious risk of suicide the patient should almost always be admitted to hospital, compulsorily if need be. It is important that a good rapport is established between the suicidal patient and the nursing and medical staff, so that the patient can feel free to articulate feelings and thoughts. The patient should be encouraged to be open at all times. Anything that may be used in a suicide attempt, such as sharp objects or a belt (which may be used as a noose) should be removed. Depending on the degree of risk that is judged to exist, the frequency of observation can be varied, for example from every 15 minutes, through an increased level of every five minutes, to the highest level of continuous observation. In this case – used when the patient is judged to be at very high risk – a nurse should accompany the patient at all times, including at night (the patient may pretend to be asleep and then get up and attempt suicide by hanging) and in the bathroom (where drowning may be attempted). It may also be useful to nurse such patients in night-clothes (without a pyjama cord, which could be used as a noose) throughout the day, so making it more difficult for them to abscond without being noticed.

Any psychiatric disorder should be treated appropriately. In particular, if the patient is suffering from a severe depressive episode, ECT may be required.

Patients with psychomotor retardation are at greater risk of suicide once their symptoms begin to improve. They now have the energy to carry out the act of suicide and they should therefore be observed carefully.

Parasuicide (deliberate self-harm)

The term parasuicide has been defined by Kreitman as referring to:

> Any act deliberately undertaken by a patient who mimics the act of suicide, but which does not result in a fatal outcome. It is a self-initiated and deliberate act in which the patient injures himself or herself or takes a substance in a quantity which exceeds the therapeutic dose (if any) of his or her habitual level of consumption, and which he or she believes to be pharmacologically active.

Thus, if a patient were deliberately to take four 300 mg aspirin tablets in one go in the belief that this is a lethal dose, this would be classed as parasuicide, even though such a dose is not usually lethal.

Methods used

Figure 9.10 shows the modes of parasuicide seen in the UK, from which it can be seen that around 90% of cases involve deliberate self-poisoning with drugs. In many cases these are prescribed drugs, such as antidepressants. It is safer to prescribe SSRIs, SNRIs, a RIMA or a NaSSA than to prescribe a tricyclic antidepressant or MAOI, as the last two are much more toxic in overdose. Paracetamol, which is freely obtainable without a prescription, is particularly dangerous, as an overdose of as little as 10 g (i.e. 20 tablets each containing 500 mg) can lead to severe hepatocellular necrosis; patients who change their minds or who had not really wished

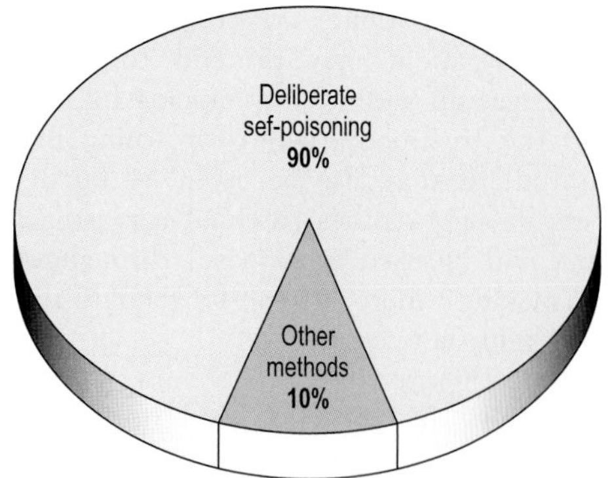

Figure 9.10 • The modes of parasuicide seen in the United Kingdom.

to die may go on to develop encephalopathy, haemorrhage and cerebral oedema within a few days, and then die. For partly this reason, in 1998, in the UK, a limit was imposed on the sale of analgesics, limiting the number of paracetamol or aspirin tablets that can be purchased at any one time at any vendor to just 16.

Epidemiology

Parasuicide is more common in women than in men and also in those under 45, particularly those aged between 15 and 25 years. Figure 9.11 illustrates how the rate rose during the 1960s and 1970s in the UK, and remained between 250 and 350 per 100 000 per year during the next two decades. The highest rates are in those who are divorced or single, teenage wives and in the lower social classes.

Parasuicide is associated with unemployment. It is more common in urban areas in which there is high unemployment, overcrowding, high social mobility, a high rate of juvenile delinquency and a high rate of sexually transmitted diseases.

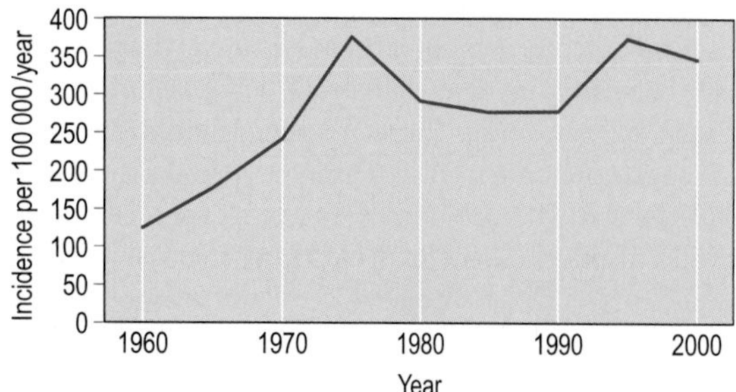

Figure 9.11 • Parasuicide rates in the UK: representative data. (Reproduced with permission from Hawley C, St John Smith P, Padhi A 2010; see Further reading)

Aetiology

Compared with the general population, life events are more common in the six months before an act of parasuicide. These include:

- the break-up of a relationship
- being in trouble with the law
- physical illness
- illness of a loved one.

Predisposing factors include:

- marital difficulties, such as infidelity
- unemployment
- physical illness, particularly epilepsy
- mental retardation
- death of one's parent at a young age
- parental neglect or abuse.

Most cases of parasuicide are associated with a psychiatric disorder, the most common being:

- depressive episodes, which may be particularly severe in middle-aged women
- dysthymia, which is more common in young parasuicides
- alcohol dependence
- personality disorder.

Assessment

It is important to note that the medical seriousness of self-harming behaviour is unrelated to the psychiatric seriousness, and that the patient's account of the medication ingested may not be reliable. When interviewing the patient after an act of parasuicide, it is important to ascertain the degree of suicidal intent that existed at the time. A high degree of such intent is indicated by the following:

- The act was *planned* and *preparations* were made, such as buying equipment or collecting medication.
- *Precautions* were taken to avoid discovery, for example doors were locked and the act timed so that the patient was unlikely to be disturbed. The act was carried out in isolation.
- The patient *did not seek help* after the act.

- The act involved a *dangerous method*, such as hanging, electrocution, shooting, jumping or drowning.
- There was a *final act*, such as making a will or leaving a suicide note.

Patients should be asked what their reactions were when they realized that they were not going to die. They should also be asked whether they want to die. A high suicide risk is indicated when patients regret not having died and still want to die.

The presence of psychiatric disorders associated with suicide should be looked for, any previous history of suicide attempts should be asked about and the patient's current problems enquired into. The social and financial support the patient can rely on should also be detailed.

Management

Following an act of parasuicide, the patient should be treated medically as appropriate and a full assessment carried out. If the patient suffers from a psychiatric disorder this should be treated appropriately.

Factors associated with a repeated attempt of deliberate self-harm include:

- a previous act of parasuicide
- previous psychiatric treatment
- dyssocial or antisocial personality disorder
- alcohol dependence
- other psychoactive substance use disorder
- criminal record
- low social class
- unemployment.

It is important to bear in mind that following an act of parasuicide the risk of committing suicide in the following year is approximately 100 times that in the general population. High-risk patients should be treated as detailed in the section on the management of suicidal patients. Factors associated with an increased risk of suicide following parasuicide include:

- high suicidal intent as elicited by the assessment
- psychiatric disorder (particularly depressive episodes), alcohol dependence, other psychoactive substance use disorders, schizophrenia and dyssocial or antisocial personality disorder
- a history of previous suicide attempt(s)
- social isolation
- age over 45
- being male
- being unemployed or retired
- chronic painful illness.

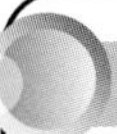

Suicide and parasuicide

- Suicide is commoner in males, over 45s, the unmarried, social classes I and V, the unemployed and retired, and is more likely to be carried out in the spring and early summer.
- Around 90% of people who commit suicide are suffering from a psychiatric disorder at the time, including depression, alcohol dependence, illicit drug use, personality disorder, chronic neurosis and schizophrenia.
- Suicide is associated with chronic painful illnesses and epilepsy.
- Following an act of parasuicide, the risk of committing suicide in the following year is approximately 100 times that in the general population.
- If there is a serious risk of suicide the patient should be treated as an inpatient, and precautions taken to prevent suicide in hospital.
- Patients with psychomotor retardation are at greater risk of suicide once their symptoms begin to improve.
- Around 90% of cases of parasuicide (deliberate self-harm) in the UK involve deliberate self-poisoning (e.g. paracetamol, antidepressants).
- Parasuicide is more common in females, the under 45s (particularly between 15 and 25 years), lower social classes and the unemployed; it is also more common in those who are divorced or single, and among teenage wives.
- Life events (e.g. the break-up of a relationship) are more common in the six months before an act of parasuicide compared with the general population.
- Most cases of parasuicide are associated with a psychiatric disorder, such as depression, dysthymia, alcohol dependence and personality disorder.
- A high degree of suicidal intent is indicated by an act of self-harm if the act was planned and prepared for, precautions were taken to avoid discovery, help was not sought afterwards and a dangerous method was used (e.g. hanging, electrocution, shooting, jumping, or drowning).

Case history: parasuicide

A 17-year-old female student was admitted to an Accident and Emergency Department having taken an overdose of 20 aspirin tablets one hour previously. Gastric emptying was carried out. A good recovery of the salicylate was achieved, with the plasma salicylate being almost zero 24 hours later. Similarly, the plasma pH, urea and electrolytes remained within the normal range 24 hours later. Therefore, fluid replacement and forced alkaline diuresis were not required.

A psychiatric assessment was carried out. The patient explained that she had not intended to die and most certainly did not want to die now. She said she had taken the overdose because on the previous day her boyfriend had suddenly announced that he was going to leave her for somebody else. She had been very upset and felt that if she took an overdose he would feel sorry for her and consider returning to her. She took the overdose at home 30 minutes before she was expecting him to meet her there to discuss the situation further. She knew he would be able to use his key to open her front door; the door had not been bolted. She had not left a suicide note. There was no previous history of parasuicide or psychoactive substance use disorder. There was no past psychiatric history and the mental state examination did not reveal any evidence of a psychiatric disorder. The overall result of the assessment was that the patient did not have a high suicide intent at the time of the overdose and did not require psychiatric treatment. She was therefore discharged home without any psychiatric follow-up arrangements.

Further reading

Griez, E.J.L., Faravelli, C., Nutt, D.J., Zohar, J. (Eds.), 2005. Mood disorders: clinical management and research issues. John Wiley, Chichester.

Hawley, C., St John Smith, P., Padhi, A., 2010. Suicide and deliberate self-harm. In: Puri, B.K., Teasaden, I. (Eds.), Psychiatry: an evidence-based text. Hodder Arnold, London.

Hawton, K. (Ed.), 2005. Prevention and treatment of suicidal behaviour: from science to practice. Oxford University Press, Oxford.

Kirsch, I., 2009. The emperor's new drugs: exploding the antidepressant myth, The Bodley Head, London.

Kreitman, N., 1988. Suicide and parasuicide. In: Johnstone, E.C., Kendell, R.E., Zealley, A.K. (Eds.), Companion to psychiatric studies. fourth ed. Churchill Livingstone, Edinburgh.

Morgan, H.G., 1979. Death wishes? The understanding and management of deliberate self-harm, John Wiley, Chichester.

Williams, C., 2006. Overcoming depression and low mood: a five areas approach, second ed. Hodder Arnold, London.

Neurotic and other stress-related disorders

Concept of neurosis

The term neurosis was first used by William Cullen (1710 – 1790) in 1777 for disorders of the nervous system for which there appeared no physical cause. The term replaced Robert Whytt's 1764 'illness of the nerves', which itself superseded the term 'vapours'.

Mental illness, which implies previous health, has been divided into psychoses and neuroses.

In *psychoses* there is loss of contact with reality and symptoms, such as delusions or hallucinations, are not understandable, nor can they be empathized with. Psychoses are regarded as severe mental illnesses and in lay terms are referred to as 'madness'.

Neuroses or *psychoneuroses*, on the other hand, have symptoms that are both understandable (reality-based) and with which one can empathize. Insight is usually maintained. They are regarded as milder and, in lay terms, are referred to as 'nerves'. They are quantitatively, but not qualitatively, different from normal, involving for instance, inappropriate or excessive anxiety. Neuroses are most usually (but not invariably) short-lived, but can be chronic and impairing, and accompanied by a change, characteristically in symptoms and often, secondarily, in behaviour.

Neuroses can be defined as abnormal psychogenic (psychologically caused) reactions. An anxiety neurosis would have predominantly anxiety symptoms; in phobic disorder there would be predominantly phobic symptoms. Neuroses typically have two components:

- a vulnerable personality
- stress factors triggering the reaction.

They can thus be seen as exaggerated forms of normal reactions to stressful events, i.e. they are inappropriate to the situation or the stress, or the reaction occurs at a greater frequency or severity than normal. Classically, a neurosis was considered to have no demonstrable organic basis and there should be no loss of contact with external reality, such as occurs in psychosis. Neurotic symptoms are thus maladaptive reactions to stress and reflect excessive and inappropriate use of psychological defence mechanisms.

Neurotic symptoms are unpleasant and lead to the individual seeking relief. They are often accompanied by a decrease in social functioning, and individuals suffering from a neurosis have an increased mortality rate, including owing to suicide and fatal head injuries.

A distinction should be made between the neuroses, which are a group of mental illnesses, and what are sometimes referred to, particularly by the lay population, as 'neurotic' individuals, who most often suffer from lifelong personality difficulties such as over-anxiousness or over-emotionality.

Epidemiology

Individual neurotic symptoms are common in the community, as well as in primary and secondary care, and thus can be regarded as normal. These include:

- inappropriate fears
- anxiety and panic
- brief bouts of depressive feelings
- tension headaches
- irritability
- sleeplessness.

Neurotic symptoms are often seen in general practice, resulting in significant societal burden. They may be the predominant symptoms in one-sixth of individuals seen there, and relevant in up to one-third. Sufferers often present with physical symptoms. Individuals suffering from neurosis are more frequently seen in a psychiatric outpatient clinic than as inpatients in a psychiatric hospital. Neurotic disorders are the most common psychiatric condition, at any one time affecting up to 10% of all individuals, and over 15% in a lifetime.

With the high incidence of neurotic symptoms in the general population, questions arise in individual cases as to whether such symptoms should be regarded as abnormal or whether such individuals are regarded as mentally ill. Should these symptoms be merely viewed as an individual's way of dealing with the problems of everyday life, or do they represent a formal mental illness? Mild neuroses, in fact, often remit spontaneously or with mild reassurance. However, individuals with neurosis are more likely to seek medical consultation, often owing to fear of physical illness, and accurate diagnosis avoids inappropriate medical investigations.

Comorbidity, especially with depression, substance misuse and personality disorder, is common. Neurotic disorders often precede the development of depression.

In the differential diagnosis of neurosis, one should ask why this particular patient is presenting at this particular time with this particular symptom. If an individual presents with neurotic symptoms for the first time after the age of 35–40 years, it is probable that they may be due to a depressive disorder or, alternatively, to underlying organic disease.

Aetiology

Predisposing factors leading to the development of neurosis are often similar to those important in the development of personality disorder. In fact, neuroses often arise in those with abnormal personalities, as these lead such individuals into social and emotional difficulties to which they overreact emotionally.

Environmental factors such as family and early background are important, but there is increasing evidence for a *genetic inherited predisposition* to neurosis.

The vulnerability of the general population to developing a neurosis under stress follows a normal distribution, as for height or weight (Figure. 10.1).

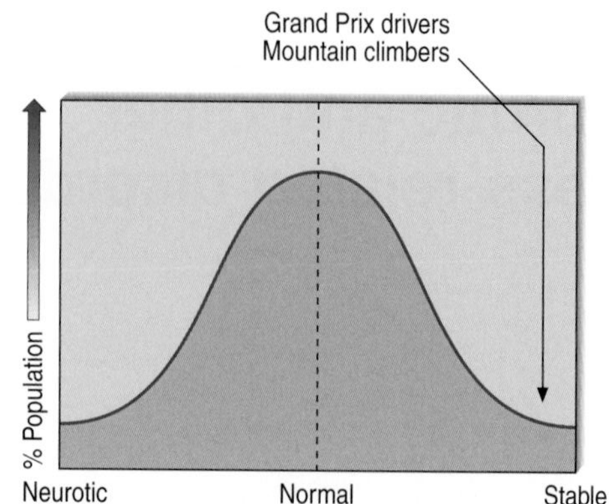

Figure 10.1 • Vulnerability to developing neurosis.

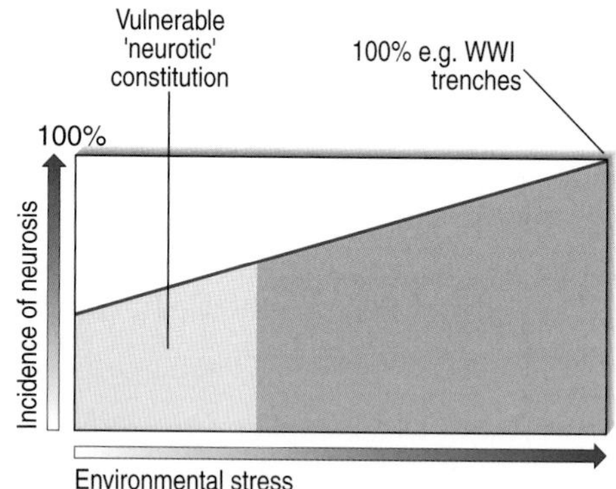

Figure 10.2 • Incidence of neurosis with environmental stress.

The incidence of neurosis rises with increasing environmental stress (Figure. 10.2). Even normal stable personalities will develop neurosis under severe environmental stress, as can be seen in individuals involved in natural disasters and in war time. During the First World War, the incidence of neurosis approached 100% in individuals in the trenches for prolonged periods, and this was similar in bomber crews during the Second World War after more than 30 missions. Although one person's stress may be another's pleasure (owing to the individual's background and personality), certain situations such as combat are experienced as stressful by over 95% of individuals. Lower percentages experience stress in examinations or public speaking, and up to 50% of the population find job interviews stressful. Although not associated with external stresses, sensory deprivation (either experimentally or as experienced by hostages kept in solitary confinement) and, to a lesser extent, boredom can also result in extreme stress and anxiety.

A number of theories have been developed to explain neuroses. In *Freudian psychoanalytic theory*, neurotic symptoms are seen as the expression of intrapsychic anxiety due to unresolved emotional conflicts dating from childhood. Freud initially proposed that anxiety represented repressed libido (mental energy or drive). Later, he considered that it reflected the birth experience, but he eventually replaced this theory with that of anxiety being a response of the ego to instinctual emotional tension. Freud differentiated the term anxiety neurosis, which he thought had a biological causation, from psychoneurosis, which included anxiety hysteria (phobic or situational anxiety), obsessive–compulsive neurosis and hysteria, all of which he saw as arising from unconscious conflicts. *Learning theory* has conceptualized the neuroses as learned maladaptive responses associated with a temporary reduction in anxiety. There is also evidence to suggest some genetic predisposition for the development of individual types of neuroses, although this may be predominantly through *genetic influence* on the development of personality.

As stated above, stress factors can be *precipitating factors* for neuroses in vulnerable individuals, and environmental factors, including family and marital factors, and social conditions such as poor housing and unemployment, may be *perpetuating factors* for such disorders. Table 10.1 summarizes factors associated with the development of neurotic and stress-related disorders.

Treatment

Evidence-based guidelines, e.g., from the National Institute for Clinical Excellence (NICE) in the UK, are now available. Each condition will be discussed in turn. Cognitive behavioural therapy (CBT) and selective serotonin reuptake inhibitors (SSRIs) are often effective. SSRIs should be continued for one year after response. However, CBT may be more effective in preventing relapse.

Table 10.1 Factors associated with development of neurotic and stress-related disorders
Lower social class
Unemployment
Divorced, separated or widowed
Renting rather than owning own home
No educational qualifications
Urban rather than rural
The homeless and prisoners have twice the risk of general population.

Prognosis

The overall prognosis in these conditions is generally regarded as good, with up to 50% of individuals recovering without treatment, and up to 70% with treatment, within two years. However, up to half of individuals seen by a GP will remain symptomatic one year later, and for those seen by a psychiatrist, about half will still be handicapped after four years. Good prognostic indicators include a stable premorbid personality and the development of acute symptoms in response to transitory stresses. Poor prognostic factors include chronic and/or severe symptoms at presentation, persisting social problems and inadequate social support. There is an excess of mortality among those with neurotic disorders, largely because of increased rates of completed suicide.

Concept of neurosis

- Neurosis is a general term for a group of mental illnesses in which anxiety, phobic, panic and obsessional symptoms predominate. The dominant symptom determines the formal diagnosis, but several commonly coexist.
- Neurotic symptoms differ from normal symptoms such as anxiety only by their intensity, not qualitatively.
- Neuroses are abnormal psychogenic (psychologically caused) reactions.
- Most neuroses are precipitated by normal life stressors and are often associated with a vulnerable personality, especially dependent and anankastic (obsessional) personality disorders.
- Neurosis is twice as common in females than in males.

Classification

ICD-10 has not retained the concept of a neurosis as a major organizing principle in classification, although it groups three types of disorder together because of their historical association with the concept of neurosis, and also their association with psychological causation. These are the neurotic and stress-related disorders (which are considered in this chapter) and the somatoform and dissociative disorders, which are described in Chapter 11. Table 10.2 summarizes neurotic and stress-related disorders on the basis of ICD-10. Mixed neurotic states are more common than the discrete syndromes. Panic disorder with or without agoraphobia and generalized anxiety disorder are the most disabling. Table 10.3 shows the frequency of neurotic conditions. DSM-IV-TR uses the term 'anxiety disorders' rather than 'neurotic disorders' and, indeed, neurosis was absent from DSM-III. Table 10.4 compares DSM-IV-TR with ICD-10 in relation to neurotic and stress-related disorders.

The basis for the current categorical classification for non-psychotic disorders has been criticized for lack of evidence and a dimensional classification, e.g., dimensions for anxiety and depression, has been proposed.

Table 10.2 Neurotic and stress-related disorders based on ICD-10

Disorders	Features
Generalized anxiety disorder	Generalized and persistent 'free floating' anxiety symptoms involving elements of: • apprehension (worries about future misfortunes, 'feeling on edge', difficulty in concentrating, etc.) • motor tension (restless fidgeting, tension headaches, trembling, inability to relax, etc.) • autonomic overactivity (light-headedness, sweating, tachycardia or tachypnoea, epigastric discomfort, dizziness, dry mouth, etc.)
Mixed anxiety and depressive disorder	Symptoms of anxiety and depression are both present but neither clearly predominates
Panic disorder	Recurrent attacks of severe anxiety (panic) not restricted to any particular situation or set of circumstances, and therefore unpredictable Secondary fears of dying, losing control or going mad Attacks usually last for minutes only and patients often experience a crescendo of fear and autonomic symptoms Comparative freedom from anxiety symptoms between attacks, although anticipatory anxiety is common
Phobic disorders	Anxiety is evoked only, or predominantly, by certain well-defined situations or objects external to the subject, which are not currently dangerous, and these are characteristically avoided or endured with dread
Specific (isolated) phobias	Restricted to highly specific situations such as proximity to particular animals, heights, thunder, flying, blood, etc.
Agoraphobia	Fear not only of open spaces but also of related aspects, such as the presence of crowds and difficulty of immediate easy escape back to a safe place, usually home May occur with or without panic disorder
Social phobias	Fear of scrutiny by other people in comparatively small groups (as opposed to crowds), leading to avoidance of social situations
Obsessive–compulsive disorder	Recurrent obsessional thoughts or compulsive acts At least one thought or act still unsuccessfully resisted Thought of carrying out the act is not pleasurable Thoughts, images or impulses must be unpleasantly repetitive
Post-traumatic stress disorder	Delayed and/or prolonged response to stressful event or situation of threatening or catastrophic nature, likely to cause distress in anyone Episodes of repeated reliving of the trauma in intrusive memories ('flashbacks'), dreams or nightmares Sense of 'numbness' and detachment from other people Avoidance of activities and situations reminiscent of trauma Usually autonomic hyperarousal with hypervigilance, an enhanced startle reaction and insomnia

Table 10.3 Relative frequencies of neurotic conditions

Condition	Frequency (%)
Mixed anxiety and depression	48
Generalized anxiety disorder	28
Depression	14
Phobia	12
Obsessive–compulsive disorder	10
Panic disorder	6

Anxiety disorders

Normal anxiety

Anxiety is a mood, usually unpleasant in nature, accompanied by bodily (somatic) sensations and occurring with a subjective feeling of uncertainty and threat about the future. The term 'fear' is used to describe a normal and appropriate mood when the danger can be perceived and defined. Most of the bodily changes seen in anxiety are caused by increased sympathetic adrenergic nervous system discharges, i.e. *Cannon's fight or flight reaction* (Figure. 10.3), which results in the release of adrenaline and other catecholamines. In our ancestral past such a reaction would prepare us to deal with a real physical threat, but today we may merely experience such reactions when under stress in everyday life, for instance in a traffic jam.

We all attempt to adjust our lives to maintain anxiety at an optimal level for us as individuals. However, like pain, anxiety is a useful warning and should not be suppressed with drugs or alcohol. It is the central nervous system's alarm system to protect us from threat, and is activated by environmental cues. There is an inverted U-shaped relationship between anxiety and performance developed by Hebb in 1955 known as the *Yerkes–Dodson law* (Figure. 10.4). This was based on an experiment on white mice being encouraged by low-, medium- and high-intensity electric shocks to learn to locate a compartment in a box. Medium-intensity shocks produced the fastest learning. Performance is reduced at low and very high levels of anxiety: thus poor examination results are obtained by those with low anxiety

Table 10.4 Comparison of ICD-10 and DSM-IV-TR neurotic/anxiety disorders

ICD-10	DSM-IV-TR
F40: Phobic anxiety disorders	
F40.00 Agoraphobia without panic disorder	300.22 Agoraphobia without history of panic disorder
F40.01 Agoraphobia with panic disorder	300.21 Panic disorder with agoraphobia
F40.1 Social phobias	300.23 Social phobia
F40.2 Specific (isolated) phobias	300.29 Specific phobia
F41: Other anxiety disorders	
F41.0 Panic disorder (episodic paroxysmal anxiety)	300.01 Panic disorder without agoraphobia
F41.1 Generalized anxiety disorder	300.02 Generalized anxiety disorder
F41.2 Mixed anxiety and depressive disorder	300.00 Anxiety disorder NOS
F42: Obsessive–compulsive disorder	**300.3 Obsessive–compulsive disorder**
F43: Reaction to severe stress and adjustment disorders	
F43.0 Acute stress reaction	308.3 Acute stress disorder
F43.1 Post-traumatic stress disorder	309.81 Post-traumatic stress disorder
F43.2 Adjustment disorders	309.9 Adjustment disorders

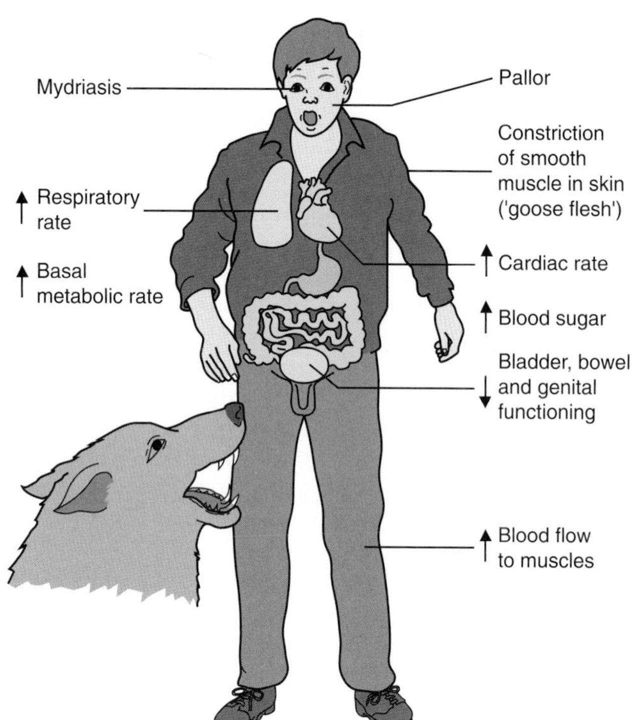

Figure 10.3 • Physiological changes in Cannon's fight or flight reaction.

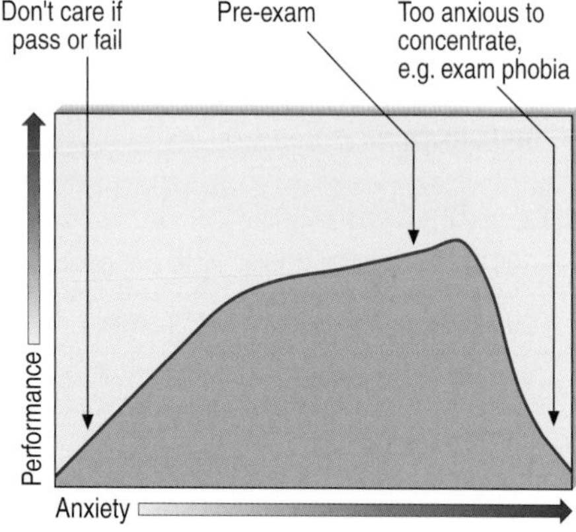

Figure 10.4 • Yerkes--Dodson law.

levels who do not care whether they pass or fail, and by those who become so highly anxious that they cannot concentrate. The Yerkes–Dodson law predicts that anxiolytic drugs reduce performance in someone with a low anxiety level, but when a deterioration in performance is caused by high anxiety, the reduction of symptoms by anxiolytic drugs should improve performance, for example in examination phobia. In assessing an individual's true level of anxiety, one should bear in mind that the complaint of symptoms of anxiety may lie anywhere along the Yerkes–Dodson curve. The individual may also be very anxious during a formal interview, but not so for long periods during the day, or vice versa. It is useful to distinguish between *trait anxiety*, which is a lifelong personality characteristic, and *state anxiety*, which is a temporal disorder with a discernible time of onset.

Anxiety is present usually where there is some possibility of choice of action. This may explain why some individuals facing execution, where there is no hope, do not appear anxious. Other factors such as depersonalization and denial may also be relevant, as may also a paranoid attitude to circumstances in that such an individual believes that others will 'get' them anyway, sooner or later.

Generalized anxiety disorder

This is also known as anxiety neurosis, anxiety state or anxiety reaction, and is characterized by unrealistic or excessive anxiety and worry, which is generalized and persistent and not restricted to particular environmental circumstances, i.e. it is '*free-floating*'.

Epidemiology

Community surveys suggest that about 1.6% of the adult population are suffering from generalized anxiety disorder at any one time, with a one-year prevalence range of 3–8% and a lifetime prevalence of 21%, with a female to male ratio of 2:1. Around 15% of patients attending GP surgeries and 25% attending medical settings in general are 'anxious'. Generalized anxiety disorder often begins in early adult life, between the ages of 15 and 25 years, but rates continue to increase after the age of 35 years. Being older than 24 years, separated, widowed, divorced, unemployed, or a 'home-maker' are associated with a higher prevalence of general anxiety disorder. Pure generalized anxiety disorder is, however, rare compared with the much more common mixed picture of anxiety and depression. Comorbidity is common, perhaps up to 90%, e.g., with panic disorder and social phobia.

Clinical features

These are summarized in Figure 10.5 and Table 10.5. Individuals will not have all the psychic (affective) and somatic symptoms, but will tend to have the same symptoms during each exacerbation, for example palpitations or trembling.

Males and individuals from lower social classes and some cultures are more likely to complain of somatic rather than psychic symptoms. It is important to understand that these are real and not merely 'all in the mind', and it is reassuring to the patient to be told this. In keeping with Cannon's fight or flight reaction, in which there is stimulation of adrenergic neurones leading to the release of adrenaline and other catecholamines, autonomic hyperactivity results in increased heart rate and palpitations and an increased rate of breathing, which results in a sensation of breathlessness. In turn, hyperventilation (sometimes referred to as the *hyperventilation*

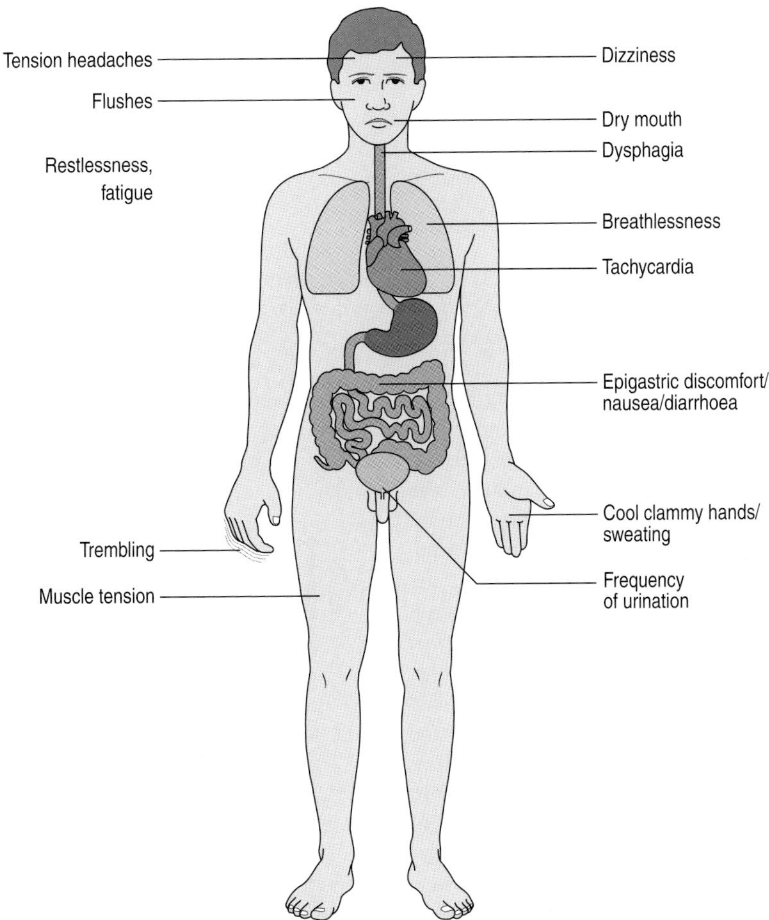

Figure 10.5 • Somatic clinical features of generalized anxiety disorder.

Table 10.5 Psychological features of generalized anxiety disorder

Symptoms	Characteristics
Psychic	Feelings of threat and foreboding Difficulty in concentrating or 'mind going blank' Distractible Feeling keyed up, on edge, tense or unable to relax Early insomnia and nightmares Irritability Noise intolerance (e.g. of children or music)
Panic attacks	Unexpected severe acute exacerbations or psychic and somatic anxiety symptoms with intense fear or discomfort Not triggered by situations Individuals cannot 'sit out' the attack
Other features	Lability of mood Depersonalization (dream-like sensation of unreality of self or part of self) Derealization (dream-like sensation of unreality of world) Hypnogogic and hypnopompic hallucinations (when, respectively, going off to or waking from sleep) Perceptual distortion (e.g. distortion of walls or the sound of other people talking)

syndrome) results in the individual excessively blowing off carbon dioxide, leading to hypocapnia, which induces peripheral vasoconstriction and a 'pins and needles' sensation (paraesthesia). This can be countered by breathing into and out of a paper bag.

It is thus easy to understand how a patient, unaware of the normal physiology of anxiety, can get into a vicious cycle of anxiety and worry about somatic symptoms. The patient may forget the original stress that precipitated the episode and become preoccupied about dying from a heart attack (sometimes referred to as *cardiac neurosis* or the *effort syndrome*). Such a fear would be increased if chest pain is also experienced owing to anxiety-induced increased muscle tension. Muscle tension is caused by increased blood flow to the muscles as well as increased tone, and contributes to the complaint of fatigue. The term *neurasthenia* (fatigue syndrome) has been used in the past to refer to a neurosis where fatigue is the predominant symptom.

Depersonalization and *derealization* are sometimes associated with generalized anxiety disorder and are disorders of self-awareness. In depersonalization, an individual has an altered or lost sense of personal reality or identity. In derealization, an individual's surroundings feel unreal. Individuals find these symptoms unpleasant and difficult to describe, and are relieved when they are acknowledged by professionals. Such feelings can occur in normal individuals, especially those suffering loss of sleep, as well as in a *primary depersonalization–derealization syndrome*. They are also seen in individuals suffering from depression, schizophrenia, alcohol and drug intoxication and withdrawal, and epilepsy. It may also be induced by prescribed medication. Although unpleasant, they are bearable compared to panic attacks, which are associated with higher levels of anxiety (Figure. 10.6).

History taking should explore the use of alcohol, caffeine and illicit drugs as possible explanations for anxiety symptoms, as well as any association of symptoms with precipitating events. The individual may have a tense and worried facial expression and posture, and may be tremulous, pale and/or sweaty. There may be overbreathing and also evidence of *agitation* (purposeless activity due to anxiety), with pacing of the floor and fidgeting. Physical examination should exclude organic causes such as thyrotoxicosis. Although investigations for thyrotoxicosis might be justified, other physical causes of anxiety, such as phaeochromocytoma, are sufficiently rare for routine investigation not to be cost-effective, unless clinically indicated.

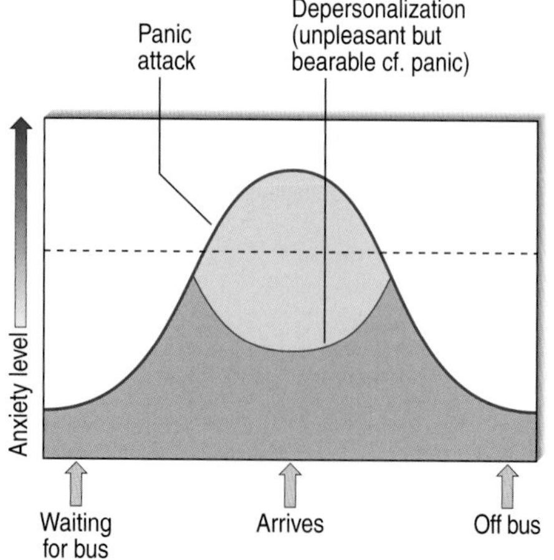

Figure 10.6 • Anxiety levels in panic attacks and depersonalization.

Differential diagnosis

Many disorders and nearly all psychiatric conditions may present primarily with symptoms of anxiety (Table 10.6). Generalized anxiety disorder very rarely begins after age 35; individuals presenting for the first time after this age are more likely to be suffering from depressive or other psychiatric disorders, but the distinction between general anxiety disorder and depression can be difficult. Rotational vertigo is not a symptom of anxiety.

Aetiology

Predisposing factors. There is some evidence of a *genetic* inherited influence on anxiety proneness associated with a vulnerability to depression, with *environmental factors* influencing presentation. Environmental factors, e.g., through social learning, are also important in themselves, e.g. anxious insecure mothers raise anxious insecure children. Individuals with a *premorbid anxious (avoidant) personality disorder* are more prone to develop a chronic generalized anxiety disorder. There is also an association with *early childhood separation* experiences, especially separation from either parent. Bowlby's attachment theory suggests that such separations result in feelings of insecurity, which are reactivated in later life.

Table 10.6 Disorders that can present primarily with symptoms of anxiety
Generalized anxiety disorder
Panic disorder
Phobic disorders
Obsessive–compulsive disorder
Depressive disorder
Schizophrenia and other paranoid psychoses
Drug and alcohol withdrawal syndromes (e.g. delirium tremens)
Early dementia (e.g. catastrophic reactions on psychometric testing)
Ictal anxiety due to epilepsy, especially temporal lobe epilepsy
Thyrotoxicosis
Phaeochromocytoma
Unexpressed complaints of physical illness (e.g. lump in breast)
Drug and alcohol abuse, dependency and withdrawal symptoms (e.g. delirium tremens, caffeinism)

Freudian psychoanalytic theory suggests that intrapsychic anxiety due to emotional conflict may be expressed directly as a generalized anxiety disorder.

Biological models of general anxiety disorder have been hypothesized, and involve:

1. Noradrenergic pathways (locus coeruleus – noradrenergic sympathetic autonomic nervous system), which are associated with fear and arousal.
2. Septo-hippocampal system and Papez circuit, which mediate anxiety and are where anxiolytic drugs act. Benzodiazepines act on $GABA_A$ receptor complexes.
3. The galvanic skin response of sweat glands to sympathetic stimulation is associated with a reduction in habituation in anxiety, but not thyrotoxicosis.

Precipitating and perpetuating factors include current stresses and life events, especially those associated with fear of loss. However, cognitive theories are now increasingly cited to explain the onset of generalized anxiety disorder.

Management

Most patients suffering from generalized anxiety disorders are treated in the primary care setting. *Counselling* alone may be very effective, for example explanation of and reassurance about somatic symptoms of anxiety, such as palpitations, which the patient may believe are indicative of an imminent heart attack, or, more generally, reassurance that the individual is not going to lose control, go mad or end up in a psychiatric hospital for life. *Self-help materials*, such as books and relaxation tapes and leaflets, reinforce counselling and can be a treatment in their own right.

Psychological treatments. There is good evidence that cognitive therapy and anxiety management techniques are effective and these should be the first choices in treatment. *Cognitive therapy* is based on the idea that thoughts and feelings are related and that anxious thinking provokes or maintains the problem. The individual is taught to recognize and re-examine his anxious thoughts in order to find alternative and more helpful ways of thinking, which are then tested out in practice. Cognitive therapy also aims to identify and modify dysfunctional assumptions or beliefs that underlie anxious thinking. The aim is to replace automatic morbid anticipatory thoughts with realistic cognitions.

A CBT approach additionally includes exposure relaxation and is superior to other forms of psychological treatment.

Anxiety management training is based on the rationale that anxiety can be managed by breaking into the vicious cycles that keep the problem going. Education is via the explanation of anxiety and its causes and consequences. Relaxation exercises and, if indicated, breathing exercises, are encouraged and new ways of coping, such as distraction and cognitive techniques, are taught.

In both cognitive therapy and anxiety management, homework assignments for the patient may be required, and the patient should be warned that temporary setbacks may occur. Both cognitive therapy and anxiety management training may also be effectively conducted in a group setting.

Relaxation techniques are based on the assumption that mental relaxation follows physical relaxation. This may involve the use of progressive muscular relaxation with or without the use of relaxation tapes. However, it is less effective than CBT.

The term *autogenic training* (e.g. by biofeedback techniques) means learning to self-monitor anxiety levels and then apply relaxation techniques to daily activities. Yoga and transcendental meditation work as relaxation techniques and can be useful in generalized anxiety disorder.

In addition to non-directive and directive counselling and supportive psychotherapy, insight-orientated dynamic psychotherapy has been used for individuals suffering from chronic generalized anxiety disorder who are unresponsive to other approaches. The technique aims to uncover and resolve unconscious emotional conflicts that result in intrapsychic anxiety, which is expressed as symptoms of generalized anxiety disorder. In particular, *brief focal psychotherapy*, which focuses on a specific problem and sets an agenda and time limits of therapy, has been found to be useful. In this technique the individual is encouraged to talk freely, but the therapist interprets the content of the talk to reveal a deeper meaning, which can be understood and accepted by the patient.

Where interpersonal conflicts and stresses underlie the generalized anxiety disorder, *marital* or *family therapy* may be required. Similarly, environmental causes, such as poor housing, may have to be tackled.

Drug treatment. In the past, most patients presenting with generalized anxiety disorder were treated with tranquillizers, mainly benzodiazepines such as diazepam (Valium). However, it is now recognized that such drugs can cause dependence and their role is limited to brief periods of use to overcome symptoms so severe that they obstruct the initiation of more appropriate psychological treatments. Acutely disabled patients may require benzodiazepine drug therapy for up to four weeks, but even in these circumstances additional counselling, self-help and support are also required. Chronic use of minor tranquillizers should generally be avoided, although evidence is emerging that antidepressants, and possibly buspirone, may have a role in the longer- term management of severe persistent forms of anxiety.

Benzodiazepines are still the first choice when a rapid anxiolytic effect (as opposed to being a first-line treatment in general) is required. They should be used in the lowest dose possible and only as required, rather than routinely. In the absence of anxiety, they may merely result in sedation and increase the risk of dependency. Benzodiazepines should not be prescribed as hypnotics for more than 10 nights, or as anxiolytics for more than two to four weeks. Diazepam and chlordiazepoxide are used as anxiolytics, whereas temazepam and nitrazepam are used as hypnotics. Diazepam is the most prescribed drug ever in the history of the world. Flurazepam has been used by astronauts in space. Longer-acting compounds, such as diazepam, are preferred to those with a shorter half-life, such as lorazepam, which have a greater risk of withdrawal symptoms. Benzodiazepines may impair the effectiveness of psychological therapies and also the performance of skilled tasks and driving; patients should therefore be warned. They should also be warned about the potentially dangerous interactions of benzodiazepines with drugs and alcohol. Benzodiazepines have a definite abuse potential, with a risk of dependence and withdrawal symptoms on discontinuing long-term use. Prescribing benzodiazepines for a period of as little as two weeks can be associated, on cessation, not only with the re-emergence of the original symptoms, which the patient may then blame on the drug, but also with *rebound anxiety and insomnia.* Thus, patients on such a short course of a benzodiazepine night sedative should be warned that they will find it difficult to sleep for a few days on stopping their medication.

Only about one-third of long-term benzodiazepine users will experience a withdrawal syndrome upon stopping their medication. Numerous symptoms have been identified as characteristic of a benzodiazepine withdrawal syndrome. These include:

- neurotic symptoms, such as panic, agoraphobia, anxiety and insomnia
- neurological symptoms, such as ataxia, paraesthesia, hyperacusis and micropsia
- other major symptoms, such as hallucinations, psychosis and, in 1%, epilepsy.

The emergence of three new symptoms on discontinuation of benzodiazepine medication, or any symptom not part of the psychiatric disorder for which it was prescribed, such as epilepsy, are indicative of dependency. It should be noted, however, that before the benzodiazepines became available, barbiturates were widely used as anxiolytics and were associated with a much greater degree of dependency, as well as being more dangerous in overdose. Benzodiazepines are rarely fatal in overdose in normal individuals, unless combined with alcohol abuse or other drugs.

Ideally the second choice of (but first-line drug) treatment of generalized anxiety disorder, if anxiety management training and cognitive treatment fail, is to use *SSRIs or serotonin–noradrenaline reuptake inhibitors (SNRIs)*, which are often better tolerated than tricyclic antidepressants or monoamine oxidase inhibitors (MAOIs), which are also effective. The combination of SSRIs and CBT may be superior to either alone.

Buspirone is a 5-HT_{1A} receptor agonist and is suitable for the short-term management of severe anxiety when a rapid onset of effect is not essential, and for the treatment of anxious patients with a history of dependence on alcohol or sedatives/hypnotics. It has a progressive onset of action. It has diminished efficacy in previous benzodiazepine users and produces the side-effects of dizziness, headache and nausea. It results in minimal sedation and psychological impairment and has no interactions with alcohol or other psychotropic drugs. It has a low or absent risk of dependence or abuse.

β-Adrenergic antagonists (β-blockers) are effective in patients with somatic anxiety symptoms caused by autonomic hyperactivity, such as palpitations, tremor and blushing. Patients may have found that blushing is also countered by cigarette smoking. β-Blockers do not affect symptoms caused by increased motor tension, such as headache, nor do they affect sweating, dry mouth, nausea, diarrhoea or frequency of micturition. They have side-effects of tiredness, occasional nightmares and possibly depression, and are contraindicated in cases of asthma and heart block. They are non-sedative and do not result in psychological impairment, abuse or dependence.

Low-dose antipsychotic medications, such as trifluoperazine or flupentixol, have also been used to some effect. Antipsychotic medication can augment a limited response to SSRIs. Although there is probably no risk of true dependence, they can produce extrapyramidal side-effects and have a risk of tardive dyskinesia.

Pregabilin, which has been used in neuropathic pain, has also more recently been found to be of use.

Course and prognosis

The more chronic the generalized anxiety disorder, the worse the prognosis. A stable premorbid personality is a good prognostic sign. Generalized anxiety disorder can be complicated by the development of agoraphobia, secondary depression and abuse of alcohol and anxiolytics. Overall the course is variable and fluctuating, but chronic.

Anxiety disorders

- Anxiety is a normal mood and, like pain, a warning.
- Anxiety is accompanied by bodily (somatic) symptoms due to Cannon's (adrenergic) fight or flight reaction.
- Primary generalized anxiety disorder is rare compared to mixed anxiety and depressive disorder.
- Anxiety is more often associated with other psychiatric disorders, such as depression, than generalized anxiety disorder, especially when the onset is after the age of 35 years.
- Cognitive therapy and anxiety management techniques are effective treatments for generalized anxiety disorder.
- Benzodiazepines should not be prescribed as hypnotics for more than 10 nights, or as anxiolytics for more than four weeks, owing to the risk of dependency.

Panic disorder (episodic paroxysmal anxiety)

Panic disorder is characterized by acute and unprovoked (spontaneous) discrete periods of intense fear or discomfort (panic attacks) owing to intense acute psychic and somatic anxiety symptoms, which are unexpected and not triggered by situations. During an attack patients experience a sudden crescendo of fear and autonomic symptoms, resulting in a usually hurried exit from wherever they are: they are unable to sit out such attacks. They may also experience feelings of impending doom or death (*'angor animus'*), and somatic symptoms such as shortness of breath, palpitations, chest pain, tremor, faintness, dizziness, choking or smothering sensations. In fact, fear of dying, going mad or losing control are cardinal features. The attacks usually last for less than 30 minutes, with a peak of intensity around 10 minutes. Nocturnal panic attacks during sleep and non-fearful panic attacks with no psychological but only physiological symptoms can rarely occur.

If panic attacks occur in a specific situation (situational), such as on a bus or in a crowd, the patient may subsequently avoid and develop a phobia (inappropriate fear) of that situation, and even generalized agoraphobia. A panic attack is often followed by a persistent fear of having another attack and of being alone. Between attacks there is comparative freedom from anxiety symptoms, although anticipatory anxiety is common and may itself precipitate an attack. Table 10.2 summarizes the ICD-10 diagnostic criteria for panic disorder. DSM-IV-TR allows for both spontaneous and situational panic disorder, i.e. with or without agoraphobia.

The frequency of panic attacks is not an accurate measure of the severity of panic disorder or the likely treatment response.

Panic disorder is maintained because the individual fears the somatic sensations associated with panic attacks. However, the only danger is subjective, due to the individual's interpretations of panic or its meaning or consequences (e.g. as threatening or dangerous). Catastrophic interpretations lead to anxious apprehension of future episodes and an increased vigilance regarding bodily sensations. Increasing autonomic nervous system arousal results and is then noted and responded to with fear, which in turn results in a further panic attack. Thus, a *conditioned fear of fear pattern* develops, with anxiety itself becoming a phobic (feared) stimulus. Individuals may stop undertaking physical exercise because this results in a raised heart rate, which sets the pattern into operation again and results in further panic attacks. The fear response may also increase muscle tension and lead to hyperventilation, exacerbating the overall experience and further aggravating the vicious cycle.

Panic disorder may also be the cause of unexplained medical symptoms.

Panic originates from the Greek god Pan, who frightened humans and animals out of the blue.

Epidemiology

Although the lifetime prevalence for isolated panic attacks without agoraphobia has been found to be up to 28%, panic disorder occurs only in 1–2% of the general population, more commonly, by two to three times, in females more than males, and may be worse premenstrually. The lifetime prevalence is around 4%, compared with 8% for panic attacks alone. The age of onset is bimodal, with the highest peak between ages 15 and 25 years and a second peak between 45–and 54 years.

Comorbidity

Agoraphobia occurs in 30–50% of cases with higher rates seen in psychiatric settings. The risk of attempted suicide is raised where there is comorbid depression (two-thirds of cases), alcohol misuse (up to one-third), or substance misuse. Comorbidity with medical conditions and bipolar disorder is also seen.

Differential diagnosis

Panic attacks can occur in established phobic disorders (situational anxiety with avoidance) in relation to the corresponding phobic situation, and also secondarily to depressive disorders, particularly in males. Some studies suggest comorbidity with depression or dysthymia may be up to 45%. They may also result from intoxication with caffeine or amphetamines or withdrawal from substances such as barbiturates.

Physical disorders such as hypoglycaemia, phaeochromocytoma and hyperthyroidism must also be considered.

Aetiology

There is evidence of a genetic inherited predisposition, with increased concordance rates for monozygotic compared to dizygotic twins. Ninety-five per cent of patients with panic disorder have been found to have a genomic duplication (DUP25) on chromosome 15, compared with 7% of the general population. Such a predisposition may result from a biological vulnerability to this disorder related to ease of autonomic arousal, a lower threshold for initial panic attacks and also ease of anxious apprehension elicited by stress. There is an increased family history of agoraphobia, depression and suicide. An association has also been found between panic disorder and childhood parental death or separation from the mother. Premorbid overanxious personalities or otherwise high levels of anxiety predispose an individual to panic disorder. Panic disorder (and agoraphobia) also follows in about 17% of cases after the implantation of a cardioversion defibrillator, increasing in rate to one in five if it has been discharged.

An association with benign joint laxity has been described, with an apparent 15 times increase in incidence. Panic attacks may also be provoked by excessive caffeine intake, injections of sodium lactate, sympathomimetic drugs and carbon dioxide inhalation. The *suffocation alarm theory* of panic disorder postulates a central carbon dioxide hypersensitivity.

Other theories include increased post-synaptic response to serotonin, increased adrenergic activity, and decreased GABA inhibitory reactive sensitivity. Pentagastrin and lactate both induce panic. It is also postulated that the amygdala, hypothalamus and brain stem areas that mediate fear may also have a role.

Management

Advances in treatment in the last decade have led to success rates of 80–100% with CBT. A success rate of 50–60% has been achieved with pharmacological treatments alone such as antidepressants and benzodiazepines.

Psychological treatments

There is good evidence for the efficacy of both behavioural methods (exposure to counter phobic avoidance, relaxation and control of hyperventilation), and cognitive methods (education about anxiety and panic and thinking errors). The *CBT* approach is the first-line treatment and involves an initial education about the nature of panic attacks and the generation of fear of fear cycles. *Cognitive restructuring* is undertaken to enable the individual to identify particular catastrophic interpretations and to substitute more adaptive cognitions in their place. This is often achieved by a question-and-answer technique to detect flaws in logic, for example asking the individual to look at the actual frequency of fainting, which is usually zero, compared to the number of panic attacks experienced.

As thoughts are difficult to change without corrective experiences, *interoceptive exposure techniques* are used to achieve a controlled exposure of the individual to somatic sensations of anxiety and panic, with the goal of habituation to such symptoms, so they can be experienced without fear. Carbon dioxide inhalation and physical exercise have been used to this end. For instance, running on the spot produces a rapid heart rate and heavy legs. Dizziness and disorientation can be produced by the individual spinning or turning the head quickly, and hyperventilation will generate blurred vision, feelings of light-headedness, tingling, numbness and hot flushes. Depersonalization can be produced by staring at a fixed object or mirror for a period. Such exercises can be practised for one to two minutes, during which the patient's catastrophic thoughts are also elicited to demonstrate that catastrophic experiences do not follow. This process is called 'hypothesis testing'.

Cognitive restructuring and interoceptive exposure can be undertaken individually or in groups, and often involve homework practice with more diverse, prolonged and natural interoceptive exposure exercises.

Secondary agoraphobic avoidance owing to panic disorder is treated by *situational exposure*, and *anxiety management techniques* and skills are taught where appropriate. For example, the patient can be instructed in muscle relaxation techniques and breathing retraining (i.e. to teach diaphragmatic and slow breathing skills to those who hyperventilate).

The CBT approach to panic disorder can be successfully completed within about 12–15 sessions, and its effect is maintained over time, as such skills can leave the individual with a sense of mastery of the condition, compared with the feelings of loss of self-control that often accompany the use of drugs. Individuals can also have occasional CBT group booster sessions from time to time.

Brief panic-focused psychodynamic psychotherapy to counter fears of being trapped and abandoned has also been used.

Drug treatments

Pharmacological treatments have proven efficacy but discontinuation difficulties arise in up to 50% of cases owing to the re-emergence of symptoms upon stopping treatment. *Antidepressants*, especially the SSRIs (the first-line drug treatment in the NICE guidelines) and also clomipramine, a tricyclic with a similar action on serotonin, are effective. Indeed, SSRIs should be regarded as the second-line treatment if CBT fails. Antidepressants may affect autonomic reactivity. They have a slower onset of action than the *benzodiazepines*, which tend to be effective only in the short term, although tolerance to anti-panic effects is said not to develop as it does with sedation, and can also cause dependency with long-term use. NICE states that benzodiazepines should not be used in panic disorder. Pharmacological treatments are currently more commonly prescribed than cognitive-behavioural approaches, which require a skilled therapist. CBT, also recommended by NICE, may be used as an adjunct to or replacement for pharmacological treatment if this alone has been unsuccessful after two to three months. Drug treatment can improve the efficacy of CBT.

Prognosis

With treatment the prognosis is good (50–60% remit with medication; 80–100% with CBT). However, a follow-up study over 20 years showed that less than 50% of patients were entirely panic panic-free. Untreated panic disorder frequently develops into other psychiatric conditions, such as depressive disorder.

Mixed anxiety and depressive disorder (or anxiety depression)

In this disorder, symptoms of anxiety and depression are both present but neither is clearly predominant. Mixed pictures of neurotic disorders are much more common than discrete entities, such as generalized anxiety disorder. Mixed anxiety and depressive disorder is frequently seen, with up to half of those with anxiety disorder meeting diagnostic criteria for depression. It is, in fact, the most common psychiatric disorder in primary care. There are many more individuals in the population who suffer from this condition but who never come to medical or psychiatric attention. Anxiety is a mood about the future, whereas depression is a mood about the past. Table 10.7 demonstrates the theoretical differential diagnosis between pure anxiety and pure depressive disorders.

Table 10.7 Differential diagnosis between generalized anxiety and depressive disorders

Generalized anxiety disorder	Depressive disorder
Common in early adult life	More common in later adult life
Onset age 20–40 years	Onset age 20–60+ years
More frequent in those of premorbid anxious personality	More frequent in those of previous stable personality
Previous episodes of anxiety	Previous episodes of depression or even mania
Panic attacks frequent	Panic attacks rare
Lack of concentration	Loss of interest (anhedonia)
Minor loss of appetite	Major loss of appetite or increased appetite
Sexual performance reduced	Reduced libido
No diurnal variation of mood	Marked diurnal variation of mood
Initial insomnia	Early morning wakening
Somatic symptoms common	Ideas of reference, guilt and hopelessness common
More related to external precipitants	Less frequently related to external precipitants
Chronic course	Episodic course

Diagnostic category often changes over time and in medical records; 90% of those with neurotic disorders will at some point be diagnosed as suffering from depression

Management

Treatment of mild mixed anxiety and depressive disorder may be best undertaken by counselling, cognitive therapy or psychotherapy, especially interpersonal therapy, but it is also frequently treated in general practice by medication. Treating the depression usually relieves anxiety symptoms. Antidepressant medication is more effective than anxiolytic medication. The SSRIs are often better tolerated than standard tricyclics. It may, however, be necessary to treat both the depression and the anxiety. In clinical practice, a common error is to misdiagnose depressive disorder or mixed anxiety and depressive disorder as merely a generalized anxiety disorder, and prescribe minor tranquillizers, such as benzodiazepines, often for long periods, with the associated increased risk of dependency. Such misdiagnosis often occurs because anxiety is present in nearly all cases of depression and may appear to be the predominant symptom.

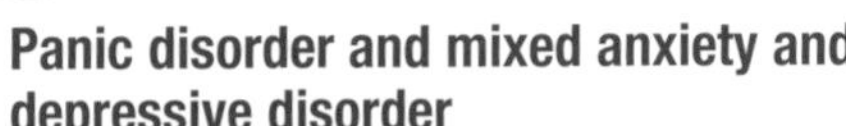

Panic disorder and mixed anxiety and depressive disorder

- Panic attacks are discrete periods of intense fear or discomfort caused by acute psychic and somatic anxiety symptoms, which are unexpected and not triggered by situations.
- Panic disorder is effectively treated by cognitive-behavioural approaches.
- Antidepressants, especially the SSRIs and clomipramine, are also beneficial in panic disorder.
- A diagnosis of mixed anxiety and depressive disorder is made when symptoms of both anxiety and depression are present, but neither set of symptoms is severe enough to justify a separate diagnosis.
- Neurotic disorders, by convention, do not now include depression if this is the predominant symptom. It is instead classified under mood (affective) disorders as a depressive episode.

Phobic disorders (phobic neurosis)

Fear is a normal prudent situational anxiety, for instance if one is under threat of attack. A *phobia* is an inappropriate situational anxiety with avoidance. The degree of avoidance is a useful measure of the severity of the disorder. The three main groups of phobic disorders and the lifetime prevalence rates are:

- specific (isolated) phobias (11.3%)
- agoraphobia (6.7%)
- social phobias (13.3%).

Table 10.2 outlines the ICD-10 diagnostic criteria for these three groups.

Specific (isolated) phobias or simple or monosymptomatic phobias

In specific phobias there is a persistent inappropriate fear of a circumscribed external object or situation, which leads to avoidance. Animal phobias occur equally in children of both sexes, but in adulthood are more common in women. An individual with a phobia of cats will develop an immediate anxiety response in their presence and will avoid them, for instance by crossing to the other side of the road. Such specific phobias often start and are statistically normal in children. They often clear in early adulthood but are still common in a mild form in adults (e.g. fears of heights, dark and spiders). For instance, half of adults are fearful of snakes. About 10% of the general population have clinically significant specific phobias, most having developed in childhood, but only a small proportion seek professional help. The resultant incapacity depends on the frequency with which the phobic situation is encountered in daily life. For instance, an individual with a flying phobia may rarely have to confront this situation, unless air journeys are important to work or social life, and treatment may not be necessary, at least for most of the year. However, avoidance of more common specific phobic objects, such as dogs and cats, may greatly interfere with an individual's daily activities, although specific phobias are less handicapping than other types of phobia. Also incapacitating is space phobia, which is a fear of falling when there is no nearby support.

Phobias of blood and bodily injury lead to bradycardia and hypotension upon exposure, in contrast to the tachycardia and increased blood pressure seen with other phobias. Such physiological changes on seeing blood could have conferred evolutionary advantage. This type of specific phobia is associated with a strong family history, often going back generations, and may be associated with a strong vasovagal reflex.

Agoraphobia

The term agoraphobia originates from the Greek for fear of the market-place, but it now has a wider meaning than just fear of open or public spaces. It also involves fear of being far from home, family and friends. The individual is fearful of being in places or situations where escape may be difficult or help unavailable if a panic attack were to occur. Individuals become anxious in anticipation of going out, particularly when unaccompanied, and this may restrict their activities. Avoidance, including an inability to enter shops, usually develops, and in its extreme form results in individuals becoming housebound. Not all individuals who develop avoidance have a history of panic attacks, but around two-thirds do. Agoraphobia can either precede or follow panic attacks. Shortness of breath is more common in panic attacks in agoraphobia. Breathlessness, dizziness, feelings of suffocation and fear of dying are common. Individuals with agoraphobia often feel worse the further they are from their home, and, when out, they may be better in the company of someone else, unlike in social phobia. In its extreme form, individuals may even be unable to open the front door to retrieve items from the doorstep.

The clinical picture often includes *claustrophobia* (fear of closed spaces), as well as of crowded places, main roads and public transport. Individuals may abuse alcohol or drugs in an effort to overcome their phobia. Others become depressed as a result of the restrictions on their lifestyle, which, in turn, further exacerbates the agoraphobia.

Although specific (isolated) phobias are the most common in the general population, 60% of the phobic patients seen by psychiatrists suffer from agoraphobia. Such individuals often have a history of childhood fears and school phobia. Over two-thirds to three-quarters are female. They are often married and have a high incidence of sexual problems. However, pure agoraphobia is rare compared with comorbid presentations with panic disorder and/or major depression.

Social phobia

Social phobia is characterized by the persistent fear of situations in which the person is subject to possible scrutiny by others and by fears that he may act in a humiliating or embarrassing way. Such situations may include eating in a restaurant or public speaking. Social phobias may be specific, such as speaking or urinating in public, or generalized, with the individual experiencing distress in any social setting, even speaking on the telephone. Symptoms may include blushing and muscle twitching.

Social phobia can be precipitated by stressful or humiliating experiences, death of a parent,

Case history: agoraphobia

Mrs A.B. was a 25-year-old married housewife. From a professional family background, she had a childhood history of enuresis (bedwetting) and excessive childhood fears of animals, such as dogs. Her father was rather passive and her mother overprotective. At the age of 11 she became increasingly reluctant to go to school and, on occasions, refused, in order to stay at home with her mother.

Mrs A.B. developed into a shy and anxious adolescent and at the age of 18 married a travelling salesman, on whom she became excessively emotionally dependent. There were some sexual difficulties in their relationship. With her husband often away with his work, she began to develop increasing anxiety on, and then fear of, going out alone. She began to experience severe anxiety and panic when using the bus or underground train and when in crowded shopping centres. She feared either losing control and making a fool of herself, or fainting when in crowded places. She felt worse the further she was from home and better when escorted by her husband. She began to abuse benzodiazepine anxiolytic drugs and alcohol to overcome her fears. She also became increasingly despondent at the limitations her condition was placing on her life.

Following the sudden and unexpected death of her father from a heart attack, her symptoms rapidly escalated such that she effectively became housebound. With much reluctance, but with the encouragement of her husband, she sought help from her GP, who referred her for a psychiatric assessment. Mrs A.B. subsequently agreed to stop abusing alcohol and was given supportive psychotherapy to help her overcome her grief at her father's death. Following a detailed assessment by a clinical psychologist, Mrs A.B., having agreed the goals of treatment, was advised to go out alone for increasing distances (a graded hierarchy). This was combined with relaxation training with the help of tapes (systematic desensitization). She was also given homework assignments to undertake, involving increasing the frequency and distance of outings from home, which also required the active participation of her husband. She was. initially prescribed benzodiazepines to get her out of the home, and subsequently the MAOI antidepressant phenelzine, which specifically relieves symptoms of agoraphobia.

In spite of some temporary setbacks with fluctuating anxiety when she went out, which she was advised she would experience, within 3 months she was again able to travel alone to shopping centres and other crowded places, including cinemas and using public transport. In fact, she developed a social life greater than she had previously experienced. Although her husband was pleased that he no longer had to restrict his work in order to either accompany his wife or to undertake shopping tasks without her, he had to adjust to her increased independence and self-confidence, which was also reflected in her regaining a normal sexual drive and sexual functioning.

separation or chronic exposure to stress, or it may have an insidious onset. Twin studies suggest a genetic vulnerability. There is little spontaneous remission and chronicity is associated with comorbidity with depression, other anxiety disorders and substance abuse in 75% of cases. Blushing is particularly characteristic of panic attacks in social phobia. Palpitations, trembling and sweating are also common.

Social phobia is more common than previously considered and occurs in 3–4% of the general population, but first-degree relatives are three times more likely to be affected. It is associated with panic disorder and other anxiety disorders, which may have led to its delayed recognition as a syndrome apart from agoraphobia. Social phobics may abuse alcohol or drugs to counter social anxiety prior to social interaction. Social phobics, who may have competent social skills, should be differentiated from those with poor social skills that lead to social anxiety. They may as children have had temperaments of behavioural inhibition. Although individuals with social phobia may well have been shy adolescents, this should be distinguished from anxious (avoidant) personality disorder, although there is comorbidity in 50% of cases of each condition. Those with avoidant personality disorder are shy and lack social confidence. Those with social phobia show marked anxiety and avoidance. Social avoidance may also be caused by depression, panic disorder, schizophrenia and physical illness. Those with schizoid personality disorder lack an interest in socializing.

Table 10.8 shows the age of onset, sex ratio, characteristics and treatment of specific (isolated) phobias, agoraphobia and social phobias. Table 10.9 shows factors relevant to the differential diagnosis of social phobia and depression; Table 10.10 shows factors relevant to the differential diagnosis of social phobia and panic disorder.

High rates of comorbidity are, however, seen in social phobia, e.g., other neurotic disorders, depression, post-traumatic stress disorder and substance abuse.

On *mental state examination* in a clinic, an individual with a phobia may appear relaxed and otherwise normal, as the phobic object or situation is not present.

Aetiology

There is some limited evidence of a *genetic inherited predisposition* to develop agoraphobia (heritability 0.30), social phobia and phobia of small animals (heritability 0.47), but not of other phenomena. In agoraphobia, there is an increased concordance for

Table 10.8 Age of onset, sex ratio, characteristics and treatment response of phobias

	Specific phobias	Agoraphobia	Social phobia
Age of onset	In childhood, three to eight years	15–30 years, most early – mid-20s	Peaks at five years and between 11 and 15 years. Presentation often delayed until late teenage/early 20s up to 35 years
	F more than M	F 2.5 : 1 M	F 2.5 : 1 M (F = M in those seeking treatment)
Feared objects	Animals (zoophobia)	Open spaces	Formal social occasions
	Thunder (tonitrophobia)	Crowded places	Eating in public
	Heights (acrophobia)	Main roads	Talking socially
	Spiders (arachnophobia)	Public transport	
	Bees (apiphobia)	Housebound syndrome	
	Birds (ornithophobia)		
CBT	+++	+	++
SSRIs or MAOIs	–	+	+

CBT, cognitive behavioural therapy; F, female; M, male; MAOI, monoamine oxidase inhibitor; SSRI, selective serotonin reuptake inhibitor.

Table 10.9 Differential diagnosis of social phobia and depression

	Social phobia	Depression
Loss of interest (anhedonia)	–	+
Energy	Normal	Reduced

Table 10.10 Differential diagnosis of social phobia and panic disorder

	Social phobia	Panic disorder
Panic attacks	In feared social situation	Unpredictable
Fear	Appearing foolish or awkward	Losing control or death
Social encounter if with friends	Little difference	Can enjoy

monozygotic compared to dizygotic twins and an increased family history of panic disorder and agoraphobia. In social phobia, there is an increased concordance rate for monozygotic compared to dizygotic female twins (24% versus 15%), whereas for simple or specific animal phobias there is evidence of increased concordance for monozygotic, compared to dizygotic (26% versus 11%), but not for situational phobias, which seem more environmentally determined. Specific phobias may originate in normal childhood fears. Even one-year-old babies are fearful of writhing and darting animals and heights, but not, for instance, of man-made dangerous objects such as guns. Such inborn fears may have been of evolutionary value.

Phobias can perhaps be best understood in terms of *behavioural learning theory* (Figure. 10.7). The *Pavlovian classical conditioning* model is illustrated by the case of Little Albert. In 1920, the American psychologist Watson caused Albert, then 11 months old, to develop a fear of his favourite furry toy rat by making a loud noise behind him when he attempted to touch it. This fear later generalized to a fear of all furry objects, and even to men with beards and his mother's fur neckpiece. Pavlovian classical conditioning with generalization might thus explain the development of a phobia, which is, in effect, the pairing of a conditioned stimulus – the phobic situation – with an unconditioned stimulus (e.g. unexpected noise) to produce the response of fear. This seems to apply in social phobias where the conditioned fear response may be environmentally determined and triggered by the social situation in which anxiety first occurred. However, only some individuals with specific animal phobias can recall their phobias being precipitated, for instance by being frightened or bitten by such animals in childhood.

Skinnerian or operant conditioning argues that the frequency of a behaviour can be altered by its consequences, such as reward or punishment. For example, avoidance of a phobic situation would be associated with a temporary reduction in anxiety, which is rewarding and thus reinforces the avoidance. This is a maladaptive learning response. The adaptive response would be to confront the phobic situation, even though this would produce a temporary increase in anxiety. The individual would then learn that such fear is excessive and inappropriate, the anxiety level would decrease and the phobia should thereafter be extinguished.

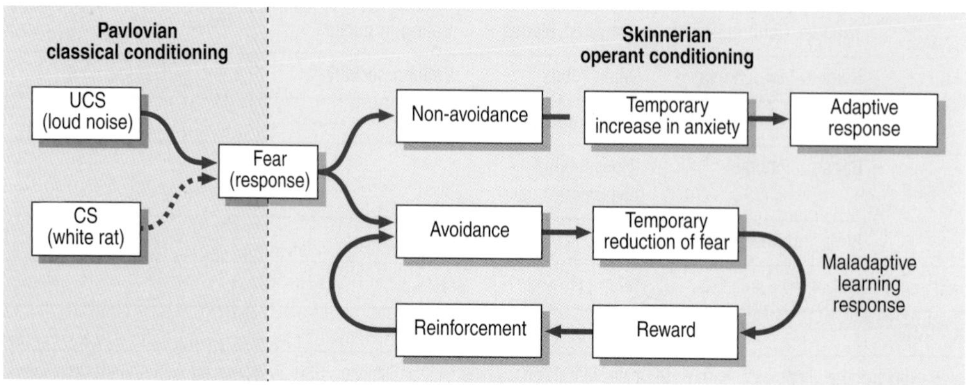

Figure 10.7 • Behavioural learning theory and the development of phobias.

In *Freudian psychoanalytic theory*, phobic neuroses arise from intrapsychic anxiety caused by emotional conflict being concentrated into a specific situation by the defence mechanism of displacement. This leaves the individual free and able to cope with other situations in life. Other defence mechanisms such as projection and avoidance may also be pertinent. In 1909, Freud described the development of a phobia of horses in a five-year-old child called Little Hans. Freud postulated that Hans' fear of his father, and specifically of castration, was displaced on to horses in general after seeing a male horse urinate in the street. Freud's assessment, however, was based on information from Hans' father and not on the basis of an interview with Hans himself. Psychoanalytic explanations conceptualize phobias as symbolic representations of conflict, frequently of a sexual nature, that prevent the individual going into a situation symbolic of that conflict. In agoraphobia, for example, a road with much traffic may represent sexual intercourse to an individual afraid of developing a sexual relationship. However, in spite of such theories, psychoanalysis is a very ineffective treatment of phobias in general.

The *'preparedness' theory* suggests that fear of some objects may be evolutionary adaptive to increase survival of the individual or species, and may thus be difficult to extinguish. An ethological theory of an evolutionary determined genetic vulnerability to unfamiliar territory has also been proposed to account for agoraphobia.

Predisposing, precipitating and perpetuating factors

The development of phobias may follow a childhood parental death. Individuals with phobic disorder are also more likely to have a dependent, emotionally immature and possibly introverted premorbid personality, but this is not invariable. In the case of agoraphobia, although it can arise spontaneously, it is frequently precipitated by traumatic events such as bereavement, illness and divorce. Social phobias tend to develop from adolescence, and more commonly in shy, anxious and avoidant individuals with low self-esteem, and also in those who have experienced parental separation, overcontrolling maternal upbringing, and childhood sexual abuse.

Phobias might be prevented by generally encouraging children to face feared situations rather than avoid them. Fears may be passed on from one generation to another within a family and, similarly, they vary according to cultural background.

Perpetuating factors may include alcohol and drug abuse, and also the collusion of family members. For instance, an agoraphobic female may obtain from her condition secondary gain from her spouse having to accompany her, or do the shopping instead of her, and he may collude in this because of his desire to have his wife dependent on him. In addition, phobic disorders get worse with intercurrent depressive episodes, which may be in reaction to the phobias and the limitations they impose on the individual, or which may coexist with them, or indeed predate them.

Management

Psychological treatment

Behaviour therapy is the treatment of choice for phobias, but requires a patient's commitment. It is most effective, in 75% of cases, for specific phobias. *Exposure techniques* are the most widely used, where the way in which avoidance maintains anxiety is explained and the individual is encouraged to face rather than avoid the phobic situation. This can be done in a graded way, tackling easier situations first and practising this repeatedly before confronting more difficult situations.

Exposure techniques developed from the behavioural technique of *systematic desensitization* (originally described by Wolpe), in which relaxation training is combined with gradual exposure to the phobic stimulus over a number of sessions. The stimulus is presented in a progressively more anxiety-provoking form (*a graded hierarchy*), either in fantasy but more effectively *in vivo*. It is based on the *principle of reciprocal inhibition*, i.e. if a response incompatible with anxiety, such as relaxation, is produced while the subject is exposed to the source of this anxiety, then the fear and avoidance response will be extinguished. Thus, a systematic desensitization programme for an individual with a phobia of spiders (arachnophobia) might involve a graded hierarchy from thinking about spiders to being in the presence of a dead spider in a room, and then a live spider being brought progressively nearer to the individual until, with agreement, the individual might tolerate actually touching and holding it. Treatment goals should be agreed with the individual, for example the goal for someone with a spider phobia might be merely to be in the same room as a spider, or it may be to hold it in the hand. 'Applied tension' may be additionally required in phobias of blood and bodily injury to counter the bradycardia and hypotension.

Flooding (implosion) is a behavioural technique where the individual is maximally exposed to the feared stimulus, under supervision, until anxiety reduction and/or exhaustion occurs. This is based on the assumption that an individual cannot maintain a maximum level of anxiety indefinitely (in fact, beyond about 40 minutes). For instance, an individual with a phobia of heights may be taken, with consent, to the top of a tower block and asked to remain there with a therapist until the anxiety subsides. Such procedures can, of course, be distressing and the individual must be physically fit enough (e.g. with no cardiac disease etc.) to tolerate them. They are probably no more effective in the long term than other exposure techniques.

In *modelling*, the individual observes the therapist engaging in non-avoidant behaviour in relation to the phobic stimulus. The idea is that the individual should later copy such behaviour. Modelling may sometimes be usefully added to exposure and other behavioural treatments.

Behavioural techniques may be undertaken in groups. For instance, a group of agoraphobic patients may be taken together to the feared situation of a town centre. Such techniques also frequently involve elements of self-help, including homework in which the family members may also have to participate. It is also of note that many sexual dysfunctions have phobic elements and can be treated behaviourally.

Where agoraphobia is accompanied by panic disorder, CBT is the treatment of choice, which uses graded self-exposure, cognitive therapy and/or behavioural experiments to test catastrophic beliefs and cease safety behaviours.

For social phobia, CBT is the treatment of choice. This involves explanation, structured exercises for recognizing maladaptive thinking, exposure to simulated situations provoking anxiety, cognitive restructuring of the patient's maladaptive thoughts, homework assignments and self-administered cognitive restructuring routines. Undertaken in groups, CBT is moderately beneficial. There is no evidence of specific benefit from social skills or relaxation training.

It is important to be aware that the behaviour of family members may reinforce the phobia and obstruct treatment, and that family members may need to be counselled accordingly.

Drug treatments

Agoraphobia and depression sometimes co-exist and antidepressant drugs are often used. *SSRIs* and *MAOIs*, such as phenelzine, are superior to placebo in specifically relieving symptoms of agoraphobia and social phobia, perhaps reflecting underlying abnormalities in the serotonergic and dopaminergic systems. *Tricyclic antidepressants* may be effective in those with depressive features. CBT is the treatment of choice for agoraphobia with panic disorder, and high-dose SSRIs are the second-line treatment, although response may not appear for six weeks and only reach a maximum level of benefit after 12 weeks.

Benzodiazepines can be used to prevent the reinforcement of fear through avoidance: diazepam, for instance, can be given one hour before an individual enters a phobic situation. However, anticipatory anxiety may sometimes be the main reinforcer of a phobia, so that benzodiazepines, for instance, taken four hours before a phobic situation, may be more effective. Benzodiazepines are, in any case, most effective when used in combination with behavioural techniques, especially in the initial stages (e.g. to allow the individual even to enter a phobic situation).

β-Adrenergic antagonists (*β-blockers*), such as propranolol, are effective if somatic symptoms predominate and reinforce a phobia, especially in specific social phobia. They do not work well in generalized social phobia. As they are non-sedative, these drugs can be particularly useful for driving tests, examinations and for those in the acting or music professions, where sedation may impair performance. β-Blockers have been used by snooker players to steady trembling arms and are certainly preferential to the use of alcohol for the same effect in professional darts players.

Although providing emotional support can be beneficial, psychoanalytic psychotherapy is considered to be very ineffective in the specific treatment of phobias.

Prognosis

Animal phobias have the best outcome. Social phobias tend to improve gradually and agoraphobias do worse, with a tendency towards chronicity.

Phobic disorders

- Fear is a normal prudent situational anxiety.
- A phobia is an inappropriate situational anxiety with avoidance.
- Specific (isolated) phobias, such as of animals, are the most common, but agoraphobia, a fear not only of open spaces but also of crowds and difficulty in making an easy escape, is most commonly seen by psychiatrists.
- Exposure techniques are the psychological treatment of choice and may involve homework assignments.
- SSRIs and MAOIs, such as phenelzine, specifically relieve symptoms of agoraphobia and social phobia.

Obsessive–compulsive disorder

Obsesssive–compulsive disorder is a *non-situational preoccupation* in which there is subjective *compulsion* despite conscious *resistance*. Such preoccupations can be thoughts (ruminations or obsessions) or acts (rituals or compulsions).

Ruminations are like having a tune stuck in one's head. The content is often absurd or alien to the individual's normal personality, such as preoccupations with sex, violence, accidents and death, although such thoughts are recognized as the individual's own (*cf.* thought insertion in schizophrenia, where there is a delusional belief that thoughts are externally inserted into the individual's mind). Ruminations may be recurrent words, thoughts, ideas or mental images that are persistent, unwelcome, egodystonic and intrusive, or which may be pointless or abstract. However, in general, sufferers do not act on their ruminations.

Rituals (Figure. 10.8) are akin to the childhood compulsion to walk between cracks in the pavement. They are repetitive and time-consuming, and usually cause distress. After an initial reduction in anxiety, rituals tend to increase anxiety further. They may involve obsessive washing or cleaning behaviour, or checking light switches or locks for example. Checking on three occasions is particularly common and has

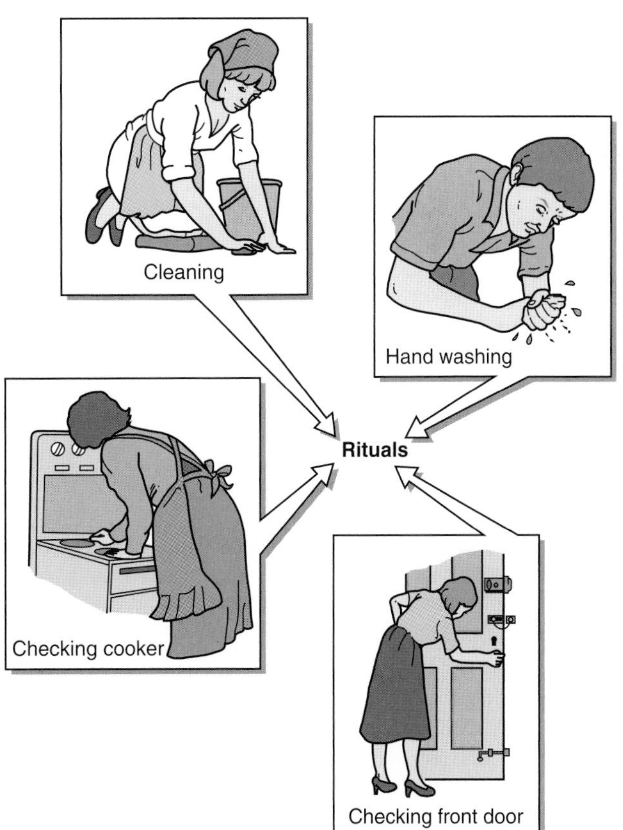

Figure 10.8 • Rituals characteristic of obsessive–compulsive behaviour.

been related to the holy trinity. Individuals may also count to a certain number before undertaking an activity. Although rituals are sometimes referred to as compulsions, both ruminations and rituals are compulsive.

In obsessive–compulsive disorder, insight is maintained in that individuals regard their ruminations or rituals as 'silly', but are unable to stop. This is in contrast to delusional ideas, which may be recurrent and preoccupying, but where insight is lost and the ideas are regarded as true. Also in contrast to rituals, stereotypies are regular repetitive non-goal-directed movements, such as foot tapping or utterances. These occur in conditions where insight is lost, such as chronic schizophrenia, infantile autism or mental handicap.

Research suggests that, particularly in chronic cases of obsessive–compulsive disorder, resistance to intrusive thoughts frequently abates and, indeed, may be absent and is therefore not an essential component of the disorder. In children, resistance is often absent. However, when conscious resistance is present it is this that helps generate the anxiety and tension, which are only relieved by again ruminating or performing the rituals.

Rituals may arise from obsessional doubts (*folie de doute*), and have been referred to as a small area of organization in the chaos of the individual's life. It is of note that when one normally checks switches or locks, one does not usually register (i.e. precisely remember) the activity, hence the capacity for obsessional doubting.

It is often helpful to individuals suffering from obsessive–compulsive disorder to point out that anxiety comes first, before the ruminations or rituals, which are seen as a defence against anxiety. The patient may otherwise regard them as evidence of madness. It should also be noted that depression and anxiety are common in obsessive–compulsive disorder.

So-called *illness phobias* can better be understood as obsessive–compulsive disorders because such individuals ruminate on whether they suffer from, for instance, cancer, AIDS or sexually-transmitted disease. These are non-situational preoccupations, as compared to a true phobia where there is an inappropriate external situational anxiety with avoidance.

Obsessions about contamination followed by washing are the most common pattern.

Individuals with washing rituals are often actually germ-phobic, but as it is not possible to see germs, they become dirt-phobic and generate washing rituals, even to the extent that they might wash up to 40 times a day.

Screening questions include enquiring about:

- worry about contamination, dirt and germs
- washing and checking excessively
- unwanted thoughts of which one cannot be rid
- doing things slowly in order to do them carefully
- over-concern about routine, orderliness and symmetry.

Extreme slowness out of proportion to other symptoms (*primary obsessional slowness*) is rare.

Case history: obsessive–compulsive disorder

Mr C.D. was a 27-year-old single man who worked as an accountant. He was devoted to his work. He had always had an anankastic (obsessive–compulsive) personality, even when he was at school, which meant he was over-conscientious and meticulous, a perfectionist, stubborn and independent. His devotion to his work was such that it prevented him developing leisure activities and friendships. He was not generous in giving time or gifts to others, towards whom he showed little affection. Although his obsessional personality traits were generally useful in his work, they also resulted in his being indecisive at times.

After making an error and being severely criticized by his superiors, Mr C.D. attempted to be even more scrupulous, meticulous and punctual at work, where he felt generally under increased stress. Before departing each morning he began repetitively to check that lights were out, windows were closed, household appliances turned off and that his street door was locked. At one level he knew such checking was silly, but he could not help it. He attempted to resist but this led to increased feelings of tension, which were only relieved by yielding to the compulsion. His checking rituals became increasingly complex, and he developed a certain order of checking things before he departed, starting upstairs with the light switches and ending by ensuring that all downstairs doors and windows were secured. He would check each object three times. His rituals developed to such an extent that it would take him 2 hours to complete them all, with the result that he was having to get up earlier to do so and was occasionally arriving late at work. This increased his anxiety and feelings of

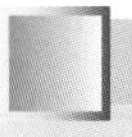

Case history: obsessive–compulsive disorder—cont'd

despondency about his life situation, and led to a worsening of his rituals.

Warned about late time-keeping, he sought help from his GP, who referred him to a psychiatrist. He was given counselling about the nature of his condition, including reassurance that the anxiety came first before the rituals, and that he was not going 'mad'. He was given a serotonin (5-HT) re-uptake inhibitor antidepressant to treat the depressive component of his disorder and referred to a clinical psychologist, who organized a behavioural programme of response prevention. This involved his being supervised at home by staff who would prevent his rituals and model behaviour without repetitive checking. He was taught self-imposed response prevention, and a relative came to stay with him initially to help him with this at home.

Mr C.D.'s improvement was such that he was able successfully to return to work, although he remained subject to exacerbations of his symptoms when under stress, especially when feeling despondent about his situation.

Epidemiology

Studies from the USA suggest that 2–3% of the population may suffer from obsessive-compulsive disorder at some time in their lives. Rates across the world are similar, although symptom themes vary. Minor obsessive–compulsive symptoms may be present in up to 17% of the population; one-month prevalence rates suggest it affects 1% of males and 1.5% of females. Males have an earlier onset. Two-thirds of individuals have an age of onset in the early 20s, before 25 years, with a mean age of about 22 years. It can even begin in childhood, with a peak age of onset of 12–14 years. Those with checking rituals have an earlier mean age of onset of 18 years, compared to other groups with a mean age of onset of 27 years. The course tends to be chronic, with exacerbations.

Differential diagnosis

Obsessional symptoms may be seen in up to 20–30% of cases of depressive disorder and also in schizophrenia, where it has been suggested that premorbid obsessional symptoms, arising even in childhood, might represent defences against psychosis. Obsessional symptoms also occur in organic psychoses, including early dementia, as well as anorexia nervosa and generalized anxiety disorder. Obsessional ruminations about harming one's baby occur as part of puerperal psychiatric disorders and, especially in cases of depression, should be taken very seriously to prevent them being acted on.

As discussed previously, delusional ideas may be recurrent and preoccupying, but insight is lost and they are regarded as true. Similarly, insight is lost in stereotypies, unlike obsessional rituals.

It is clinically useful to distinguish between the compulsions of obsessive–compulsive disorder and the *impulsive behaviour* of those with low impulse control and lack of resistance, such as individuals suffering from psychopathy or eating disorders, or those with disorders of sexual preference or gamblers.

Aetiology

The aetiology of obsessive–compulsive disorder is some way from being understood, and it is probable that its aetiology is different from other neurotic disorders. There is an increased genetic predisposition in first-degree relatives (3–7%) and a greater concordance between monozygotic (50–80%) and dizygotic twins (25%). However, types of rumination and ritual are not always the same in different affected family members. These is also a genetic association between *Tourette's syndrome*, chronic motor tic disorder and obsessive–compulsive disorder. Indeed, up to 20% of individuals with obsessive–compulsive disorder may have tics, which, in turn, are suggestive of basal ganglia disorder.

There is an increased incidence of obsessive–compulsive disorder in those who have suffered brain injury, for example owing to head injuries, encephalitis, including encephalitis lethargica, or syphilis. Neuropsychological studies show abnormalities in executive function. Evidence for a neurobiological basis has been accrued from positron emission tomography (PET) and functional magnetic resonance imaging (fMRI) techniques, in which orbito-frontal and cingulate cortices and basal ganglia abnormalities have been found. Reductions bilaterally in the size of the caudate nuclei and retrocallosal white matter have been found in structural MRI studies. There is also evidence for abnormalities in serotonin transmission or in its interaction with dopamine in the central nervous system. Some children and adolescents develop obsessive–compulsive disorder and motor tics after β-haemolytic streptococcal infections, suggesting a cell-mediated autoimmune aetiology against basal ganglia peptides affecting the cortico-striatal-thalamic-cortical circuits.

A premorbid *anankastic (obsessive–compulsive) personality disorder* is said to predispose to the subsequent development of obsessive–compulsive disorder, but is present in only about 15–35% of cases. Some studies suggest that a majority of sufferers have a premorbid anankastic personality, whereas others suggest that it is only a minority who do. Those with an anankastic personality are characteristically obsessional, rigid, orderly, punctual and stubborn. However, they do not resist their obsessionality and their thoughts are not alien to them. Certain obsessional personality traits, such as conscientiousness, can be useful unless they result in insecure dithering and indecisiveness.

In Freudian psychoanalytic theory, anankastic personality disorder originates at the anal training stage of development (e.g. due to harsh toilet training). Obsessive–compulsive disorder is seen as a regression back from the Oedipal to the anal-sadistic phase of development. Magical thinking (the belief that thinking about an event can cause it) is also cited (omnipotence of thought). Obsessional symptoms are considered to arise from intrapsychic anxiety due to emotional conflicts being expressed via the defence mechanisms of displacement, reaction formation and undoing (e.g. checking to feel secure). Obsessive–compulsive disorder may represent a defence against anxiety associated with sexual and aggressive impulses, and also a defensive regression to the anal stage of development.

Learning theory cannot fully account for obsessive–compulsive disorder, but does inform CBT. Anxiety comes first; obsessions follow. The latter give rise to more anxiety, which leads to compulsions to reduce the feared consequences of the obsession and level of anxiety, but this is only short-lived and serves only to reinforce the compulsion.

Management

In the treatment of obsessive–compulsive disorder, any depressive component or other comorbid intercurrent mental illness should also be effectively treated. The most common cause of ruminations is depression, not primary obsessive–compulsive disorder.

Psychological treatment

Supportive psychotherapy may be of value in pointing out to the individual that he or she is not going mad, and that anxiety comes before symptoms, which are seen as a defence against anxiety. However, psychoanalytic psychotherapy is ineffective as such patients show poor free association and may unprofitably ruminate during therapy, although anankastic personalities may benefit. This ineffectiveness may be further evidence in favour of a neurobiological basis for the condition.

CBT is effective. This involves graded self-exposure and self-imposed response prevention of the 'undoing' of obsessions through compulsions, and/or cognitive therapy.

In general, rituals are easier to treat than ruminations. One behavioural approach for rituals is *exposure and response prevention*, whereby individuals learn to cope with the increasing tension associated with resistance when they are prevented from undertaking their rituals. Prevention is by distraction, discussion and, occasionally, mild physical restraint. Inpatient treatment may be required for such treatment to be effective. Modelling can also be useful.

An alternative to response prevention is *mass practice*, in which the individual is told to keep repeating the rituals to a degree beyond that even he would wish to undertake voluntarily, until the anxiety reduces and the compulsion subsides.

Ruminations are less easy to treat. The technique of *thought stopping* can, however, be helpful. In this, an individual is asked to relax and ruminate, whereupon the therapist will shout 'Stop!', at which point the patient must alter the content of those thoughts. Shouting of the word 'Stop' is later replaced by the individual merely thinking of it. The technique is repeated until the individual can learn such thought control and to employ the technique as required. Smelling salts have also been used as an aversion technique to achieve thought stopping. An adjunctive method to thought stopping involves the additional use of snapping a well-fitting rubber band placed around the wrist whenever the individual has an obsessional thought. Individuals have also been taught to restrict their ruminating to a fixed period each day, and otherwise get on with their everyday lives.

Drug treatments

SSRIs at high doses are the drug treatment of choice and developed from the observation that the tricyclic antidepressant clomipramine (the tricyclic with the most powerful 5-HT reuptake inhibition) was helpful over months, e.g., 8 – 16 weeks, in 40–60% of cases. Their beneficial effect is not dependent on their antidepressant properties. They are superior to other tricyclic antidepressants, although these too have produced improvement, perhaps because they treat the often-associated depression. Clomipramine causes significant antimuscarinic (anticholinergic) side-effects and sexual difficulties, and can produce seizures at high doses. Clomipramine may be marginally superior, but SSRIs are better tolerated. MAOIs have also been used successfully.

Low-dose atypical antipsychotic medication appears to be more effective than benzodiazepines, possibly because of effect on conditioned responses. However, its use is as an adjunct to cases resistant to SSRIs, not as a monotherapy. Benzodiazepines may be helpful in the short term.

Placebo response rates in studies are low (about 5%) compared to other psychiatric disorders.

Overall, for severe cases of obsessive– compulsive disorder, it is usual in the UK to combine CBT with SSRIs or to use an SSRI alone, but the combination may be superior.

Psychosurgery

In severe, intractable, chronic and incapacitating cases, where all other treatments have failed, stereotactic site-specific brain surgery has been reported to be successful, although there is a lack of adequate trials and such procedures carry stigma. Radioactive yttrium implants and, more recently, non-invasive proton, electron and X-ray techniques have been used.

Anterior cingulotomy, capsulotomy and limbic leucotomy have been found to be effective in 25–30% of such cases. Cingulotomy carries a 1% risk of epilepsy. All involve a separation of the frontal cortex from deep limbic structures. A prerequisite for any such surgery is a stable premorbid personality, as those with a history of antisocial behaviour and alcoholism may be further disinhibited in their behaviour as a result of such procedures. In England and Wales, under the Mental Health Act 1983, Section 57, neurosurgery for this condition requires both the consent of the patient and the agreement of a second opinion to that of the patient's responsible clinician (consultant psychiatrist). It is banned for this purpose in some countries.

Prognosis

Obsessive–compulsive disorder can now be effectively treated in up to 70% of cases. The prognosis tends to be worse the more reasonable the preoccupation, for example checking that the house is locked before leaving home has a poorer prognosis than pointless rituals such as walking between cracks in the pavement. Other poor prognostic factors include early age of onset, the co-existence of obsessions and rituals, low social functioning at baseline, magical obsessions, and rituals.

Table 10.11 summarizes the treatments for generalized anxiety disorder, panic disorder, phobic disorders and post-traumatic stress disorder.

Obsessive–compulsive disorder

- Non-situational preoccupations with subjective compulsion despite conscious resistance.
- Can be thoughts (ruminations/obsessions) or acts (rituals/compulsions).
- Insight is maintained: 'It's silly but I can't stop it'.
- Obsessional symptoms are common in depressive disorder and any depressive component should always be adequately treated.
- CBT treatments include thought stopping for ruminations and response prevention for rituals
- SSRIs and clomipramine specifically treat obsessional symptoms.

Neurotic disorders in the elderly

In those over the age of 65 years, the incidence and prevalence of neurotic disorders is reduced (generalized anxiety disorder 4%, simple phobia 4%, agoraphobia up to 8%, social phobia 1%, and obsessive--compulsive disorder up to 0.8%). The onset of panic disorder in old age is unusual and depression and underlying physical disorders should be excluded. In the elderly, anxiety symptoms are often associated with depression, and may be

Table 10.11 Treatment of neurotic and stress-related disorders (treatment of choice given in italics)

Neurosis	CBT	Drugs
Generalized anxiety disorder	*Cognitive therapy*	SSRIs or SNRIs
	Anxiety management	Benzodiazepines, e.g. diazepam
	Applied relaxation techniques	β-Adrenoceptor antagonists
Panic disorder	*CBT*	SSRIs
Phobic disorder		
Specific phobia	*Behavioural therapy* with graded self-exposure and cessation of safety behaviours	
Agoraphobia	*CBT*	SSRIs
Specific social phobia	*CBT*	β-Adrenoceptor antagonists
General social phobia	*CBT*	SSRIs
Obsessive–compulsive disorder	*CBT*	
	Thought stopping	SSRIs
	Ritual prevention	Clomipramine
	Mass practice	
Post-traumatic stress disorder	*CBT* *EMDR*	SSRI or mirtazapine

NICE guidelines recommend the following:
Psychological therapy is more effective than pharmacological therapy, and should be used as first-line treatment. Pharmacological therapy is effective. Most evidence supports the use of SSRIs.
Generalized anxiety disorder. Benzodiazepines should not be used beyond two to four weeks. A SSRI is the first-line treatment. Self-help based on CBT principles should be encouraged.
Panic disorder. Benzodiazepines should not be used. A SSRI should be used as first-line treatment. Self-help based on CBT principles should be encouraged.
Obsessive–compulsive disorder. Use a SSRI or intensive CBT. Combine these if response to single strategy is sub-optimal. Use clomipramine if SSRIs fail. If response is still sub-optimal, consider adding an antipsychotic.

CBT, cognitive behavioural therapy; EMDR, eye movement desensitization processing; SNRI, serotonin–noradrenaline reuptake inhibitor; SSRI, selective serotonin reuptake inhibitor.

secondary to physical disorder, and also to prescribed drugs. Hypochondriacal symptoms are prominent.

Reactions to severe stress and adjustment disorders

ICD-10 provides a classification for a group of disorders that are a direct consequence of exceptionally stressful life events, producing *acute stress reactions*, or of significant life changes leading to continued unpleasant circumstances, which result in *adjustment disorders*. Whereas psychosocial stresses can precipitate the onset or contribute to the presentation of many psychiatric conditions, the disorders in this group would not occur without the impact of such stresses. They can be regarded as maladaptive responses to severe or continued stress in that they interfere with successful coping mechanisms and lead to impaired social functioning. Acts of self-harm, most commonly self-poisoning by a prescribed medication, may be associated closely in time with the onset of either an acute stress reaction or an adjustment disorder.

Acute stress reaction/disorder

Acute stress reaction in ICD-10 or acute stress disorder in DSM-IV-TR is a transient disorder that develops in an individual with no other apparent mental disorder in response to exceptional physical and/or mental stress; it usually subsides within hours or days. The stress may be an overwhelming traumatic experience involving serious threat to the subject or loved ones, or an unusually sudden and threatening change in their social position and/or network, such as multiple bereavement, a domestic fire, etc. The risk of developing this disorder is increased if physical exhaustion or other organic factors are present. Clearly, individual vulnerability and coping capacity are important, as not all those exposed to exceptional stress develop such a disorder. There is a mixed and usually changing picture of symptoms, typically including an initial state of 'daze', followed by depression, anxiety, anger, despair, over-activity (flight reaction or fugue) or withdrawal. No one symptom predominates for long, and the condition resolves rapidly within a few hours at most with removal from the stressful environment. When the stress continues or cannot be reversed, symptoms usually begin to diminish after 24–48 hours, and are usually minimal after three days.

This disorder was originally introduced into DSM-IV in 1994 to help identify those who would develop post-traumatic stress disorder. However, only about half of cases do so and the condition may be removed from DSM-5.

Post-traumatic stress disorder

Post-traumatic stress disorder (PTSD) is a common reaction of normal individuals, usually within six months, to an extreme trauma ('an exceptionally threatening or catastrophic experience'), which is likely to cause pervasive distress to almost anyone, such as natural or man-made disasters, combat, serious accidents, witnessing the violent death of others, being the victim of torture, terrorism, rape or other crimes. Man-made disasters are more likely to cause post-traumatic stress disorder than natural disasters. Although predisposing factors, such as personality traits or a previous history of neurotic or affective illness, may lower the threshold for the development of the syndrome or aggravate its course, they are neither necessary nor sufficient to explain its occurrence. The syndrome is characterized by five elements:

- experience of a major trauma
- intrusive recollections in the form of thoughts, nightmares and flashbacks
- sense of numbness and emotional blunting, which represents an attempt to avoid reminders of the trauma
- increased arousal and hypervigilance, with an enhanced startle reaction and insomnia
- the onset follows the trauma with a latency period of a few weeks to months, but not more than six months, and the condition lasts for at least one month.

Note that incomplete memory of the trauma can occur but is not characteristic.

The condition is seen as arising from the overwhelming and overloading of normal emotional processing. Emotional numbing/dissociation following traumatic events is predictive of post-traumatic stress disorder at six months.

Epidemiology

The lifetime prevalence has been estimated as 8% in the USA, with women twice as commonly affected as men. It occurs after a traumatic event in 8–13% of men and 20–30% of women. The exposure rates for significant traumatic events is much higher (61% of men and 52% of women).

Neurobiology

Abnormalities in the hypothalamo-pituitary-adrenal axis, including hypocortisolaemia and super-suppression in the dexamethasone suppression test, the opposite of what has been found in some studies of depression, together with abnormalities in regional blood flow in the basal ganglia and orbitofrontal cortex, as seen in obsessive compulsive–disorder, have been found, as have increased noradrenergic and serotonergic central activity.

Reduced hippocampal volume was reported in Vietnam War veterans with PTSD. The hippocampus mediates conscious memory, including of traumatic events, whereas the amygdala mediates unconscious memories, e.g., autonomic aspects of trauma. Decreased medial pre-frontal and anterior cingulate areas have been found in neuro-imaging studies, which correlate with increased activity in the amygdala, resulting in hypersensitivity to external threats, which is seen in PTSD.

Comorbid psychiatric diagnoses are present in up to 80% of sufferers. Anxiety and depression are commonly associated, and suicidal ideation may also occur. Both major depression and dysthymia may develop. The condition may be complicated by drug or alcohol abuse. Rarely, there may be dramatic acute episodes of fear, panic or aggression, triggered by stimuli that arouse a sudden recollection and/or a re-enactment of the trauma, or of the original reaction to it. Simple phobias, agoraphobia and social phobia may also develop.

PTSD, although not always referred to by that term, has been recognized throughout history. During the First World War, it was known as shell-shock, but it was the Vietnam War that provided the major impetus for research into and description of the condition, and since 1980 a number of natural disasters have led to its increasing recognition.

Prevention

Primary prevention has been attempted through stress inoculation in high-risk groups (e.g. exposure to dead bodies). Secondary prevention strategies that have been found to be of value in aiding early emotional processing include early meetings of groups of survivors, within one to two days if possible, where group discussion can set the individual's emotional reactions within the normal range, and *critical incident debriefing*. The long-term efficacy of such measures is, however, unproven, and inappropriate and ill-timed interventions or interventions which lead to inappropriate rumination on the trauma can be harmful. NICE in the UK does not recommend brief single session interventions.

Management

Many cases go undetected owing to the individual's reluctance to discuss symptoms and seek help. A high level of clinical suspicion is therefore required. Making the diagnosis can be reassuring to the individual, who often feels that no one can understand what he or she has been through. Specific treatment is indicated where symptoms have persisted for more than six months and social handicaps are significant. Self-help and mutual support groups, such as Rape Crisis Centres, can be of benefit. Central to most treatment approaches is the *rehearsal of the 'trauma story'*, either in a cognitive- behavioural approach, which may include imaginal or *in vivo* exposure, and which may be combined with adjunctive anxiety management, or in a technique called *'testimony'*. The aim is to rehearse the trauma and reawaken associated emotions, but in a way that can be tolerated and processed without leading to avoidance. Verbal recall represents behavioural exposure to a traumatic event and the aim is to achieve habituation to it. Audio-tape desensitization, using the individual's own account of the trauma, may also be of value. For torture survivors, the pain is often compounded by guilt and fear, for instance over actions they may have been forced to carry out. They are encouraged to reframe their thinking and to see that such actions were due not to their betrayal of others, but to the conditions to which they were subjected.

In the UK, NICE has made recommendations for sequential treatment in primary and secondary care settings, and recommended either a CBT approach or eye movement desensitization processing (EMDR). EMDR involves rapid and rhythmic eye movements induced by the patient visually tracking the therapist's finger moving back and forward for about 20 seconds, during which the patient focuses on the traumatic image and associated negative emotions, sensations and thought, and discusses such associated emotions. Once the distress begins to reduce, reference to positive thoughts for the event are encouraged. However, eye movement may not, in fact, be necessary, with the effectiveness of the procedure merely owing to inducing and facilitating desensitization.

Antidepressant medication, though not recommended as a routine first-line treatment, has also been found to be effective in the management of PTSD, treating the commonly associated depression, facilitating sleep and reducing intrusive memories. SSRIs have been cited as especially beneficial for core symptoms of PTSD at high doses for five to eight weeks. Tricyclic antidepressants help the intrusive symptoms and associated anxiety and depression. However, the MAOI phenelzine may be better than the tricyclic imipramine. Response may be delayed for up to eight weeks. NICE recommends the noradrenergic and specific serotonergic antidepressant (NaSSA) mirtazapine or the SSRI paroxetine. Benzodiazepines should be avoided because of their high dependency potential, but especially in the first two weeks following the trauma as this may interfere with the memory processing necessary to reduce symptoms.

Hospital disaster plans should also take into account the psychological responses of victims.

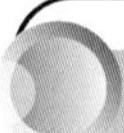

Post-traumatic stress disorder

- A reaction of normal individuals to a major trauma.
- Intrusive recollections, emotional numbing, increased autonomic arousal and hypervigilance occur.
- Meetings of groups of survivors and critical incident debriefing within one to two days may be preventative.
- Self-help and mutual support groups are helpful.
- Psychological treatments include rehearsal of the 'trauma story', such as 'testimony'.
- Antidepressant drugs are effective, although their main effect may be on the associated depressed mood.

Adjustment disorder

Adjustment disorders are states of emotional distress and disturbance, usually interfering with social functioning, arising in a period of adaptation to a significant life change or stressful life event such as bereavement or separation. Onset is usually within one month of the event and the symptoms do not usually last more than six months. In contrast to an acute stress reaction, individual predisposition or vulnerability plays a greater role in the risk of developing such a disorder and in shaping its manifestations. However, it is assumed that the condition would not have arisen without the stress. There may be a brief or prolonged depressive reaction, a mixed anxiety and depressive reaction or disturbance of conduct, for example in adolescence. Other predisposing factors include culture shock and hospitalization in children. As a condition, it has been little researched. Its management has been informed by the treatment of other conditions with similar symptomatology. It may respond better to antidepressant medication than major depression.

in the USA than in the UK. It can be iatrogenic if reinforced during psychotherapy.

Reflecting the influence of culture, *dissociative trance* or *possession disorder* is more common in the East.

Predisposing and precipitating factors

Predisposing factors include severe childhood emotional trauma and abuse (often sexual), and a borderline personality disorder. The condition is usually triggered by severe psychological stress.

Conversion disorders

Conversion disorders are characterized by loss of or alteration in bodily function arising from psychological conflict or need, not explicable by a medical disorder. Symptoms are typically neurological, affecting the voluntary nervous system. Typically, one or two neurological symptoms are seen. They are not, however, under voluntary control, as the individual is not conscious or aware of their psychological basis, i.e. the individual is not intentionally producing symptoms or otherwise malingering. Such symptoms arise via the unconscious defence mechanism of displacement. This group of disorders was central in the history of the development of psychoanalytic theory.

Classically, symptoms in dissociative (conversion) disorders are of symbolic significance and have an unconscious motivation or *primary gain*, such as relief from intolerable intrapsychic conflict or the reduction or loss of anxiety, which may present as a calm acceptance (*la belle indifférence*) of what appears to be a serious disability. Internal conflicts are kept away from awareness. The gain is primarily psychological, not financial, legal or social. Thus, an individual who is fearful both of battle and of being thought a coward may solve this conflict unconsciously by developing paralysis of the lower limbs, symbolizing the conflict. Similarly, individuals who unconsciously do not wish to see or hear what is going on may develop hysterical blindness or deafness. In the past 'hysterical fits' (dissociative seizures) in females were related to sexual 'frigidity'. Such individuals may also achieve *secondary gain* from their symptoms, such as attention, care and affection from others, including relatives, by the manipulation of relationships and by avoiding unwanted everyday tasks or situations, i.e. adopting the advantages of the sick role.

Theoretically, in dissociative and conversion disorders the motivation is unconscious, whereas in malingering it is conscious. In clinical practice, however, such a differentiation may be less clear cut and it is often better to assess the degree of unconsciousness of motivation, which itself may vary over time.

Family and early background, as well as cultural factors, may determine the choice of hysterical symptoms, which may be modelled closely on symptoms experienced during a childhood illness, when the rewards of attention resulting from the sick role may have been learnt. Similarly, an individual may develop a conversion symptom when a close relative develops similar symptoms, such as paralysis of one side as the result of a stroke.

In the past hysterical fainting by females was common, but is now a rare event. Similarly, in developed countries, gross paralysis of the limbs is now less common, whereas more subtle neurological conversion symptoms are more apparent. Gross conversion symptoms, however, still occur frequently in some developing countries.

Neurophysiological studies show that although an individual with a conversion disorder may say that no feeling in an area is experienced, corresponding cortical evoked responses to tactile stimulation may be detected in the brain using an electroencephalogram.

Individuals with conversion disorder (e.g. with limb paralysis) are suggestible and may 'take up their beds and walk' on suggestion from a respected other. Alternatively, they may respond to physiotherapy, thereby unconsciously saving face.

Epidemiology

The age of onset is usually in adolescence or early adulthood, but it may appear for the first time during middle age or even later. However, it should be emphasized that symptoms suggestive of a conversion disorder occurring in middle age or beyond are very likely to be caused by organic illness. Although conversion disorder was considered common several decades ago, it is now much more rarely encountered and is considered to be more common in women than in men. Most cases are seen in neurological or orthopaedic practice, or in military settings, especially at times of war, and it may be more common in lower socioeconomic groups. The incidence is falling in developed countries, but remains high in developing countries.

Clinical features

To summarize the above, symptoms have a primary gain, which reduces anxiety and helps resolve emotional conflict. They may be associated with secondary gain (e.g. the attention of others), and symptoms may be symbolic and determined by, or modelled on, cultural, family or early background factors. Classically, symptoms may be calmly accepted (*la belle indifférence*), although in practice this is not frequently seen. However, the diagnosis is not dependent on the demonstration of gain or indifference. There is usually only one conversion symptom present in one episode of conversion disorder. Symptoms include:

- *Sensory symptoms*. These are incompatible with peripheral or central nervous system disorders and may include anaesthesias and paraesthesias, especially of the extremities. For example, it can produce 'stocking and glove' anaesthetic areas of the hands and feet (Figure 11.1), but it should be noted that this particular presentation can also result from certain organic causes, notably diabetic neuropathy and treatment with amiodarone.
- *Special sense organ symptoms*. These may include deafness and either unilateral or bilateral blindness or tunnel vision.
- *Motor signs* are summarized in Figure 11.2.

Conversion symptoms may be distinguished from organic symptoms by their variability, their nature – which often reflects an individual's concept of anatomy and physiology – and by their inconsistency with known anatomy and physiology. For example, individuals with hysterical aphonia are able to use the same muscles to cough that they would normally use to speak. Individuals with hysterical blindness may avoid colliding with objects. Areas of anaesthesia may be increased by suggestion from a doctor during an examination. Apparently paralysed extensor muscles of one leg may contract when the individual is asked to lie supine and raise the opposite leg.

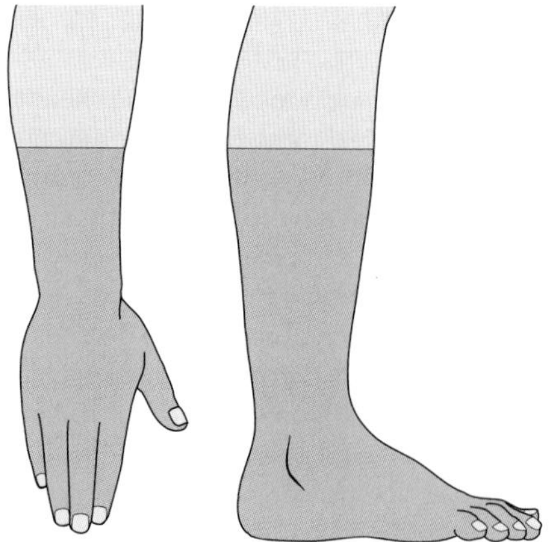

Figure 11.1 • Typical areas of sensory loss in conversion disorders.

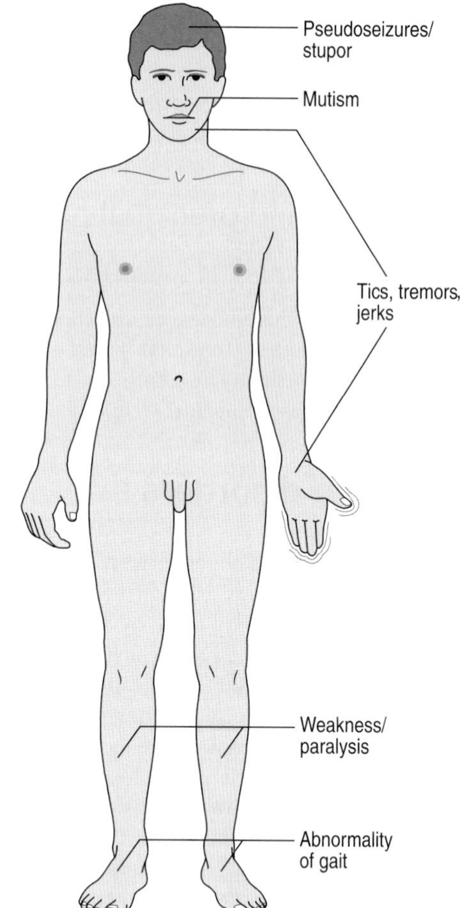

Figure 11.2 • Common motor symptoms of conversion disorders.

History taking should concentrate on eliciting precipitating stress factors, and a close relative or acquaintance should also be interviewed, as this may help elucidate, among other matters, the individual's use of the sick role. Physical examination and investigations should be completed quickly and, if normal, the physical symptoms themselves thereafter ignored.

Differential diagnosis

This includes any undiagnosed physical disorder, especially one that presents with vague multiple somatic symptoms, such as *systemic lupus erythematosus* or *multiple sclerosis*. Undiagnosed physical disorders may be either difficult to diagnose (e.g. haemangioblastoma of the cerebellum or tumours of the foramen magnum) or not routinely considered (e.g. *myasthenia gravis* or *acute intermittent porphyria*). Recent studies, in contrast to some of those in the past, have found low rates of development of neurological disorders (range 1–3%).

Conversion symptoms can occur in *somatization disorder* and, more rarely, in schizophrenia. Other diagnoses to be considered include *hypochondriacal disorder*, and also *malingering* where symptoms are consciously produced.

Aetiology

Predisposing factors

There is little evidence in favour of a genetic predisposition to conversion disorders.

It was Freud who initially used the term conversion. He had observed the French neurologist Charcot producing conversion hysteria in susceptible individuals by the use of hypnosis and even suggestion. The mechanisms underlying this condition have been unsatisfactorily sought since. Freud saw these disorders as arising from mental or psychological energy and anxiety being repressed and converted into physical symptoms, which were often suggestive of a neurological disease, and which resulted in avoidance of emotional conflict and thus a reduction in intrapsychic anxiety. The conflict is between instinctual impulses, e.g. aggressive or sexual, and inhibition against their expression.

A premorbid histrionic, dependent, passive-aggressive or antisocial personality disorder may be present in up to one-fifth of cases. Traits of suggestibility and increased capacity to dissociate may predispose towards the development of conversion symptoms.

Learning theory explains conversion disorders in terms of classical conditioning.

Either previous physical disorders and/or exposure to such disorders in others may be a predisposing factor by providing a model for the choice of conversion symptom. For instance, dissociative convulsions (pseudoseizures) are more likely to occur in those who suffer from epilepsy, as this provides a model for their symptoms and also they have learnt the advantages of the sick role as a result.

The increased incidence of conversion disorder in the young and immature may reflect the fact that they have only recently emerged from the privileged dependent state of childhood. Similarly, it has been suggested that the greater proportion of women sufferers apparent in the past perhaps reflected their overall greater dependence on men. In keeping with this theory, the ratio of female to male sufferers has fallen considerably in recent decades.

Precipitating and perpetuating factors

Precipitating factors include severe stress, such as the recent death of a close relative, whose physical symptoms may be modelled by the patient, and at times of war. In fact, experience of warfare suggests that everyone is capable of developing a conversion disorder. Head injury and temporal lobe epilepsy have also been suggested as precipitating factors. Impaired action generation with decreased activity in the left dorso-lateral pre-frontal cortex has also been found.

The condition is perpetuated by secondary gain and the advantages of the sick role (see above).

The possibility of financial gain, such as in *compensation neurosis*, may also perpetuate the disorder. Table 11.4 summarizes the aetiology of conversion disorders.

Table 11.4 Aetiology of conversion disorders

Predisposing factors	Childhood experience of illness
Precipitating factors	Physical illness, e.g. epilepsy, Guillain–Barré syndrome
	Negative life events
	Relationship conflict
	Modelling of others' illness
Perpetuating factors	Behavioural responses, e.g. avoidance, disuse, reassurance seeking
	Cognitive responses, e.g. fear of worsening, fear of serious disease

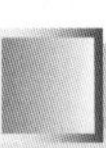

Case history: conversion disorder

A 25-year-old married woman, Mrs A., presented with paralysis of her left hand and left leg, which had come on abruptly over the course of 2 days. As a child, Mrs A. had undergone a number of orthopaedic operations on her left lower limb owing to congenital dislocation of the hip and club foot, which had necessitated her spending several periods in hospital of up to a month's duration. Four months prior to her presenting with symptoms of paralysis her own father had had a cerebrovascular accident (stroke), resulting in left hemiparesis, on which she may have unconsciously modelled her own symptoms.

She herself had developed into an extroverted, overemotional woman, who, behaved overdramatically under stress and was very suggestible. She had married 3 years earlier, mainly to move away from her parents who, she felt, restricted her lifestyle and were overprotective. However, the marital sexual relationship was never good, and at times her husband would beat her if his needs were not immediately met. He was profusely apologetic afterwards. At times she would attempt to hit him back. Meanwhile, she had developed a relationship with a man at the firm where she worked as a personnel assistant, who had asked her to leave her husband and live with him; however, she remained ambivalent about this. Her left-sided paralysis came on following a verbal row between her and her husband when she threatened to leave him.

After being assessed by her GP she was admitted to a general hospital neurology ward. At assessment, however, she appeared comparatively unconcerned about her physical condition (*la belle indifférence*). Neurological examination showed a weakness in her left hand to be of glove distribution. This was inconsistent with known neurological lesions, as was the fact that when she was asked to lie supine and raise her right leg, her paralysed left thigh muscles contracted. Investigations revealed no evidence of an organic medical illness and she was advised that there was nothing gravely medically wrong with her and that her symptoms would remit. She was given reassurance, and prescribed relaxation exercises and physiotherapy for her left hand and left leg.

Mrs A. was diagnosed as suffering from a conversion disorder, the primary gain of which was considered to be related to her conflict over whether or not to leave her husband. Her choice of symptoms was symbolic of this conflict and appeared to be modelled on her father's recent cerebrovascular accident.

After initially making good progress, it became clear that she was obtaining *secondary gain* from the attention of staff and her family, which was in marked contrast to her then marital situation. Acknowledging that there was a possible connection between the stresses in her marital relationship and the onset of her physical symptoms, she reluctantly agreed to discuss her situation with a psychiatrist. He saw her regularly to help her gain insight into the psychological origins of her disorder, and she increasingly recognized that psychological stresses had been important in precipitating her condition. With her agreement, her husband and other family members were interviewed, including in her presence, to further elucidate the psychological causes of her condition. Eventually her progress was such that she felt able to leave hospital. She initially went to live with her parents, with a view to later being seen with her husband for joint marital therapy. Within a month her physical symptoms had remitted fully. In the longer term she and her husband decided to separate, at which time there was a temporary relapse in her condition.

Management

Most cases remit with non-specific supportive measures, particularly if suggestion is used. To prevent secondary gain, chronicity or relapse, early resolution of symptoms is important. Physical investigations should only be undertaken if indicated, not merely as reassurance. In the absence of any abnormalities the patient should be firmly reassured that there is no serious medical illness present, and that the symptoms are familiar to the doctor and will remit. Any associated psychiatric disorder should, of course, be treated in its own right. Relaxation training, hypnosis and anxiolytics may also be of value.

If the symptoms do not remit, or precipitating or perpetuating factors continue, then it is necessary to help the patient recognize these and take action to counter them in order to prevent chronicity. Cognitive behavioural therapy (CBT) has been found to be the most effective specific treatment. Cognitive, behavioural and physiological factors interrelate. Therefore, cognitive-behavioural treatments can result in physiological changes. Behaviour therapy alone has clinically been found to be effective. Psychotherapy may be indicated to gain insight into and explore the origins of the symptoms (e.g. by linking them to mood). However, the severe stresses may prevent the individual from being able to discuss these problems.

Abreaction may also be indicated. This is the recall to consciousness of the underlying and causative repressed trauma, with the simultaneous re-experiencing of the emotion that originally accompanied it. Methods of achieving abreaction (catharsis) include psychotherapy alone, hypnosis and the use of drugs, most safely with intravenous diazepam, but intravenous barbiturates or amphetamines have also been used.

Secondary gain may need to be countered by behavioural therapy and environmental manipulation. The advantages of the sick role should be minimized and those of health maximized. The involvement and help of family and other individuals important to the patient may have to be enlisted.

Prognosis

In general, the prognosis for most cases is good, with complete and rapid recovery either spontaneously or on removal of the precipitating factors. Good prognosis is associated with acute onset and a clear and resolvable emotional conflict. If the condition persists after one year, the course is likely to be more intractable. Intractability is also associated with personality difficulties and poor motivation. About one-quarter will have another conversion symptom within six years.

The prognosis is also better for a sustained disabling conversion disorder, such as paralysis, than the intermittent use of symptoms such as dissociative convulsions (pseudoseizures), or where the symptom produces little disability in everyday life.

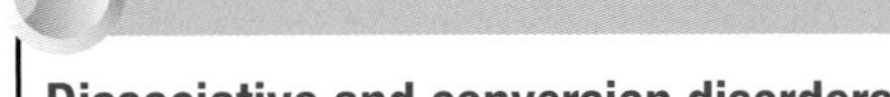

Dissociative and conversion disorders

- In dissociative states, such as amnesia or fugue (unexpected journeying with amnesia), there is partial or complete loss of normal integration between two or more mental processes.
- In conversion disorders there is loss or change in bodily function, usually affecting the voluntary nervous system, such as paralysis or anaesthesia.
- Dissociative and conversion disorders have an unconscious motivation to resolve intrapsychic conflict, and may show the following features:
  - primary gain (to resolve conflict or reduce anxiety)
  - secondary gain (e.g. the attention of others)
  - symptom choice may be symbolic of the conflict and reflect modelling of symptoms either the individual or others have experienced
  - *la belle indifférence* (calm acceptance of symptoms).

Somatoform disorders

ICD-10 divides the somatoform disorders into somatization disorder, hypochondriacal disorder and persistent pain disorder (see Table 11.5). DSM-IV-TR

Table 11.5 Somatoform disorders as described in ICD-10

Disorder	Characteristics
Somatoform disorder	At least two years of multiple and variable physical symptoms for which no adequate physical explanation has been found
	Persistent refusal to accept the advice or reassurance of several different doctors that there is no physical explanation for the symptoms
	Some degree of impairment of social and family functioning attributable to the nature of the symptoms and resulting behaviour
Hypochondriacal disorder	Persistent belief in the presence of one or more serious physical illnesses underlying the presenting symptom(s), despite strong evidence to the contrary, or a persistent preoccupation with a presumed disfigurement
	Persistent refusal to accept the advice or reassurance of several different doctors that there is no physical illness underlying the symptoms
Persistent pain disorder	Severe and distressing pain, which cannot be explained fully by a physiological process or physical disorder
	Occurs in association with emotional conflict or psychosocial problems sufficient to allow the conclusion that they are the main causative influences
	Usually results in marked increase in support and attention

Table 11.6 Somatoform disorders as described in DSM-IV-TR
Somatization disorder
Undifferentiated somatoform disorder
Body dysmorphic disorder
Conversion disorder
Hypochondriasis

(Table 11.6) also includes conversion disorder, which has already been described, and body dysmorphic disorder (dysmorphophobia).

Hypochondriacal disorder (hypochondriasis or hypochondriacal neurosis or severe health anxiety)

This is characterized by a persistent belief in the presence of one or more serious physical illnesses underlying the presenting symptom or symptoms, even though repeated examination and investigations have identified no adequate physical explanation. There is a persistent refusal to accept the advice and reassurance of doctors that no such physical illness exists.

Hypochondriacal disorder can thus be defined as an excessive concern about having a serious disease and morbid preoccupation with one's body or state of health, which is out of proportion to actual medical morbidity and is present a major part of the time. Characteristic features are:

- somatic (bodily) symptoms without medical explanation
- disease conviction (belief in an occult medical illness, which is, in fact, not present)
- disease fear
- bodily preoccupation.

N.B. The term hypochondriasis is also used to refer not only to a primary independent disorder, but also to a personality trait or a symptom in a number of psychiatric disorders (e.g. depression). Hypochondriacal symptoms are, in fact, most often seen as a feature of depressive disorder. The term hypochondriasis originates from the ancient belief that it was associated with actual physical disorder of the organs below (*hypo*) the cartilage (*chondros*) of the costal margin.

Epidemiology

This disorder can begin at any age, but most commonly between the ages of 20 and 30 years. It occurs slightly more commonly in males, or at least equally to females, in contrast to other somatoform disorders, which are more common in women. Its exact prevalence in the general population is unknown, and this is compounded by the fact that hypochondriacal complaints more commonly occur as part of another psychiatric syndrome, such as depressive disorder. Although hypochondriacal disorder is commonly seen in general medical practice (estimates of 4–15%), such individuals often refuse referral to mental health services, and so are not frequently seen in psychiatric facilities.

Primary hypochondriacal disorder is said to occur more often in lower social classes, the very young, the elderly, Jews, and those associated with disease, including medical students. It may be more common in non-European cultures where depressive disorder presents more commonly with hypochondriacal or somatic features.

Clinical features

Individuals experience symptoms that strongly suggest disease to them, but not to their examining doctors. Even if organic disease is present, symptoms will be disproportionate and typically refer to a number of anatomical locations and organs. Individuals are very concerned as to the exact significance of the symptoms and their aetiology, and also with their authenticity being accepted by others. They are convinced that they suffer from a serious disease, which is yet to be detected, and they cannot be persuaded otherwise, in spite of adequate reassurance, negative investigation results and a benign course of their condition over time.

Sufferers have a disease fear that is intense and persistent. They are vigilant to the slightest indication of illness, which alarms them greatly. Their bodily preoccupation is profound and extends to their general health status. They scrutinize themselves intensely. They habitually visit GP and hospital clinics and accumulate a long history of medical contact. Ultimately, they always remain dissatisfied by their contact with the medical profession, whom they often criticize and blame for their continuing complaints, and a deteriorating doctor–patient relationship is common.

Differential diagnosis

This includes true organic disease, especially the early stages of neurological disorders such as multiple sclerosis, endocrine disorders such as thyroid or parathyroid disease, and also disorders that frequently affect multiple body systems such as systemic lupus erythematosus. The presence of true organic disease does not, however, rule out coexisting hypochondriacal disorder.

Hypochondriacal symptoms are most often seen, in up to 80% cases, in depressive disorder. *Somatic delusions* of physical disease may be present in psychotic disorders, including depression and schizophrenia. In hypochondriacal disorder, beliefs are characteristically not of delusional intensity, in that the individual will accept the possibility that the disease may not be present, although such distinctions may be difficult to make, especially initially. Hypochondriacal concerns may also be present in generalized anxiety disorder, panic disorder and somatization disorder. In somatization disorder, the preoccupation is with the symptoms rather than the fear of having a specific disease or diseases.

Aetiology

Hypochondriasis is a polythetic disease, i.e. has numerous interacting causes. It has been argued that it is a variant form of other mental illnesses, e.g. depression or anxiety disorder, rather than a primary neurotic disorder. However, the validity of primary hypochondriasis has been accepted.

Predisposing factors. Past experience of true organic disease, especially in childhood, in either oneself or a family member, predisposes to the development of this disorder (e.g. by modelling or reinforcement). Illness may have been a particular focus of attention and source of concern for family members of such patients.

Case history: somatization disorder

A 25-year-old woman, Mrs B., had a history of multiple physical complaints which persisted for 3 years. They totalled 16 in number and included vomiting, pain in the extremities of her limbs, difficulty swallowing, burning sensations in her genitalia and rectum, and painful menstruation. As a result she was attending the gastrointestinal, neurology and gynaecological outpatient clinics of a general hospital.

Her father was a labourer and had a history of alcoholism and law involvement. He had been physically abusive towards her when she was a child and during her adolescence. She had two elder brothers, who also had a history of drug abuse and of having served custodial sentences for acquisitive offences. She had one elder sister who, like Mrs B., had a number of physical complaints for which no organic cause had been found.

Mrs B. had shown conduct disorder as a child, including at school. She had had a disturbed adolescence, during which she abused alcohol and shoplifted. She had had dysmenorrhoea from her menarche. She had had a number of unstable and unsatisfactory sexual relationships from an early age, associated with significant sexual difficulties, including pain on intercourse. Her interpersonal relationships were generally stormy and, at the time of presentation, she was in her second marriage, to a man who was violent to her. She had two children, both of whom were unplanned, towards whom she was rather neglectful and inconsistent in discipline. She was also a poor domestic organizer. Although she had worked in a clerical capacity for a local business in her late adolescence, over the last 2 years she had been unable to work due to her physical complaints. She would spend at least 8 days a month in bed. She often felt anxious and despondent and had taken a number of overdoses because of discord with her husband.

Mrs B. had been to a number of GPs and many hospital departments, often simultaneously, in an effort to resolve her physical complaints. Numerous organic diagnoses had been considered at various times by various hospital specialists, but no significant medical disorder had ever been found. Analgesic and psychotropic medication had been ineffective and only produced complaints from her of side-effects.

Mrs B. was very reluctant to take up the suggestion that she seek psychiatric help. Her GP, however, sought the advice of a consultant psychiatrist, who advised the GP about the nature of somatization disorder and outlined some treatment goals with the aim of avoiding further unnecessary medical or surgical interventions. He encouraged the GP to see the patient regularly and to build up a long-term supportive relationship with her, during which he should attempt to increasingly turn her attention from her somatic complaints to the problems in her life. Although her physical complaints remained chronic and fluctuated in severity, over time her florid symptoms were less in evidence and she became less intent on doctor shopping and seeking further investigative procedures. However, in spite of this, every year or so she obtained a specialist hospital opinion about her physical complaints.

Psychodynamic theory holds that hypochondriacal symptoms and associated suffering are assumed to have an unconscious meaning and gratification for an individual. Hypochondriacal disorder has been viewed as a somatic expression of oral dependency needs, including nurturing, attention, physical contact and sympathy. It has also been viewed as a transformation, through repression and displacement, of aggressive and hostile wishes arising from the past towards other people in the present, to whom such individuals make numerous and persistent physical complaints.

Hypochondriacal disorder has been seen as a hypochondriacal personality disorder. It has also been viewed as a non-verbal communication from individuals with interpersonal problems. For an individual feeling overwhelmed by apparently insoluble problems, such complaints may represent a request to be placed in the sick role, in order to avoid normal obligations, postpone unwelcome events and attract support and sympathy with no implications of blame.

Precipitating and perpetuating factors. Precipitating factors are usually significant psychosocial stresses. The condition is perpetuated by the persistence of such stresses, unresolved psychodynamic conflicts and the advantages of the sick role.

Management

This is usually undertaken by a GP, as such individuals often do not find psychiatric referral acceptable. Clearly, organic disease should be excluded and any primary psychiatric disorder, such as depression, vigorously treated.

Specific psychiatric treatment may be of benefit if the individual can acknowledge emotional difficulties underlying the physical complaints. Psychiatric treatment is better undertaken in a non-psychiatric medical setting, with an emphasis on the reduction of psychosocial stresses and education about the role of psychological factors in the development of symptoms, and how to cope with such symptoms. The psychodynamic meaning of the symptoms should be sought, as should their relationship to the family and social situation. However, one should be cautious if it is clear that the symptoms are acting as a last-ditch powerful psychological defence.

CBT is the specific treatment of first choice. Misinterpretations should be identified and challenged and realistic interpretations substituted. Graded exposure to illness cues and illness related situations with response prevention should be undertaken, and core illness beliefs modified. Such an approach can result in up to 75% symptom reduction.

Antidepressant medication, particularly selective serotonin reuptake inhibitors (SSRIs), is recommended by some for all such patients, particularly as most hypochondriacal symptoms in the general population are secondary to depression, which may explain the response. Antidepressant treatment is certainly the second-line treatment of choice if CBT fails or if there is significant comorbidity or severe symptoms.

Group psychotherapy is the psychotherapeutic approach of choice, although the aim primarily is usually supportive rather than curative. The evidence for this and of individual insight-orientated psychotherapy is lacking.

Overall, it is worth remembering that the patient is symptomatic for psychological and social reasons, and no specific medical or surgical intervention will cure the need to be sick. The aim is to concentrate on the person as a whole. The patient should be seen regularly and attention given to any social and personal factors from which the complaints are considered to arise.

Specific medical interventions should be kept to a minimum, for example a simple physical examination. The main treatment is the physician's personal attention. Elaborate and invasive diagnostic therapeutic procedures should only be undertaken when there is objective evidence for their use, and incidental abnormalities and equivocal findings should not be treated.

Prognosis

The prognosis is often poor, with individuals having chronic mild disability most of their adult life. The prognosis is worse the more chronic the condition. Where symptoms are associated with depressive or generalized anxiety disorder, the prognosis is better.

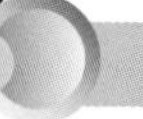

Hypochondriacal disorder

- Disease conviction in spite of medical reassurance.
- Intense persistent fear of disease.
- Profound preoccupation with body and health status.
- Abnormally sensitive to normal physical signs and sensations, and tendency to interpret them as abnormal.
- Hypochondriacal symptoms are most frequently secondary to depressive illness.

Somatization disorder (Briquet's syndrome; St Louis hysteria)

This is a chronic syndrome of multiple somatic (physical) symptoms, which have persisted for several years with no adequate medical explanation, associated with psychosocial distress, impairment and medical help seeking. There is no autonomic overstimulation. The alternative terms of Briquet's syndrome or St Louis hysteria arose from Briquet's 1859 concept of hysteria, which was revived by psychiatrists at Washington University, St Louis.

The ICD-10 description of somatization disorder is given in Table 11.5. It will be seen that at least two years of multiple and variable physical symptoms are required for diagnosis. DSM-IV-TR criteria for somatization disorder indicate that the disorder should begin before the age of 30 years, must be of several years' duration and that it is not caused or fully explained by organic disease, medication, illicit drugs or alcohol, and has caused the individual to seek treatment or resulted in significant impairment of social, occupational or other important areas or functions. For the diagnosis to be made the individual must have had:

- two gastrointestinal symptoms, e.g. vomiting
- four pain symptoms, e.g. pain in extremities
- one sexual symptom other than pain
- one pseudoneurological symptom, e.g. amnesia or difficulty in swallowing.

These symptoms must not be intentionally produced or feigned (as in, respectively, factitious disorder or malingering).

Epidemiology

This disorder is very rarely diagnosed in males. For females, prevalence rates of up to 2% have been found. Women have been found to outnumber men with this condition 5–20 fold. Symptoms usually begin in the teenage years or, rarely, in the 20s, usually before the age of 30.

Clinical features

Such individuals have long and complicated medical histories, with many diagnoses having usually been considered. Even if some benign organic disorders have been diagnosed, the complaints and disabilities are excessive and the individual is severely disabled. The majority are unable to work, and may spend up to one-quarter of each month in bed. They may consult a number of doctors, at a number of institutions, even at the same time.

Associated features include:

- anxiety, depression, threats of suicide and parasuicide attempts
- an increased incidence of antisocial personality disorder, and alcohol and drug abuse
- interpersonal discord.

History taking often reveals poor childhood adjustment, school difficulties, a disturbed adolescence, menstruation difficulties and dysmenorrhoea from menarche, sexual activity from an early age with sexual problems common, interpersonal discord, unstable relationships, a number of marriages and inconsistent or neglectful parenting of any children.

Differential diagnosis

Physical disorders should be ruled out, particularly those with vague, multiple or confusing somatic symptoms, such as hyperparathyroidism, porphyria, multiple sclerosis and systemic lupus erythematosus. Multiple physical symptoms of late onset in life are almost always due to physical disease. In somatization disorder, there is an early onset of multiple symptoms involving a number of body systems, and a long but benign cause without the development of serious medical illnesses.

Unlike hypochondriasis, in somatization disorder there is less disease conviction, less disease fear and less bodily preoccupation. In addition, somatization disorder primarily affects females, whereas in hypochondriacal disorder males are at least equally affected.

The differential diagnosis also includes conversion disorder, depressive disorder, panic disorder and schizophrenia with multiple somatic delusions. Such disorders may coexist with somatoform disorder, particularly depression, and increase physical symptoms and negative appraisal of them.

Aetiology

Genetic and *environmental factors* probably both have a role. Monozygotic compared with dizygotic concordance rates in somatiform disorders were found to be 29:10 in one study. Somatization disorder occurs in 10–20% of first-degree female relatives. First-degree male relatives, however, have an increased incidence of alcoholism, drug abuse and antisocial personality disorder. Such genetic predisposition is in contrast to its absence in conversion disorder. Abnormal regulation of the cytokine system has also been hypothesized. Parental example may lead to behavioural learning of this condition, and physical illness in childhood may result in somatic rather than emotional responses for attention, care and countering hostility in adulthood.

Management

Ideally the diagnosis should be made early and unnecessary organic investigations and interventions avoided, as these are likely to result in further complaints arising from complications of the procedures, side-effects of medication and iatrogenic disease. Medical practitioners are reluctant to diagnose somatoform disorder but are inclined to search for rare medical illnesses. Gallbladders, uteri, appendices and teeth may all be needlessly removed. The aim should be to direct attention to the associated psychosocial stresses in the patient's life and away from the symptoms. 'Doctor shopping' should be discouraged and instead an attempt should be made to engage the patient in a long-term supportive therapeutic relationship with the GP, who can be advised, as required, by a psychiatrist as to the nature of the disorder and the feasible goals of treatment. Although the goal is to move the patient beyond somatization, a complete elimination of symptoms is unlikely and general support and care of the patient is more important. Specific CBT may assist by leading to the reattribution of physical symptoms, for example through behavioural experiments with hyperventilation. Fixed beliefs by patients that their physical symptoms are due to environmental hypersensitivity and candida are, however, difficult to alter. Psychodynamic psychotherapy has also been used. Psychotropic medication and analgesics tend not to be effective and such patients often concentrate on resulting side-effects.

Prognosis

This is generally poor with a chronic course, with repeated recurrences of symptoms, and disability persisting for most of life. Symptoms do tend to be more florid in early adult life but the course is often fluctuating. However, spontaneous remission is very rare. It is unlikely that such individuals will go more than two years without medical attention.

Towards a unified model of medically unexplained symptoms

In recent years, attempts have been made to integrate dissociative, conversion and somatization disorders into a unified model of medically unexplained symptoms, including with a view to adopting a unified treatment approach.

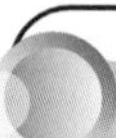

Somatization disorder

- A chronic syndrome of multiple physical symptoms not explainable medically.
- Increased incidence in first-degree female relatives.
- First-degree male relatives have an excess of alcoholism, drug abuse and antisocial personality disorder.
- Unlike hypochondriacal disorder, there is less disease conviction, less fear of disease and less bodily preoccupation.
- Occurs primarily in females, compared to the, at least, equal incidence in males of hypochondriacal disorder.
- Onset usually before 30 years, and long course without serious medical illness emerging.

Persistent somatoform pain disorder (psychogenic pain)

The essential feature of this disorder is the preoccupation with persistent, severe and distressing pain in the absence of adequate physical findings to account for the pain or its intensity. Pure psychogenic pain is, in fact, rare compared to psychological elaboration of pain associated with existing or previous injuries.

Pain always has a psychological component to it and has been defined as an unpleasant sensory and emotional experience associated with actual or potential tissue damage. Psychiatric consultation is often requested for those with chronic pain, which is not an uncommon complaint. Although many may have a past history of injuries, they often show no current evidence of tissue or nerve damage. In normal circumstances healing takes place within three months, or more rarely up to six months, and the correlation between pain and injury is poor after that period.

Epidemiology

The disorder is considered to be common in general medical practice, and is diagnosed almost twice as frequently in females as in males. Onset can occur at any age, but is most frequent in the 30s and 40s.

Clinical features

The normal course is for pain to appear suddenly and increase in severity over a few weeks to months. Such pain is inconsistent with the anatomical distribution of the nervous system. Characteristically it is continuous for much of the day, may cause difficulty in getting off to sleep but does not cause wakening, and has symbolic significance, for example chest pain in an individual who had a relative die from a heart attack.

The common sites of pain are summarized in Figure 11.3. There is limited insight into associated psychological factors, and patients characteristically respond less well to analgesics than to psychotropic medication. Persistent pain disorder may be accompanied by local sensory and motor changes, such as paraesthesias and muscle spasm. Doctor shopping and excessive use of analgesics without relief are often seen. A past history of conversion symptoms is common, as is an associated depressive disorder.

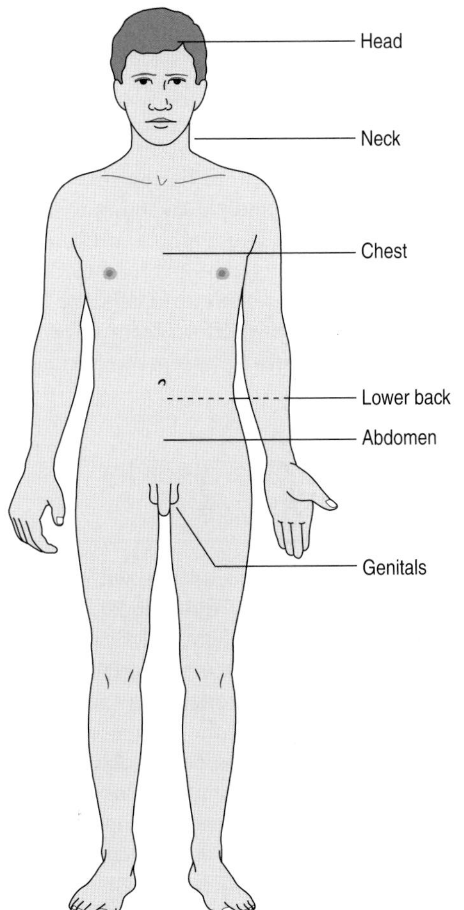

Figure 11.3 • Common sites of psychogenic pain.

The pain solves a psychological problem for the patient and may be ameliorated by psychological and environmental changes. It also corresponds to ideas held by the patient about the condition. The degree of resulting disability reflects these beliefs, rather than the severity of any previous injury or organic disease. The more uncertain the patient is of the cause of this pain, or the greater the belief that the pain will endure, the worse the disability and the associated demoralization. The complaint often increases following extensive investigations with negative results, which merely frustrate the patient.

The history may reveal a vulnerable hypochondriacal personality with a low pain threshold. Getting a history from an informant is also useful and previous hospital records will need to be examined. The previous psychiatric history may reveal similar episodes, including similar causes and precipitants.

Physical examination is required, not only to exclude organic disease but also to gain credibility in the patient's eyes and to more fully appreciate the complaints. Persistent pain disorder is characterized on examination by overreaction to the examination itself, diffuse superficial tenderness and weakness of all muscle groups in the region.

Investigations might also include requesting the patient to complete a diary of pain and associated behaviour and activities. This may reveal, for instance, that the pain is worse if the spouse is present and being sympathetic. Following assessment, it may be harmful to continue with a diary, as this may merely increase the patient's attention to the pain.

Differential diagnosis

True organic pain may be dramatically presented, particularly in those with a histrionic personality. A physical cause is suggested if it is characteristically described as 'sore, boring or nagging', and wakes the patient at night, and also if it is localized to a particular dermatome.

Atypical facial pain, which may be as severe as trigeminal neuralgia, should be differentiated from tempero-mandibular joint (TMJ) syndrome. In atypical facial pain, the pain usually lasts minutes to hours, sometimes being continuous. The pain is aching, dull, burning, or crushing, although occasionally sharp or knife-like. In the TMJ syndrome, there is focal tenderness of a TMJ, aggravated by talking, chewing or lateral jaw movement, and requires referral to an oral surgeon.

Other psychiatric illnesses should be excluded, in particular depressive disorder and somatization disorder, but pain rarely dominates the clinical picture of these conditions, although patients often complain of aches and pains. Some psychotic individuals, such as those suffering from schizophrenia, may have a *delusional pain syndrome*. Generalized anxiety disorder may present with muscle pain due to tension and tension headaches. Malingering should also be excluded. Individuals dependent on narcotics may complain of pain to obtain opioids.

Aetiology

Predisposing factors. Those with this disorder are more likely to have begun working at an unusually early age, held jobs that were physically strenuous or overly routinized, or were workaholics and rarely took time off. In many cases, however, the pain is shaped by organic, psychological, personal and cultural factors.

A *pain-prone personality* profile has been proposed. Such personalities court injuries and unsuccessful surgery. However, such a profile, for example the inverted V profile on the Minnesota Multiphasic Personality Inventory (MMPI) (high scores for hypochondriasis and hysteria and a low score for depression), is often secondary to the impact of chronic pain.

A further theory suggests that such individuals come from an *abusive parental family background*, where the child is subject to physical abuse from parents who subsequently show remorse and comfort him, so that the child grows up associating parental love with pain and suffering. However, such a background is infrequently seen in clinical practice, although an *increased history of childhood physical and sexual abuse* has been identified. Some *ethnic and cultural groups*, such as Asians, are said to somatize problems more frequently.

Precipitating and perpetuating factors. These include physical trauma, which occurs in about half of cases, and also dissatisfaction with employment prior to injury.

A background of litigation with a view to compensation makes the resolution of the pain very unlikely while litigation is in progress. Even after a satisfactory legal settlement, a number of patients will continue to complain of chronic pain.

This disorder has also been considered as a variant of depressive disorder.

Management

Organic disease should be excluded and, if it cannot, a full evaluation of the degree and extent of physical pathology and its contribution to the presentation of pain should be made.

Clearly, adequate medical treatment of any organic basis to pain is essential. Multidisciplinary pain clinics, with an anaesthetist, psychiatrist and physician present, may facilitate management. Current psychosocial stresses will need to be resolved. Antidepressants such as amitriptyline, which affect both serotonin and noradrenaline reuptake, are more effective than those that act mainly on noradrenaline uptake. Tricyclic antidepressants also have an analgesic action of faster onset than, and independent of, their antidepressant effects. Cognitive behavioural methods of treatment have also been found to be of value.

Prognosis

In most cases the symptom has persisted for many years by the time the individual comes to the attention of psychiatrists. Those who express emotional distress with physical symptoms tend to do poorly, whereas those who are able to accept the pain and appreciate that their own efforts to improve the quality of their life are of the utmost importance tend to do better.

Body dysmorphic disorder (dysmorphophobia)

This is a distressing preoccupation with some imagined or slight defect of appearance in a normal-appearing person. If a slight physical anomaly is present, the person's concern is grossly excessive. However, there is no correlation between body dysmorphic disorder and the degree of deformity. The belief in the defect is not of delusional intensity, although in clinical practice this distinction is often difficult to make and may not be valid, as the belief may vary from an overvalued idea to a delusion. The term dysmorphic originates from the Greek word for ugliness of face. Although such patients do often fear ridicule, and even fear upsetting others and thus show avoidance, the European term dysmorphophobia is not used in the American DSM-IV-TR as it is argued that there is no pure phobic avoidance. In ICD-10, both dysmorphophobia and body dysmorphic disorder are included under the category of hypochondriacal disorder.

Epidemiology

The most common age of onset is from adolescence through to the third decade. Psychiatrists see only a small proportion of cases and the disorder may actually be more common than has previously been thought. Women are affected slightly more often than men. Such patients are more likely to go to plastic surgeons and dermatologists than to a psychiatrist. Studies of US college students have suggested that a quarter may meet DSM-IV-TR criteria for body dysmorphic disorder.

Clinical features

The most common imagined defects are of the face, including wrinkles, the shape of the nose, excessive facial hair and facial asymmetries. More rarely, the complaint involves the feet, hands, back, breasts and genitals. Any preoccupation with genitals and breasts must be more than is normal. Women are more preoccupied with breast and legs and are more likely to use make-up as camouflage and check their appearance in the mirror. Men are more preoccupied with their genitals, height and excess body hair. There is never a disturbance of the whole body image, as is seen in anorexia nervosa, but more than one imagined defect in appearance may occur at one time, or a series may occur over time. The disorder can be markedly disabling, resulting in repeated visits to plastic surgeons or dermatologists in an effort at correction. There is avoidance of social or occupational situations because of anxiety and fear of attention. Worry, dysphoria and depressive disorder frequently occur. Comorbidity is frequent. In women, this is often with generalized anxiety disorder, panic disorder and bulimia. In men, there is a lifetime comorbidity increase in bipolar disorder. Such individuals' whole lives may be affected: they become socially isolated, restrict their activities and are usually unmarried. They may frequently check their appearance in the mirror and may often change their hairstyle to alter their appearance.

Feeling grossly disfigured, such individuals often fear seeking help or will present to a plastic surgeon or dermatologist before a psychiatrist. They may also fear being viewed as vain about their appearance. They are very sensitive to and feel confused about their internal, ideal and actual self-image. They may become socially isolated, unemployed, and suicidal. A quarter attempt suicide.

Differential diagnosis

Anorexia nervosa or transsexualism do not fulfil the diagnostic criteria for body dysmorphic disorder, as these two conditions are characterized by a disturbance of the whole body image and not some imagined defect in appearance. Concern about minor defects in appearance, such as acne, is common in normal adolescence but not grossly excessive. An individual may exaggerate defects in appearance in major depression, as may those with an anxious (avoidant) personality disorder and social phobia, but such symptoms are not the predominant disturbance.

In delusional disorders, an individual's belief in a defect of appearance is of delusional intensity, which by definition is not the case in body dysmorphic disorder. Studies have suggested that up to 50% of those complaining of a large nose and requesting plastic surgery are 'neurotic', but an increased incidence of schizophrenia and depression has also been found.

Aetiology

There is little definitive information on predisposing factors of body dysmorphic disorder. In psychodynamic theory, body dysmorphic disorder has been considered to represent an unconscious displacement onto body parts of sexual or emotional conflicts, or more general feelings of inferiority, poor self-image or guilt. Alternatively, the disorder may be used to explain the individual's failures with, and suffering in relation to, the opposite sex. In Freud's classic case history of the Wolf Man, the patient is described as neglecting his daily life and work because of his perception of a defect in the appearance of his nose.

Some individuals have a sudden onset of body dysmorphic disorder precipitated after distressing experiences, including abandonment by their spouse.

Increased family history of affective disorder and obsessive–compulsive disorder and high comorbidity with depressive disorder is seen. The pathophysiology may involve serotonin, given the response of the condition to SSRIs.

Relationship with other psychiatric disorders

A relationship between body dysmorphic disorder and a number of other psychiatric disorders has been postulated, including mood disorder, obsessive–compulsive disorder and schizophrenia. It has been suggested that body dysmorphic disorder may, in fact, be only a non-specific symptom of such conditions. The links appear to be greatest with obsessive–compulsive disorder, but in that disorder preoccupying thoughts are more intrusive and unnatural than in body dysmorphic disorder.

The condition may also be related to delusional disorders, although, by definition, the defect is not of delusional intensity in body dysmorphic disorder. Where the belief is of delusional intensity, the terms *monosymptomatic hypochondriasis* or *monosymptomatic hypochondriacal psychosis* have been used. In fact, the delusional intensity of such beliefs can vary with time and thus the clinical picture overlaps with body dysmorphic disorder.

Management

Although CBT and psychodynamic psychotherapy have been described as being of benefit, and CBT is the first-line treatment of choice, with proven benefit over two years, it appears that the best results have been obtained by using SSRIs. Surgery is not generally effective, as individuals often express dissatisfaction with the results, requesting and obtaining repeated operative procedures. However, where there is a slight physical anomaly and the defect in appearance is well circumscribed, some studies have shown good results from plastic surgery alone (e.g. rhinoplasty for a big nose).

Prognosis

The course is often chronic, persisting for several years, and often worsens over time in spite of treatment.

Other associated concepts

Undifferentiated somatoform disorder

This category, included within the somatoform disorders in DSM-IV-TR, is for individuals whose clinical picture does not meet the full criteria of somatization disorder. There may be either single circumscribed symptoms, such as difficulty in swallowing or, more commonly, multiple physical complaints, such as fatigue, loss of appetite and gastrointestinal problems. The duration of disturbance must be at least six months for this diagnosis to be made. The main categories of somatoform disorders are narrow and most patients in clinical practice will be in this residual subcategory, a reflection of the current unsatisfactory classification, or, alternatively, suffer from another primary psychiatric disorder, such as depression or anxiety.

Medically unexplained physical symptoms

Most patients in clinical practice with such symptoms will, as previously described, have either undifferentiated somatoform disorder or suffer from another primary psychiatric disorder, such as anxiety, producing real somatic anxiety symptoms due to autonomic hyperactivity, or depression, for example producing facial pain (a depressive equivalent that is sometimes considered psychodynamically to equate to an emotional 'slap in the face'). The various terms used to refer to symptoms with no organic cause are listed in Table 11.7. Such terms are often used loosely and overlap.

Table 11.7 Terms applied to medically unexplained symptoms
Hysterical
Hypochondriacal
Neurasthenia
Postviral fatigue syndrome
Chronic fatigue syndrome (CFS)
Myalgic encephalomyelitis (ME)
Functional overlay
Psychophysiological reaction
Psychosomatic reaction
Factitious
Münchausen (hospital addiction) syndrome
Malingering

About one in five new consultations in primary care will be with medically unexplained symptoms. This latter term avoids making assumptions about their cause. Many symptoms are transient but one-third persist and cause distress and disability. They result from interactions between biological, psychological, social and cultural factors. All patients should be asked about low mood and biological symptoms of depression, what their beliefs are about their symptoms (e.g. fear of cancer), why they are seeking help now and the relationship between symptoms, mood and social factors with a view to the patient reattributing the cause of their symptoms (for instance relating overbreathing to anxiety, and lower pain threshold to depression). The reality for patients of their symptoms should be accepted and an explanation of these should be provided if possible.

CBT can be of benefit, as can antidepressants for chronic pain and associated poor sleep even in the absence of depression.

Somatization and medically unexplained symptoms

Somatization, from the Greek word for body, *soma*, is a helpful concept in understanding patients with medically unexplained symptoms. It is a tendency to experience physical distress and symptoms unaccounted for by pathological findings, to attribute them to physical illness, to communicate them and to seek medical help for them. It may be an earlier phenomenon than psychologization, which is especially prevalent in developed countries.

Individuals in general may characteristically view symptoms as having physical, psychological or external causes. There may be a spectrum in the way individuals experience stress (Figure 11.4): at one extreme this may be with pure psychic symptoms, such as worry about the stress; further along the spectrum certain individuals may have free-floating anxiety, with both psychic and somatic symptoms, and at the other extreme individuals experience only somatic symptoms, which may be anxiety or depressive equivalents. The latter do not perceive such symptoms as having a psychological basis, which leads to their resisting psychological help and to their seeking a medical explanation. Somatization may be facultative, and cease when help is received, or chronic true somatization of psychosocial distress.

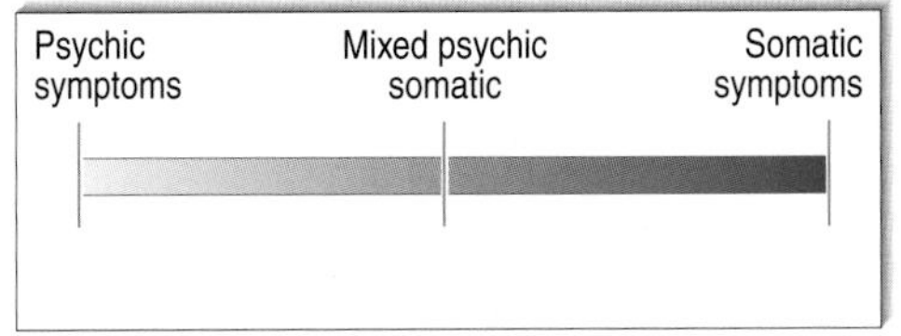

Figure 11.4 • Spectrum of stress response.

Autonomic hyperactivity accounts for the genuine somatic anxiety symptoms. In conversion disorders, physiological changes can be demonstrated in the voluntary nervous system. In hypochondriacal disorder, individuals are abnormally sensitive to normal sensations in the body.

Patients with medically unexplained physical symptoms exert disproportionately high financial and service burdens on health and social services. In any week 60–80% of healthy people experience bodily symptoms but only a small proportion of these will attend their GP; in 20% the physical symptoms will be due to minor emotional disorders. Patients who visit their GP may be referred to hospital specialists, despite no abnormal physical findings on examination. Up to 40% of cases seen by hospital medical specialists have medically unexplained physical symptoms and receive no organic diagnosis.

Such patients are resistant to any psychological interpretation, which they perceive as implying that their symptoms are not real but all in the mind. However, it is important to remember that the causes of such symptoms do not have to be either physical or psychological, i.e. if no organic disorder is found, it does not therefore have to be assumed to be a purely psychological problem. A medical model of disease does not, and should not, have to be restricted to organic or biological causes alone. Often, psychiatric disorder is not looked for if any possible organic causative factor is found. In contrast, another investigation can always be proposed if no causative organic factor has been identified.

It is always important to consider not only the symptoms but also the patient's understanding of the illness and anxieties about it (i.e. thoughts) and the way the patient's daily life is affected by the symptoms (i.e. behaviour). A good doctor–patient interaction can only be achieved if the patient feels understood. With this in mind it is possible to work with such patients' thoughts and behaviours via cognitive behavioural therapy.

Pathophysiological mechanisms proposed for specific medically unexplained symptoms (Figure 11.5)

Emotional arousal may lead to increased paravertebral muscle tension, which can be detected by an electromyogram, and results in *chronic low back pain*. Pelvic vein dilatation may result in *pelvic pain* in females. Hyperventilation, with resetting of respiratory control mechanisms to a reduced Pco_2, may result in *breathlessness*, or the *hyperventilation syndrome (HVS)* (also known as da Costa's Syndrome, cardiac neurosis, effort syndrome and circulatory neurasthenia). About one-quarter of patients with HVS have symptoms of panic disorder, and 50–60% of those with panic disorder or agoraphobia have symptoms of HVS. Inactivity, which reduces the capacity for further activity, and increased muscle tension may result in *fatigue*. Psychological stress produces irregular contractile activity of the smooth muscle in cases of *altered bowel habit*.

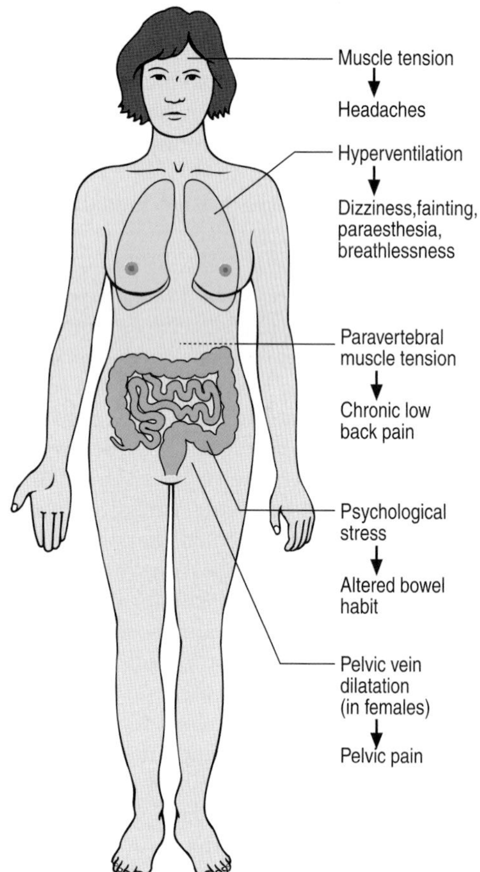

Figure 11.5 • Pathophysiological mechanisms proposed for specific medically unexplained symptoms.

Table 11.8 outlines the interactions between psychiatric and physical illness. Table 11.9 gives some examples of the factors influencing a patient's response to a physical illness.

Psychological defensiveness, such as having a repressive coping style, may be associated with lower rates of psychopathology and psychiatric disorder, but this is counterbalanced by a restriction in self-awareness and interpersonal and social functioning, and a trade-off in physical ill health, for example increased blood pressure and heart rate reactivity, reduced cell-mediated and humoral immunity responses, and possibly even progression of certain tumours, such as breast cancer.

Myalgic encephalomyelitis (ME) or chronic fatigue syndrome (CFS)

Myalgic encephalomyelitis (ME) or chronic fatigue syndrome (CFS) is characterized by the onset of unexplained physical and often mental fatigue, and heightened awareness of this, lasting for over six months and not related to ongoing exertion nor alleviated by rest. Prevalence is about seven per 100,000. It usually presents between 20 and 50 years of age. Biopsychosocial factors contribute to the aetiology. There is strong evidence of genetic influences and of genetic subtypes. There is evidence of structural and chemical changes in the brain; brain levels of choline-containing compounds have been found to be increased in ME subjects. Many subjects relate the onset to an infection, which may indeed trigger the condition. There is some evidence that patients with ME might be more likely to have been infected with viruses, such as xenotropic murine leukaemia virus-related virus (XMRV). In some cases it may be a variant of the less chronic postviral infection fatigue. Some cases follow immunization. Evidence of Epstein–Barr virus infection is present in 10% of cases. Most severe viral infections are associated with immunological abnormalities, especially in T cell-mediated immunity.

Sixty per cent of patients have no previous psychiatric history, but a half to two-thirds have a current comorbid psychiatric disorder, especially minor depression in 40–50% of these cases, anxiety and somatization disorder. Diagnosis is primarily based on clinical history. The differential diagnosis includes depression. Comorbidity with depression may result from primary depression or depression secondary

Table 11.8 Interaction between psychiatric and physical disorders

Organic mental disorders
Physical illness has direct effect on brain function • delirium/acute confusional state/organic psychosis, e.g. liver failure • dementia/chronic organic psychosis • postoperative psychosis
Maladaptive psychological reactions to illness
Depression, e.g. amputation, mastectomy (owing to loss)
Guilt, e.g. fear of burden on relatives
Anxiety, e.g. before operation, unpleasant procedure
Paranoid reaction, e.g. if deaf, blind
Anger
Denial
Preoccupation with illness
Prolongation of sick role (fewer responsibilities, more attention)
Psychosomatic disease
Multiple (i.e. biopsychosocial) causes. For example, life events/stress on physically and emotionally vulnerable leads to changes in nervous and endocrine systems, etc. and disease, e.g. bereavement may precipitate a heart attack, or stress may precipitate asthma, eczema, peptic ulcer
Psychiatric conditions presenting with physical complaints
Somatic (physical) anxiety symptoms due to autonomic hyperactivity, e.g. palpitations
Conversion disorders (via voluntary nervous system)
Depression leading to facial pain, constipation, hypochondriacal complaints and delusions, e.g. of cancer, sexually transmitted disease
Hypochondriacal disorder: excessive concern with health and normal sensations
Somatization disorder
Monosymptomatic hypochondriacal delusions, e.g. delusions of infestation or smell; and other psychotic disorders, e.g. schizophrenia
Münchausen (hospital addiction) syndrome
Alcoholism leading to liver disease
Self-neglect
Physical conditions presenting with psychiatric complaints
Depressive disorder precipitated by cancer, e.g. of pancreas
Anxiety in hyperthyroidism
Postviral depression, e.g. posthepatitis, glandular fever, influenza
Medical drugs leading to psychiatric complications
e.g. antihypertensive drugs leading to depression
corticosteroids leading to depression, euphoria
Psychiatric drugs leading to medical complications
e.g. overdoses
chlorpromazine leading to jaundice
Coincidental psychiatric and physical disorder

Table 11.9 Factors influencing response to physical illness
Patient
Personality (e.g. overanxious, obsessional)
Illness behaviour (e.g. at what severity does the patient present)
Illness
Meaning and significance of illness (e.g. cancer)
Social environment
Threat to finances and employment
Welcomed if resolves conflict (e.g. marital)

to chronic fatigue syndrome itself. Some argue that the condition is synonymous with the ICD-10 diagnosis of neurasthenia. However, patients and family frequently fear the stigma of a psychiatric diagnosis.

The condition is exacerbated, often a day or two later, by increased activity and also by alcohol consumption. The essence of the treatment recommended by NICE in the UK is early paced activity management, avoiding over- or underactivity, and gradual rehabilitation with emotional support. CBT, incorporating a rehabilitation approach and graded exercise, can be offered as a more formalized approach, and has been recommended by NICE. However, these NICE recommendations have been questioned by those who favour a predominantly organic, rather than psychiatric/psychological, causation. Biofeedback approaches, self-help groups (attendees at these have a poorer prognosis), and psychodynamic therapy have also been used. Patients are sensitive to drug side-effects but low doses of tricyclic antidepressants can be helpful in improving sleep and alleviating pain. SSRIs, in contrast, may not be helpful unless depression is present. There is some evidence that treatment with essential fatty acids may be beneficial. At the time of writing, there are several ongoing biologically based treatment studies, including the use of antiviral agents. Poor outcome is associated with personality disorder and prolonged convalescence.

Psychosomatic disorders

Rheumatoid arthritis, ulcerative colitis, bronchial asthma, essential hypertension, thyrotoxicosis and peptic ulcer have all been described as psychosomatic disorders, a category developed in the 1950s by analysts in the USA. These are physical disorders aggravated or precipitated by psychological factors. Past theories that there are direct causal links between specific unconscious conflicts, psychological methods employed by individuals in coping with them and the development of specific organic diseases have now fallen into disrepute, e.g. asthma, and a more general theory has evolved, linking psychological stress in people with vulnerable personalities and an inherent vulnerability of certain of their bodily systems, leading to autonomic, endocrine and/or immunological changes, which, in turn, precipitate an organic disease to which they are predisposed. For instance, life events may precipitate a myocardial infarction, although the underlying coronary artery disease would already have been present. An increased vulnerability to cardiovascular conditions has been demonstrated in the first year after the death of a spouse. A link has also been suggested between coronary heart disease and type A personality (ambitious, aggressive and competitive, with a chronic sense of time urgency). Some also regard obesity and anorexia nervosa as psychosomatic disorders.

Other concepts and disorders related to physical complaints

These are described here for comparison, but are not by definition somatization disorders.

Monosymptomatic hypochondriacal psychosis

Those conditions where hypochondriacal delusions occur may take various forms. There may be a delusion of insect infestation of the skin (*Ekbom's Syndrome*), delusions of lumps under the skin, delusions of internal parasitosis and a delusion that the individual is emitting a foul smell. Delusionally believing that there is a physical cause, the patient attempts to gather evidence for this and seeks multiple medical opinions, to whom they may suggest bizarre treatments. Although such patients may become paranoid and angry towards their doctors, there may be an otherwise encapsulated systematized hypochondriacal delusional system. Such individuals are difficult to manage and may be resistant to treatment, although the antipsychotic oral medication pimozide has been found to be especially effective. Some cases have also been reported to respond to antidepressant medication; in other cases the disorder is part of a paranoid psychosis, depressive disorder or organic brain disorder.

The sick role

This was described by Parsons in 1951 and derived from learning and role theories. If an individual adopts the sick role, there are two rights (exemption from normal social responsibilities and not being held responsible for one's condition) and two obligations (the obligation of wanting to recover and an obligation to seek appropriate help, usually from a doctor, and to cooperate with such help). An individual is liable to find the sick role attractive and adopt it when its advantages outweigh its disadvantages. For instance, an individual may be unable to respond adequately to the demands of daily life, or may otherwise feel that adopting the sick role is the only way to receive sufficient sympathy, attention and love. Those who as a child had indulgent parents may find the sick role particularly attractive, due to their having learned that status and power can be achieved by manipulative behaviour strategies. Individuals may be especially prone to adopt the sick role at times of increased responsibility and stress (see also Chapter 4).

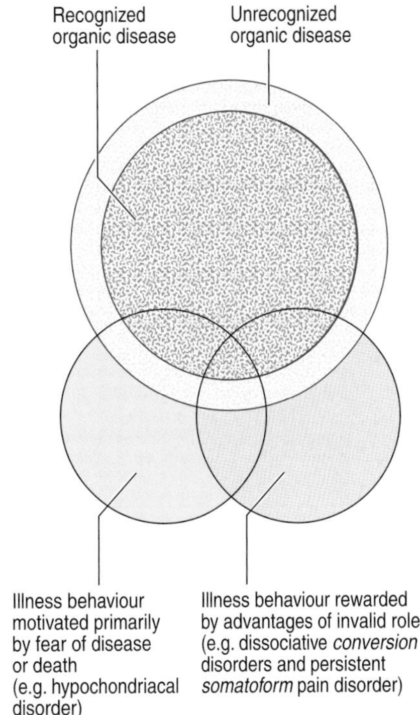

Figure 11.6 • The relationship between organic disease and illness behaviour.

Illness behaviour

Illness behaviour is the way in which symptoms are perceived, evaluated and acted on. Factors such as religion and social class affect how an individual responds to these symptoms, for example the tendency to seek, and the threshold for seeking, medical advice. Such behaviour may be judged inappropriate, given the individual's degree of disability and the situation. It may then be referred to as *abnormal illness behaviour*. Figure 11.6 illustrates the suggested relationship between organic disease and illness behaviour.

Accident neurosis

This condition overlaps with *post-traumatic neurosis*, which is itself often used to refer to neurotic symptoms following head injury (*postconcussional syndrome*). True malingering is uncommon following head injury. Gross 'neurotic' symptoms are inversely related to the severity of the head injury and most often occur when the cause of the injury is perceived by the individual as someone else's fault, or if financial compensation is possible. It is more likely to occur in males of lower social class following industrial injuries. Sexual dysfunction may be marked. It is now realized that even in cases of so-called compensation neurosis, symptoms may persist independent of seeking and achieving compensation, and that the resulting disability is often underestimated. However, the longer disputes about compensation continue, the worse the prognosis.

Factitious disorders

Factitious means not genuine, real or natural, and such disorders are characterized by physical or psychological symptoms that are intentionally produced or feigned, associated with a psychological need to assume the sick role, as evidenced by the absence of external incentives for such behaviour such as economic gain, better care or physical well-being. This contrasts with malingering, where symptoms are also produced intentionally but for an external goal that is obviously recognizable when the environmental circumstances are known, e.g. financial compensation. Examples of physical symptoms in factitious disorders include self-inflicted injuries to the skin or symptoms arising from the acceptance of medication, despite the individual being aware of having an abnormal sensitivity to the drug. It usually begins before the age of 30 years. The main treatments

Table 11.10 Difference between somatoform, conversion, dissociative and factitious disorders and malingering

	Physical symptoms	Psychological symptoms	Unconscious motivation	Conscious motivation	Voluntary production of symptoms	Involuntary production of symptoms
Somatoform disorders	+++	–	+	–	–	+
Conversion disorders	++	–	+	–	–	+
Dissociative disorders	–	++	+	–	–	+
Factitious disorders	++	+	+	–	+	–
Malingering	++	+	–	+	+	–

used have been psychological, either confrontatory or non-confrontatory. Table 11.10 summarizes differences between somatoform, conversion, dissociative and factitious disorders and malingering.

Münchausen syndrome (hospital addiction syndrome)

This is the best-studied form of factitious disorder with physical symptoms, and was described by Asher in 1951 and named after Baron von Münchhausen (sic), Raspe's 1785 fictitious French cavalry officer who lied harmlessly about his exploits. Such individuals feign illness to bring about repeated hospital admissions, investigations and operations for no obvious gain. Although symptoms are consciously produced, motivation is largely unconscious but directed to achieving the sick role. It is an abnormal illness behaviour, a disorder of both illness behaviour and sick role. The patients simulate symptoms suggestive of serious physical illness and deceive medical staff. Men appear to be affected more than women. Their histories are often plausible but overdramatic. They may inflict injuries on themselves or simulate symptoms in a bizarre way, such as swallowing needles. Abdominal symptoms are the most common. Pathological lying (*pseudologia fantastica*) is often present. Variants include presenting with psychiatric complaints, including false histories of bereavement. Patients may seek analgesic drugs and, more generally, attention. The condition is conceptualized as histrionic or hysterical behaviour in a severely disordered, sometimes masochistic, personality. Such individuals become impostors as a defence against feelings of inferiority and may masochistically play out a game with staff involving aggressive and sexual elements, perhaps to counter unconscious guilt and the psychological disintegration of the individual. Their behaviour may induce a sadistic response from staff. However, physical illness may predispose, coexist with, or result from Münchausen syndrome.

When their feigning comes to light, such individuals may abscond from hospital, but travel to another hospital (*peregrination*) and present with the same clinical scenario. They frequently change their name and the hospitals they approach, and they have a characteristic lack of visitors. Consistent management is thus made very difficult with considerable associated costs, morbidity and even mortality. Those who wander usually have longer histories, are more often men, unemployed, or frequently change jobs, are more likely to present with abdominal or psychological symptoms, to have abused drugs and alcohol, and to have criminal convictions. Non-wanderers tend to be female, to be more stable socially, to be nurses, and to have less dramatic symptoms.

Aetiological factors may include parental abuse, neglect, early experience of chronic illness or hospitalization, paramedic employment, and experience of medical mis-management with an associated grudge. Organic mental disorder should be excluded.

Treatment of coexisting depressive disorder may sometimes be of benefit. Psychological treatment is the ideal treatment of choice, either non-confrontatory or confrontatory.

A further variant is *Münchausen by proxy*, in which physical symptoms are intentionally produced in others, for instance by a mother in her child. Such children do not show symptoms when in the care of others or when the mother is supervised. There may be a similar history of unexplained symptoms or even death in a sibling of the child. The mother may have medical experience such as being a nurse and an emotionally distorted relationship with her spouse. Through her behaviour she becomes the centre of attention and herself receives care, which may underlie the motivation for such behaviour. Such mothers rarely ever admit to having produced physical symptoms in their children, often due to underlying feelings of deep humiliation.

Malingering

This is the conscious production of physical or psychiatric symptoms for external gain, e.g. to avoid prison, to obtain benefits or to avoid military service. It is not a mental disorder in ICD-10 or DSM-IV-TR, although the latter describes it as an *'additional condition that may be the focus of clinical attention'*.

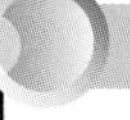

Body dysmorphic disorder and other associated concepts

- In body dysmorphic disorder (dysmorphophobia), there is a preoccupation with some imagined defect in appearance in a normal-appearing person, which is not of delusional intensity.
- In clinical practice, most medically unexplained symptoms are due to undifferentiated somatoform disorder or are due to another primary psychiatric disorder, e.g. somatic anxiety symptoms, facial pain in depression.
- Somatization is the tendency to experience somatic (physical) symptoms unaccounted for by organic causes, to attribute such symptoms to physical illness and to seek medical help.
- Psychosomatic disorders are physical conditions aggravated or precipitated by psychological factors, e.g. bronchial asthma, peptic ulcer or ulcerative colitis.
- In monosymptomatic hypochondriacal psychosis, there are hypochondriacal delusions, such as skin infestation by insects or of an emission of a foul smell.
- Adopting the sick role exempts an individual from normal responsibilities and from being held responsible for his/her condition.
- Illness behaviour refers to the way symptoms are perceived and acted on by an individual.
- Accident neurosis overlaps with post-traumatic neurosis. Postconcussional syndrome refers to neurotic symptoms following a head injury.
- In cases of compensation neurosis, symptoms may persist after compensation.
- In malingering, symptoms are consciously produced for an obvious goal, which is lacking in factitious disorders.
- Münchausen (hospital addiction) syndrome is a factitious disorder where patients repeatedly present at and get admitted to hospitals with feigned symptoms suggestive of serious physical illness.

Psychiatry of menstruation and pregnancy

Introduction

Psychiatric disorders are more common in women. Genetic, social and cultural theories have been put forward to explain these findings. Table 12.1 shows psychiatric disorders for which the prevalence is different between men and women. The lifetime risk of developing bipolar mood disorder or schizophrenia is, however, equal in males and females.

Premenstrual syndrome (PMS) (late luteal-phase dysphoric disorder)

PMS consists of emotional, physical and behavioural symptoms, which occur regularly during the second half of each menstrual cycle (i.e. between ovulation and menstruation), subside during menstruation and are completely absent between menstruation and ovulation.

Epidemiology

Most women experience some premenstrual symptoms, but of these only 20–40% consider them severe enough to seek medical help. For about 6% these symptoms are considered incapacitating. The syndrome does not improve with age or parity. Although PMS is found more often in those with other psychiatric disorders, it may be that these sensitize such women to the additional premenstrual changes.

Clinical features

Over 150 symptoms of PMS have been described. Among the most common are *psychological symptoms* such as tension, irritability, depression, fatigue and poor concentration. Physical symptoms are shown in Figure 12.1.

During the premenstrual period there is an increase in parasuicidal acts, suicide, accidents, violent crimes, shoplifting and poor academic performance. Migraine and skin disorders worsen during this period. Mothers are also more likely to take their children to see their GP. Mental hospital admissions are increased premenstrually, suggesting that PMS exacerbates pre-existing psychiatric disorder.

Investigations and diagnosis

Diagnosis depends predominantly on confirming the timing of symptoms in relation to menstruation, i.e. symptoms begin in mid-cycle, they increase in number and severity to maximum intensity the day

Table 12.1 Psychiatric disorders more common in men or women

More common in men	More common in women
Alcoholism (eight times)	Senile dementia
Mental retardation	Dysthymia
Criminal behaviour, especially violence	Unipolar psychotic depression
Completed suicide	Anxiety and phobic disorders
	Dissociative (conversion) disorders
	Anorexia nervosa (nine times)
	Bulimia nervosa
	Deliberate self-harm

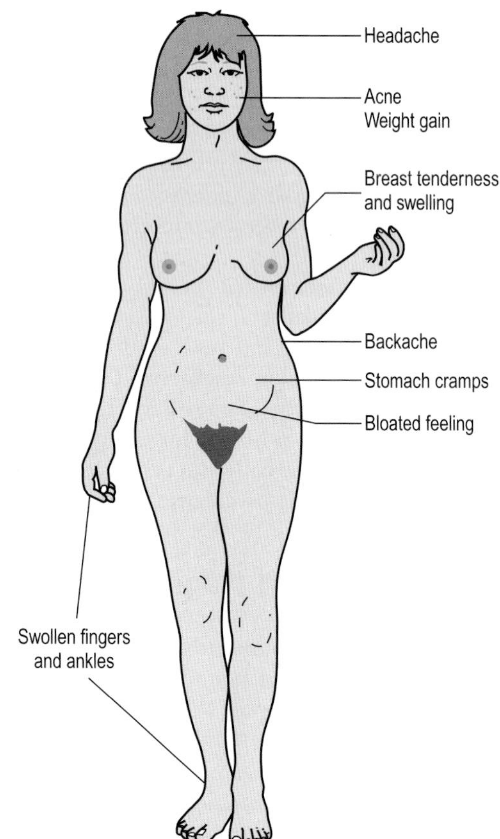

Figure 12.1 • Physical symptoms of premenstrual tension.

before the onset of menstruation, and this is followed by rapid and complete resolution of symptoms. The woman should be advised to keep a diary for at least two months of daily ratings of common menstrual cycle symptoms, using a standard symptom record chart (Figure 12.2) to help confirm the diagnosis.

Differential diagnosis

There is at least a seven-day symptom-free phase after menstruation in PMS. This distinguishes PMS from merely premenstrual exacerbation of other psychiatric disorders, such as depressive disorder or panic disorder and physical disorders. In *dysmenorrhoea* (painful menstruation), the symptoms occur with menstruation, whereas in premenstrual syndrome the symptoms are worst premenstrually.

Aetiology

The exact cause of PMS is unknown and different factors may be important in the development of different symptoms. Genetic factors have been suggested, as there is an increased incidence in monozygotic compared to dizygotic twins. Psychological factors may also have a role. A correlation of PMS with neuroticism has been suggested.

Physiological factors have also been suggested. Luteal-phase changes in hormones are likely to be important, for example a relative deficiency of progesterone, or a rise in oestrogen levels. Alterations in the renin–angiotensin system resulting in excessive aldosterone secretion and fluid retention, pyridoxine deficiency and alterations in monoamine neurotransmitters with increased monoamine activity have also been suggested.

Management

For many no medical treatment is required, other than information giving, explanation of the development of symptoms and reassurance, including supportive psychotherapy. For those more severely affected, target symptoms should be identified and treated, for example with *analgesics* if the predominant symptoms are headache or pain, or evening primrose oil or danazol for cyclical breast pain.

Pyridoxine (vitamin B_6) may provide some benefit.

Epidemiology

One in five to one in ten women develop a non-psychotic depressive disorder in the postpartum period. This is more likely to occur in those of increased age and lower social class. However, fewer than 1% see a psychiatrist and most receive treatment from their GP or no treatment at all.

Clinical features

These are similar to those seen in depression at other times, but may be mistaken for normal physiological changes following childbirth, e.g. reduced energy, sleep and libido.

Despondency, tearfulness and irritability are typically seen. Fatigue, anxiety and phobias also frequently occur. Mothers develop fears about their ability to cope with their newborn baby and their own and the baby's health. Feelings of inadequacy, difficulty in sleeping and concentrating, feeling 'confused', a poor appetite and decreased libido are also common. Guilt feelings can develop over their irritability and their perception of being inadequate mothers. Decreased libido, which may be the main symptom, has been related to falling hormone levels.

The degree of depression itself may be relatively mild or masked and somatic symptoms may be more prominent. Migraine may be worsened.

Symptoms are often worse at night. A vicious cycle of worry and insomnia may be set up. The presentation is often one of '*atypical depression*'. Mothers painfully contrast their despair with others' observations of how lucky they are to have a newborn child.

Individuals who develop postnatal depression may be more likely to have high levels of anxiety in the first three months of pregnancy, and also during the last trimester, which may then also be associated with admission to hospital for psychosocial reasons, although often ostensibly on clinical grounds, for instance with proteinuria, oedema and/or hypertension.

At interview, the mother's mood should be assessed, depressive (including suicidal) ideas elicited, and her feelings for and attachment to her baby explored. Fleeting or intrusive thoughts of harming the baby are present in 40% of postnatally depressed women but rarely acted on.

Investigations

It is always advisable to visit the family home to assess the home circumstances and to interview the husband or partner.

The Edinburgh Postnatal Depression Scale (EPDS) is a 10-item self-report screening questionnaire; a score of more than 11 or 12 out of 30 is suggestive of postnatal depression.

Aetiology

This condition seems predominantly related to the psychological demands of infant care. There is little evidence for biological or hormonal factors. The risk is, however, doubled by a *previous psychiatric history of depressive disorder* or an *absence of personal social support* from husband, family or friends.

Some cases may represent mild puerperal psychosis. However, overall there is little evidence for genetic factors. Individuals do not differ from controls in relation to their previous psychiatric history or family history of psychiatric disorder. They also do not differ in their parity. There is an increased history of previous menstrual problems and severe maternal 'blues'. Hormonal effects on tryptophan metabolism have been suggested, but not proven, and even adoptive mothers can develop postnatal depression. A study of national fish intake in 19 countries found a significant negative correlation between the prevalence of postpartum depression and average fish consumption per person. Countries with a high intake include Japan and Singapore, whereas countries with a low intake include New Zealand and the United Arab Emirates (Figure 12.5).

An association with physical problems during the pregnancy or the postnatal period has been found, especially with caesarean section. Lack of a confiding supportive relationship with the partner or other members of the family may predispose towards the development of depression, and this may be associated with social, financial and marital changes consequent on the birth of a child.

Those with postnatal depression are more likely to have had four or more unpleasant significant *stressful life events* (e.g. bereavement or illness) shortly before or during pregnancy. They are also more likely to have had chronic difficulties in their life (e.g. poverty, poor living conditions and physical ill health) and a poor quality of social support (e.g. from husband or partner, parents, parents-in-law, friends) and a poor social network. These chronic difficulties are present at other times, but the burden of a newborn child may induce helplessness against this background and precipitate postnatal depression.

It is said that individuals with postnatal depression are in general more neurotic and introverted.

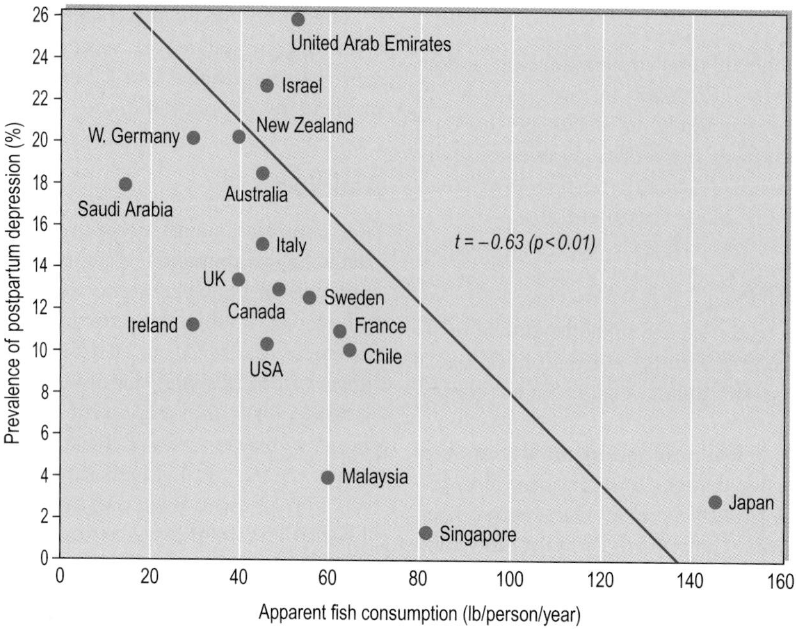

Figure 12.5 • Relationship between point prevalence of postpartum depression in 19 countries and the apparent consumption of fish in the same countries. (Reproduced with permission from Hibbeln JR 1999 LCPUFAs in depression and related conditions. In: Peet M, Glen I, Horrobin DF (eds) Phospholipid spectrum disorder in psychiatry. Marius Press, Carnforth)

Also, postnatal depression may be more common in women with *rigid, obsessional personalities*; those with low self-esteem; those who are less keen on stereotypical female behaviour and see little of value in a newborn child after a long pregnancy; those who are *emotionally immature* who may marry too young; and those with *overdependent personalities*, particularly if they are in a mutually overdependent relationship with their spouse. The birth of a child may reactivate a mother's unresolved conflicts, such as with her own mother and over her own dependency needs, and bring home to both parents their overdependency on each other. Such a mother may have difficulty caring for a newborn child. There may also be covert hostility to the child.

Mothers who develop this disorder may be more anxious during pregnancy, for instance if it was the first birth, or if they have a past history of infertility.

A *disturbed mother–infant relationship* may be causal or caused by postnatal depression. Bonding with a newborn child may be important in preventing postnatal depression. This can be facilitated by the husband or partner being present at delivery, which also decreases the mother's isolation. Research shows that 15 minutes' breastfeeding on delivery is associated with increased eye contact with the child and bonding months later. Postnatal depression is associated with demonstrable disturbance of mother–child interaction, whatever the cause, which then produces a vicious cycle of worsening interactions and further exacerbation of the mother's mental state (Figure 12.6). Jealousy of the newborn child may lead to *behavioural disturbance in the siblings*, and thus additional stress for the mother.

A mother may develop postnatal depression during one pregnancy and not another because the

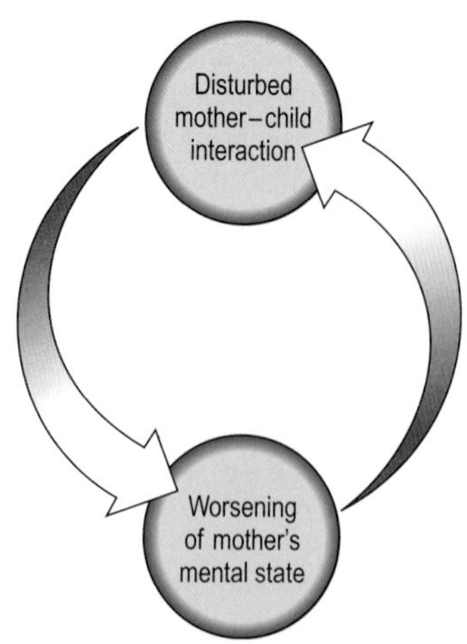

Figure 12.6 • The vicious cycle of postnatal depression.

relationship between her and her husband or partner is changed: each successive pregnancy represents a tightening bond in the marriage. Also, one child may be temperamentally more difficult to manage (e.g. crying more and sleeping less), although this may be due to the circular relationship of the mother's anxiety causing the child to feel insecure.

Management

It is said that postnatal depression is, for 90% of those suffering from it, a self-limiting condition often lasting less than a month, even without treatment.

However, *preventative interventions* are important and include education about postnatal depression, good antenatal care with attention to risk factors for postnatal depression, treatment of depression during pregnancy and support during labour, childbirth and after the baby is born, e.g. for breastfeeding.

Supportive psychotherapy, e.g. non-directive counselling, and reassurance are of value, as is specific brief psychological therapy, e.g. cognitive behavioural therapy. Also helpful are facilitating the involvement of the husband or partner in the newborn's care and providing practical help to overcome the mother's difficulty in coping. The involvement of a health visitor can also be of much benefit. A group of mothers with similar problems may also be of value. If the depression lasts for longer than a month, antidepressants are indicated and some mothers may respond better to monoamine oxidase inhibitors (MAOIs) than to tricyclic antidepressants or selective serotonin reuptake inhibitors (SSRIs). However, overall most respond to standard antidepressants. These are secreted in breast milk but are rarely detectable and have not to date been found significantly to affect infants adversely. Nonetheless, clinicians should always consider the potential risks as well as benefits of such treatment for both mother and infant. Chronic marital difficulties may require marital therapy.

Prognosis

Many recover spontaneously within three to six months without treatment, but one-third to one-half still have features of postnatal depression at six months and 10% at one year. Overall, it is said that 60% are fully recovered within one year. Others have residual symptoms and go on to develop a chronic or recurrent mood disorder. Research, however, suggests that only 1% see a psychiatrist and that many cases are missed; as a result such women may continue to suffer from mild depression, with loss of libido often prominent. This sometimes explains why some women state that following pregnancy they are 'never the same again'.

Among primaparae, 30% develop depression after a subsequent birth. The rate is increased where the first episode of postnatal depression represents the first-ever depressive illness, suggesting that the postpartum period is a specific risk factor.

Maternal postnatal depression in the absence of adequate fathering or substitute mothering may result in an increased incidence of emotional disturbance in the mother's children and adverse effects on the next generation of parents and their parenting capacities. Postnatal depression can affect the emotional and cognitive development of the child, especially among boys and in lower social class families. It results in insecure emotional attachments at 18 months and frank behavioural disturbance in boys aged five years.

Given the high rates of undetected and treatable postnatal depression, extra vigilance is necessary from primary care services, i.e. health visitors, midwives and GPs, to ensure early recognition.

Case history: postnatal depression

A 35-year-old successful but rigid, obsessional business woman, Mrs A., had been unable to return to work after giving birth to her first baby six months earlier. She complained of increasing depression, severe fatigue and irritability. She felt unable to cope with her baby, which was born prematurely and initially required nursing in an incubator. Under pressure from her husband she had been seen by her GP, who had referred her to a psychiatrist for advice.

The psychiatrist interviewed the woman and then her husband alone, and subsequently saw them together. As a result of his assessment the psychiatrist ascertained that the woman's mother had also suffered from severe depression, Mrs A.'s pregnancy had been unplanned and that Mrs A. felt ambivalent about having a baby and in conflict between her wish to resume her employment and her new responsibilities as a mother. She was also concerned about the financial implications for her and her husband if she had to be away from work for a prolonged period. She found it difficult to confide her feelings to her husband.

Continued

Case history: postnatal depression—cont'd

The psychiatrist enquired as to whether Mrs A. had thoughts of harming her child or herself, and excluded a diagnosis of puerperal psychosis due to the absence of psychotic symptoms and of a course characteristic of puerperal psychosis, i.e. there was no early and rapid onset of symptoms following a lucid and then a prodromal phase. The history was more in keeping with the slow progression of increasing depressive symptoms seen in postnatal depression.

The psychiatrist arranged for Mrs A. to be admitted with her child for inpatient psychiatric treatment on a mother and baby unit. This increased the bonding between them. Mrs A. received antidepressant medication, on which she was subsequently discharged home. By this time her husband and family had been mobilized to provide her with emotional and practical support and her own mental state had much improved. She had also been seen jointly with her husband for marital therapy to improve the communication between them.

With the improvement in her postnatal depression, and as a result of the supervision and help in caring for her new baby that she had received on the mother and baby unit, Mrs A. again felt able to look after her child with the support of her husband and family. Six months later, after enlisting the help of a childminder, she returned first part-time and then subsequently full-time to her employment, satisfied more in her own mind about the balance she would need to strike between the care of her baby and her own needs.

Postnatal depression

- Onset is usually after postpartum maternity blues and puerperal psychosis, characteristically in or after the third week postpartum.
- There is a slow progression of symptoms of fatigue, insomnia, anxiety, irritability, restlessness and loss of libido.
- Feelings of inadequacy about caring for the baby are common.
- Aetiological factors include ambivalence towards baby, previous history of termination, lack of social support and chronic marital and social difficulties.
- Depressive symptoms may be masked. Early recognition is important.
- Management is by supportive psychotherapy, social support and antidepressants.

Postpartum maternity 'blues'

Epidemiology

Following delivery, half to two-thirds of women have a short-lived disturbance of emotions, commencing between three and five days and lasting for one to two days, but not beyond 10 days. It is more common following the birth of the first child and those with a history of premenstrual tension.

Clinical features

These are characterized by episodes of weeping, feelings of depression, anxiety, irritability, feeling separate and distant from the baby, mild hypochondriasis, difficulty in sleeping and poor concentration.

Aetiology

It is assumed that postpartum 'blues' have a biochemical and hormonal basis, which is associated with the findings of weight loss, reduced thirst and increased renal sodium secretion. It has also been related to normal exhaustion after a climactic delivery following a prolonged pregnancy. The onset after three days has also been related to the euphoria of delivery being replaced by the reality of having to look after and feed the baby. High neuroticism scores on personality assessment have also been found to be more common.

Management

This requires only reassurance and explanation to the mother and her partner, as the condition is self-limiting within 10 days of delivery.

Other concepts relating to pregnancy and childbirth

Couvade syndrome

This is a dissociative (conversion) disorder in which the prospective father himself develops symptoms characteristic of pregnancy, such as morning sickness, gastrointestinal disturbance and food craving. These symptoms are associated with anxiety and tend to develop either in the first trimester or at the end of pregnancy.

The syndrome can be seen as understandable anxiety in an overanxious husband. Often there is a strong bond between the couple and overidentification by the male with the future mother. There may also be elements of unconscious envy of the woman and her role in childbearing, which may be tinged with hostility. It may also reflect the woman being preoccupied with the pregnancy and less interested in the man. Up to 10% of expectant fathers may develop gastrointestinal symptoms at some stage during their wife's pregnancy.

Management requires only reassurance, and symptoms usually clear completely following the delivery.

Use of psychotropic drugs during pregnancy and lactation

Psychotropic drugs may:

- have a *teratogenic effect* on the developing fetus
- result in *withdrawal symptoms* in a newborn baby, if taken by the mother at the end of the pregnancy
- be present in breast milk fed to the child.

The most up to date information should be consulted before prescribing any medication to a pregnant patient. One excellent source of such information is the latest edition of the *British National Formulary*.

Mother–infant relationship

Breastfeeding on delivery is associated with increased eye contact with the child and bonding months later. Maternal feelings for a newborn child may normally be delayed for up to three weeks, and this may need explaining to a mother and husband to avoid feelings of rejection towards the child. For the first three to four weeks a mother may feel tired, insecure and find managing the child unrewarding and hard work. A baby's smile often first elicits maternal feelings. By three months mothers feel pangs of guilt when they leave their baby.

Stillbirth

Both mothers and fathers undergo the bereavement process following a stillbirth. The psychological effects of stillbirth and the need for counselling have been increasingly recognized. Mothers are now encouraged to see and handle stillborn babies, particularly as their imagined perception of the stillborn is usually worse than the reality. Fifty per cent of mothers become pregnant again within one year, mostly on a planned basis to replace the lost child. Compared with those who become pregnant after one year, they show more anxiety during pregnancy and more depression and anxiety in the year following delivery, perhaps reflecting insufficient grieving of the stillbirth or other vulnerabilities, including that of personality.

Oral contraception

In spite of earlier concerns that oral contraception was associated with, precipitated or exacerbated by severe mental illnesses (such as depression) and reduced libido, more recent research has found only a mild increase in psychiatric symptoms in those with a past psychiatric history, and then only in the first month of oral contraception use. Pyridoxine deficiency was found to be associated with depression in a small number on the pill, and thus oral pyridoxine was recommended for administration with oral contraception.

Sterilization

Where the woman is properly assessed and counselled beforehand, sterilization generally results in an improvement in her mental state, well-being, marital and sexual relationships and social adjustment. Overall, there is no increase in psychiatric symptoms, but individuals who are younger, with a small family and are under pressure to be sterilized are most at risk.

Other concepts related to childbirth and pregnancy

- Couvade syndrome is a hysterical disorder in which the prospective father develops symptoms characteristic of pregnancy.
- Maternal feelings for a newborn child may normally be delayed for up to three weeks.
- Breastfeeding increases bonding with a newborn.

Menopause

There is no evidence that severe mental illness is more common in women around the time of the menopause. Previous descriptions of a distinct depressive disorder – involutional melancholia – specifically linked to the menopause have not been confirmed. The clinical picture described then probably merely reflected the characteristic presentation of depressive disorder at that age. The menopause may psychologically alter the woman's perception of herself, and often occurs at a time when other major life events are also taking place (e.g. children leaving home, retirement, parents dying).

Ninety per cent of women do experience hot flushes and excessive sweating for one to two years after the cessation of periods, due to reduced ovarian activity causing vasomotor changes. These respond to oestrogen treatment. However, in the year following the menopause up to one-third of women experience anxiety, irritability, fatigue and headaches, which is 10% greater than at other times. Such mild affective (mood) disorder during the menopause does not respond to oestrogen therapy any better than placebo.

Hysterectomy

Although psychiatric referral following a hysterectomy is greater than for other abdominal operations, particularly where no physical pathology was found at operation, research has shown that such individuals had a high level of preoperative psychiatric morbidity, which the operation reduces but to a level still higher than in the general population. It has been suggested that psychiatric disorder may be associated with menorrhagia (heavy periods), which leads to the operation.

Amenorrhoea

This can occur following psychological stress and in psychiatric disorders such as depression and anorexia nervosa. Conventional (first-generation) antipsychotic medication may increase prolactin levels and thus cause amenorrhoea.

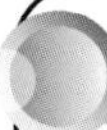

Menopause/hysterectomy/amenorrhoea

- During the year following menopause up to one-third of women experience a 10% greater frequency of anxiety, irritability, fatigue and headache, but not a distinct depressive disorder.
- Psychiatric referral following a hysterectomy is greater than for other abdominal operations; such individuals also have a high level of preoperative psychiatric morbidity.
- Amenorrhoea can follow psychiatric stress and occurs in psychiatric disorders such as depression and anorexia nervosa.
- First-generation antipsychotics can increase prolactin levels, resulting in amenorrhoea.

Psychiatry of sexuality

Introduction

Psychosexual disorders can be divided into *disorders of sexual preference* and *disorders of sexual functioning*. The forensic aspects of the former are addressed in Chapter 21.

Disorders of sexual preference are strongly culturally determined. For example, in the early part of the 20th century *masturbatory insanity* was an accepted diagnosis derived from the observation of incarcerated 'lunatics and mental defectives'. This term was dropped when, first, the malign influence of sensory deprivation in increasing the likelihood of repetitive behaviours was realized, and secondly when masturbation became more accepted as a part of 'normal' human sexuality in Western culture. Similarly, homosexuality was included in the ninth International Classification of Diseases but is not in ICD-10.

Disorders of sexual functioning were not properly identified until the pioneering work of Masters and Johnson in the USA examined human physiological responses during sexual behaviour, and put forward a four-stage model of sexual arousal.

Sexual response

Before considering the sexual response it is important to be familiar with the anatomy of the human genitalia. The important structures are depicted in Figures 13.1 and 13.2. It must be remembered, however, that sexual responsiveness is not confined to the genitalia but can and does involve the whole body. Indeed, this is an important consideration in some of the treatments for sexual dysfunction.

The four phases identified by Masters and Johnson are excitement, plateau, orgasm and resolution. Kaplan proposed instead a three-phase model of desire, excitement and orgasm. Kaplan introduced desire (also referred to as libido, or sexual interest) as an additional concept because of her clinical observations in the treatment of people with sexual dysfunction that problems could remain despite normal physiological responses in the other phases. Excitement and orgasm phases were distinguished because of their predominant mediation by the parasympathetic and sympathetic nervous systems respectively.

In Masters and Johnson's model:

- *Excitement phase* – arousal develops in response to sexual stimulation (fantasy as well as actual). In the female there is rapid vaginal lubrication, expansion and distension of the inner part of the vagina, swelling and elongation of the clitoris, some elevation of the uterus and, in some women, nipple erection. In the male there is erection of the penis, thickening of the scrotal skin and some elevation of the testes. In both sexes there is some increase in blood pressure and pulse.
- *Plateau phase* – an intensification of excitement from which orgasm can occur. In the female there is breast and areolar enlargement, swelling of the outer third of the vagina, withdrawal of the clitoral head and shaft into the clitoral hood, and a reddening of the labia minora. In men there is some colour change of the penis head and enlargement and further elevation of the testes. In both sexes there is an increase in muscle tension, pulse and blood pressure. In some there is a 'flush' across the front of the trunk and head on some occasions.

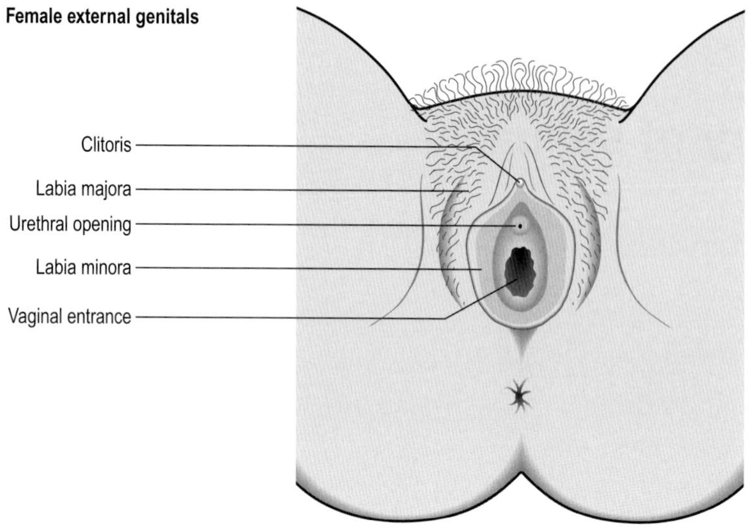

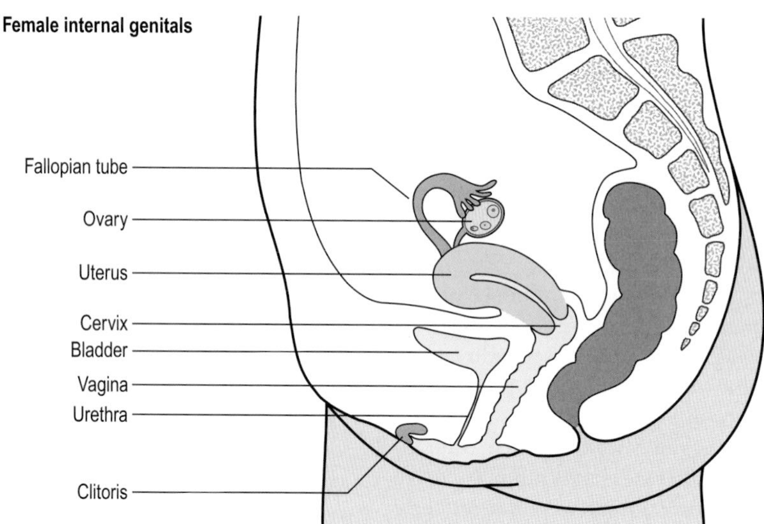

Figure 13.1 • Female genitalia.

- *Orgasm phase* – involuntary release of sexual tension. In the female there is rhythmic contraction of the outer third of the vagina and contractions of the uterus. In the male there is ejaculation of the prostate, seminal vesicles, etc. to produce seminal fluid (ejaculatory inevitability), followed by rhythmic contractions of the urethra to expel the semen. In both sexes maximal pulse, blood pressure and respiration are produced.
- *Resolution phase* – in which the bodily status returns to normal. In women the cervix is lowered to the vaginal floor and there is some gaping of the cervical os. The resolution phase may occur without orgasm or plateau phases.

The relative timings of each of these phases are shown in Figure 13.3. In females there may be rapid response to reach orgasm (e.g. during masturbation). In either sex there may be excitement and plateau without orgasm, although this is much more common in the female. In males there is a refractory period after orgasm during which a further orgasm cannot occur. The length of this increases with age.

Male external genitals

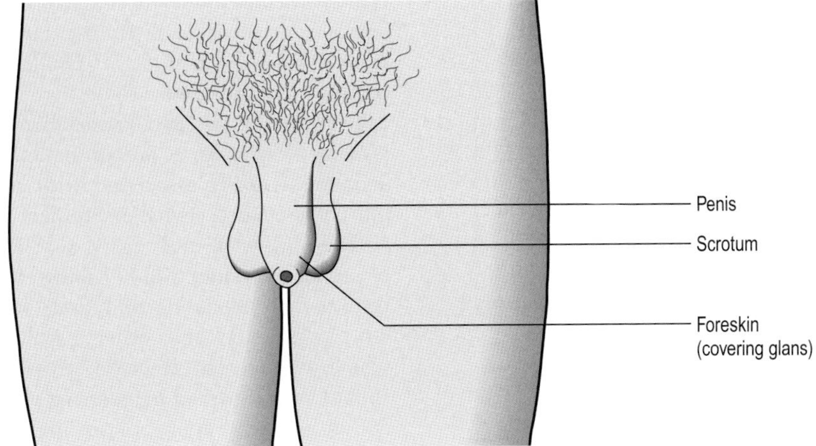

Male internal genitals

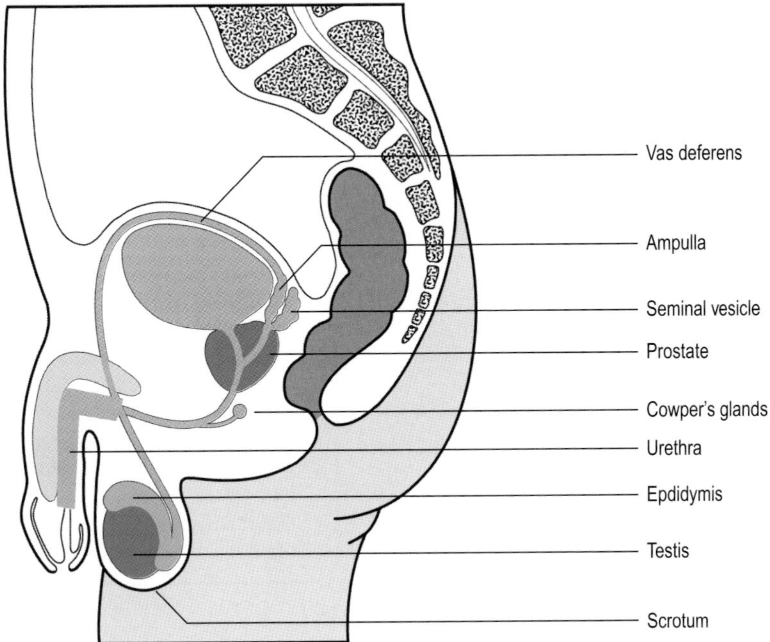

Figure 13.2 • Male genitalia.

Classification and diagnosis of sexual disorders

The ICD-10 category for *disorders of sexual preference* is shown in Table 13.1 and the DSM-IV-TR category for paraphilias in Table 13.2. These may variously be referred to as *paraphilias*, *perversions* or *sexual deviances*, although the latter two labels have become regarded as stigmatizing in many circles, perhaps because of the overlap between these disorders and *sexual offences* (see Chapter 21). Disorders of sexual preference are characterized by sexually arousing fantasies, urges and/or activities, which are not part of normative sexual functioning *and* which interfere

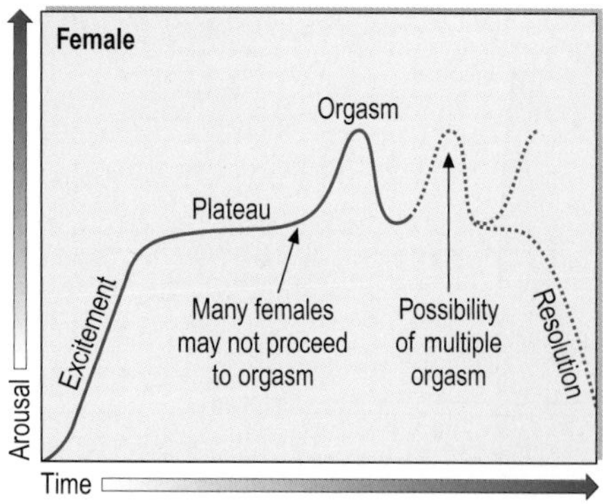

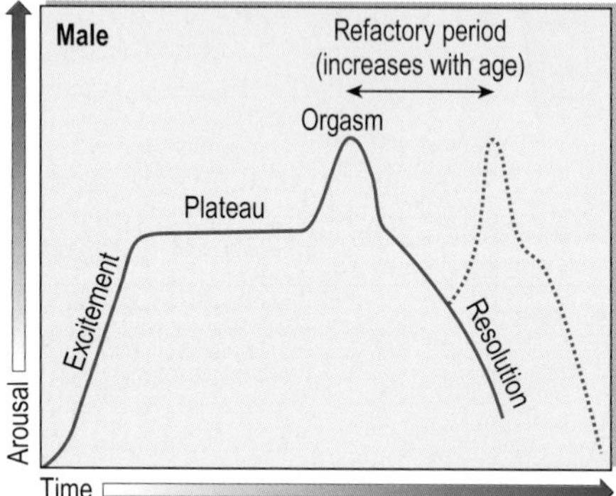

Figure 13.3 • Relative timings of Masters and Johnson's phases of the sexual response.

with reciprocal affectionate activity. Some of these activities are illegal, but this can vary between jurisdictions. Some of the activities, such as voyeurism and exhibitionism, can present to a lesser degree in 'normal' sexuality, but are not persistent or preferred. Mental illness may be associated with the disorder of sexuality and should be diagnosed if present.

Gender identity disorders are classified in ICD-10 under category F64, and include transsexualism, dual-role transvestism and gender identity disorder of childhood. *Transsexualism* is a desire to live, function and be accepted as a member of the opposite sex. There is a conviction that 'wrong' gender assignment has occurred and a sense of discomfort with anatomical sexual characteristics. This leads to pursuit of hormonal treatment and surgery to make the external appearance as congruent as possible with the preferred sex. Such features usually are present from childhood, but must be present persistently for at least two years before the ICD-10 diagnosis can be made. Psychiatrists are usually extensively involved in assessment where gender reassignment surgery is being contemplated. *Dual-role transvestism* is the wearing of clothes of the opposite sex for part of the time without the wish permanently to change sex and without sexual excitement (*cf.* fetishistic transvestism, F65.1). *Gender identity disorder of childhood* is rare, and refers to a child's desire to be the opposite sex, typically from the preschool years but certainly before puberty. There is a preoccupation with activities and dress usually associated with the opposite sex but no associated sexual excitement.

The ICD-10 and DSM-IV-TR classifications of sexual dysfunction (Tables 13.3 and 13.4) refer to disorders of normal sexual functioning. Anxiety, depression and other psychiatric disorders, which all have an effect on sexual responsiveness, should be considered in assessing sexual dysfunction and diagnosed if appropriate. The anergia of schizophrenia can include a reduction in sexual drive.

Sexual dysfunction may be *primary* (no previous satisfactory sexual functioning) or *secondary* (following a period of satisfactory sexual functioning).

Introduction

- Psychosexual disorders can be divided into disorders of sexual preference and disorders of sexual functioning.
- Disorders of sexual preference can, in part, be culturally determined and may have forensic implications.
- Masters and Johnson identified a four-phase model of sexual arousal in humans: excitement, plateau, orgasm and resolution. Kaplan added desire as an additional component.
- Other psychiatric disorders may have an effect on sexual behaviour and should be diagnosed where they occur.
- Disorders of sexual functioning refer to abnormalities of normal sexual functioning.

Disorders of sexual preference

Epidemiology

Reliable statistics on the levels of these disorders in the community are difficult to obtain because of the social and legal stigmas and hence the reluctance of individuals to participate in surveys of sexual activity. There are figures for convictions for those disorders that include behaviours that are against the law, but it

Table 13.1 I CD-10 classification: F65 Disorders of sexual preference
F65.0 Fetishism
Reliance on some non-living object as a stimulus for sexual arousal, e.g. articles of clothing, particular texture such as rubber or plastic
F65.1 Fetishistic transvestism
Wearing of opposite-sex clothes for sexual excitement
F65.2 Exhibitionism
Recurrent or persistent tendency to expose the genitalia to strangers (usually of the opposite sex) or to people in public places
F65.3 Voyeurism
Recurrent or persistent tendency to look at people engaging in sexual or intimate behaviour such as undressing
F65.4 Paedophilia
Sexual preference for children, usually prepubertal or early pubertal
F65.5 Sadomasochism
Preference for sexual activity that involves bondage or the infliction of pain or humiliation. Preference to be the recipient is masochism, to be provider is sadism
F65.6 Multiple disorders of sexual preference
Most common combination is fetishism, transvestism and sadomasochism
F65.7 Other disorders of sexual preference, e.g.
Frotteurism: rubbing up against people for sexual stimulation in crowded public places Necrophilia: preference for sexual activity with corpses Zoophilia: preference for sexual activity with animals (bestiality) Scotophilia: arousal from viewing of sexual scenes and genitalia (as with viewing of pornography) Telephone scatalogia: making of obscene telephone calls

Table 13.2 DSM-IV-TR Paraphilias
302.40 Exhibitionism
302.81 Fetishism
302.89 Frotteurism
302.20 Paedophilia
302.83 Sexual masochism
302.84 Sexual sadism
302.3 Transvestic fetishism
302.82 Voyeurism
302.9 Paraphilia NOS
NOS, not otherwise specified

is reasonable to assume that these are only a small proportion of the population figures. Also, conviction levels will be affected by many factors other than population prevalence, such as the level and type of law enforcement arrangements.

Fetishism

In fetishism, sexual excitation arises from inanimate objects or features of objects (e.g. material or colour). Fetishism may be compulsive or symptomatic, i.e. an individual may be impotent unless a fetish object is present. Various theories have arisen to account for fetishism: from ethology (a young child 'imprints' on mother's shoes, for example); from learning theory (sexual responses are conditioned to the fetish object); and from object relations theory

Table 13.3 ICD-10 classification: F52 Sexual dysfunction, not caused by organic disorder or disease

Table 13.3 ICD-10 classification: F52 Sexual dysfunction, not caused by organic disorder or disease
F52.0 Lack or loss of sexual desire
Normal sexual responsiveness but sexual activity less frequent and less wanted
F52.10 Sexual aversion
Strong negative feelings or anxiety associated with prospect of sexual activity with subsequent avoidance
F52.11 Lack of sexual enjoyment
Sexual activity occurs but is not enjoyed. More common in women
F52.2 Failure of genital response
In males, erectile dysfunction. In females, vaginal dryness (rarely complained of)
F52.3 Orgasmic dysfunction
Lack or delay of orgasm. More common in women
F52.4 Premature ejaculation
Inability to control ejaculation sufficiently to allow both partners to enjoy sex. May occur before vaginal penetration or in the absence of erection
F52.5 Non-organic vaginismus
Spasm of perivaginal muscles so that penile penetration is painful or not possible
F52.6 Non-organic dyspareunia
Pain on intercourse. Not diagnosed if other primary cause present (e.g. F52.5 or F52.2)
F52.7 Excessive sexual drive
Usually in late teens or early adulthood. May be secondary to mania or early dementia, in which case these diagnoses should be used
F52.8 Other sexual dysfunction, not caused by organic disorder or disease
F52.9 Unspecified sexual dysfunction, not caused by organic disorder or disease

(the fetish object is symbolic of early psychological conflicts). Fetishism can lead to recurrent convictions for theft of objects such as underwear from clothes-lines ('snow dropping'). In these circumstances the fetishist values the thought that such items have been used.

Exhibitionism

Exhibitionism is a recurrent or persistent tendency to expose one's genitalia to another person, usually of the opposite sex. Indecent exposure is the most common single sexual offence in the UK (over 3000 convictions per year in England and Wales). Most offenders are aged 20–40 years, with only a quarter being older than this (i.e. the 'dirty old man' is not usually old); 60% of offenders are married. Most are of normal intelligence, although up to 5% may suffer from psychosis or have some learning disability. The offence occurs most frequently in daylight, midweek (especially Tuesday) and is more likely in summer than in winter. Clinically two types of indecent exposer can be identified:

- *Type 1* (80% of cases) are usually inhibited young men who struggle against their impulse to expose, but find it irresistible and subsequently feel anxious, guilty and humiliated. They expose a flaccid penis, do not masturbate and derive little pleasure from the act. Such behaviour is related to lack of assertiveness and offenders describe enjoying the feeling of being in control of their transactions with females at the time of exposure. A response of annoyance, fear or even amusement is valued more than no response at all. The offender's intention is not usually to have sexual intercourse with the victims.

Table 13.4 DSM-IV-TR classification of sexual dysfunctions

Sexual desire disorders
302.71 Hypoactive sexual desire disorder
302.79 Sexual aversion disorder
Sexual arousal disorders
302.72 Female sexual arousal disorder
302.72 Male erectile disorder
Orgasmic disorders
302.73 Female orgasmic disorder
302.74 Male orgasmic disorder
302.75 Premature ejaculation
Sexual pain disorders
302.76 Dyspareunia (not due to a general medical condition)
306.51 Vaginismus (not due to a general medical condition)
Specifiers: lifelong type/acquired type; generalized type/situational type; due to psychological factors/due to combined factors

- *Type 2* (20% of cases) is less inhibited and more psychopathic/sociopathic (see Chapter 15) than Type 1. They expose in a state of sexual excitement, with an erect penis, and often masturbate while exposing. They obtain pleasure from the act, which is often sadistic, and show little guilt. The act may be combined with indecent suggestions, and may be accompanied by fantasies of more active assault. The behaviour may escalate in seriousness over time to indecent assault or rape.

Late onset of indecent exposure is associated with an increased likelihood of the presence of a major psychiatric disorder, such as alcohol dependence syndrome, depression or dementia.

Eighty per cent of indecent exposers do not reoffend after their first court appearance (especially those in the Type 1 group). There is a small recidivist group whose offending tends to decrease in frequency from the age of 40. These may be helped by behavioural techniques such as covert desensitization (exposure to anxiety-provoking situations in imagination), group therapy with similar individuals, or individual supportive psychotherapy, which includes some measure of social skills training and attempts to improve self-esteem. Antilibidinal drugs, such as cyproterone acetate, may also be helpful, particularly as a temporary expedient.

Exhibitionists are not usually physically dangerous, except for a few Type 2 individuals whose offending may escalate in seriousness. A good prognosis is associated with good general social relationships, mature heterosexual experiences, including marriage, and a good work record.

Paedophilia

This is a sexual preference for children, usually of prepubertal or early pubertal development, and usually for one or other rather than both sexes. Identification of paedophiles is problematic because of the strong taboo against sexual behaviour with children in Western society, even among other sex offenders. Those who are caught are likely to be unrepresentative, although this may be changing because of society's attempts to empower children to disclose abuse. The unpleasant stranger ('sex monster' beloved of tabloid journalism) is not at all typical, as paedophiles are often extremely skilful at interacting with children and are more often than not well known or related to their victims. Paedophiles may find it more difficult to relate to other adults. Alcohol abuse may be a precipitating factor to offending. Female victims are most frequently aged 6–11 years, but children of all ages may be abused, including babies.

Paedophiles may be classified by their own characteristics, by their relationship to their victims and by the sex of the victims:

- Offenders
  - Adolescents who are socially or emotionally immature and whose offending often amounts to 'immature investigation'. In these circumstances the offenders may kill their victims in panic. It must be noted that retrospective studies of adult paedophile sex offenders find that most started their offending behaviour in adolescence. Unlike other groups of offences, adolescents 'grow into' rather than 'out of' their offending behaviour.
  - Middle-aged males with marital problems (although on occasion this may be effect rather than cause) who are maladjusted in other areas and may be handicapped in normal adult relationships.
  - Elderly males who are lonely, isolated and have a fear of impotence.
- Relationship with the child
  - Where the sexual relationship arises in the context of a more general relationship. Paedophiles are also known to target somewhat inadequate single parents towards

whom they act in a protective manner. Also, paedophiles tend to gravitate towards employment or voluntary organizations concerned with children. Emotionally deprived children longing for affection can be more open to strangers and thus more often victims.
  - The child is merely a source of sexual gratification and is usually a stranger to the abuser. The paedophile activity may be in the context of non-aggressive seduction (e.g. with sweets or money) or there may be threats or actual harm to the child or children, or there may be a combination of both.
- *Sex of the victim*: heterosexual paedophiles are often married and have a lower conviction rate than homosexual paedophiles, who are more likely to be single.

Finkelhor has proposed a four-factor theory of the aetiology of child sexual abuse, which is compelling as it incorporates all the research findings relating to paedophilia. This is illustrated in Figure 13.4.

Convicted paedophiles are usually imprisoned, particularly in the absence of available treatment. However, there is evidence to suggest that the tendency to segregate such prisoners together for their own safety results in a swapping of information and prejudice, which at the least sustains the likelihood of repeating the offending behaviour and at worst increases the skills of individual paedophiles in entrapping children and avoiding discovery. Recently, various group programmes, both in prison and in the community, have claimed some success in treating paedophiles. Such programmes are highly selective and demand an extremely high level of motivation, often with the added threat of further legal sanctions if not continued. Cognitive behavioural techniques have been used, as has antilibidinal medication. Some have suggested that specific serotonin reuptake inhibitors (SSRIs) reduce deviant sexual fantasies and behaviour, although others regard any helpful effect as part of the overall reduction in libido associated with these drugs. Overall paedophilia is extremely difficult to treat successfully.

Disorders of sexual preference

- Disorders of sexual preference are characterized by sexually arousing fantasies, urges and/or activities that are not part of normative sexual functioning *and* that interfere with reciprocal affectionate activity.
- They are, in part, culturally determined and the legality of particular activities may vary between jurisdictions.
- They must be distinguished from gender identity disorders, which are, to different degrees, desires to take on the characteristics of the opposite sex and are not specifically to do with sexual arousal.
- Treatment depends to great extent on good motivation, but even then the results can be disappointing.

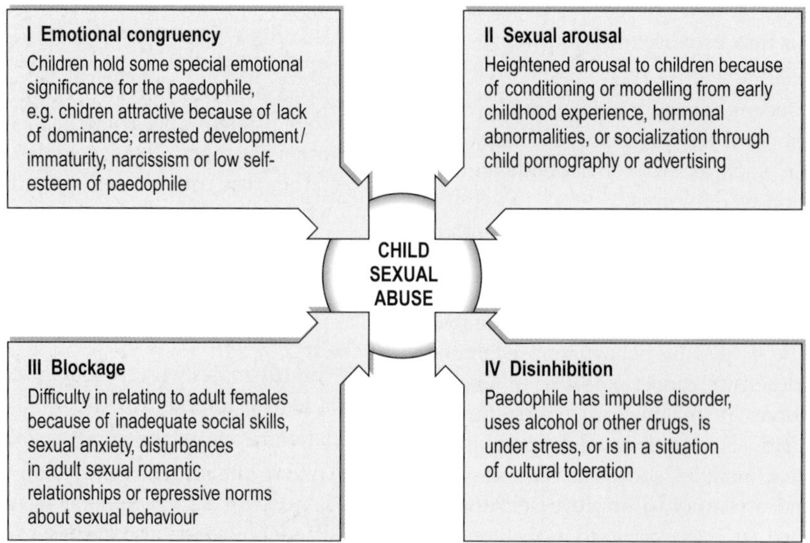

Figure 13.4 • Finkelhor's four-factor theory of the aetiology of child sexual abuse.

Disorders of sexual functioning

Epidemiology

Over half of men referred to sexual dysfunction clinics complain of erectile dysfunction; over half of women complain of impaired sexual interest. The next most frequently referred problems are orgasmic dysfunction in women and premature ejaculation in men.

Community surveys of sexual dysfunction are bedevilled by unrepresentative samples, poor response rates and inconsistent coverage of the full range of sexual dysfunctions. Kinsey and colleagues' pioneering work in the 1940s has recently been questioned on the basis of reports that samples were not representative of the community, including, for example, large numbers of prisoners. The Hite report on female sexuality was based on only 3000 completed questionnaires out of 100 000.

Despite this, it is apparent from these studies and the demand for sex therapy that the prevalence of sexual dysfunction in the community is significant. Studies suggest that sexual dysfunction is more common among women (or at least women admit it more often) and possibly in the lower social classes. The prevalence in women (including lack of interest) has been put at between 35% and 60%, with complete anorgasmia in 10–15%. Men have been questioned less frequently (this may well be cultural), but some degree of dysfunction has been proposed in 40%.

Aetiology

As the sexual response involves a complex interplay of physical and psychological factors, it is not surprising to find that the aetiology of sexual dysfunction is similarly a combination of *psyche* and *soma* (mind and body). Aetiological factors are often multiple and interact in a non-linear fashion. For example, inability to achieve erection or orgasm when under the influence of alcohol may well set up subsequent performance anxiety, which itself contributes to further erectile or orgasmic dysfunction.

There are many physical causes for sexual dysfunction, most of which become more frequent with age. Medical conditions, surgery and drugs may affect sexual functioning, and in many cases physical causes may interact with psychological causes. SSRIs are a common cause of altered orgasm (most often reduced or delayed, but occasionally multiple).

Psychological causes of sexual dysfunction are summarized in Table 13.5.

Table 13.5 Psychological causes of sexual dysfunction

Predisposing factors
Restrictive upbringing
Disturbed family relationships
Inadequate sexual information
Traumatic early sexual experiences
Early insecurity in psychosexual role
Precipitants
Childbirth
Discord in the general relationship
Infidelity
Unreasonable expectations
Dysfunction in the partner
Random failure
Reaction to organic factors
Ageing
Depression and anxiety
Traumatic sexual experience
Maintaining factors
Performance anxiety
Anticipation of failure
Guilt
Loss of attraction between partners
Poor communication between partners
Discord in the general relationship
Fear of intimacy
Impaired self-image
Inadequate sexual information; sexual myths
Restricted foreplay
Psychiatric disorder

(Reproduced with permission from Hawton K 1985; see Further reading)

Assessment

The assessment will first establish the presence or absence of sexual dysfunction; second will elucidate the nature of the dysfunction and some indication of aetiology; and third will assess suitability for treatment. Table 13.6 summarizes those situations in which sex therapy is unsuitable. These are not absolute contraindications, but require attention and/or resolution before therapy is likely to be helpful. Physical causes are not in themselves reasons for not providing appropriate counselling and therapy, as it is often the case that there is an exaggeration of symptomatology because of anxiety or lack of understanding.

After initial introductions it is advised that the couple (if indeed it is a couple seen) are seen both separately and together. This provides opportunities for individual exploration of issues such as other sexual liaisons or different expectations, but also allows the assessor to gauge the relationship between the couple. The effectiveness of the individual interviews may be compromised by the patient's uncertainty regarding confidentiality. It is therefore essential that each of the partners is reassured regarding what will and will not be disclosed to the other, and that each gives permission for anything disclosed.

Sensitivity towards the patient's embarrassment must be balanced against the need to obtain accurate and full information: it may well be that the most embarrassing topics are those that are important to an accurate formulation. It is also well established in general medical interviewing that the doctor's level of comfort in discussing sexual matters is correlated with the amount of information obtained. Many medical schools now address this issue with relevant courses but, if not, supervision by and possibly even role-play practice with an experienced clinician is recommended.

Table 13.6 Reasons for unsuitability for sex therapy
One partner having other sexual liaisons
Severe psychiatric disorder in one or other partner
Alcohol abuse
Pregnancy
Poor general relationship
Poor motivation

A full family, social, medical and background history is required, including attitudes to sexuality in the upbringing and both appropriate and inappropriate sexual experiences. Not all relevant information may be forthcoming in the initial interview, but may only arise in the course of therapy.

As usual (see Chapter 4) open questioning should precede more specific interrogation. Physical examination may well be appropriate, although this will depend on the source of referral and previous investigations.

Treatment

Treatment begins in all cases with a discussion of the likely causes of the development of the problem. This elucidates matters, allows additional information to be given and provides a basis for explaining the rationale of treatment. The following emphasizes the psychological treatment of sexual dysfunction. The reader is referred to Chapter 3 and urological and medical texts for more information on physical treatments (e.g. the use of oral sildenafil or of intracavernosal injection).

'Sex therapy' consists of a series of relatively closely spaced appointments (no less than weekly) at which treatment is discussed and homework tasks are set to be carried out between appointments. Fears by patients that they will be expected to 'perform' in the clinic need to be allayed at this point. The homework tasks are a series of progressively more intimate interactions leading eventually to full sexual intercourse, which is *prohibited* at the outset, although there is no restriction on masturbation without the partner present. An important principle is that progression to the next stage of intimacy should not be prescribed until both partners are comfortable with it. The progression through different stages will also be modified by discussion of individual preferences. Difficulties with a particular homework task must be seen as opportunities to clarify further the formulation of the dysfunction, and not as failure. Figure 13.5 illustrates a standard progression of homework tasks.

It may be seen that different homework tasks will be particularly problematic for particular dysfunctions. For example, failure of genital response in males may occur at the point of vaginal containment if the main aetiological factor is performance anxiety.

For *premature ejaculation* the *stop–start* technique was developed by the improbably but appropriately

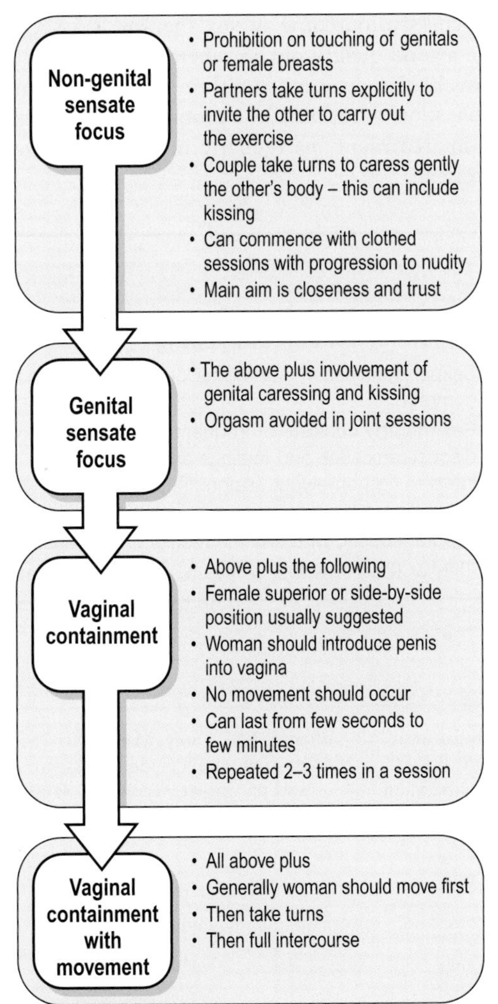

Figure 13.5 • Progression of homework assignments in sex therapy.

named Semans in the 1950s. Both this and the *squeeze* technique are based on the premise that premature ejaculation occurs because of excessively rapid male arousal and lack of identification of the point of ejaculatory inevitability. The techniques are usually introduced at the genital sensate focus stage (Figure 13.5). The stroking of the penis to the point of high arousal before ejaculatory inevitability occurs in both techniques. In the stop–start technique the arousal is allowed to subside by cessation of the caressing, whereas in the squeeze technique the glans penis is squeezed to delay ejaculation. This is repeated a number of times before masturbation to ejaculation. For more details of this and the other techniques mentioned here the reader is referred to a manual of sex therapy (see Further reading).

For female orgasmic dysfunction *masturbation training* is required, starting with the woman practising on her own and progressing to inclusion in the genital sensate focus stage (see Figure 13.5).

Non-organic vaginismus requires a sensitively paced programme of increasing vaginal contact and penetration, again progressing from solo homework to involving the partner. Increasing sizes of vaginal dilators have been used, but these are not absolutely necessary and can introduce an added complication, which may be inappropriate.

It must be emphasized that all the above techniques will only work if the anxieties and feelings associated with tasks are properly and comprehensively explored. If the primary problem is one of marital discord then this must be addressed first, by *marital therapy*.

Sexual phobias (see Table 13.3, F52.10) will usually be tackled by the progressive homework assignments, but where there is a very specific item or activity about which an individual becomes excessively anxious, a progressive desensitization programme may be necessary.

Individual therapy may be required where one or other partner has problems because of prior traumatic sexual experiences. Features of post-traumatic stress disorder (flashbacks, nightmares, etc.; see Chapter 10) may well be apparent.

Case history: sexual dysfunction

Joy (25) and Frank (29) presented with problems 'to do with their sex life'. The main complaint was that Joy never initiated sex and seemed to Frank to be unresponsive during intercourse. The couple had three children, the youngest being six months old.

On individual interview Joy said that she felt panicky and under pressure from Frank, if he made any advances to her. Frank, when seen on his own, complained bitterly about his wife's 'frigidity', saying that it had not been the same before marriage (although it later transpired that sex had occurred infrequently before marriage, and usually under the influence of alcohol). Joy was well made-up and somewhat coquettish in her presentation to the male interviewer. Frank was blunt, gruff, but rather reticent to talk about his 'sex life'.

After three sessions in which one reason or another was put forward for not attempting the non-genital sensate focus exercise, the couple failed to attend (the only attempt at the exercise had resulted in full intercourse, much to Joy's dismay). Three years later the therapist learned that Frank had been imprisoned for sexual offences against his own children, Joy had revealed that she had been sexually

Continued

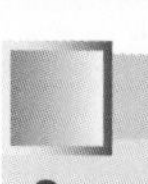

Case history: sexual dysfunction—cont'd

abused as a child by her stepfather. The therapist, in assessing Joy for depression, found she was still experiencing the same sexual dysfunction with her new partner.

Course and prognosis

Between a third and two-thirds of couples who participate in sex therapy programmes report a major improvement or resolution of their difficulties. The best results are found for vaginismus and erectile dysfunction (both around 80%). Follow-ups tend to show that the improvements are sustained.

Spontaneous improvement in sexual dysfunction is not well researched.

Successful outcome of sex therapy is associated with: a good quality of the general relationship; lack of psychiatric disorder in either partner; high motivation; short duration of the problem; and early progress in treatment, particularly in the sensate focus exercises.

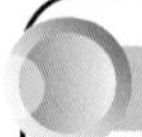

Disorders of sexual functioning

- Sexual dysfunction is a matter of expectation and is common.
- Sex therapy consists of frequent appointments to discuss anxieties and feelings associated with intervening homework assignments.
- Disorders of sexual functioning do not usually resolve spontaneously, whereas the results of successful therapy are sustained.

Further reading

Bancroft, J., 2008. Human sexuality and its problems, third ed. Churchill Livingstone, Edinburgh.

Hawton, K., 1985. Sex therapy: a practical guide. Oxford Medical Publications, Oxford.

Treasaden, I., 2010. Paraphilias and sexual offenders. In: Puri, B.K., Teasaden, I. (Eds.), Psychiatry: an evidence-based text. Hodder Arnold, London.

Wincze, J.P., Carey, M.P., 2001. Sexual dysfunction: a guide for assessment and treatment, second ed. Guildford Press, New York.

Sleep disorders

Normal sleep

Sleep is usually described as a series of phases characterized by changes in physiological variables, most notably the electroencephalogram (EEG), as illustrated in Figure 14.1. There is usually a typical body posture (associated with good thermoregulation); physical inactivity; more stimulation required to arouse than during wakefulness; a specific site or nest for this behaviour; and regular daily occurrence. The progression between the phases can be shown by means of a 'hypnogram' (Figure 14.2). There are a number of theories regarding the function of sleep (listed in Table 14.1). Evidence is accumulating for each, suggesting that sleep serves a number of functions. Sleep has been found to facilitate mathematical insight, as shown in Figure 14.3.

With less than three hours sleep in 24 hours, humans show increased irritability and a decreased attention span. Long periods of sleep deprivation result in poor concentration, deterioration in general performance, increased suggestibility and, later, hallucinations, paranoia and even seizures. The prominence of psychological effects suggests to some that sleep specifically restores brain functioning.

Normal sleep-dependent consolidation of memory is disrupted in schizophrenia. This is illustrated in Figure 14.4.

Length of time asleep

Humans spend, on average, 25% of their lives asleep. There is variation in sleep time, both in individuals during the course of development and the life cycle, and also between individuals (Figure 14.4). The individual differences within and between subjects are particularly noticeable in infancy. The mean daily sleep length in the first week of life is 16 hours (SD two hours). There is a gradual reduction in mean daily sleep length throughout infancy and middle childhood (Figure 14.5). Most infants wake at least once each night but, apart from babies who need feeding (more often those who are breastfed), they usually drop off to sleep again by themselves. Parents are not normally aware of this unless they themselves are having problems sleeping. Adults will also wake briefly during the night but often will not remember. Frequency of waking increases with age.

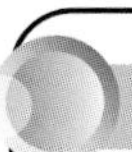

Normal sleep

- Normal sleep consists of a series of phases 1–4 of increasing depth, interspersed with short periods close to wakefulness during which there are rapid eye movements (REM).
- Each phase of sleep has a characteristic EEG.
- There is a wide range of individual differences in sleep length but there is generally a decrease with age.

Classification of sleep disorders

Sleep disorders may be divided into those primarily of emotional origin and those with an organic basis. The ICD-10 and DSM-IV-TR categorizations

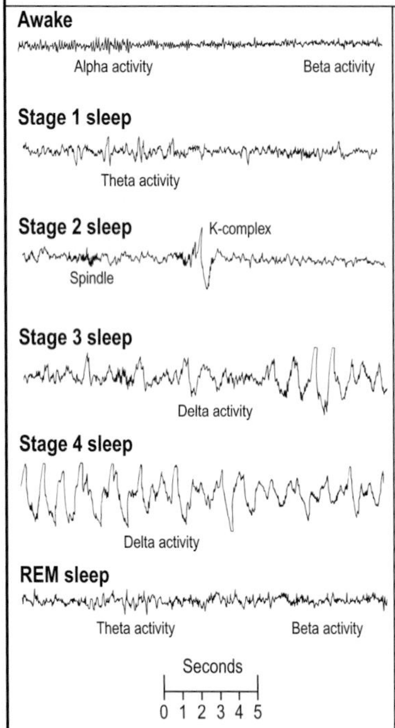

	EEG	% sleep (young adult)	Ease of arousal	Temperature	Heart rate	Respiration	BP	Other
Awake	Alpha activity, Beta activity	n.a.	n.a.	Normal	Normal	Regular		
Stage 1 sleep	Theta activity	5%	Easy	Normal	Normal	Irregular		Eye rolling Eyelids opening and shutting
Stage 2 sleep	K-complex, Spindle	45%	Transition	Dropping	Dropping slightly	Transition		
Stage 3 sleep	Delta activity	7%	Difficult	Decreased slightly	↓	Regular some slowing	↓	• Myosis • ¬ Sweating • Loss of galvanic skin responses
Stage 4 sleep	Delta activity	13%	Difficult	Decreased slightly	↓	Regular some slowing	↓	
REM sleep	Theta activity, Beta activity	30%	Difficult	Increase in brain thermoregulation otherwise poor	↑	Very variable	↑	• Rapid eye movements • Penile erection • Loss of muscle tone especially in neck

Seconds 0 1 2 3 4 5

Figure 14.1 • Physiological concomitants of the stages of normal sleep.

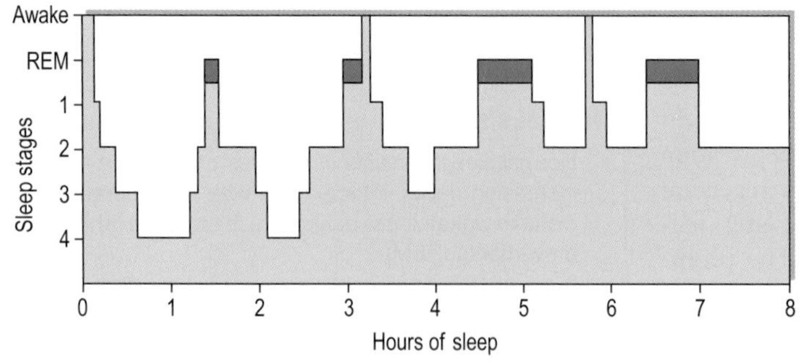

Figure 14.2 • A hypnogram of sleep stage changes of the night in normal young adults. (Reproduced with permission from Horne J 1985 Why we sleep. Oxford University Press, Oxford.)

of sleep disorders are shown in Tables 14.2 and 14.3 respectively. This chapter will cover predominantly those sleep disorders with a psychiatric basis. However, sleep disorders with organic causes are important differential diagnoses and interactions with psychological factors are usual. Also, sleep disorders are often a component or complication of other psychiatric disorders.

Insomnia

Insomnia is a disorder in which there is insufficient quantity or quality of sleep. The diagnosis may be used at any age (previously sleep disorder in childhood was classified separately). Insomnia may be transient (a history of only a few days or weeks) or chronic (an unremitting history over months or years).

Table 14.1 Theories of sleep

Conservation of energy – energy use decreases to between 5–% and 25% of waking level
Restorative – sleep allows the body to 'mend itself' after the ravages of the day. Anabolism/catabolism ratio increases. Increased growth hormone release
Consolidation of memory **Vestigial** – sleep is the remnant of a mechanism useful at an earlier stage of evolution
Safety – superficially similar to death, sleep may discourage predators from attack, but those animals more at risk of attack sleep less
Social bonding – the clustering of humans at sleep time may be useful in keeping a social group together
To dream – the function of dreaming is not clear, but if artificially suppressed (e.g. with drugs) there is a significant increase on the cessation of suppression. This suggests that dreaming may serve an important function
Behavioural – sleep occurring because of the absence of stimulation and the lack of anything better to do
Humoral – due to accumulation of sleep-inducing substances in the brain during wakefulness

Epidemiology

The complaint of sleeplessness is far more common than any other complaint about sleep. Prevalence estimates in adults vary from 15% to over 40%, and increase in the elderly. Many more people experience intermittent insomnia than complain to their GP, despite this being a common surgery complaint.

In childhood it is not usually the child who complains. As many as 14% of children have sleep difficulties at three years of age. This can mean a complicated mixture of settling problems and evening and night-time waking.

It has been shown that sleep problems occur in as many as 50–80% of children with learning disabilities. This may be due to different sleep architecture in the profoundly learning disabled. In Down's syndrome there is also an increased incidence of obstructive sleep apnoea, which can disrupt sleep.

Clinical features

True insomnia, in adults as well as in children, results in tiredness throughout the day. It is important to distinguish lack of sleep from difficulty settling (particularly in children), although this may also reduce the length of time asleep. It is also important to identify the pattern of insomnia, i.e. difficulty staying asleep, early waking, phase-shift disorders.

Variations in sleep requirements mean that it is unwise to prescribe an ideal amount of sleep during childhood. However, insufficient sleep due to late bedtimes will most often result in morning tiredness, with difficulty rising, daytime sleepiness and unscheduled napping. Other children may show irritability, increased activity and impairment of concentration when tired. The times when sleeps are taken, and the amount of 'napping' and 'microsleeps' (a few seconds of light sleep during reduced activity) vary during a lifetime. Short sleeps may increase in frequency in old age.

Differential diagnosis

Insomnia is a prominent feature of both depression and mania, and can also occur in anxiety disorders. Where history and examination show other symptoms of these disorders, then the predominant diagnosis must be of the mood or neurotic disorder rather than the sleep disorder. Similarly, insomnia may be secondary to many organic disorders (see below), and again the primary diagnosis should be made. In schizophrenia, there may be a day/night reversal in sleeping pattern.

Aetiology

The causes of insomnia are summarized in Table 14.4.

Predisposing factors

The complaint is more common in lower socioeconomic groups. Individual differences in body temperature, skin resistance and corticosteroid excretion have been associated with variation in frequency of insomnia. Family attitude to sleep may also determine the degree to which an individual complains of insomnia.

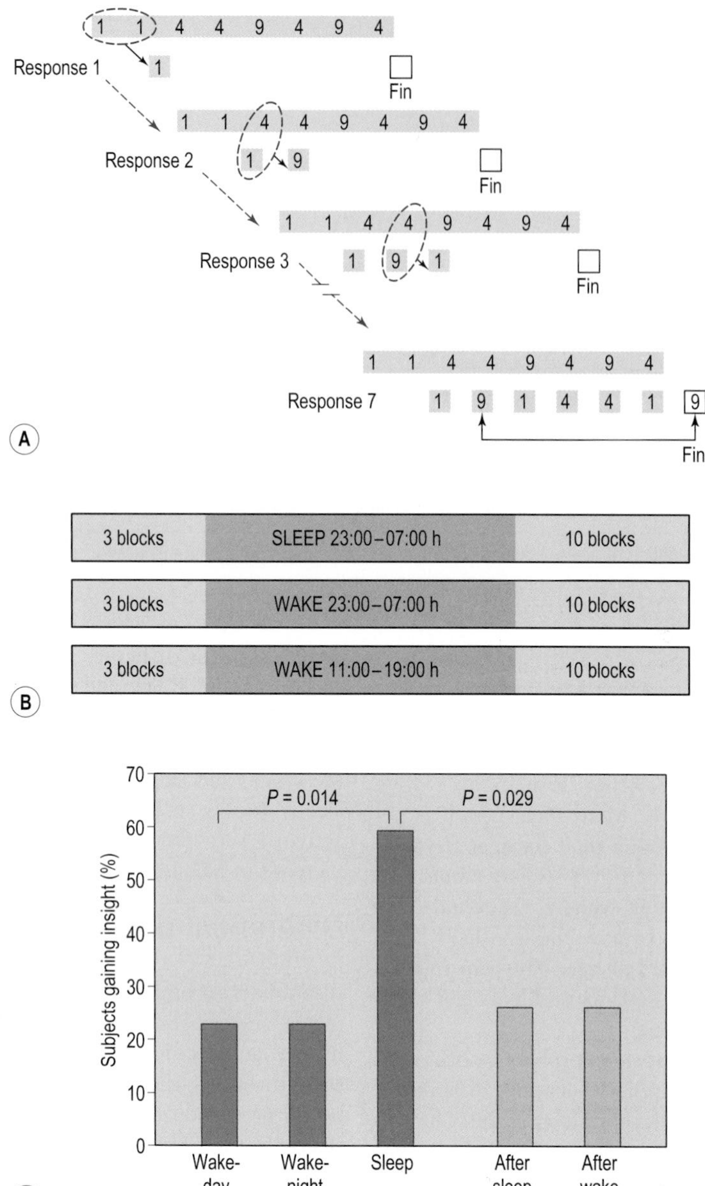

Figure 14.3 • Facilitation of mathematical insight by sleep. • (a) Number Reduction Task (NRT), illustrated by an example trial. On each trial, a different string of eight digits was presented. Each string was composed of the digits '1', '4', and '9'. For each string, subjects had to determine a digit defined as the 'final solution' of the task trial (Fin). This could be achieved by sequentially processing the digits pairwise from left to right according to two simple rules. One, the 'same rule', states that the result of two identical digits is just this digit (for example, '1' and '1' results in '1', as in response 1 here). The other rule, the 'different rule', states that the result of two non-identical digits is the remaining third digit of this three-digit system (for example, '1' and '4' results in '9' as in response 2 here). After the first response, comparisons are made between the preceding result and the next digit. The seventh response indicates the final solution, to be confirmed by pressing a separate key. Not mentioned to the subjects, the strings were generated in such a way that the last three responses always mirrored the previous three responses. This implies that in each trial the second response coincided with the final solution (arrow). Subjects who gain insight into this hidden rule abruptly cut short sequential responding by pressing the solution key immediately after the second response. (b) Experimental design (main experiment). An 8-h period of nocturnal sleep, nocturnal wakefulness, or daytime wakefulness separated an initial training phase (three blocks) from later retesting (ten blocks). (c) Columns indicate percentage of subjects gaining insight into the hidden rule in the three experimental conditions of the main experiment (grey), in which subjects either slept (at night) or remained awake (at night or during daytime) between initial training and retesting, and in two supplementary conditions (hatched), where subjects were tested after nocturnal sleep or daytime wakefulness in the absence of initial training before these periods. (Reproduced with permission from Wagner U *et al* 2004 *Nature* 427:352–355)

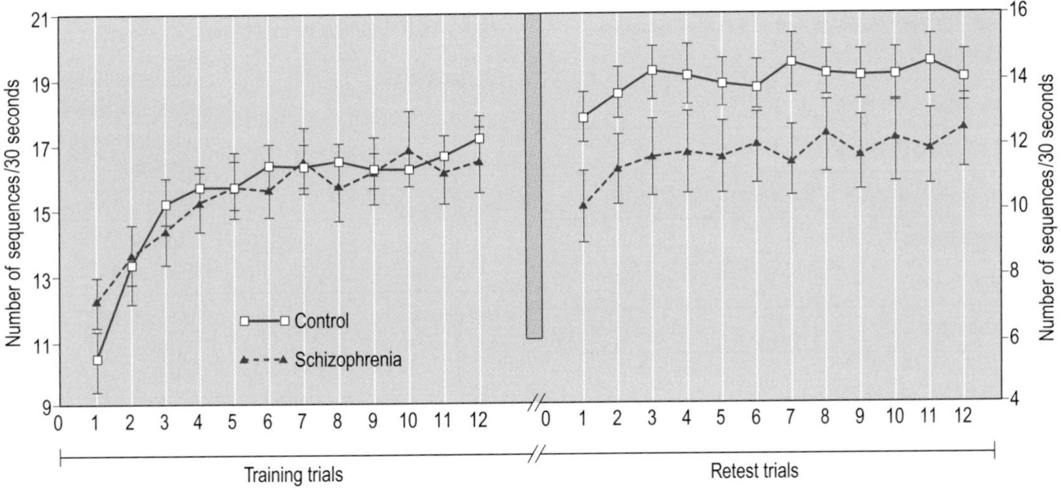

Figure 14.4 • Sleep-dependent consolidation of memory. • Fourteen healthy controls (open squares) and 20 schizophrenia patients (closed triangles) were asked to learn a motor skill (typing a sequence of digits). The vertical axes represent the number of correct sequences typed in each 30-second trial. Note that the these axes are scaled separately for control subjects (left) and patients (right) to illustrate better the qualitative similarity of learning curves on day 1 and the failure of overnight improvement in the schizophrenia group only. The dashed line is positioned at the mean value of the last three training trials for both the control and patient groups. The shaded bar represents the passage of 24 hours, including a night of sleep. Patients and control subjects did not differ in the amount of learning during training, but only control subjects showed significant overnight improvement. (Reproduced with permission from Manoach DS *et al* 2004 *Biological Psychiatry* 56:951–956.)

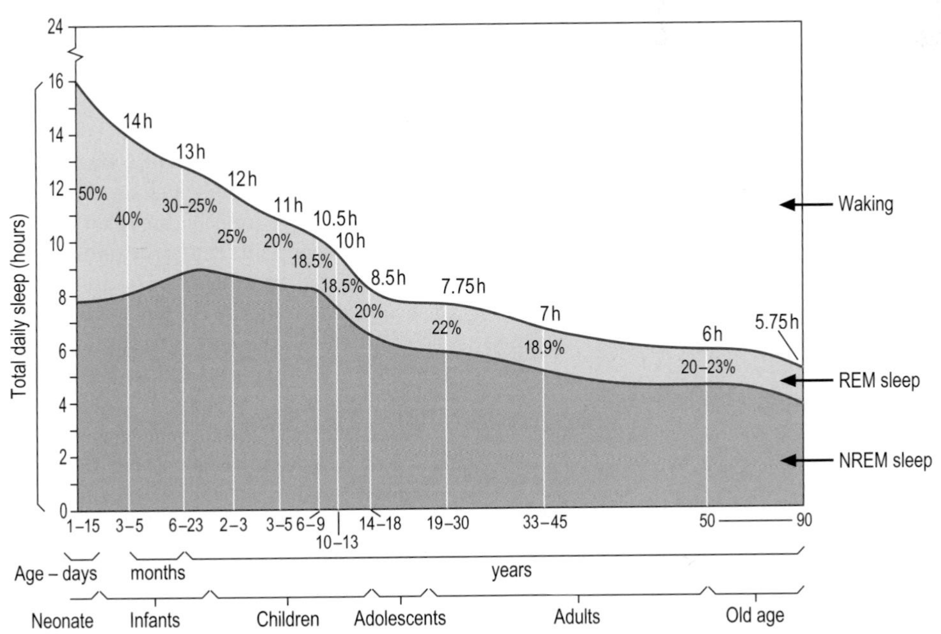

Figure 14.5 • Changes with age in total amounts of daily sleep and daily REM sleep. (Reproduced and modified with permission from Roffwarg *et al.* 1966 Science 152: 604–619.)

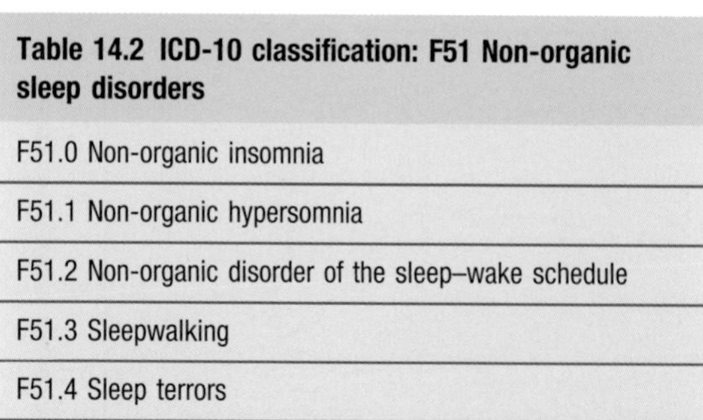

Table 14.2 ICD-10 classification: F51 Non-organic sleep disorders
F51.0 Non-organic insomnia
F51.1 Non-organic hypersomnia
F51.2 Non-organic disorder of the sleep–wake schedule
F51.3 Sleepwalking
F51.4 Sleep terrors
F51.5 Nightmares

Table 14.3 DSM-IV-TR Sleep disorders	
Primary sleep disorders	
Dyssomnias	
307.42	Primary insomnia
307.44	Primary hypersomnia
347	Narcolepsy
780.59	Breathing-related sleep disorder
307.45	Circadian rhythm sleep disorder (*Specify type:* Delayed sleep phase type/jet lag type/shift work type/ unspecified type)
307.47	Dyssomnia NOS
Parasomnias	
307.47	Nightmare disorder
307.46	Sleep terror disorder
307.46	Sleepwalking disorder
307.47	Parasomnia NOS
Sleep disorders related to another mental disorder	
307.42	Insomnia related to. . .(indicate Axis I or II disorder)
307.44	Hypersomnia related to. . .(indicate disorder)
Other sleep disorders	
780.xx	Sleep disorder due to. . .(indicate general medical condition)
.52	Insomnia type
.54	Hypersomnia type
.59	Parasomnia type
.59	Mixed type
—.—	Substance-induced sleep disorder (code as Substance related disorder)

NOS, not otherwise specified.

Table 14.4 Causes of insomnia	
Environmental	Poor sleep hygiene Change in time zone Change in sleeping habits Shiftwork
Physiological	Natural short sleeper Pregnancy Middle age
Life stress	Bereavement Exams House move, etc.
Psychiatric	Acute anxiety Depression Mania Organic brain syndrome
Physical	Pain Cardiorespiratory distress Arthritis Nocturia Gastrointestinal disorders Thyrotoxicosis
Pharmacological	Caffeine Alcohol Stimulants Chronic hypnotic use
Parasomnias	Sleep apnoea Sleep myoclonus

Precipitating factors

Transient insomnia is usually the result of some environmental change or a change in the work–rest pattern, and is frequently due to an emotional crisis such as bereavement. It may be one of the first signs of distress due to outside pressure. There appears to be no direct relation between the type of experience and the likelihood of insomnia, but this will depend on the significance to the individual of a stressful event.

There are individual preferences in noise level, light and temperature levels for sleep. A move to a quieter area may evoke insomnia in someone who is used to the noise of the city, and vice versa. Generally sleep is likely to be disturbed at a temperature of more than 24°C. A change in temperature may also evoke an episode of insomnia.

Ingestion of pharmacologically active foods and drinks, especially caffeine and alcohol, may disrupt sleep. Some drugs, particularly stimulants, may cause insomnia either directly or as a result of side-effects (e.g. akathisia (restless legs) with chlorpromazine and related phenothiazine drugs).

Withdrawal from alcohol or hypnotics may also reduce sleep or produce alterations (e.g. increased rapid eye movement (REM) sleep) that increase waking. The use of very-short-acting hypnotics may produce rebound waking in the middle of the night.

Shiftwork changes require changes in circadian rhythm that take several days to achieve, and transient insomnia may result. If shifts are frequently changed then even more disturbed sleep may occur.

Although most chronic insomnias are related to medical, psychiatric or behavioural problems, some people experience prolonged poor sleep without any obvious disturbance in any of these areas. This may be labelled 'primary chronic insomnia', and can occur with daytime sleepiness and/or impairment of mood and well-being. It is thought that this is either associated with as yet undetected changes in sleep architectures or as part of the range of individual differences.

The main cause of chronic insomnia secondary to organic factors is any condition that involves pain (see also Table 14.4).

Perpetuating factors

Clearly, if any of the underlying factors is missed then insomnia continues. Transient insomnia may progress to chronic insomnia if there is poor sleep hygiene (see below), or if a vicious cycle is set up of worry about the lack of sleep leading to anxiety symptoms, which lead to further waking and difficulty settling.

In childhood insomnia, increased parental agitation, anxiety and irritability (having been frequently woken) can produce increased arousal in the child and consequently less sleep. Also, such parental exhaustion can disrupt the most competent individuals, making them less likely to achieve their normal level of appropriate management.

Inadequate or inappropriate management of insomnia may also perpetuate the problem.

Management

Sleep hygiene

Sleep hygiene is the basis of a preventive strategy for insomnia and is the approach of first choice once a full assessment has eliminated primary psychiatric or medical disorders. The basic features of sleep hygiene are shown in Figure 14.6.

Figure 14.6 • Features of sleep hygiene.

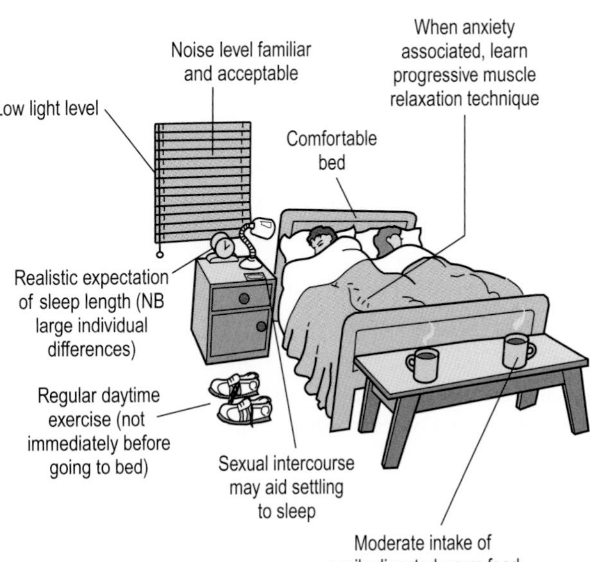

Hypnotics

Hypnotics, especially benzodiazepines (and previously barbiturates), have been prescribed in large quantities over recent years but are now under something of a cloud because of substantial problems of dependence and withdrawal symptoms with long-term usage. Tolerance develops within 3–14 days. For these reasons, hypnotics should only be prescribed rarely, for short periods (preferably for only a few days but certainly less than a month) and intermittently. Those who are dependent on benzodiazepines can experience significant rebound insomnia on withdrawal, with vivid dreams and increased REM sleep.

Longer-acting benzodiazepines (see Chapter 3) such as diazepam or nitrazepam may be helpful where the insomnia is associated with daytime anxiety, but not when the anxiety is part of a depressive or other psychiatric disorder. In the elderly, such long-acting drugs are contraindicated as they can build up over a relatively short time to produce dangerous levels of drowsiness, unsteadiness and confusion.

Shorter-acting benzodiazepines are preferred in order to avoid the morning 'hangover' effects seen with those benzodiazepines with a longer half-life.

Chloral hydrate is effective and cheap but can cause gastric irritation and rashes, can result in dependence and is lethal in overdose.

The newer hypnotics zopiclone, zolpidem and zaleplon (see Chapter 3) may be better, although zopiclone produces an unpleasant metallic taste in some patients. In the UK, the pineal hormone melatonin is licensed for the short-term treatment of insomnia in adults over 55 years of age.

Behavioural approaches

Behavioural approaches are the treatment of choice for children. Drugs are rarely indicated, although they can be used sometimes for a very few days in order to break a cycle of night-time waking or provide rest for exhausted parents.

The keys to successful treatment are:

- a thorough assessment of the settling–sleep–wake pattern
- a clear understanding of the wishes and views of carers in order for a partnership to management to be achieved.

The first of these requirements is achieved by a combination of careful history taking and the carers keeping a diary of settling, sleeping and waking with their responses (Figure 14.7). If the waking is frequent or the settling period is lengthy, the diary not only provides a record to monitor therapy but also reminds the carer of what has happened. Behavioural treatment approaches to children's sleep disorders can be roughly divided into:

- those that emphasize not giving the child attention when they wake or when they are showing distress about wishing not to settle (quick, but very traumatic for all concerned)
- those that take a much more gradual approach to teaching the child to settle (see Further reading).

Course and prognosis

As noted previously, transient insomnia can become chronic if various perpetuating factors are in place, if measures are not taken to manage it appropriately or if the underlying cause is a chronic condition. Chronic insomnia may occur throughout adult life. It is usually the consequence of old age, medical, behavioural or psychiatric problems.

Insomnia

- Insomnia is insufficient quantity or quality of sleep, and may be transient or chronic.
- Sleeplessness is the most common complaint about sleep. Prevalence varies from 14–40%.
- It is important to distinguish insomnia from difficulty settling, and also to identify the pattern.
- Causes of insomnia are many and may be multiple and interacting. Transient insomnia is usually due to some environmental change.
- 'Sleep hygiene' is the basis for prevention and treatment of insomnia.
- Hypnotics should be prescribed only rarely, for short periods.

Case history: insomnia

Helen, aged five, came downstairs at 10-minute intervals throughout the evening until her mother went to bed. This behaviour started a few weeks after her parents had separated and the day after she had

Case history: insomnia—cont'd

witnessed them having a particularly noisy argument. At first she was rather tearful and responded warmly to her mother's hugs, but more recently she had protested vigorously when returned to bed, only to come down a few minutes later with a further enquiry, request for a drink, etc. Helen's mother had felt sorry for her at first, but latterly could only keep her temper for a brief time before getting into a lengthy and heated discussion with her daughter about why she should be in bed. Helen's mother herself was finding it difficult to get off to sleep, and was waking early. She admitted that sometimes she found it reassuring to have Helen's company in the evening, and let her stay to watch a favourite TV programme or play a short game.

Helen was getting increasingly irritable during the day and conflicts with her three-year-old sister Sophie were becoming more frequent. After a full background assessment (see Chapter 16) including individual interviews with both mother and daughter, it was agreed that Helen's mother would try a simple tactic of returning Helen to bed with minimum discussion and no loss of temper on her part. It was agreed that a simple diary would be kept of the number of times Helen came down, with a note of her reaction on each occasion. The assessing psychiatrist considered the possibility of Helen's mother's sleep disturbance being a symptom of depression, but decided against this on balance, preferring to keep the possibility under review.

The new arrangements were explained to Helen. A telephone call to the family home a week later determined that, although Helen had shown distress the first night, she was, after three nights staying in her room, asleep all evening and all night. Her mother also commented that Helen seemed more settled during the day.

Hypersomnia

Clinical features

Hypersomnia is a condition of excessive daytime sleepiness and sleep attacks, which occurs on a regular basis or recurrently for short periods, and causes a disturbance of social or occupational functioning. In ICD-10, the diagnosis *non-organic hypersomnia* (F51.1) is used to distinguish a condition in which excessive daytime sleepiness is the predominant symptom (although most likely part of another mental disorder) and in which there is no organic basis for the symptomatology (see below).

In the UK, perhaps 1–3% of road traffic accidents, and maybe 10% of serious accidents and 20% of motorway accidents, are associated with drowsiness in the driver.

Epidemiology

In questionnaire and sleep laboratory studies, daytime drowsiness has been found to occur in between 0.3 and 4% of the population. (Narcolepsy occurs in between 0.01 and 0.09% of the adult population.) A 1981 study estimated a UK prevalence of 4000 sufferers from idiopathic hypersomnolence.

Differential diagnosis

Hypersomnia must be distinguished primarily from narcolepsy (see Table 14.5). Although narcolepsy can consist of sleep attacks only, other symptoms, including cataplexy (sudden loss of muscle tone when arousal abruptly increased, e.g. when surprised), sleep paralysis and hypnagogic hallucinations, are usually present. The most common combination is of sleep attacks and cataplexy. Narcolepsy is no more associated with psychiatric disorder than would be expected for any chronic illness.

Psychogenic hypersomnia must also be distinguished from the daytime sleepiness associated with sleep apnoea. In this, apnoeic episodes are observed on a frequent basis while the individual is asleep, and there is characteristic snoring (periods of slowing frequency of snoring until apnoea occurs, followed after a while by a snort, more rapid snoring, which again slows, and so on). There may also be hypertension, impotence, cognitive dulling, extreme restlessness and daytime irritability (or overactivity in children). Other symptoms may be related to the cause of the apnoea (central or obstructive).

Other causes of daytime drowsiness are organic and are distinguished both by clinical evidence of the cause of clouding of consciousness and by appropriate investigation (see Chapter 6). Hypersomnia must also be distinguished from fatigue states (either normal, or as in chronic fatigue syndrome) and circadian rhythm disturbances (see below). Kleine–Levin syndrome is a rare disorder of hypothalamic activity with onset in adolescence, a male preponderance, excessive eating and episodic hypersomnia.

NAME: *Rebecca Smith* AGE: *5*

Date	Time to bed	Time settled	Time woke	Time settled	Notes
6-11-10	7.45	8.30			Got up 6 times– drink, tummy hurts, "what are you doing?"; "don't forget..." "what's that noise?" etc. Returned to bed.
			10.30	10.50	Shouted– told to shut up and go to sleep.
			2.10	2.50	Shouted– ignored. Changed to crying.
			3.15	3.45	Crying in bed. Went in. Told to go to sleep.
			4.30	4.50	Came into my room– I was exhausted so took her into my bed.
			6.45		Got up.
7-11-10	7.30	8.10			Got up 5 times. Excuses as usual. Got really cross and smacked her. Went up crying.

Figure 14.7 • Sleep diary showing a typical pattern of waking, and responses before a programme is initiated.

Table 14.5 Differences between hypersomnia and narcolepsy

	Hypersomnia	Narcolepsy
Duration of attack	> one to two hours	< one hour
Onset	Gradual	Sudden
Control	Resistible	Irresistible
Diurnal variation	Worse a.m.	Worse evenings
Place	Rarely in unusual places	Often in unusual circumstances
Night-time sleep	Prolonged, deep	Interrupted
EEG	Non-REM onset (sleep-onset REM when depression or drug withdrawal)	Typically sleep-onset REM
Other symptoms	None (except when part of another disorder)	Cataplexy, sleep paralysis, hypnagogic hallucinations

EEG, electroencephalogram; REM, rapid eye movement.

Table 15.1 ICD-10 classification of personality disorders

Personality disorder	Main characteristics
Paranoid	Oversensitivity, tendency to bear grudges, suspiciousness, misconstrues neutral or friendly actions of others as hostile or contemptuous
Schizoid	Emotional coldness, preference for fantasy, introspective reserve, little interest in having sexual experiences with others, lack of close, confiding relationships
Anxious (avoidant)	Pervasive tension and apprehension, self-consciousness, hypersensitivity to rejection, enters into relationships only if guaranteed uncritical acceptance
	Exaggerates potential dangers and risks in everyday situations and avoids certain activities, leading to restricted lifestyle
Dependent	Encourages or allows others to assume responsibility for major areas of individual's life; subordinate to, compliant with and unwilling to make demands on those on whom they depend
	Perceives self as helpless, fears being abandoned and alone, devastated when close relationships end
Anankastic (obsessive–compulsive)	Indecisiveness, perfectionism, excessive conscientiousness, pedantry and conventionality, rigidity and stubbornness, plans all activities far ahead in immutable detail
Histrionic	Tendency to theatricality, overemotional, suggestible, shallow and labile affectivity, craves attention, manipulative
Emotionally unstable	
Impulsive type	Emotionally unstable, lack of impulse control, outbursts of violence or threatening behaviour common
Borderline type	Unclear or disturbed self-image, intense and unstable relationships, which may lead to repeated emotional crises that may be associated with a series of suicidal threats or acts of self-harm
Dissocial	Irresponsibility, cannot maintain relationships, low tolerance of frustration and low threshold for discharge of aggression, including violence
	Incapacity to experience guilt and to profit from experience (including punishment), blames others or offers plausible rationalizations for antisocial behaviour

- the antisocial personality (dramatic, emotional, flamboyant and erratic) (DSM-IV-TR cluster B)
- the dependent personality (anxious and fearful) and the inhibited personality (DSM-IV-TR cluster C).

The differences in the onset and course of these three clusters are illustrated in Figure 15.2.

Individuals with personality disorders may or may not regard their personalities as desirable (i.e. respectively egosyntonic or egodystonic). However, most are dissatisfied with the resulting difficulties they experience in everyday life and in sustaining interpersonal relationships. This frequently results in depression or anxiety, which may be the main complaint that leads an individual to seek psychiatric contact.

Withdrawn personality

Paranoid personality disorder

Those with a paranoid personality disorder tend to interpret the actions of others as being deliberately demeaning and threatening. They are oversensitive, suspicious, jealous, 'make mountains out of molehills', blame their own failures on others (projection) and overvalue their own abilities. They hold grudges and can be litigious. In this latter context they may be seen more frequently by those working within the legal system than in the health service. Occasionally they champion others. Inevitably this personality disorder leads to impairment in their occupations, particularly in dealing with fellow workers and authority figures. Those with this personality disorder have

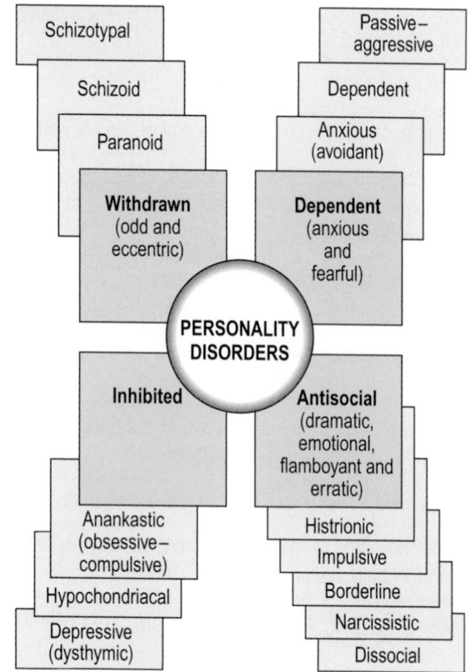

Figure 15.1 • Clustering of personality disorders.

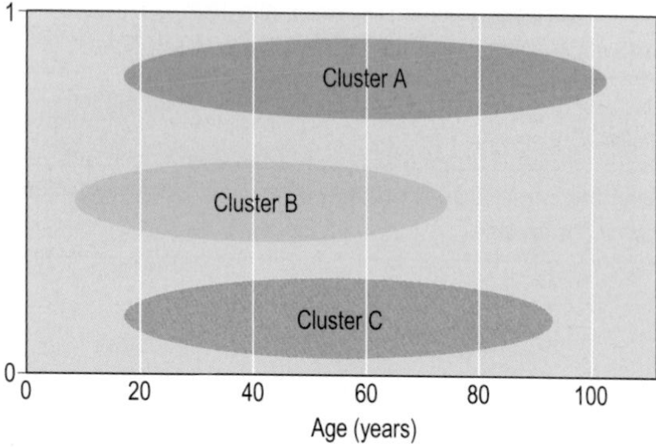

Figure 15.2 • Differences in onset and course of clusters of personality disorders. (Reproduced with permission from Tyrer P 2010; see Further reading)

been leaders of cults and fringe groups, fanatics and dictators who collect 'yes' men around them and attempt to isolate those with whom they do not agree. It is more common in males. Under extreme stress, such individuals can develop transient paranoid psychotic symptoms such as paranoid delusions (e.g. that people are persecuting them) and hallucinations (e.g. voices of others saying derogatory things about them). Such individuals may also be predisposed to more prolonged episodes of paranoid psychosis.

Schizoid personality disorder

Those with schizoid personality disorder are indifferent to social relationships. They have a restricted range of emotional expression and experiences. Reserved, shy, introspective and eccentric, they become loners and possibly vagrants or hermits. They resent being pushed into social situations such as parties. They may have an eccentric interest, for instance in flat earth theory or the search for the Loch Ness monster. They may have a preference for numbers rather than people and may function well as mathematicians or with computers. However, their isolation may make them prone to depression. There may be some overlap of this condition with Asperger's syndrome, sometimes referred to as a schizoid disorder of childhood or autistic psychopathy, and which may include cases of mild autism without delays in language or cognitive development.

Schizotypal personality disorder

Another personality disorder included in the withdrawn (odd and eccentric) group is the schizotypal. This is characterized by peculiarities and anomalies in ideation, appearance, speech and behaviour (which may be eccentric), as well as deficits in interpersonal relationships. The schizotypal personality disorder is more common in first-degree biological relatives of those suffering from schizophrenia, and is now seen as part of a genetic spectrum of schizophrenia.

Dependent personality

Anxious (avoidant) personality disorder

The anxious personality disorder is common and is characterized by social discomfort and self-consciousness, fear of rejection and negative evaluation, and timidity. Such individuals have a restricted lifestyle and may avoid certain activities because of their excessive fears. It is associated with depression, anxiety, the development of specific phobias and social phobia, and anger at oneself for failing to develop social relationships.

Dependent personality disorder

Dependent personality disorder, also referred to as *inadequate*, *passive* or *asthenic* (Greek for inadequate) personality disorder, is characterized by dependency on others, submissive behaviour and resourcelessness. Individuals adopt a passive role and let relatives and others decide on important life issues. They fear being alone, have a low self-esteem and may refer to themselves as 'stupid'. This personality disorder predisposes such individuals to dysthymia and depressive disorder.

Passive–aggressive personality disorder

This is a related condition, characterized by passive resistance to demands for adequate social and occupational performance, procrastination, childish obstruction and sulkiness. Such individuals tend to work slowly on tasks that they do not wish to perform, and often believe they are doing a better job than others think.

Case history: dependent personality disorder

Mrs A.B. was a 40-year-old woman who was often separated from her parents during her childhood. Her father was frequently away at sea and her mother in and out of hospital. Mrs A.B. herself was an anxious child, fearful of the dark and of going to school. She lacked self-confidence. After school she began working as a typist, which went well as long as she was not expected to work independently. She married during her adolescence. In the marriage she assumed the passive role, allowing her spouse to decide where they should live, where she should work and with whom they should be friendly. She would generally only take everyday decisions following advice from her husband and would easily feel hurt by his criticisms. She had no close friends outside her marriage. When her husband left her for another woman, she found it very difficult to adjust and became increasingly depressed and began drinking excessive amounts of alcohol. Feeling 'stupid' and unable to cope with the demands of everyday life, she took an overdose of paracetamol tablets. The severity of Mrs A.B.'s dependent personality disorder had thus been revealed by her separation from her husband. She was admitted to a general hospital, where she was assessed by a psychiatrist as being dependent on alcohol. She was transferred to a psychiatric hospital for alcohol withdrawal and subsequently followed up as an outpatient by a psychiatrist, on whom she became very dependent. Using supportive psychotherapy, the psychiatrist encouraged her to become more independent. She was also given a course of a tricyclic antidepressant for depression which had persisted following her withdrawal from alcohol, on

Case history: dependent personality disorder—cont'd

which she made a fair response. She was able to return to work and increasingly took over making day-to-day decisions in her life that others had previously made for her.

Inhibited personality

Anankastic (obsessive–compulsive) personality disorder

The term anankastic is derived from the Greek for compulsion. This personality disorder is characterized by perfectionism and inflexibility. Obsessional personalities, although insecure, may be conscientious and hardworking professionals. They may make good subordinates and have bureaucratic capacities. Alternatively, they may be obsessional ditherers. They may wish others would be as efficient as they see themselves, and may become angry when their rigid views are challenged. Unlike those suffering from obsessive–compulsive neurosis, they show no resistance to their obsessional behaviour and may become bogged down in details rather than take a broad view. This personality disorder corresponds to the Freudian anal personality, i.e. fixated at the anal stage of development, with their obsessionality reflecting the symbolic collection of faeces. Such individuals lack fantasy. It is more common and more frequently diagnosed in males. In general, medical practice obsessional personalities may circumstantially describe their symptoms at great length in an effort not to miss out any detail. They may pick up at an early stage any body changes, for instance in bowel function, and they react poorly to any doubt as to diagnosis. They are more prone to develop depression, obsessive–compulsive disorder or neurosis, hypochondriasis, anorexia nervosa, migraine and duodenal ulcer. Anankastic personality disorder is more common among first-degree biological relatives of those who suffer from it.

Two related conditions include *hypochondriacal personality disorder* (health conscious, disease fearing) and *depressive (dysthymic) personality disorder*, characterized by longitudinal depressed mood, pessimism and low self-esteem.

Cyclothymic or cycloid personality disorder (cyclothymia)

Cyclothymia is characterized by persistent instability of mood, with numerous periods of mild depression and mild elation. It is said to predispose to bipolar mood disorder.

Antisocial personality

Histrionic personality disorder

Histrionic personality disorder is characterized by excessive emotionality, attention seeking and overdramatic behaviour. It corresponds to the Freudian phallic personality, fixated at the Oedipal stage (the five-year-old child being seductive towards the parent of the opposite sex). Insecurity results in such individuals attempting to become the focus of attention, for instance everyday events are described as 'just fantastic' and greetings to others are 'over the top'. Such individuals may act out the role of victim or superstar, but can nevertheless be entertaining and the centre of the party. They are often empathic and sexually flirtatious, although sometimes frigid. Histrionic personality traits may be useful in acting and may explain the stereotype descriptions of actresses. Interpersonal relationships are often stormy and ungratifying for such individuals: they may select spouses who are 'doormats'. It is diagnosed more commonly in females than in males, which may, in part, reflect sexual stereotyping, as males with identical case histories may be diagnosed as suffering from antisocial personality disorder instead. Previously, histrionic personality disorder was generally referred to as hysterical personality disorder. However, the behaviour is conscious in histrionic personality disorder and should be distinguished from hysterical dissociative or conversion disorder (neurosis), where symptoms are unconsciously produced, and also from mass hysteria. Those with histrionic personality disorders are more liable to take overdoses of medication under stress and to develop conversion and somatization disorders.

Emotionally unstable personality disorder

Impulsive type. The impulsive type of emotionally unstable personality disorder (also referred to as explosive or aggressive personality disorder) is characterized by episodic loss of control of aggressive impulses, resulting in serious assaultative acts or destruction of property disproportionate to any precipitating psychosocial stresses. Such individuals have a short fuse, with a liability to outbursts of anger and violence under stress. They may subsequently show genuine regret for and self-reproach about such behaviour. Such individuals may batter their spouse and children, from which they may at the time derive feelings of power, countering those of inadequacy. It is more common in males than females, and may be more common in the first-degree biological relatives of those suffering from such a disorder.

Borderline type. The borderline type of emotionally unstable personality disorder is characterized by instability of self-image, interpersonal relationships and mood. Such individuals may have chronic feelings of emptiness and boredom, and their liability to become involved in intense and unstable relationships may cause repeated emotional crises and may even be associated with a series of suicidal threats or acts of self-harm, such as self-cutting. Primitive defence mechanisms, such as splitting and projective identification (see Chapter 4), are seen.

Under extreme stress, transient psychotic symptoms may develop in such individuals. Borderline personality disorder was originally described in individuals undergoing psychoanalysis, and the term is sometimes loosely used to describe individuals with severe personality disorder on the 'borderline' of psychosis. More common in females than in males, such individuals are prone to dysthymia, depressive episodes, psychoactive substance abuse and brief reactive psychosis.

Reflecting diagnostic overlap among those with personality disorder, 95% of those with borderline personality disorder meet criteria for a second personality disorder and 50% for a third.

Narcissistic personality disorder

Narcissistic personality disorder is characterized by grandiosity, in fantasy and in behaviour, hypersensitivity and lack of empathy. Such individuals react poorly to disfigurement due to physical illness or surgery.

Dissocial or antisocial personality disorder

Dissocial personality disorder is characterized by irresponsible and antisocial behaviour in individuals at least 18 years of age, who have a history of conduct disorder such as truancy from the age of 15. Such individuals are prone to drug and alcohol abuse, and are more likely to die prematurely by violent means. Features of this disorder are shown in Table 15.1. Included in this category is *psychopathic* or *sociopathic personality disorder*.

Psychopathic personality disorder

During the 19th century it was recognized that there was a group of individuals who suffered from neither mental illness nor mental retardation, but who showed abnormally aggressive, antisocial, seriously irresponsible or inadequate behaviour from an early age, with which society felt impelled to deal. In 1801, Pinel, the humanitarian psychiatrist who first unlocked the chains from patients in the French psychiatric hospital Bicêtre, coined the term *manie sans délire* to describe this group of patients. Not all the patients he described appeared to be what we would nowadays call psychopathic. A typical case, however, was that of a man, spoiled by a weak mother, who killed any animal who 'offended' him. He was found to be intellectually normal and was able to run his own estate, but had thrown a woman who was abusive to him down a well.

In 1835, the psychiatrist and anthropologist Pritchard coined the term *moral insanity* for this group of patients, the term 'moral' at that time meaning psychological more than ethical. His cases also included individuals suffering from manic-depressive psychosis. In 1891, Koch used the term *psychopathic inferiority*, in 1909, Kraepelin used the term *psychopathic traits* and, in 1927, Schneider the term *psychopathic personalities*. In 1930, the term *sociopathy* was used by Partridge in the USA, which indicated and emphasized the social malfunctioning of such patients. The term *psychopathy* originally included all personality disorders, which still applies on the European continent. The term became restricted in the USA to antisocial personality disordered people and was imported to the UK with that meaning by Henderson in 1939. He distinguished three kinds of psychopathic personality:

- the predominantly aggressive
- the predominantly inadequate (pathological liars or pseudologia phantastica, swindlers, conmen – who are themselves the most easily conned, etc.)
- creative psychopaths, who have high ability combined with their severe personality disorder, such as Lawrence of Arabia and the Renaissance sculptor Cellini.

The term psychopathic disorder was incorporated first into the England and Wales Mental Health Act in 1959, and, in the 1983 Mental Health Act, it is defined as a persistent disorder or disability of mind (whether or not including impairment of intelligence), which results in abnormally aggressive or seriously irresponsible conduct on the part of the patient. As a legal diagnosis it can be used to detain those suffering from all clinical personality disorders. However, to detain an individual on such grounds, it must be stated that the condition is treatable. There is no legal diagnosis of psychopathic disorder in the current Mental Health Acts of Scotland or Northern Ireland.

The equivalent of the clinical diagnosis of psychopathic disorder in DSM-IV-TR is antisocial personality disorder, and in ICD-10 it is dissocial personality disorder, although some psychopathic individuals are best described by the category 'emotionally unstable personality disorder, impulsive type'. The term psychopath is also used clinically in a pejorative sense to describe unreliable, uncooperative and often difficult male patients. The definition of psychopathy has also been used in a circular fashion, i.e. antisocial behaviour is presumed to be due to psychopathy, yet psychopathy is presumed present from the behaviour.

Case history: psychopathic or dissocial personality disorder

Mr C.D. was born to an alcoholic father with an extensive criminal record who was frequently violent to Mr C.D's mother. Following his parents' separation during his childhood, Mr C.D. was taken into care. Until 11 years of age he wet the bed. At school he frequently became involved in fights, would lie, be destructive and also set fires. At secondary school he began to truant excessively. In his early teens he began abusing alcohol and drugs and getting involved with others in taking and driving away cars and burglary. As he became older, his offending increased in seriousness to include robbery and possession of a knife (at the age of 19). His offending appeared to be impulsive and he showed no guilt. He had a number of sexual relationships but did not sustain these, being basically affectionless. He would be violent to his girlfriends, especially when drunk. He was unable to sustain regular work and accumulated debts. His continued offending resulted in his receiving a number of prison sentences, which did not deter him from reoffending upon release. At the age of 27 years, while intoxicated with alcohol, he killed his then-girlfriend, with whom he was living, when she told him she was leaving because of his alcohol abuse and violence to her. Following the offence, no evidence of mental illness was found. He stated

Continued

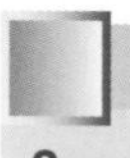

Case history: psychopathic or dissocial personality disorder—cont'd

that she had deserved what had happened to her and he showed little guilt. He was not considered to be amenable to psychiatric treatment and was convicted of murder and sentenced to life imprisonment.

Differential diagnosis

The differential diagnosis of personality disorder includes deterioration in personality and social functioning and/or disinhibition of behaviour due to *severe mental illness* (e.g. schizophrenia). Hypomania, with its associated increase in irritability, disinhibited behaviour and increase in sexual drive, can be misdiagnosed as dissocial personality disorder, especially when mild and chronic. The differential diagnosis also includes *drug and alcohol-induced states* and *organic psychoses*, including brain damage resulting from focal or diffuse brain disorder and from toxic, infective, metabolic or neoplastic causes. In particular, *frontal lobe syndrome* may present with pseudopsychopathic personality change with disinhibition. *Seizure disorder*, with or without brain damage, may be associated with personality change, particularly in temporal lobe epilepsy.

The classic features of psychopathic personality are shown in Table 15.2.

As classically described, a 'primary' psychopath would rarely seek assistance from a clinician and is most likely to be found within the penal system. 'Secondary' psychopaths, however, are described with higher levels of anxiety or tension, hidden guilt and regret, and low self-esteem. They may impulsively harm themselves under stress, seek assistance from psychiatric services and may have a better prognosis. Contrary to popular belief, psychopaths do not make good soldiers as they are too impulsive and do not work cooperatively, although they can on occasion undertake breathtaking and heroic acts. The general characteristic of psychopaths – the seeking of immediate gratification of needs – may result in sexual offending.

Table 15.2 Clinical features of psychopathic disorder

	Clinical feature
Classically	Affectionless
	Impulsive
As a result	Egocentric and lacks empathy
	Lacking in shame; totally guiltless/no regret
	No ability to profit from experience, including punishment
	No life plans, as lacks normal drive or motivation
	Viciousness
	Unable to sustain emotional relationships, but may present as initially articulate and charming
Other features	Very low anxiety/tension
	Breathtaking escapades
	Autonomic nervous system abnormalities, with slower conditioning
	Rarely seeks assistance
	Untreatable in pure form
Negative features	Lack of psychosis
	Lack of intellectual deficit
	Lacks criminal motive

Enduring personality changes

ICD-10 also refers to a category called enduring personality changes, which are not attributable to gross brain damage or disease and develop in persons with no previous personality disorder, following a severe psychiatric illness, excessive prolonged stress or a catastrophic experience. Examples of catastrophic stress cited include concentration camp experiences, torture, terrorism (including hostage situations) and post-traumatic stress disorder.

Epidemiology and clinical features

- About 10% of the outpatient psychiatric population and 5% of the inpatient psychiatric population may be diagnosed as suffering from personality disorder.
- More commonly diagnosed in those aged 18–35 years, in males and in lower social classes.
- Personality disorders tend to cluster in four groups
  - withdrawn (odd and eccentric)
  - dependent (anxious and tearful)
  - inhibited
  - antisocial (dramatic, emotional, flamboyant and erratic).
- Psychopathic personality disorder is characterized by:
  - affectionlessness
  - an incapacity for love or feeling
  - impulsivity
  - egocentricity
  - the seeking of immediate gratification without regard for the consequences
  - lack of guilt
  - antisocial and violent behaviour
  - failure to learn from experience, including punishment.

Personality disorder may be an additional diagnosis to other psychiatric disorders, and not necessarily merely an alternative. Problems attributable to personality disorder should have been persistent since adolescence, not episodic as can be the case in mental illness.

Aetiology

Personality disorders are thought to result from a number of predisposing factors, for example:

- hereditary
- constitutional
- psychological.

Hereditary factors

Genetics

Twin studies for personality traits have shown concordance is greater for monozygotic (MZ) than dizygotic (DZ) twins for extroversion, introversion, neuroticism and psychopathy (where concordance rates demonstrated for MZ:DZ = 52%:22%). In Danish adoption studies, criminality in adoptees was 36% where biological and adopting fathers were both criminal, 21% where the biological father only was criminal and 10% where neither father was criminal. An analogy of the role of genetic factors may be with sporting proficiency, where genetic predisposition requires experience, for example to 'hard wire' the cerebellum by playing sport from an early age. Particular genetic traits (e.g. sensation seeking) can also increase exposure to particular environmental factors. There is also an increased incidence of personality disorder, especially schizotypal, in the biological relatives of those who suffer from schizophrenia.

Chromosomal abnormalities

It has been suggested that individuals with XYY chromosomal abnormality may show evidence of increased criminality independent of low IQ and socioeconomic status.

Infant temperamental differences

Temperamental differences are not entirely caused by genetic factors but are seen between babies from birth, even within families. Differences are observed in emotionality, activity, sociability and impulsivity. Temperament has a large influence on the child's interaction with parents, especially where there is a mismatch between the child's temperament and the personality and coping skills of the parents. Overall, temperamentally difficult children are vulnerable to later developing behavioural and personality disorders.

Autonomic nervous system activity

Psychopaths have underactive autonomic nervous and reticular activating systems and are accordingly underaroused, resulting in sensation-seeking behaviour and poor behavioural conditioning. This is considered to have an inherited genetic basis.

Neuropsychophysiological factors

Electroencephalography (EEG) studies have shown immature traces, such as posterior slow (theta) waves (Figure 15.3), in psychopaths who have also been shown in studies to have both reduced evoked potentials and contingent negative variation.

Among those with psychopathic personality disorder, studies have shown abnormalities in the frontal and temporal cortices and their connections. Functional magnetic resonance studies have also shown difficulties in processing and understanding emotional material compared with control subjects. The amygdala in the limbic system, which is responsible for emotional processing of fear and of other individuals' faces, may be abnormal. However, it remains unclear if these abnormalities are primarily biological or secondary phenomena.

Constitutional factors

Prenatal effects

The possibility of intrauterine effects and hormones on personality development is suggested by animal experiments and in isolated human cases (e.g. the masculinization of the behaviour of female offspring by testosterone). In humans, impaired nutrition during pregnancy (as well as in the postnatal period), hypoxia at birth, low birthweight and birth complications are all associated with the development of children with lower IQ and behavioural abnormalities (maladjustment). Minor congenital defects, such as squints, minimal brain damage and deafness, are also associated with impaired development of personality.

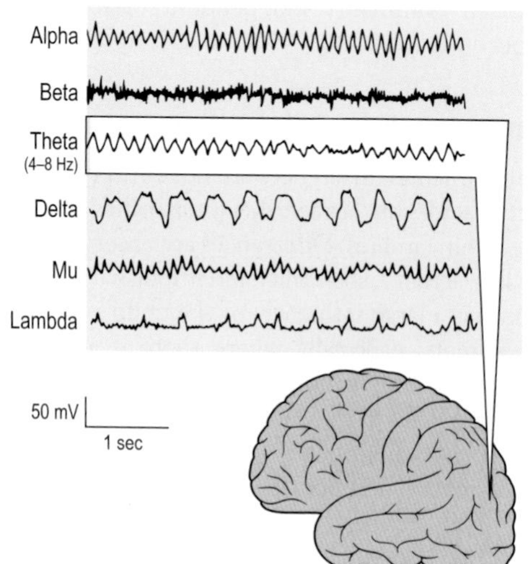

Figure 15.3 • EEG study showing posterior slow (theta) waves in a psychopath. (Reproduced with permission from Swash M, Kennard C 1985 Scientific basis of clinical neurology. Churchill Livingstone, Edinburgh)

Psychological factors

Psychological factors are currently considered to be probably the most important aetiological factors.

Psychoanalytic theories

Personality develops from an entirely egocentric baby to, ideally, an altruistic mature adult, and requires the formation of attachment bonds. Personality disorder may develop as a result of disruption of the development process, which may be halted at particular stages, for example at the Freudian oral, anal or phallic stages.

Classically, fixation at the Freudian oral stage results in dependent personality disorder, at the anal stage in an anankastic personality disorder, and at the phallic stage in a histrionic personality disorder. Psychopathic disorder is considered to be related to a weakly formed superego (the conscious).

Psychopathic personality disorder is also associated with lack of parental affection, poor parenting and *maternal deprivation* in the first three years of life (as described by Bowlby), as well as child abuse, removal from the parental home and the absence of paternal figures. Borderline personality disorder is associated with a history of childhood sexual abuse.

Learning theory

Behavioural psychological learning theory considers that personality disorder is a result of maladaptive conditioning and modelling in childhood and adolescence (e.g. in social relationships). An individual may be 'trained' to antisocial standards by family discord, violence and criminality. Alternatively, an individual may be 'untrained' due to inconsistent, neglecting or rejecting parents.

Other early background factors

Brain damage in early life due to head injuries, encephalitis or other causes may result in psychopathic disorder. Chronic physical illness and childhood separation anxiety disorder predispose to dependent personality disorder. Social sensitivity (avoidant) disorder of childhood and disfiguring physical illness during childhood may predispose to avoidant personality disorder. Hyperkinetic disorder and conduct disorder in childhood are also associated with the development of psychopathic personality disorder. The causes of psychopathic personality disorder may be multifactorial and include social and environmental factors, such as poor social conditions, overcrowding in the family home (with the resulting reduced parental contact), differential association with delinquents, other subcultural influences and labelling.

Precipitating and perpetuating factors

Although personality disorders are by definition lifelong and enduring, they may be revealed by stress or by the removal of support through the death of, or separation from, a spouse or parents. Such individuals may present with depression, anxiety, drug or alcohol abuse, self-harm or other psychiatric disorders. These 'symptoms' may result from the individual's dissatisfaction with personality difficulties and the limitations these place on social functioning and the ability to sustain interpersonal relationships.

Again, although personality disorders are by definition lifelong, they may be perpetuated through, for example, social reinforcement, subcultural expectations and labelling.

Differential diagnosis and aetiology

- Personality disorder may be emulated by:
  - severe mental illness, e.g. schizophrenia, hypomania
  - organic psychosis, e.g. brain damage
  - drug and alcohol-induced states.
- Personality disorders arise from family and early background factors, including:
  - psychological factors, e.g. early attachments, maladaptive learning
  - constitutional factors, e.g. prenatal factors
  - hereditary factors, e.g. genetic predisposition or chromosomal abnormalities such as XYY.

Management

Assessment

History

Personality disorder is a clinical judgement: the diagnosis rests on evidence of persistent personality traits and associated behavioural abnormalities from childhood, which should be clearly independent of mental illness or any other psychiatric disorder. A detailed history is therefore required, not only from the patient but also from other independent sources such as parents, relatives or other informants and, if possible, schools. It is important to differentiate personality disorder from normal personality variation. Evidence should be sought for lifelong general personality and social malfunctioning. Particular attention should be paid to the patient's interactions with others, ability to sustain work and tolerate stress, and characteristic mood (Table 15.3). An independently verified account of consistent patterns of behaviour provides more objective evidence

Table 15.3 Personality assessment at interview – possible areas to be explored
Introversion/extroversion
Shyness, introspection, fantasy
Oversensitivity, suspiciousness, paranoid attitude to others
Overanxiousness
Impulsivity
Obsessionality, rigidity
Histrionic
Dominant or submissive
Low tolerance of stress with a liability to temper and/or violence
Antiauthoritarian attitude
Characteristic mood and capacity for enjoyment
Low self-esteem
Ability to sustain interpersonal relationships and work
Interests. Religious beliefs
History of alcohol consumption, drug abuse, cigarette smoking and law involvement

of personality disorder than a patient's own account of personal aims and goals. One should try to establish not only the weaknesses but also the strengths of each individual's personality, and also the relative importance of the social context.

Examination

In severe personality disorder it is rare to find no abnormalities on mental state examination, as individuals with personality disorder often do not present unless they are additionally suffering from, and complaining about, depression, anxiety, tension and other problems. Physical examination may reveal evidence of alcohol or drug abuse, and possibly evidence of associated organic factors, including brain damage.

Investigations

Although well-established personality inventories such as the EPI and the MMPI are available, they are mainly of use as indicators of personality variation in a normal population. In personality disorder, especially in the presence of mental illness, the EPI is of little clinical use, although the MMPI is considered by some to be of some validity and reliability (Figure 15.4). Theoretically, those with psychopathic disorder should score high on extroversion and neuroticism on the EPI due to underarousal of the reticular activating and autonomic nervous systems. In practice, clinicians do see psychopaths who are introverted. Hare's Psychopathic Checklist (PCL-R) is also widely used in diagnosing psychopathy. Structured interview schedules, such as the Standardized Assessment of Personality and the Personality Assessment Schedule, can partially overcome the problem of distinguishing personality from current mental illness, including using an informant in assessing premorbid personality. Prolonged acquaintance with the patient still provides the most accurate assessment of personality. If there is a question of an organic component, an EEG (for example in suspected seizure disorder) or computed tomography (CT) or magnetic resonance imaging (MRI) brain scan may be indicated.

Treatment

Reasons for treatment include the fact that personality disorder increases vulnerability to, and worsens prognosis and treatment response of, mental illness. Personality disorder is also associated with high rates of self-harm and suicide and expensive use of Accident and Emergency (Casualty) departments and psychiatric services. It can also lead to the next generation of those with personality disorder.

However, personality disorder is generally regarded as resistant to specific psychiatric treatment, although in the absence of systematic studies one should not make this assumption. In any case, the medical profession is often compelled to deal with such individuals as they often present to them in crisis, for instance either threatening or following self-harm, or threatening violence to others. As previously discussed, those with a personality disorder often do not present until they have become additionally depressed, anxious and/or tense. One should be aware, however, that an apparent improvement

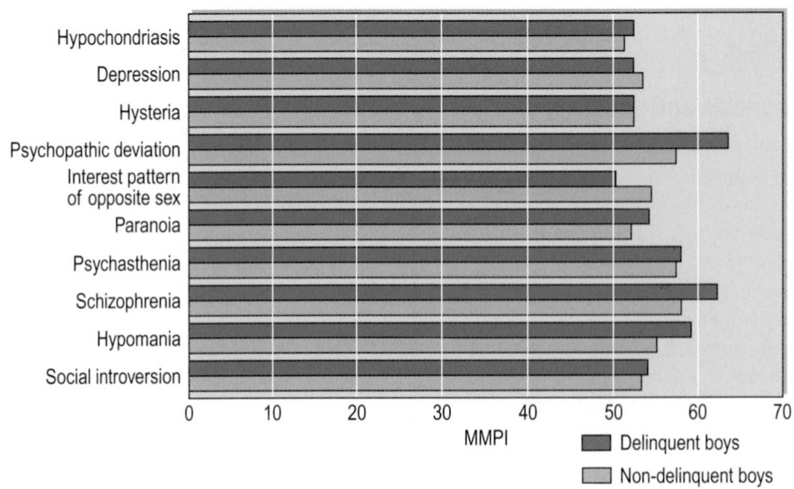

Figure 15.4 • Personality profiles of male delinquents and non-delinquents as measured by the MMPI.

often reflects merely the spontaneous improvement in (or treatment of) associated mental illness. One must anticipate that treatment of personality disorder will have to be prolonged and that full recovery is unlikely, which is consistent with the definition of personality disorder as being a lifelong abnormality. Patients may be difficult and unrewarding to manage, and they easily engender negative countertransference reactions in those attempting to help them (see Chapter 4). This may facilitate their rejection from treatment. Although attempts at limit-setting of such patients' behaviour while in treatment may have to be made, they may additionally be unreliable in keeping appointments and in complying with treatment. They may act out to relieve feelings of tension or to ensure attention.

However, individual or group psychotherapeutic and psychological treatments, including behaviour modification, cognitive behavioural therapy and drug therapy, have all been used. Drugs are not usually appropriate unless to treat superimposed mental illness, such as depression or transient psychotic symptoms, or to reduce feelings of tension in a crisis. Manipulation of the social environment can also be beneficial. Increasing the patient's adaptation to his social situation, rather than fundamental personality change, may be the only realistic goal.

Organic factors should be excluded and, if possible, treated when present, as should any additional psychiatric disorder. This includes mental illness and drug and alcohol abuse or dependency.

Treatment will usually be on an outpatient basis and involve counselling and supportive psychotherapy, with a view to helping the patient avoid and/or deal with stressful life circumstances. A relationship with one therapist over a long time is often beneficial, as it provides emotional security and the therapist may be the only person with whom the individual has ever sustained a relationship. Cognitive behavioural techniques may be utilized as indicated, for instance *social skills training* and *anger management*. One should avoid provoking patients who make threats to harm themselves or others into acting on such threats by rejecting them on grounds of untreatability. However, it is also helpful to realize the limitations of what can be offered by way of treatment and accept that the prognosis may be poor.

Those with a personality disorder usually benefit little in the long term from inpatient treatment in conventional psychiatric units. However, short-term hospital admission may tide such patients over crises and allow 'cooling off'. Longer term milieu therapy in a *therapeutic community* (pioneered by Maxwell Jones in the UK), such as at the Henderson Hospital in Surrey, UK, may be helpful.

As an overall guide it may be best to aim to treat only those with intercurrent mental illness in a conventional psychiatric hospital, and to provide those with inadequate personality disorders with support in the community, including from the social services. For aggressive psychopaths the only option may be to let the law take its course if they behave antisocially, with the likelihood that they may end up in prison.

Withdrawn personality disorders

Individuals with withdrawn personality disorders (odd and eccentric) seldom present for treatment. They mistrust and blame others, including the medical profession, and will easily resort to threatening legal action. They tend to do badly in any form of group setting, and if they are to receive psychotherapy this should generally be on an individual basis. An object relations psychotherapeutic approach is recommended, based on the theory of Winnicot (i.e. that satisfaction is sought by individuals in relationships). Such patients are often reluctant to receive drug treatment but may benefit from low doses of antipsychotic drugs, in either oral (e.g. flupentixol) or depot injection form.

Dependent personality disorders

Individuals with dependent personality disorders (anxious and fearful) may become very reliant on their doctor, to whom they easily develop positive transference feelings. Therapeutically, this may be more important than any other psychological or drug treatment offered and should be utilized in attempts to help the patient find independent ways of functioning. Occasionally, self-help groups may be of value. Behaviour therapy has been found to be of value in those with anxious (avoidant) personality disorder. When anxiety and depression are significant, benefit may be obtained from conventional tricyclic antidepressants. Such patients are at risk of becoming dependent on, and long-term users of, anxiolytic and sedative benzodiazepines.

Inhibited personality disorders

Individuals with an inhibited personality disorder, such as anankastic (obsessive–compulsive) personality disorder, may not regard this as their main problem, but instead blame their problems on others and their disorganization. This is unlike those suffering from obsessive–compulsive neurosis, who complain of their symptoms. Psychodynamic psychotherapy can be used to break down defences, which are maladaptively attempting to preserve the individual's sense of security in life. Cognitive therapy may be used to point out the inconsistencies between the patient's view of the world and reactions to others. Behavioural treatment may aim to prevent the patient undertaking obsessional activities, which are attempts to avoid anxiety and uncertainty. This is usually through the process of gradual exposure (desensitization). Unlike in obsessive–compulsive neurosis, the patient may not recognize these obsessional activities as a handicap and may therefore be much less motivated to change. If obsessional neurotic symptoms or mood disturbance, such as panic, anxiety or depression, are also present, treatment with antidepressant drugs (especially clomipramine) can be effective.

Antisocial personality disorders

In the antisocial group of personality disorders it may be difficult to engage the patient in treatment. Low stress tolerance may also lead the patient to make insistent demands for treatment (including drugs) and for instant results from such treatment, upon threat of self-harm or harm to others. Patients may often stop treatment themselves, unless they are forced to receive it while detained under a Mental Health Act or are encouraged to do so during a custodial sentence. They may do best with younger therapists, whom they perceive as being less authoritarian. However, such patients often lack motivation for treatment.

Group therapy is usually preferable to individual psychotherapy. This may be undertaken within a *therapeutic community*, where the patient lives with other patients and staff and where the consequences of antisocial behaviour are immediately apparent, which contrasts with the delayed punishment for such behaviour given by the legal system. In therapeutic communities there is open communication and shared examination of problems between patients and staff in a democratic and communal environment, with regular feedback (*reality confrontation*) given to individuals about their behaviour. This allows social learning to take place. Severely handicapped personalities may, however, be unable to tolerate the stress of such a regime and may act out. They may benefit from a more paternalistic authoritarian approach. Therapeutic community treatment is offered at the Henderson Hospital in Surrey, UK, where research shows subsequent decreases in levels of hospitalization and criminality and also cost savings in subsequent care, and, for those non-mentally ill personality disordered individuals who are serving a custodial sentence, at both Grendon Underwood and Wormwood Scrubs prisons in England.

Among those with borderline personality disorder, interpersonal group therapy and dialectical behaviour therapy have been shown to be effective, the latter reducing parasuicidal behaviour.

Depression, suicidal impulses and general impulsivity and aggression may be countered by low-dose antipsychotic medication, in either oral or depot injection form. The latter helps overcome the usually poor compliance with oral drug treatment in this group. However, as such treatment is usually required on a long-term basis, there is a risk of tardive dyskinesia. Brain levels of serotonin have been shown to be low in the brains of impulsive, self-harming and aggressive personalities, and thus antidepressants, especially selective serotonin reuptake inhibitors (SSRIs), may also be of benefit, as may lithium carbonate, which also raises serotonin levels, because of its anti-aggressive as well as mood-stabilizing properties. The anticonvulsant carbamazepine is regarded as a stabilizer of the limbic system and is promoted as a treatment for the 'dyscontrol syndrome'. Benzodiazepines should be avoided, as they may release paradoxical aggression.

Aggressive psychopaths are generally not admitted to Medium Secure Units in England and Wales. Those with a legal diagnosis of psychopathic disorder may be detained in 'special hospitals' such as Broadmoor, where treatment may do little more than keep such individuals out of the community, free from drugs and alcohol and away from potential victims during the years of their greatest risk to others, while their personality matures naturally with age.

The new Mental Health Act for England and Wales includes controversial proposals for the preventative detention of those with 'Dangerous Severe Personality Disorder', whether or not they have yet offended, in existing prison and secure hospital facilities.

Nidotherapy

This is a new form of therapy pioneered by Professor Peter Tyrer. It is based on the systematic adjustment of the environment to fit the patient. It is useful for personality disorders that are resisting treatment. Its use in such patients has been supported by a recent randomized controlled trial. The reader is referred to the excellent book on nidotherapy in Further reading.

Course and prognosis

Accurate personality assessment in general helps predict subsequent behaviour (e.g. reaction to physical illness) and helps in giving a prognosis. Those with personality disorder, especially antisocial and other high emotion personality disorders, tend to improve naturally with age and maturation. This is less true for anankastic (obsessive–compulsive) and low emotion, odd and eccentric, and especially schizotypal personality disorders. Normal individuals become less emotional and impulsive and more cautious and careful with age. Those with antisocial personality disorders are usually most destructive in their early life. They are diagnosed most frequently between the ages of 30 and 35, and tend to 'burn out' after then, becoming less antisocial, although family difficulties (including battering of spouse and babies, divorce, alcohol and drug abuse, depression and self-blame) may persist. There is also a higher incidence of death by violence or suicide.

The presence of personality disorder also predicts impairment of both the course and response to treatment of mental illnesses. The prognosis generally is improved if the individual establishes a stable domestic relationship with another person.

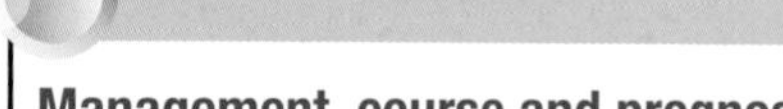

Management, course and prognosis

- Personality disorder is often difficult to manage.
- Individual or group psychotherapeutic, therapeutic community, cognitive and behavioural techniques have been used.
- Drugs are not usually appropriate unless to treat superimposed mental illness, such as depression or psychosis, or to reduce feelings of tension.
- Nidotherapy, in which the patient's environment is systematically adjusted, can be beneficial, particularly for personality disorders resisting treatment.
- Tendency to improve naturally with age and maturation.
- Normal individuals become less emotional and impulsive, and more cautious and careful with age.

Further reading

Sampson, M.J., McCubbin, R.A., Tyrer, P. (Eds.), 2006. Personality disorder and community mental health teams: a practitioner's guide. John Wiley, Chichester.

Tyrer, P., 2010. Personality disorders. In: Puri, B.K., Treasaden, I. (Eds.), Psychiatry: an evidence-based text. Hodder Arnold, London.

Tyrer, P., 2009. Nidotherapy: harmonising the environment with the patient. The Royal College of Psychiatrists, London.

Child and adolescent psychiatry

This chapter covers those psychiatric disorders in which onset usually occurs in childhood, and also addresses the specific variations in adult disorders seen in children and adolescents. A section on child psychiatric disorder in general is followed by sections on particular disorders.

Child psychiatric disorder

Definition and classification

The ICD-10 classification of 'Behavioural and emotional disorders with onset usually occurring in childhood and adolescence' (F90–98) is shown in Table 16.1. In general, if the criteria for one of the other 'adult' disorders (such as depression) are met, then such a diagnosis should be made rather than a 'childhood-onset' diagnosis. Recognition of different dimensions of childhood functioning has led the WHO to develop a multiaxial framework for the diagnosis of child psychiatric disorder (Table 16.2). DSM-IV-TR disorders usually first diagnosed in infancy, childhood or adolescence are outlined in Table 16.3.

Rutter has pointed out that the majority of child psychiatric disorder is a *quantitative* deviance from the norm, with *suffering and/or handicap*. In other words, most children show some of the 'symptoms' of child psychiatric disorder at some point in their development (generally at a roughly similar time). These are usually of a certain intensity and duration and resolve with appropriate environment and management (e.g. tantrums are common in two to three-year-olds but might be considered a disorder in a nine-year-old). It is important to emphasize that a deviance on its own is not sufficient to constitute a disorder: consequent suffering and/or handicap is also required (although not necessarily to the child). The example given by Rutter is of a child who has a high level of intelligence: the child is quantitatively deviant from the norm, but would not suffer unless this was out of step with social expectations, or if the child was not provided with appropriate educational opportunities.

As with all generalizations there are exceptions, both to this view of child psychiatric disorder (such as the pervasive developmental disorders, which are qualitatively different) and to the converse description of adult psychiatric disorder as a qualitative deviance (e.g. depressive disorder without psychosis may be regarded as a more severe or prolonged form of normal misery).

There is a high level of comorbidity seen in children and adolescents. This perhaps reflects the above and also the essentially descriptive nature of most diagnoses.

In child and adolescent psychiatry it is essential to have a clear knowledge of the *normal development* of all aspects of behavioural and psychological functioning. Detailed accounts of childhood development may be found in paediatric texts and developmental psychology books. Table 16.4 shows an outline of various developmental milestones, and includes references to various different theories of psychological development. It must be noted that these theories are ways of conceptualizing development, each designed to explain and predict, with implications for management and treatment. They are not the literal truth and are by no means mutually exclusive. Only brief outlines of the theories can be given here.

Table 16.1 ICD-10 classification: F90–F98 Behavioural and emotional disorders with onset usually occurring in childhood and adolescence

F90	**Hyperkinetic disorders**
	F90.0 Disturbance of activity and attention
	F90.1 Hyperkinetic conduct disorder
	F90.8 Other hyperkinetic disorders
	F90.9 Hyperkinetic disorder, unspecified
F91	**Conduct disorders**
	F91.0 Conduct disorder confined to the family context
	F91.1 Unsocialized conduct disorder
	F91.2 Socialized conduct disorder
	F91.3 Oppositional defiant disorder
	F91.8 Other conduct disorders
	F91.9 Conduct disorder, unspecified
F92	**Mixed disorders of conduct and emotions**
	F92.0 Depressive conduct disorder
	F92.8 Other mixed disorders of conduct and emotions
	F92.9 Mixed disorder of conduct and emotions, unspecified
F93	**Emotional disorders with onset specific to childhood**
	F93.0 Separation anxiety disorder of childhood
	F93.1 Phobic anxiety disorder of childhood
	F93.2 Social anxiety disorder of childhood
	F93.3 Sibling rivalry disorder
	F93.8 Other childhood emotional disorders
	F93.9 Childhood emotional disorder, unspecified
F94	**Disorders of social functioning with onset specific to childhood and adolescence**
	F94.0 Elective mutism
	F94.1 Reactive attachment disorder of childhood
	F94.2 Disinhibited attachment disorder of childhood
	F94.8 Other childhood disorders of social functioning
	F94.9 Childhood disorders of social functioning, unspecified
F95	**Tic disorders**
	F95.0 Transient tic disorder
	F95.1 Chronic motor or vocal tic disorder
	F95.2 Combined vocal and multiple motor tic disorder (Gilles de la Tourette's syndrome)
	F95.8 Other tic disorders
	F95.9 Tic disorder, unspecified

Continued

Table 16.1 ICD-10 classification: F90–F98 Behavioural and emotional disorders with onset usually occurring in childhood and adolescence—cont'd

F98	**Other behavioural and emotional disorders with onset usually occurring in childhood and adolescence**
	F98.0 Non-organic enuresis
	F98.1 Non-organic encopresis
	F98.2 Feeding disorder of infancy and childhood
	F98.3 Pica of infancy and childhood
	F98.4 Stereotyped movement disorders
	F98.5 Stuttering (stammering)
	F98.6 Cluttering
	F98.8 Other specified behavioural and emotional disorders with onset usually occurring in childhood and adolescence
	F98.9 Unspecified behavioural and emotional disorders with onset usually occurring in childhood and adolescence

Table 16.2 ICD-10 Multiaxial framework

Axis One	Clinical psychiatric syndromes
Axis Two	Specific disorders of psychological development
Axis Three	Intellectual level
Axis Four	Medical conditions
Axis Five	Associated abnormal psychosocial situation

Some aspects of Freud's psychoanalytic theory are described in Chapter 4. Erikson saw development as a series of stages or psychosocial crises that must be overcome to make proper relationships at each stage in life. The stages relate to a widening and narrowing social world (see Chapter 2).

Piaget produced a theory of cognitive development based on careful observation of a relatively small number of children. Others have subsequently refined and modified Piaget's theory, on the basis of psychological experimentation and further observation. The sensorimotor stage (zero to two years, approximately) is a process of distinguishing the self and others through sensory inputs and motor manipulation of objects. The preoperational stage (approximately two to seven years) is a period of development of appreciation of symbols for outside objects, but the rules connecting them are primitive and developing. The child's view of the world is very self-centred (egocentric). At the concrete operational stage (approximately seven to 12 years), categorization and development of hierarchy of concepts (e.g. volume over height) occurs. At the formal operational stage (age 12 onwards) there is even more development of the internal world, with the ability to see another's viewpoint being developed further and hypothesizing by manipulation of internal concepts occurring.

Epidemiology

Preschool

A study in the early 1970s showed a 7% prevalence for moderate to severe problem behaviour, and another 15% with mild behaviour problems in a population study of an outer London borough with a social class distribution similar to the whole country (Waltham Forest). There were strong continuities of behaviour and language disorders over the early school years. The disorder was as reported by parents and showed a strong relation to psychosocial adversity.

School-age children

In 1999, the Office for National Statistics of the UK with Dr Robert Goodman and colleagues carried out face-to-face interviews with 10 500 parents of children aged five to 15 and also with 4500 children and adolescents aged 11–15. The sample was derived randomly

Table 16.3 DSM-IV-TR disorders usually first diagnosed in infancy, childhood or adolescence

Learning disorders	
315.0	Reading disorder
315.1	Mathematics disorder
315.2	Disorder of written expression
315.9	Learning disorder NOS
Motor skills disorder	
315.4	Developmental coordination disorder
Communication disorders	
315.31	Expressive language disorder
315.32	Mixed receptive–expressive language disorder
315.39	Phonological disorder
307.0	Stuttering
307.9	Communication disorder NOS
Pervasive developmental disorders	
299.00	Autistic disorder
299.80	Rett's disorder
299.10	Childhood disintegrative disorder
299.80	Asperger's disorder
299.80	Pervasive developmental disorder NOS
Attention-deficit and disruptive behavioural disorders	
314.xx	Attention-deficit/hyperactivity disorder
.01	Combined type
.00	Predominantly inattentive type
.01	Predominantly hyperactive–impulsive type
314.9	Attention-deficit/hyperactivity disorder NOS
312.xx	Conduct disorder
.81	Childhood-onset type
.82	Adolescent-onset type
.89	Unspecified onset
313.81	Oppositional defiant disorder
312.9	Disruptive behaviour disorder NOS
Feeding and eating disorders of infancy or early childhood	
307.52	Pica
307.53	Rumination disorder
307.59	Feeding disorder of infancy or early childhood

Continued

Table 16.3 DSM-IV-TR disorders usually first diagnosed in infancy, childhood or adolescence—cont'd

Tic disorders	
307.23	Tourette's disorder
307.22	Chronic motor or vocal tic disorder
307.21	Transient tic disorder (115) (*Specify if* Single episode/recurrent)
307.20	Tic disorder NOS (116)
Elimination disorders	
—.—	Encopresis
787.6	With constipation and overflow incontinence
307.7	Without constipation and overflow incontinence
307.6	Enuresis (not due to a general medical condition) (*Specify type:* Noctumal only/diurnal only/nocturnal and diurnal)
Other disorders of infancy, childhood, or adolescence	
309.21	Separation anxiety disorder (*Specify if* Early onset)
313.23	Selective mutism
313.89	Reactive attachment disorder of infancy or early childhood (*Specify type:* Inhibited type/disinhibited type)
307.3	Stereotypic movement disorder (*Specify if* With self-injurious behaviour)
313.9	Disorder of infancy, childhood, or adolescence NOS (134)

NOS, not otherwise specified

Table 16.4 Childhood development and developmental stages

Age	Milestones	Freudian stage	Piagetian stage	Ericksonian stage
Zero to six months	Vocalizes up to double-syllable sounds, rolls over, objects – palmar grasp, hand to hand and to mouth, smiles and laughs	Oral	Sensorimotor	Trust vs. mistrust
Six months to one year	Crawls, stands with support, sits unsupported, pincer grasp present, stranger shyness	Oral	Sensorimotor	Trust vs. mistrust
One to two years	Walks, runs, builds up to two to three word sentences, feeds self with spoon, parallel play, beginning to attain continence	Anal	Sensorimotor	Autonomy vs. shame and doubt
Early infancy	Attains continence, cooperative play, draws a man, much questioning, speech increases in fluency, learns to skip and hop and to dress and undress	Phallic	Preoperational	Initiative vs. guilt
Late infancy to middle childhood	Increasing involvement with peer group, schooling, increased autonomy	Latency	Concrete operational	Industry vs. inferiority
Adolescence	Moves towards independence, relates mostly to peer group	Genital	Formal operational	Identity vs. confusion

from address records. This produced an average prevalence of psychiatric disorder of around 10%.

Among five to 10-year-olds the prevalence was 10% in boys and 6% in girls. In the 11–15-year age group, the proportions were 13% boys, 10% girls. Marked differences in social class distribution were seen. Children of parents with unskilled occupations had three times the rate of psychiatric disorder compared with children of professional parents. For parents who had never been in paid work the multiplier was four.

This large study confirms earlier epidemiological studies in the Isle of Wight (1960s), London, UK (1970s); Canada; Blackburn, UK and Dunedin, New Zealand. These studies generally found a doubling of disorder in urban as opposed to rural contexts. Increased levels of parental discord and parental psychiatric disorder in cities could account for this difference.

Clinical features

The first general point to note is that it is relatively unusual for the child or adolescent to be the one initiating psychiatric contact. This is more usually a parent or other carer, school, social services or the court. Arising from this, and confirmed by population studies as above, is the observation that there are often considerable discontinuities in a child's presentation in different circumstances (in particular school and home, but also with different people). This of course has considerable implications for assessment (see later).

Although there are exceptions, in general collections of symptoms or disorder classifications are not closely correlated with particular aetiologies. In other words, different children will produce different disturbances in the same predicament, and some may show no disturbance at all.

Aetiology

In child and adolescent psychiatry *multifactorial aetiology* is the rule. This is not simply in the sense of many factors contributing to a given predicament, but in the interaction of such factors at all levels of a child's or adolescent's functioning, either adding to or subtracting from the risk (Figure 16.1). Such interactions may be circular rather than simply linear. There is also a variation in effect, according to the development level of the child, the family's stage in the life cycle and the particular resilience and vulnerability factors operating in an individual situation.

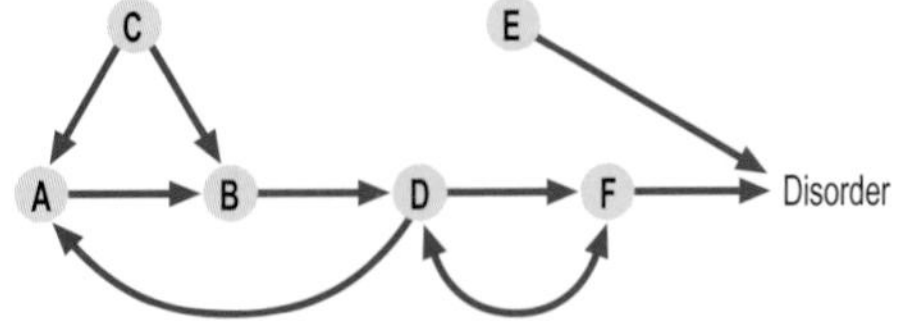

Figure 16.1 • Interactive multifactorial aetiology.
• A,B,C etc. are aetiological factors.

Aetiological factors according to biopsychosocial level are summarized in Figure 16.2.

Level of individual self-esteem is an issue that can influence the persistence or otherwise of behavioural disturbance. A child with low self-esteem will take longer to respond to positive reinforcement of wanted behaviour, and may feel more comfortable with failure and a reputation as rather bad, to the extent of sabotaging success. (This latter point is often difficult for parents to understand, and may be seen as 'ungrateful'.) Low self-esteem develops where there is repeated criticism or failure without balancing praise and/or success.

'Attachment' is an important concept in psychiatry as it encompasses both early social relationships and subsequent patterns of interaction with others. It must be emphasized that attachment is a *relationship variable*, not a personal characteristic. Quality of attachment to one carer does not predict type of attachment to another. The cardinal features of attachment are shown in Figure 16.3. The quality of attachments has been explored, most notably by Ainsworth, who devised an experimental procedure (the strange situation procedure) in which a child goes through a series of short separations and reunions with both carer and a stranger in an unfamiliar room. Responses were classified to produce three 'types' of attachment (Table 16.5).

Other researchers have questioned the utility and predictive validity of this descriptive schema, but follow-up studies have shown that those infants designated as 'securely' attached later show greater social competence and better peer relationships. Conversely, children reared in institutional environments who have had a lack of consistency of carers, and where emotional links may not have been encouraged, showed increased levels of emotional and behavioural disorder throughout childhood and into adulthood – in particular showing disturbed relationships. Parenting ability of adults who as children were designated as 'insecurely attached' was mitigated where there was a supportive spouse. In clinical practice, assortative mating (where people choose partners with similar backgrounds) may lessen the

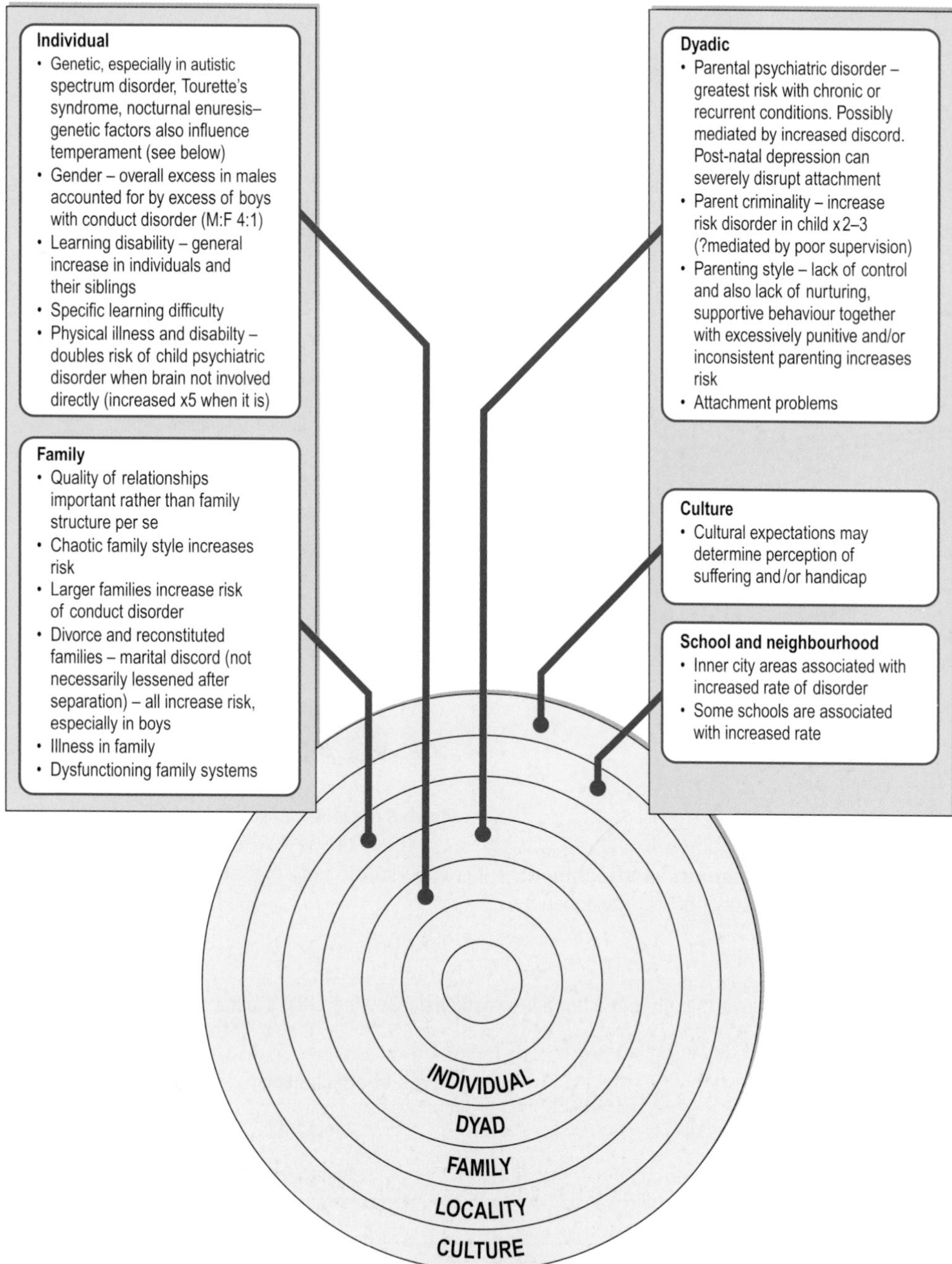

Figure 16.2 • Aetiological factors for child psychiatric disorders.

likelihood of this situation occurring. Similarly, clinical observation of families in whom there is inconsistency and neglect of parenting shows clinginess, overfriendliness and inappropriate attention-seeking in the children. Adoption studies confirm the strong influence of environment in determining levels of difficult behaviour in children.

Brief separations of children from their carers in families with healthy relationships and functioning show little persisting disturbance in the children. However, where family relationships are dysfunctional (see below) child psychiatric disorder can arise subsequently. If the change is to another family where parenting is more appropriate to the

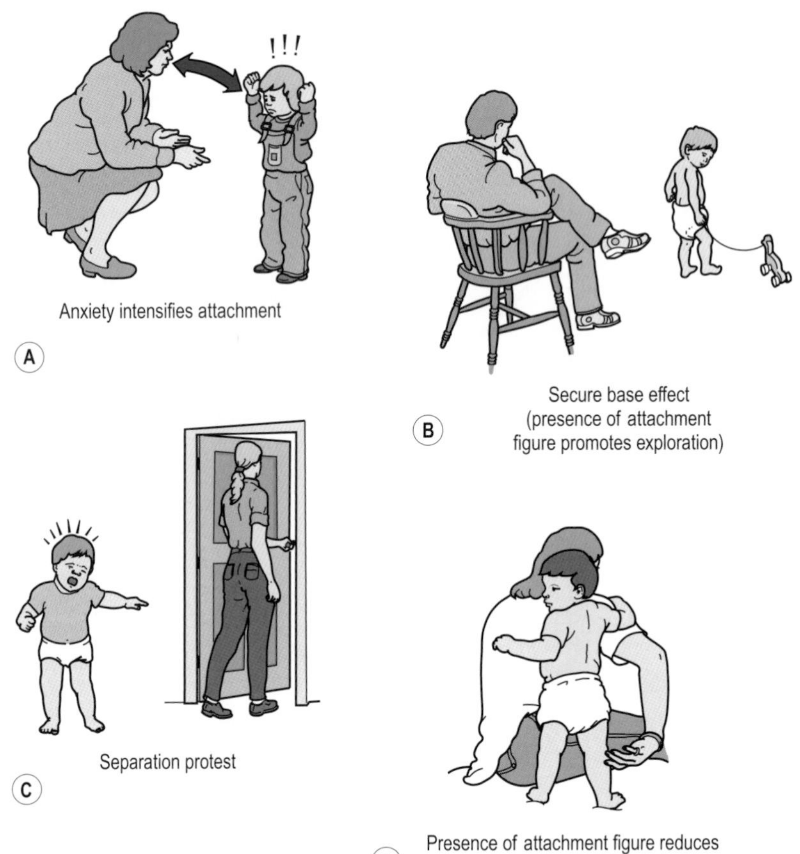

Figure 16.3 • The cardinal features of attachment. • It is important to note that attachment occurs in *dyadic* relationship and is only one aspect of that relationship.

Table 16.5 Attachment: Ainsworth's strange situation procedure (showing child's behaviour seen in different situations)

	Type of attachment		
Situation	Normal	Avoidant	Anxious
With parent	Exploratory	Aggressive	Clingy
When separated	Upset	Undisturbed	Upset
When rejoined	Comforted easily, greets actively	Avoids, ignores	Angry, clingy

child's need, then the child is likely to do well, despite the separation. Response to separation for hospital admission is complicated by the anxieties associated by a family with such an admission (and hence the reasons for admission). Generally, though, single short admissions have little lasting effect, whereas repeated admission does increase the risk for psychiatric disorder (although again this is confounded with the reason for such multiple admission).

Research confirms an increase in emotional and conduct disorders after divorce (particularly in boys), which usually resolves within two years, especially if discord between the parents has subsided and the quality of relationship of the child with individual parents is adequate. The structure of families is much less important than the quality of the relationships between parents and children.

All behaviour arises in the context of relationships. Taking a family perspective raises interactional issues that may be aetiologically important in a given case. Minuchin and others have described particular features of families with a child with a 'psychosomatic' complaint (enmeshment, rigidity, inappropriate parent–child alliances). Most papers have been descriptive of the therapeutic approaches of a particular 'school of family therapy', although there is considerable overlap between these. A linear view of causality is generally not helpful in considering families and the wider system: a circular model is preferable. Changes in one part of the system will require other parts to adjust to take account of this, or alternatively act in such a way to maintain the status quo. An example would be where a particular child is taking all its parent's attention by naughty behaviour: this relieves the pressure on the siblings, who may act to 'wind up' the identified child if their naughtiness then appears to be reduced. There are many similar features of family systems that may trigger, maintain or predetermine a presenting complex of symptoms. Table 16.6 summarizes the areas that must be considered, though research is difficult and scanty in determining the relative importance of these different variables.

Children in local authority care are at increased risk of suffering a psychiatric disorder. This factor is confounded with the reasons for the child being looked after.

Some characteristics of schools, regardless of catchment area, influence the level of child psychiatric disorder (Table 16.7). Epidemiological studies have further emphasized that there is a discontinuity between a child's presentation in school and at home. Children spend a large part of their formative years in school. Poor relationships between home and school can be significant in maintaining an undesirable symptom complex.

Culture may determine whether a behaviour is seen as handicapping, and also has some bearing on parenting style (e.g. the amount of physical chastisement that is socially permissible varies considerably). Cross-cultural studies have shown variations in level of conduct disorder and in sleep disorder, but these studies have also included some socioeconomic confounding factors.

Table 16.6 Elements of family functioning

Interactional patterns	Who is in the family?
	Biological and marital relationships
	Communication patterns
	Hierarchical structure
	Pattern of alliances
	Clarity or otherwise of intergenerational boundary
	Control or authority systems
	Relationship with the outside world
Sociocultural context	Economic status
	Social mobility
	Migration status
Location of the family on the life cycle	Number of transitions
	Requirements for adaptation
Intergenerational structure	Experiences of parents as children
	Influences of grandparents and extended family
Significance of symptom for the family	Symbolic meaning?
	Implications?
	Factors rewarding or inhibiting symptom
Family problem-solving skills	Family style
	Previous experience

(Derived from Dare C 1985 Family therapy. In: Rutter M, Hersov L (eds) Child and adolescent psychiatry: modern approaches. Blackwell Scientific, Oxford.)

Management

Assessment

As will be apparent from the above, a full assessment is a complex procedure, starting from the moment of consideration of the referral. The initiator of the referral is rarely the child and may often not even be the family (or alternatively may be one parent, but not the other). Other agencies that impinge on

Table 16.7 Features of a school associated with a lower level of child psychiatric disorder (independent of catchment population)

- Reasonable balance between intellectually able and less able
- Ample use of rewards and praise by teachers
- Pleasant, comfortable and attractive school
- Children involved in running of the school (children given responsibility, e.g. prefect system)
- Appropriate emphasis on academic matters
- Good modelling by teachers
- Appropriate group management skills in classroom
- Firm leadership involving all staff
- Cohesion provided by mutual support

children include: education; other parts of the health service (e.g. paediatric medicine); social services; the courts; solicitors; the probation service; and so on. Determining whose idea it was to refer a child to a psychiatry service is an important first step, and will influence the approach taken.

Studies of referred populations of children show that child psychiatric disorder is not necessarily a prerequisite for a referral: the child's symptomatology may reflect disorder elsewhere in their environment, with the child reacting normally to this. Paradoxically, nor is child psychiatric disorder a sufficient reason for referral: most children with such disorders are not seen by psychiatrists or psychiatric services. The question 'Why now?' or perhaps 'What led to you being referred to us?' usually reveals some additional stimulus, such as school complaints on a background of conduct problems, police involvement or, in the case of divorce, disputes between parents over finances. More simply, a parent may feel at the end of their tether (although additional pressures often contribute to this too).

The next question is, 'who to invite to the assessment?' Some idea of the child's family context is essential, so the family is usually requested to attend. Some child psychiatric teams request prior knowledge of family compositions so as to avoid misunderstanding or extra alienation by making assumptions. It may also be important to see other, non-related, members of the household or members of other agencies working with a family.

At the first assessment appointment a considerable amount of information is required to obtain a sufficiently wide view of the presenting problem (Table 16.8). Studies suggest that an active probing style produces more detailed information than does a 'free-form' dialogue, but it is important to start with open questioning before proceeding to more specific queries.

A standard child psychiatric assessment comprises

- *introductory phase* – in which the structure, purpose and length of the interview are explained to the family, any queries are clarified and apprehensions addressed
- *a whole-family interview* – in which individual members' views of the referral are explored and family interaction is encouraged and noted
- *interview with the parents or carers* – allowing 'adult' issues to be considered and any extra information that may not be known to the children (e.g. about prior marriages, parental childhood trauma or abortions) to be aired

Table 16.8 Information to be amassed in a child psychiatric interview

Source and nature of referral

- Who made referral?
- Who initiated referral?
- Family attitudes to referral

Description of presenting complaints

- Onset, frequency, intensity, duration, location (home, school, etc.)
- Antecedents and consequences
- Ameliorating and exacerbating factors
- Specific examples
- Parental and family beliefs about causation
- Past attempts to solve problem

Continued

Table 16.8 Information to be amassed in a child psychiatric interview—cont'd

Description of child's current general functioning
• School: — behaviour and emotions — academic performance — peer and staff relationships • Peer relationships generally • Family relationships
Personal/developmental history
• Pregnancy, labour, delivery • Early developmental milestones • Separations/disruptions • Physical illnesses and their meaning for parents • Reactions to school • Puberty • Temperamental style
Family history
• Personal and social histories of both parents especially: — history of mental illness — their experience of being parented • History of family development: — how parents came together — history of pregnancies — separations and effects on children • Who lives at home currently • Strengths/weaknesses of all at home • Current social stresses and supports
Information from observation of family interaction
Structure, organization, communication, sensitivity
Information from observation of child at interview
Motor, sensory, speech, language, social relating skills
Mental state, concerns, and spontaneous account if age appropriate
Results of physical examination
Plan for future investigation and management

(Reproduced with permission from Eminson M 1993 In: Black D, Cottrell D (eds) Seminars in child and adolescent psychiatry. Gaskell, London.)

- *an interview with the 'identified child'* – this may not strictly be an interview, depending on the age of the child, but may include free play and/or drawing as aides to communication and anxiety reduction
- *possibly interviews with siblings or others attending* (e.g. grandparents, social workers).

With adolescents it is developmentally appropriate to take account of their need to individuate (and possibly to model this to the family!) and spend rather longer seeing them on their own. With younger children a greater proportion of time is spent with the whole family. It is not essential to see very young children (under three years) on their own, although this needs to be judged with reference to their parents. It is not justified to insist on separation where this causes significant distress in the child, although behaviour on separation and reunion is important to note as an indicator of attachment.

Assessment of a child's mental state must also include some view of developmental level, both global and specific. This will both inform the approach taken to the child and the significance given to particular psychological phenomena and behaviours (e.g. 'obsessional' rituals are common in middle childhood and usually resolve spontaneously).

The child's individual interview is a forum for the child to discuss confidentially views of themselves and the family. In addition, the assessor is better able to gauge the child's degree of suffering from symptoms, and the degree to which this poses a handicap. In some cases the child may disclose abuse. The question of confidentiality is one that may vex parents or carers, but it is usually sufficient to explain that the child is unlikely to feel confident enough to disclose issues he or she feels uncomfortable about discussing with the parents if such matters are subsequently passed on by the interviewer. Where there is a clash between the interests of the child and those of the adults involved, the child's needs are paramount. In the case of disclosure of abuse, local child protection procedures must be followed. It is essential not to guarantee confidentiality to parents or child, but to be open and clear about the occasions when this will not apply.

Beyond the initial assessment (which may take more than one session), the child's wider environment requires exploration. Usually the minimum requirement is for contact with the school, by standard questionnaire, telephone or face-to-face discussion. Other professionals in the system may also be contacted. Such wider discussions require the consent of both the child's carers and (depending on age) the child, although again, exceptions occur when the child is perceived to be at risk of significant harm.

A further consideration in the initial assessment is that the therapeutic process should already be under way, with modelling of age-appropriate interactions and ventilation of feelings and views, both individually and in the family context. In some cases the assessment interview may be the only chance to make a therapeutic impact (or may be all that is required).

Physical examination

Although, ideally, this should always take place, the degree to which it is appropriate will vary considerably from case to case, in some situations jeopardizing the rapport built up with a child and in others (e.g. anorexia nervosa) being essential. The timing of an examination and the personnel involved can be arranged so that any concerns about the effect on relationships, etc. can be minimized.

Psychometric testing

This can be helpful in quantifying any specific or general cognitive difficulties indicated from less formal assessment. An experienced psychologist will put the results of testing in an appropriate context. In some instances they will already be available from a formal educational assessment. It is important for the medical practitioner to be familiar with the limitations of psychometric testing in predicting performance and outcome.

Laboratory tests

Physical tests (biochemistry, chromosomal testing, electroencephalogram, diagnostic imaging, etc.) should be arranged if there are indications from the history and examinations, as in any other medical context.

Course and prognosis

Most child psychiatric disorder *does not* progress to adult psychiatric disorder. Conversely, however, a significant proportion of adult psychiatric disorder is preceded by childhood problems. This varies from condition to condition. Schizophrenia in adulthood may be preceded by non-specific atypical behaviour in childhood (there is no significant association with any particular behaviour pattern, including that of schizoid-type behaviour). Childhood parental loss has been associated with later depression. Depression in childhood shows a later association with adult depressive disorder. In only some cases do childhood anxiety disorders lead on to later neurosis. There is a strong continuity for obsessive–compulsive disorder between childhood and adulthood. Conduct disorder in the early years is associated with later adverse functioning.

Management

Interventions in specific disorders are covered below. In general it is important to note that appropriate and effective input may include consultation and/or training with other professionals or agencies with or without direct contact with the family.

Child psychiatric disorder

- Child psychiatric disorder is a quantitative deviance from the norm, with suffering and/or handicap.
- Child and adolescent psychiatric disorder occurs in 5–20% of the child population, being higher in urban than rural areas (2×) and varying according to the severity of the disorder.
- There are discontinuities in presentation in different settings.
- Multifactorial aetiology is the rule.
- Child psychiatric disorder must be assessed in the context of the child's family systems, the wider environment impinging on the child and the child's developmental level.
- Most child psychiatric disorder does not progress to adult mental illness, but there is a higher than expected history of childhood problems in adult psychiatric patients.
- Treatment approaches will be chosen according to hypothesized aetiology, parental and child preference, and practical issues such as availability and ease of access.

Specific conditions

'Adult' diagnoses in childhood

As noted above, if a diagnosis other than F90–98 can be made, then it should be. The reader is referred to the other chapters of this book for details of these. Below are points of difference that occur in childhood and adolescence.

Psychotic disorders

The difficulty in distinguishing affective psychosis from other psychotic disturbance (in particular schizophrenia) is even more marked in adolescence, and there is a notable mutability from one set of symptoms to another. It is therefore difficult to predict course and outcome from initial psychotic episodes. Early psychotic symptomatology can occur for long periods (up to several years) before diagnosis or indeed any contact with specialist services. Research in adults has suggested that the longer the symptoms have persisted before diagnosis of psychosis, the poorer the prognosis, especially for the development of 'negative' symptoms (see Chapter 8).

Psychosis as understood in adulthood is rare in children before puberty. ICD-10 refers to the group of childhood disorders that were formerly known, confusingly, as 'childhood psychoses' (autism, Asperger's syndrome, etc.) as *pervasive developmental disorders* (F84). This is to distinguish these qualitatively different conditions from adult psychosis, as there is no evidence of continuity between them.

Mood disorders

Mania is generally thought to be rare before puberty. However the diagnosis, together with adult style pharmacological management has become more common in North America. Depressive disorder is not rare. Its point prevalence in prepubertal children is estimated to be 1–2%, and in adolescents it is 3–8%. A depressed mood state is common and occurs in approximately 20% of 14-year-olds at any one time. A cross-sectional view (e.g. a single interview) will often mistake a depressive *state* for a disorder in adolescence. A longitudinal perspective is therefore essential. Suicidal ideation must be sought in a single interview; however, as the risk of a suicide *attempt* while in a depressed mood is high in this age group (although not in the younger child). It must be noted that an individual interview with the child or young person is essential, as it has been shown convincingly that even adults close to them will significantly underestimate the presence of low mood or misery.

Depressive *disorder* is distinguished by the sustained, pervasive nature of the lowered mood state, with prolongation well beyond the apparent provocation. There is significant anhedonia (loss of pleasure) in all areas of functioning, and there may be increased irritability. Deterioration in school performance and withdrawal from social activities is often seen. Sleep disruption may occur, but it is more usually a difficulty in settling than the adult pattern of early morning wakening.

Investigation should include tests for glandular fever and other chronically debilitating conditions.

Treatment may include the variety of measures described in Chapter 9, depending on presentation. CBT is helpful in mild to moderate depression in adolescence. The risk–benefit ratio does *not* support the use of SSRIs, or mirtazapine or venlafaxine in individuals under the age of 18 years. The 58th edition of the BNF warns: 'The use of antidepressant has been linked with suicidal thoughts and behaviour; children, young adults, and patients with a history of suicidal behaviour are particularly at risk.

Where necessary, patients should be monitored for suicidal behaviour, self-harm, or hostility, particularly at the beginning of treatment of if the dose is changed.'

Personality disorder

Personality disorder (see Chapter 15) is rarely diagnosed in childhood. This is because

- during development the personality is still amenable to change
- labelling a child can be a self-perpetuating exercise, which removes hope from all concerned
- most children with the symptom complexes that are retrospectively associated with personality disorder do not go on to develop such a disorder. As Wolff has written for dissocial personality disorder and conduct disorder, 'The association between childhood symptoms and adult personality . . . is strong looking backwards but not looking forwards.'

Stability of personality characteristics in childhood has been described in Chapter 2 under the label of 'temperament'. Constitutional shyness has been shown to be a particularly stable characteristic at the extreme end of the spectrum and has been associated with anxious (avoidant) personality disorder in adulthood (F60.6). Activity level is also a stable personality characteristic. The continuity here is with dissocial personality disorder, but only where there is associated conduct disorder in childhood, especially where this includes aggressiveness.

Schizoid or schizotypal personality disorder of childhood (Asperger's syndrome) comprises a set of personality traits of social aloofness and stereotyped interests without the cognitive or language delay of autism. This is one circumstance where a diagnosis of personality disorder may be justified so that appropriate management and educational provision may be made. Having noted this, in ICD-10 the guidance against making a personality disorder diagnosis excludes Asperger's by classifying it as 'pervasive developmental disorder.'

Delirium, dementia and other organic disorders

Delirium occurs in childhood as it does in adulthood and requires the same precautions and treatment of the underlying cause. There are also a number of deteriorating conditions of childhood that include a dementing process. For details of these, the reader is referred to a paediatrics textbook.

Hyperkinetic disorders (ADHD)

Diagnosis

The cardinal features of hyperkinetic disorder are *impaired attention*, *impulsivity* and *overactivity*, which occur in more than one environment (i.e. not just at home or at school), are of early onset (under six years of age) and of long duration. Associated features that are not necessary for the diagnosis include social disinhibition, recklessness and impulsive flouting of social rules (butting in, poor turn-taking). There is an increased incidence of learning difficulties and clumsiness, but these should be coded separately.

There is some controversy regarding the subdivision of hyperkinetic disorders, but the main prognostic factor is the presence or absence of associated dissocial behaviour (see above). Differential diagnosis is from pervasive development disorders, conduct disorder and anxiety disorder.

The equivalent DSM-IV-TR diagnosis is 'attention-deficit hyperactivity disorder' (ADHD). This is generally regarded as a somewhat wider category than hyperkinetic disorder (HD) as it also includes those children who have attention problems but no overactivity. The 'combined type' of ADHD is probably equivalent to HD.

Epidemiology

A number of studies indicate that the point prevalence of ADHD in primary school age children is around 5% (and around 1.5% for HD). The condition is much more frequent in boys, declines with age and increases with social adversity.

Clinical features

Impaired attention means premature breaking off of one activity to 'flit' to another: research has not shown undue distractibility. *Overactivity* is a high level of restlessness (wriggling and fidgeting in particular) with extreme difficulty in sitting in one place. This is made worse or is more apparent in structured situations such as the classroom. It is important to make sure that the low attention span and level of activity are exceptional for the situation and for the child's age and developmental level.

Aetiology

Hyperkinetic disorders are thought to have a constitutional or genetic basis, with a significant contribution from brain abnormality, as evidenced by the increased frequency in children with such abnormalities; however, no specific defects have been found. More detailed brain imaging techniques may help with this in the future. At present, although there is disagreement, HD is regarded as one extreme of a continuum rather than a discrete entity.

Diet and food allergy have been suggested as causes of overactivity. A diet high in caffeine-containing drinks (such as cola) and artificial colourings may increase activity and irritability.

Management

It is important in a full assessment to evaluate the extent of the attention deficit and increased activity in as many different settings as possible, with some estimate of variation over time. Observation in one setting has poor predictive value. Other coexisting disorders should be identified (e.g. conduct disorder or depression).

Once the diagnosis has been established and discussed with the family, psychometric assessment may be helpful in determining whether there are specific deficits or global delay that will affect the response to any management strategy. General advice and support is very important.

Behavioural management approaches of different kinds have been advocated as effective in these disorders, but depend on relevant individual and family dynamics (including the level of self-esteem) being taken into account, as these may seriously help or hinder any approach taken.

Drug treatment with stimulant medication (methylphenidate, dexamfetamine) has been found to be very effective in reducing restlessness and increasing on-task activity. Side-effects can include reduced growth, insomnia and loss of weight. The non-stimulant atomoxetine is an alternative (see Chapter 3). Other drugs, such as the tricyclic antidepressants and haloperidol, have been shown to reduce excess activity but these and phenothiazine tranquillizers should definitely be regarded as second-line drugs reserved for the more refractory cases and prescribed only in specialist centres.

Liaison with other agencies, especially education, is extremely important. Advice regarding management, particularly for more individual and small group teaching, can be direct or via agency support services, depending on local arrangements.

Prognosis

Outcome is largely determined by the presence or absence of other concurrent disorders, such as conduct disorder. Restlessness and reduced attention span do, on average, improve with development, but the poor self-esteem secondary to repeated failures and disturbed family relationships, especially if there is associated conduct disorder, remain to give a potential adverse effect on personality development. This emphasizes the need to address all these issues in management, rather than simply the hyperkinetic symptoms.

Some individuals continue with symptomatology into adulthood. The degree of handicap or associated disruption is less because of the possibility of finding a niche that fits, and the greater likelihood of individual or small group training.

Conduct disorders (F91)

Diagnosis

Conduct disorders consist of a repeated and persistent pattern of dissocial, aggressive or defiant behaviour that exceeds the normal expectations for the child's age. It does not include toddler tantrums or isolated episodes of dissocial behaviour. Examples of behaviours that come under this category are listed in Figure 16.4. For diagnosis the duration of the disorder should have exceeded six months.

Overlap with hyperkinetic disorders and emotional disorders occurs. In the former, hyperkinetic disorder should be diagnosed instead, and, in the latter, a mixed disorder should be diagnosed (F92).

A diagnosis of conduct disorder confined to the family context (F91.0) requires that there should be no behavioural disturbance outside the home, and that the home-based behaviour should be seriously dissocial or aggressive. Although there may be disruption of the parent–child relationship, this in itself is not sufficient grounds for the diagnosis.

F91.1 and F91.2 distinguish between *unsocialized* and *socialized* conduct disorder. In the former, there is poor, if any, integration into the child's peer group, and misbehaviour is generally solitary. Socialized conduct disorder is diagnosed when there are sustained relationships between the child and others of that age group who may or may not also be involved in dissocial activity.

Oppositional defiant disorder is distinguished from other subcategories of conduct disorder by the absence of behaviour that violates the law or the rights of others. Typically, this is a diagnosis of middle childhood and may lead on to the other diagnoses above in adolescence.

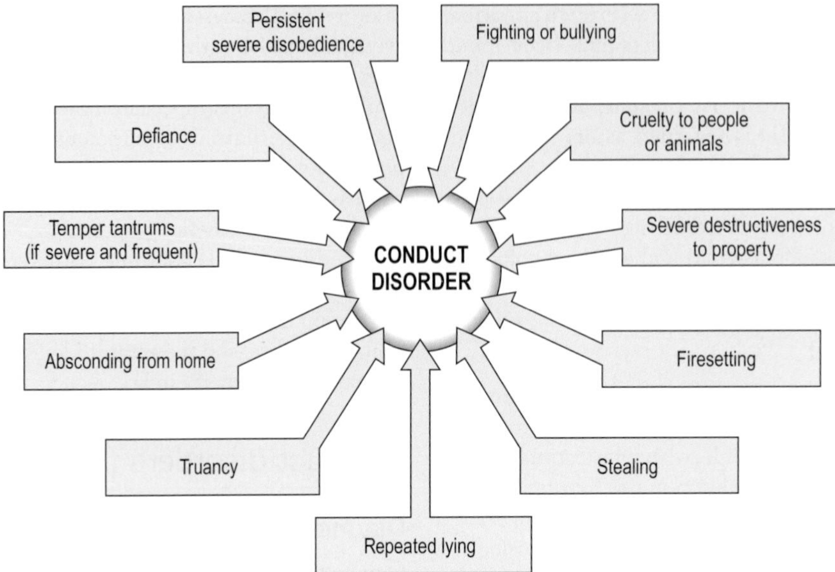

Figure 16.4 • Behaviour that may be part of a conduct disorder.

Delinquency is a sociolegal label and not a psychiatric category, and requires that a person be above the age of 'criminal responsibility' (10 years in the UK) and have committed a crime.

Epidemiology

In the Goodman *et al.* UK study, conduct disorder was identified in 4.6% of children aged five to 10 and 6.2% aged 11–15 years. The rates in inner city areas are significantly higher. Boys show higher rates than girls. Younger children tend to show aggressive rather than antisocial symptoms.

It has been estimated that 22% of the male population will obtain a criminal conviction before the age of 21, and those convicted are more likely to have further convictions. The equivalent figure for females is 4.7%. Self-report studies show that breaking the law in adolescence and young adulthood is the norm, although persistent repetitive delinquency is not, and is usually associated with conviction.

Clinical features and aetiology

Antisocial behaviour may take different forms with increasing age and sophistication. Temper tantrums (or outbursts, as they tend to be known in older children), for example, may be a typical complaint in early or middle childhood, whereas oppositional defiant behaviour becomes more evident in older children, and wider ranges of inappropriate activity are seen in adolescence. Cognitive deficits may modify this. Parents also vary in their tolerance and consistency of management. Both extremely punitive and extremely lenient responses (or varying mixes of both) to misdemeanours may be seen.

Although similar behaviours may be seen in different contexts, the degree to which they are complained of may be totally at odds, because of the different expectations. The psychiatry service may inadvertently be drawn into disagreements between school and home in such situations. Attempts at making a judgement between the two settings should be avoided, and mediation skills employed.

Parents may often describe behavioural problems as 'attention-seeking' and withdraw attention, so that behaviours escalate until attention is unavoidable. In such circumstances, if prolonged, the child's self-esteem suffers, they may identify themselves as 'the naughty one' and then act accordingly, as this is familiar to them: they have a role.

In divorce, children may pick up on and 'play out' continuing tensions between their parents. Contact with the non-custodial parent can be a time of particular stress associated with increased behaviour problems. If parents incorporate this into a dispute between them, the behaviours may worsen and not resolve until the parents sort out their differences. The child psychiatrist, again, must be sensitive to the dangers of becoming allied with one or other adult party and concentrate on the needs of the child.

The child's own concern about such behaviour is not easily or accurately elicited in the family context, as this can be strongly influenced by the expectations of the rest of the family. Frequently, no response is produced: this is not too surprising, as remorse may be followed by 'Well why do you continue doing it then?' and defiance by 'There, you see what he's like!'. Such negative responses only confirm the child's view of him or herself.

Aetiology

Aetiological factors of conduct disorder are summarized in Figure 16.5.

Management

As usual, a thorough assessment is required, addressing all areas of a child's functioning and placing these in the family, social and cultural context.

In some families advice regarding parenting approach will be sufficient, or even simply providing a forum in which to discuss such issues, either as parents, in the family or in groups of parents. An educational approach discussing behavioural management, with plenty of opportunity for discussion has been used successfully. To see that different children respond differently to different parenting styles may be instructive. Parents' own confidence in their ability may have taken something of a battering by the time they reach the child psychiatry service, and so efforts to reverse this are important. Frequently, however, parents will have had a surfeit of advice and will report that 'nothing works'. Careful exploration of the approaches tried will often reveal that many have been abandoned without a reasonable trial.

Behavioural management techniques can be helpful, but need close supervision. They can be enhanced by group work with parents. Careful scrutiny of a child's areas of success is required, for which positive attention can be given. Record keeping by parents is important as, for example, ten tantrums a day may

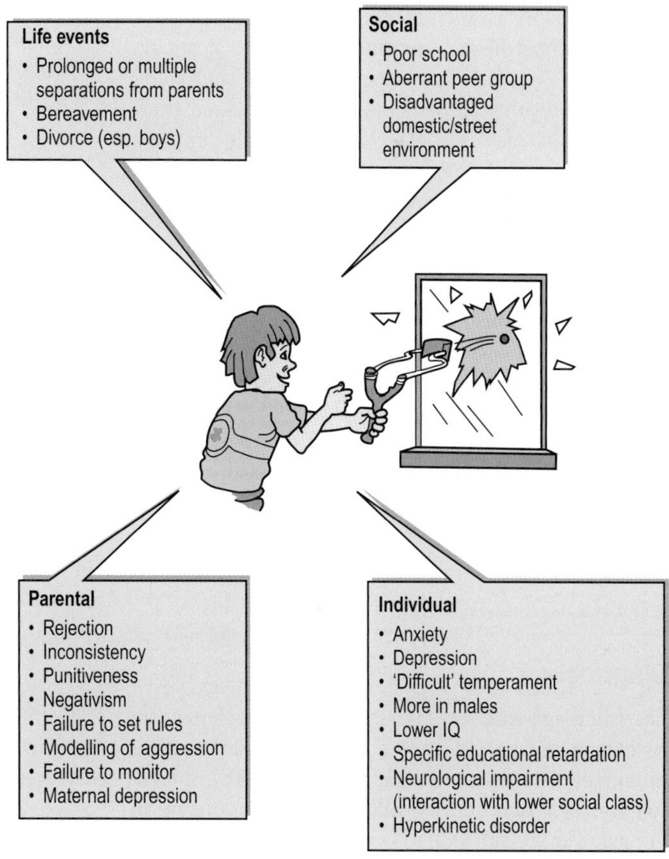

Figure 16.5 • Aetiological factors in conduct disorder.

not feel very different from 15 to a harassed carer, although it is a significant reduction in frequency.

Cognitive therapy may be useful in older children, particularly in anger management, but only if they are motivated to change.

Where there is evidence of interactional variables within the family triggering or perpetuating unwanted behaviours, then *family therapy* may be indicated.

Groups for children, which focus on methods to build up self-esteem and self-confidence, can be helpful in supporting the above measures. Conduct can be improved by giving a child or young person the opportunity to talk through worries (e.g. about divorce or bereavement) in a group or individual setting.

Work with the wider *system* is essential where the conduct disorder extends outside the family. This includes school and court work.

In adolescence, conduct disorder may become part of a habitual way of behaving, later to be termed a personality disorder. The psychiatrist needs to be sensitive to the danger of perpetuating poor behaviour by offering therapy to teenagers, who may paradoxically take this as a signal that they are 'mental' and thus do not need to take responsibility for their actions. However much it is pointed out that there is no mental disorder, the action of referral to a psychiatric service is a much stronger message. If such individuals are motivated to change their behaviour, then work on this may be better carried out in another setting (e.g. probation, juvenile justice service).

Course and prognosis

Robins' classic follow-up studies of children with antisocial behaviour showed that although preschool aggressive behaviour was not associated with later sociopathy, such behaviour in middle childhood was, particularly if accompanied by poor academic attainment. Fifty per cent of highly antisocial children are antisocial as adults; 60% of adult sociopaths have a childhood history of highly antisocial behaviour, with a further 30% displaying moderately antisocial behaviour as children.

Emotional disorder (F93)

Diagnosis

The full diagnostic label is 'Emotional disorders with onset specific to childhood'. This is to distinguish them from the 'Neurotic disorders' (F40–48), which can also be diagnosed in childhood and should be if the criteria are fulfilled. The emotional disorders:

- mostly do not develop into neuroses or other mental disorders in adulthood
- are exaggerations of normal developmental trends
- may result from different mechanisms from neuroses
- are relatively less clearly demarcated than the F40–48 diagnoses.

In *separation anxiety disorder of childhood* (F93.0), anxiety occurs in response to real or imagined separation from attachment figures. This label does not include symptoms that arise *de novo* in adolescence. Many examples of school refusal occur under this category, but only when there are no particular concerns or upset regarding school. (It must be noted that school non-attendance alone is a sociolegal, not a psychiatric issue. It is only where there is a demonstrable mental disorder that the child mental health team needs to be involved.)

Phobic anxiety disorder of childhood (F93.1) is distinguished from 'adult' phobias by its development at the appropriate time (e.g. fear of dogs in two to four-year-olds) but accompanied by a greater than usual level of anxiety. Similarly, *social anxiety disorder of childhood* (F93.2) is that which occurs before the age of six (i.e. the time of normal fear of strangers) and is of an excessive degree. In *sibling rivalry disorder* (F93.3), the negative behaviour towards the sibling should date from its birth.

Clinical features

The features of 'emotional disturbance' that occur in emotional disorders may range from apathy and withdrawal to tantrums, including anxiety symptoms, misery, sleep disturbance and general worrying. How this is classified depends on the circumstances in which these upsets occur, as described above.

Epidemiology

The level of emotional disorder in children has been found to be 2.5%, with increases in large towns and cities, and in adolescence. There is an approximately 1:1 male:female ratio before adolescence, with a shift to a female preponderance (as with the neurotic disorders) in the teenage years.

Management

For most of the emotional disorders, *behavioural management techniques* based on behavioural principles, but embedded in an approach of *support* and *empathy* for the child and family, are the approaches of choice. No parent or carer likes to see a child upset, and may therefore have shied away from taking a firm, kind approach to the anxiety- or upset-provoking situation. To insist on a 'flooding' approach straight away (i.e. rapid introduction of upsetting stimulus) may work quickly (see sleep disorders). It is also a high-risk strategy, which may fail because the parent or carer cannot sustain it for long enough to be effective, or the child may 'shut off', run away or psychologically dissociate, which does not allow him/her to learn. Parent and child alike may prefer a more gradual approach. The different 'talking therapies' may form a part of a treatment programme, to allow anxiety reduction by ventilation of upsetting stimuli. The different talking therapies may form a part of the treatment programme. Reduction of anxiety by ventilation of upsetting stimuli may be helpful in these approaches but this must be carefully monitored and adjusted to be age-appropriate.

In the case of sibling rivalry disorder, measures such as making a special time for the affected child, and involving the child in a positive way in care for their sibling, can be helpful. Where there are fundamental relationship difficulties between the affected child and the carer, however, such simple measures are unlikely to work without considerable extra support and input, for example in a *parent and child group*.

Prognosis

Most emotional disorders of childhood do not proceed to adult disorders. If there is a subsequent disorder it is almost invariably one of the neuroses. However, the symptom pattern may well have varied over time. Most childhood emotional disorders improve or disappear over time (only about one-third still have a disorder five years after diagnosis).

Disorders of social functioning (F94)

This section describes three patterns of social functioning, which differ from the norm. This group of categories is distinguished from the pervasive development disorders (F84) by the capacity to function socially at other times, and in other situations.

Selective mutism (previously known as elective mutism) is a resistant and powerful symptom in which a child does not speak in selected situations (often school), but converses normally in other places or at other times. A consistency and persistence about where and when the child will not speak is required for this diagnosis. Although socially normal speech is present, in a substantial minority there are or have been speech difficulties in articulation or speech production (comprehension must be normal).

Reactive attachment disorder of childhood (F94.1) and *disinhibited attachment disorder of childhood* (F94.2) are patterns of functioning familiar to child protection agencies because of their association with abuse and neglect. Evidence of such is not sufficient or necessary for these diagnoses. Some children do not show these patterns of functioning despite extreme abuse. The clinical features of these disorders are shown in Figure 16.6.

Epidemiology

Selective mutism occurs in six to eight cases per 1000 children. It is more common in girls (55–65% of cases; as high as 75% in community studies). The attachment disorders are more common and are particularly seen in the field of child protection investigation. Children who respond quickly to normal environmental stimulation will not come to psychiatric notice unless expert evidence is required for court proceedings. Reliable figures for frequency are difficult to find, partly because of controversy about the limits of the diagnostic labels.

Figure 16.6 • Clinical features of attachment disorders of childhood.

Reactive attachment disorder
- 'Frozen watchfulness'
- Fearfulness
- Hypervigilance
- Lack of response to comforting
- 'Radar gaze'
- Misery
- Withdrawal
- Aggressive responses to own or others' distress
- Failure to thrive
- Possibly signs of physical abuse
- Improves with 'normal' parenting

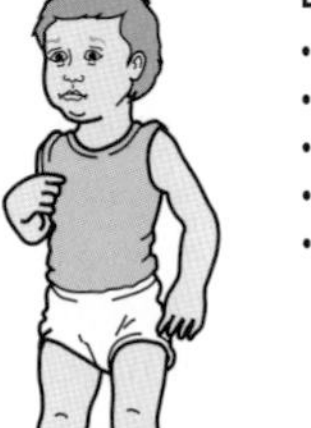

Disinhibited attachment disorder
- Clinginess
- Attachment diffuse
- 'Attention seeking'
- Indiscriminate friendliness
- Poor modulation of peer interactions

Starts under age 5

Aetiology

Selective mutism is associated with a sulky or difficult personality in the child and an increased frequency of aggressive behaviour in both the child and the carer. Higher levels of psychiatric disorder in parents than in the general population have been reported. The intelligence of the child is usually in the normal range. It is likely that, having once discovered the powerful effect of mutism, the child continues and then finds it difficult to 'get out of'. These observations dictate the approach to management.

The aetiology of attachment disorders includes any factor that can interfere with the relationship between the child and the carer. Inconsistency of response, either from an individual carer or because of frequent changes of carer (e.g. in a succession of institutional care placements) is particularly likely to result in the disinhibited attachment disorder of childhood. As this is by no means inevitable, research continues into the features that predict resilience in children. Studies so far find high intelligence to be a protective factor.

Child factors such as difficult temperament, perinatal complications and disabilities can all interfere with relationship with carers. Physical or mental health problems in parents or guardians can interfere significantly with normal parenting. Parents' own experiences of parenting, if inadequate or inappropriate for whatever reason, may make it difficult to relate adequately to an individual child.

Management

For *selective mutism*, a combination of behavioural approaches to reduce the payback for lack of speech, and 'ways out' of the situation (e.g. using telephone or tape-recorder messages) will be successful in a proportion of children. Others may benefit from non-verbal therapies such as play therapy or art therapy. Attention needs to be paid to whether there are any speech abnormalities. Where there are family interaction issues, these can be addressed using family therapy.

The *attachment disorders* may benefit from work on the relationship between carers and child, with an emphasis on consistency, firmness, kindness and positive interaction. This can occur in family or group settings and may form part of a *family centre* programme, which also works with carers on other coping skills. The child may require individual *psychotherapy* to attain a more normal development trajectory, although this is only likely to be helpful once the environment is appropriate. Sometimes it is apparent that an improvement in relationships is unlikely to occur in time for the child's developmental needs, and alternative family placement is required, arranged either statutorily or voluntarily.

Prognosis

The long-term prognosis for selective mutism is good, although the concurrent presence of other disorders will modify this. It has been found that other behaviour problems may improve with resolution of the selective mutism.

The attachment disorders may interfere with future relationships to an extent that perpetuates the pattern in future generations. Lack of appropriate stimulation and consistency can lead to behavioural abnormalities, which can interact with a low self-esteem in a vulnerable child to produce a spiral of failure that manifests itself in adult psychiatric or personality disorders.

Tic disorders

Diagnosis and clinical features

Tic disorders are complex neurodevelopmental disorders that may be diagnosed in psychiatric, paediatric or neurology clinics. A tic is an involuntary, rapid, recurrent, non-rhythmic motor movement or vocal production that is of sudden onset and serves no specific purpose. It usually disappears during sleep, but it may not. Tics may be voluntarily suppressed, but sufferers (referred to as 'ticqueurs') often report that after a period of suppression the tic frequency increases, as though to compensate for having had to 'miss some'. Tics can also be reproduced voluntarily. Although non-purposive, tics usually involve particular muscle groups, for example those involved in eye blinking, shoulder shrugging, head shaking and facial grimacing. Vocal tics can be grunts, squeaks, barks, sniffs and coughs.

The above are examples of *simple tics*. More complex motor tics include hopping and tapping, and in extreme cases copropraxia (obscene gestures). Complex vocal tics can include the explosive utterances of words. When the words are obscene this is called *coprolalia*. There can be some imitation of gestures (echopraxia) and of words (echolalia).

Tics must be distinguished from the purposive repetitive movements of obsessive–compulsive disorder. Also, the manneristic stereotyped repetitive movements of people with learning disability and/or pervasive developmental disorder must not be confused with tics, which tend to be less rhythmical.

Although ICD-10 separates a number of different tic disorders (see Table 16.1), it is probably more helpful to view them as a continuum. The spectrum is from simple tics, which occur commonly in middle childhood and most of which resolve spontaneously, to the complex *Gilles de la Tourette's syndrome*, which involves complex vocal and motor tics and other associated features.

Epidemiology

Between 10% and 24% of children will manifest tics at some point during development, but the majority are simple and transient. Tourette's syndrome has a lifetime prevalence of 0.01–1.6%, depending on the study. Boys are affected with tic disorders more commonly than girls, although the male:female ratio tends to be <2:1 in most community surveys. In the Isle of Wight study published in 1970, around 6% of boys and 3% of girls were reported as suffering from twitches, mannerisms, or tics of the face or body. The average age of onset is seven years (range two to 15 years). The age of diagnosis of Tourette's syndrome is usually later, probably because it can often start with simple motor tics; 40% of patients with Tourette's also show symptoms of obsessive–compulsive disorder. The prevalence of Tourette's syndrome currently varies between 2.9 and 299 per 10 000.

Aetiology

In common parlance, the word 'tic' is frequently preceded by 'nervous'. Although clearly nerve impulses are involved, and tics are also usually worse with increased arousal and can be associated with emotional disturbance, it is probably incorrect to attribute tics to underlying neurosis.

Environmental pressures can modulate the expression and frequency of tics, in particular parental anxiety or irritation.

Hypothesized aetiological factors are shown in Table 16.9.

Table 16.9 Aetiology of tics

Family	Family clusters reported, especially Tourette's
	Prevalence of multiple tics in 14–24% of first-degree relatives of patients with Tourette's
	Increased family psychopathology in families of ticqueurs, although may be cause or effect
Individual	No gross neurological abnormalities
	Increased incidence of 'soft' neurological signs and 'non-specific' EEG changes
	Some verbal – performance discrepancies in functioning
	Some neuroleptic medications effective in controlling tics
	Tics exacerbated by dopamine agonists
	Wide range of psychological mechanisms proposed for tic disorders, from the psychoanalytic to the classically behavioural
	Tic movements have been shown to mimic involuntary startle responses to sudden stimulus

Management

It is first essential to establish the correct diagnosis from the history. Physical examination and neurological investigations, as noted above, are usually inconclusive. There is currently no diagnostic 'test' that confirms a tic disorder – the diagnosis is a clinical one.

Once this has been done, it is necessary to reassure the patient and family about the nature of the disorder. Contact with the school is essential in order to avoid unnecessary castigation of the child by teachers and peers. A child with a serious tic disorder may need some help in dealing with teasing, in addition to work on self-esteem and clarification of educational needs, possibly by psychometric testing.

Specific psychological treatments have been used with variable success. 'Massed practice', in which the tic is repeated frequently at convenient points in the day, has been helpful in some, but does not usually produce sustained improvements. Similar results have been found for other behavioural techniques. Methods that can produce a change in arousal level, such as relaxation and hypnotherapy, may be more useful.

Pharmacotherapy can be startlingly successful in abolishing or reducing tics. Haloperidol has been the most widely used, although more recently sulpiride and some of the SSRIs such as fluoxetine have been used successfully. The second-generation antipsychotic risperidone has been shown to have superior efficacy to placebo in four trials to date.

Risperidone is much less likely to cause extrapyramidal side-effects than is the first-generation antipsychotic haloperidol. Also, haloperidol is sedative and there is evidence of an association with decreased academic performance in children taking it. Drug withdrawal after a number of months is not necessarily associated with resumption of the tic. Continual revision of drug use is therefore necessary.

Prognosis

The natural history of tic disorders is one of variation in type, intensity and frequency, hence the difficulty in determining true treatment efficacy. The majority of children's tics will be transient, disappearing spontaneously after a few weeks or months. Some, however, will show a downwards progression to involve all the limbs and the trunk, and the addition of vocal tics to produce a picture of Tourette's syndrome. In one-third of cases of Tourette's syndrome, the presenting symptom is of vocal tics (6% coprolalia). Improvement in the majority of cases occurs in adolescence, although the degree is related to the severity of the condition.

Elimination disorders

Non-organic enuresis (F98.0)

Diagnosis and clinical features

Non-organic enuresis is the voiding of urine in inappropriate places, at inappropriate times, at an inappropriate age. It may occur during the day or at night during sleep (nocturnal enuresis). It may be 'primary' (continence never achieved) or 'secondary' (wetting resumed after a period of continence of more than a month). This diagnosis is not used if there is any organic reason, such as neurological or structural abnormality of the urinary system or infection (although infection can occur secondary to continued wetness, especially in girls). In general, enuresis is not diagnosed in children aged less than five years, or where there is evidence of general developmental delay.

Enuresis may or may not be associated with emotional disorder (see below). *Deliberate wetting* (e.g. on the outside of the bedcovers) is usually part of a wider emotional or conduct disorder and should be coded as such. In these cases, however, care should be taken to exclude automatism occurring as part of a sleep or epileptic disorder.

Epidemiology

The prevalence of enuresis at different ages is shown in Figure 16.7. Relapse into wetness occurs most commonly around the ages of five to six and is rare after age 11. The male:female ratio increases from 1:1 at age five to nearly 2:1 in adolescence. Boys are twice as likely to develop secondary enuresis. Combined day and night wetting is associated with a higher level of disturbance.

Aetiology

There are many theories and explanations for enuresis, perhaps suggesting there is no single cause. These are summarized in Figure 16.8.

Management

Assessment should include enquiry for evidence of a physical cause, such as frequency, haematuria, dysuria and urgency. Microscopy and microbiological analysis of the urine is necessary, but may have been carried out by the GP before referral. Evidence of other psychiatric disorders should also be sought.

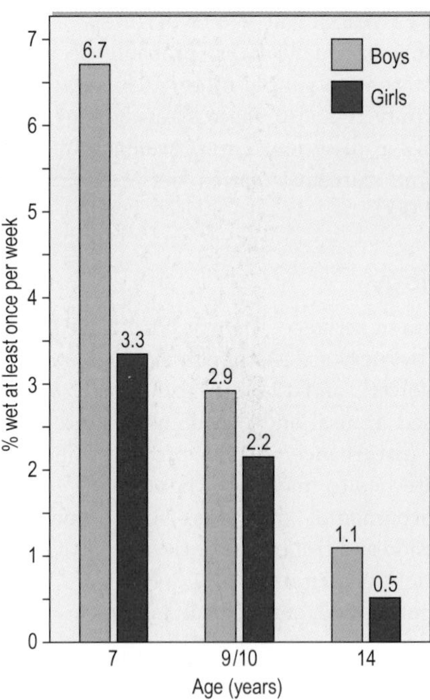

Figure 16.7 • Prevalence of enuresis (% with at least once per week) by age and sex. (Derived from Rutter *et al.* 1973 Enuresis and behavioural deviance: some epidemiological considerations. In: Kolvin I *et al.* (eds) Bladder control and enuresis. Clinics in Developmental Medicine Nos. 48/49, Heinemann, London, pp 137–147.)

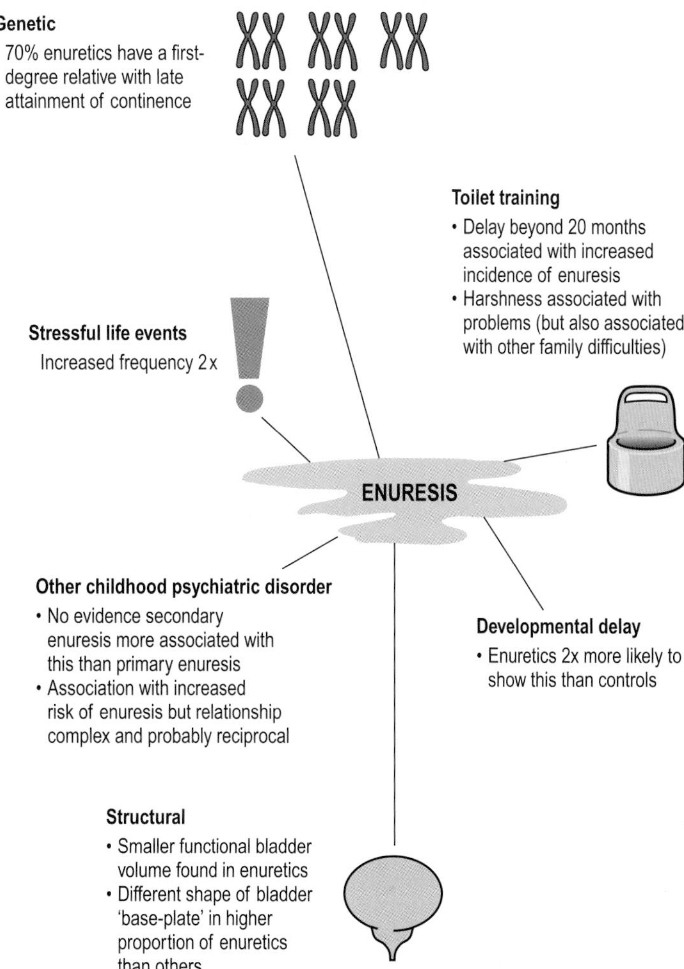

Figure 16.8 • Causes of non-organic enuresis.

Choice of treatment may be influenced by:

- home circumstances (may cause practical difficulties for some treatments)
- parent–child relationship (some treatments require a high degree of patience and persistence, with a non-judgemental approach)
- parental attitude to treatment (some parents find drugs unacceptable, for example)
- age of child (understanding of the approach)
- availability to supervise (some treatments may fail through lack of adequate supervision of the programme).

A period of observation should precede any treatment. This can usefully be monitored using a *star chart*, with the child getting a star for each dry bed. Care must be taken that wet beds are not recorded by some other symbol, otherwise the reinforcement for dry beds is cancelled out. Each dry bed should be accompanied by social praise. This process should persist for at least two weeks, and continued if the frequency of dry beds is increasing.

The next stage, if this has been negotiated, is to use the treatment of choice: *the pad and buzzer* (or in older children the pants alarm). This is an arrangement that warns of a wet bed or wet pants by an audible alarm. At the alarm the parent and child should go to the toilet and then change the bed. Most 'failures' occur because the method is not properly supervised, the parent is not committed to carrying it through, the family get fed up with false alarms, the child turns the alarm off or the method is used for too short a time (less than three months).

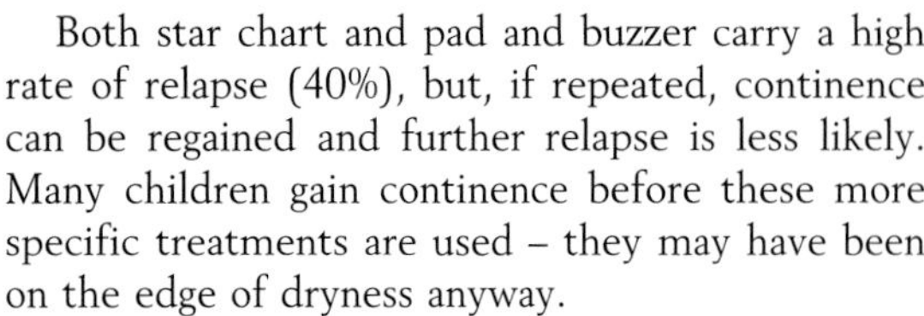

Both star chart and pad and buzzer carry a high rate of relapse (40%), but, if repeated, continence can be regained and further relapse is less likely. Many children gain continence before these more specific treatments are used – they may have been on the edge of dryness anyway.

Small doses of tricyclic antidepressants are effective in enuresis, although the mechanism is unclear. The effect occurs immediately, but there is a very high relapse rate on discontinuation of the treatment. However, they can be useful for short periods such as school trips or holidays away from home.

In recent years, desmopressin, a synthetic version of vasopressin, administered as a nasal spray, has been shown to help some children with enuresis by reducing urinary output.

Exercises designed to increase the functional capacity of the bladder have been used to try to correct the theoretical small functional capacity in some children.

Daytime wetting can be treated by 'habit' training, i.e. frequent toileting with rewards for success. Where the wetting is deliberate, attention paid to individual and family dynamics will be more appropriate.

Prognosis

The vast majority of physiologically normal children with healthy individual and family relationships will respond to one of the above programmes. Where there are complicating factors, the result is less certain. Military conscription discovered a number of young men who still wet the bed at 18 years old. In clinical practice, adults occasionally report the cessation of bed wetting coinciding with sharing a bed on marriage or cohabitation. With these caveats the general prognosis for enuresis is very good.

Non-organic encopresis (F98.1)

Diagnosis and clinical features

Table 16.10 summarizes the different ways in which encopresis can present. The key feature is the inappropriate deposition of faeces. This may range from simply in the child's pants to bizarre placements such as in a visitor's luggage (as described by Taylor, discovered when the luggage was opened by a Customs Officer). Faeces may be smeared on the child or over furniture and walls. There may be accompanying anal fingering or masturbation. The differential diagnosis should include organic disorders such as aganglionic megacolon, spina bifida or, more commonly, anal fissure or gastrointestinal infection. The more common disorders may trigger or maintain non-organic encopresis. If there is associated emotional or conduct disorder then these should be coded. If enuresis is present with encopresis, the latter should be the main diagnosis.

Table 16.10 Presentation of faecal soiling (encopresis)

Consistency of faeces	Normal, loose or constipated
Place deposited	In pants, hidden or in 'significant' places (e.g. in a particular person's cupboard)
Development	Never continent (continuous), after period of continence (discontinuous) or regression (in various contexts – see below)
Activity	Smearing, anal fingering or masturbation
Context	Power battle, upsetting life events (e.g. sexual abuse, divorce) and/or other psychiatric disorder
Physical	With soreness, anal fissures, etc., or with normal anus

A child presenting with encopresis may appear 'unconcerned' when seen with parents and this may be reported by the family with some irritation. This lack of concern is usually not so apparent when the child is seen alone – embarrassment may be the more prominent feature.

When bowel control has never been achieved, this is termed *continuous encopresis*. When there has been a period of normal bowel control, this is called *discontinuous encopresis*.

Epidemiology and aetiology

The frequency of soiling in boys is three to four times that in girls. At age five, the average rate of encopresis is 1.5%. The Isle of Wight study found figures of 1.3% for boys and 0.3% for girls age 12. Table 16.11 summarizes the causes of encopresis.

Management

A careful history should give an indication of the various factors contributing to an individual child's predicament. Co-working or close liaison with paediatric colleagues is essential. Chronic constipation and consequent megacolon can be difficult to detect by physical examination alone, even if rectal examination is performed. Behavioural or other treatment techniques will not be effective if such physical problems are not resolved.

Table 16.11 Causes of encopresis	
Congenital	Constitutional variability can include bowel control
Individual	Developmental delay
	Physical trigger • anal fissure • constipation (low-roughage diet) • other bowel disorders
Parent–child	Coercive toilet training
	Emotional abuse or neglect
	'Battleground' for relationship problems
Wider environment	Sexual abuse
	Family disharmony

Careful attention must be paid to both family relationships and home circumstances, particularly those for toileting (e.g. is the toilet a cold uncomfortable place?). The assessor must look for signs that there is a 'power battle' between child and carer over toileting. Any successful treatment approach will have to 'defuse' this.

Education of the carers regarding the mechanics of defecation can be helpful in designing a programme of regular toileting, with small rewards and social praise for success. 'Success' may need to be defined as a series of steps towards continence (e.g. sitting on the toilet rather than successful bowel movements there; or clean pants rather than successful defecation). Work focused on building up the child's *self-esteem* may also be required. There are other 'externalizing' approaches derived from family therapy practice that similarly engage the child with the family in beating the problem by labelling it as something outside normal family life (e.g. Michael White's 'sneaky poo' approach).

Drugs to soften stools or promote gastrointestinal motility may be helpful in encouraging bowel actions at regular intervals where there is constipation. *Individual and family therapy* are appropriate where there is accompanying conduct and/or emotional disorder.

Triggering of the appropriate child protection procedures should occur if child sexual abuse is discovered.

An intense behavioural programme carried out in hospital may be successful where other methods have failed, but unless the carers are involved there is a great danger of lack of generalization to home.

Most approaches may be lengthy, so this must be emphasized to families at the outset.

Prognosis

All reports of programmes to tackle encopresis show a high degree of success, although none, even followed up to late teens and early adulthood, is 100% successful.

Feeding disorders

This includes F98.2 *Feeding disorder of infancy of childhood* and F98.3 *Pica*. The former is an exaggeration of normal childhood faddiness, where there is normal food availability and a competent carer. Such concerns were expressed by the parents of 12% of preschool children in one study. Assessment should include a measure of calorie intake, as the child may be grazing on snacks or milk between meals and simply not eating at mealtimes.

Pica is the persistent eating of non-nutritive substances, especially soil and paint chippings. This is more common in children with learning disability. Anaemia can be associated. Correction of the anaemia can improve the behaviour.

Stereotyped movement disorders (F98.4)

These are voluntary, repetitive, non-functional movements, which are not part of any of the other disorders, such as obsessive–compulsive disorder or autism, which often include such movements. In isolation the behaviours may be self-injurious (Figure 16.9).

Such behaviours occur more commonly in understimulated children, especially where there is some learning disability or sensory impairment. Treatment includes distraction techniques and attention to appropriate stimulation. Some psychotropic drugs are said to help self-injurious behaviour in certain circumstances.

Specific speech disorders (F98.5–6)

Stuttering is a prolongation or repetition of certain parts of speech, usually syllables or words. This is commonly a transient phenomenon in childhood. This coding should be used if stuttering persists. Speech therapy may be helpful.

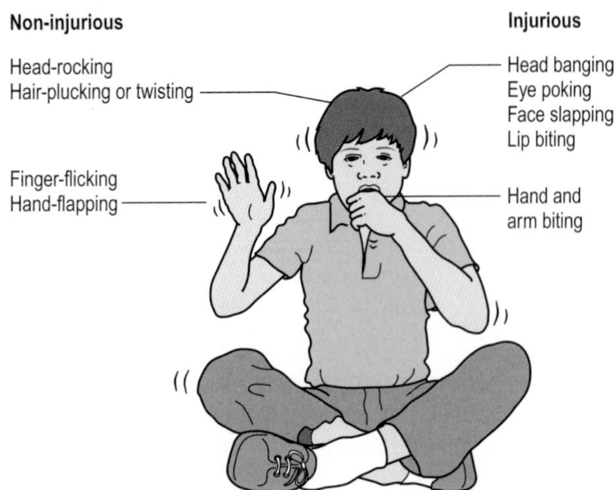

Figure 16.9 • Behaviours of stereotyped movement disorder.

Cluttering is a rapid rate of speech with a breakdown in fluency. This should only be coded where it is an isolated phenomenon and not part of either a neurological or a psychiatric disorder. Child psychiatrists rarely see the problem, as direct referral to speech therapy is usual.

Specific conditions

- Where 'adult' psychiatric disorder occurs in childhood and adolescence there may be clinical differences from the typical adult presentation.
- Hyperkinetic disorders are characterized by impaired attention and overactivity, but not distractibility.
- Behavioural treatment of the symptoms of hyperkinetic disorder are of short-term efficacy; drug effects are more sustained, but have significant adverse side-effects.
- The nature of conduct disorder changes with increasing age, progressing from aggression to oppositional defiant behaviour to more sophisticated misbehaviour in adolescence.
- Conduct disorder in childhood is strongly associated with later personality problems, especially when the symptoms include aggression.

Specific conditions—cont'd

- Emotional disorders should only be diagnosed when there is no definite neurotic disorder.
- Emotional disorders in general have a good prognosis.
- Attachment disorders of infancy are commonly seen by child protection agencies in situations of inappropriate parenting.
- Tics occur in 10–24% of children, but the majority are simple and transient.
- Non-organic enuresis is more common in boys, reduces in frequency with age and responds to a range of behavioural and pharmacological treatments.
- Non-organic encopresis is the inappropriate deposition of faeces. The context and physical factors are key parts of the assessment. Defusing any power battle is important in the success of any treatment approach.
- Pica is the persistent eating of non-nutritive substances. Other feeding disorders of infancy are common.
- Stereotyped movement disorders must be diagnosed only if *not* part of a disorder such as autism.
- Specific speech disorders include stuttering and cluttering.

Further reading

Cheng, K., Myers, K. (Eds.), 2010. Child and adolescent psychiatry: the essentials. second ed. Lippincott Williams and Wilkins, Philadelphia.

Rutter, M., Bishop, D., Pine, D., Scott, S., Stevenson, J., Taylor, E. et al., (Eds.), 2008. Rutter's child and adolescent psychiatry. fifth ed. Blackwell Publishing, Oxford.

Psychiatry of disability

This chapter considers the psychiatric concomitants of disability. The reader is referred to the rest of this book for consideration of the disabling effects of psychiatric disorder.

Definitions

It is important at the outset to distinguish impairment, disability and handicap. The World Health Organization (WHO) definitions are as follows:

- An *impairment* is a loss or abnormality of psychological, physiological or anatomical structure or function.
- A *disability* is a restriction or lack (resulting from an impairment) of ability to perform an activity in the manner or within the range considered normal for a human being. More recently, the WHO has preferred to connote this positively by referring to *activity* as the nature and extent of functioning at the level of the person.
- A *handicap* is a disadvantage resulting from an impairment or disability that limits or prevents the fulfilment of a role that is normal (depending on age, sex and cultural factors) for a given individual. This could be construed as a question of biopsychosocial level (see Chapter 2 and Figure 17.1). Handicap has similarly been turned round and replaced with the concept of *participation*, being the nature and extent of a person's involvement in life situations in relation to impairment, activities, health conditions and contextual factors.

Using these concepts, the WHO has devised a complex quantitative classification system that can be applied to any individual to designate their level of functioning, or problems faced. This is called the International Classification of Impairments, Activities and Participation. It is designed to be complementary to ICD-10.

Many terms were used in the 20th century to describe people with learning disabilities. As each set of terms has been imbued with stigma and negative connotations a new set has been introduced, in the hope that attitudes towards such people will be more positive as a result, thus lessening the potential for handicap. The use of terms in successive UK mental health legislation illustrates this (Figure 17.2), as does the alteration in WHO labels. Different cultures also currently use different terms. A search of the literature for 'learning disability' (current UK term) would need to use 'mental retardation' or 'developmental disability' in the USA, or 'mental handicap' in other Western countries. In the USA, 'learning disability' encompasses 'specific developmental delays' (F81 – see Table 17.2).

Equivalent terms for physical disability, including sensory disabilities, have also varied over the years. It is only relatively recently that people with disabilities themselves have participated fully in this debate, either directly or via advocacy schemes. Medical terms with more specific meanings, such as 'spastic', have been used as a generic description and have also been imbued with stigma.

In ICD-10, the categories F70–79 cover 'mental retardation' (Table 17.1). Whether a behaviour difficulty is also present can be specified for each level of disability. It must also be noted that, where possible, the syndrome or organic aetiology for the mental retardation should be coded (e.g. Q90 Down's syndrome). Labels such as those in section F70–79

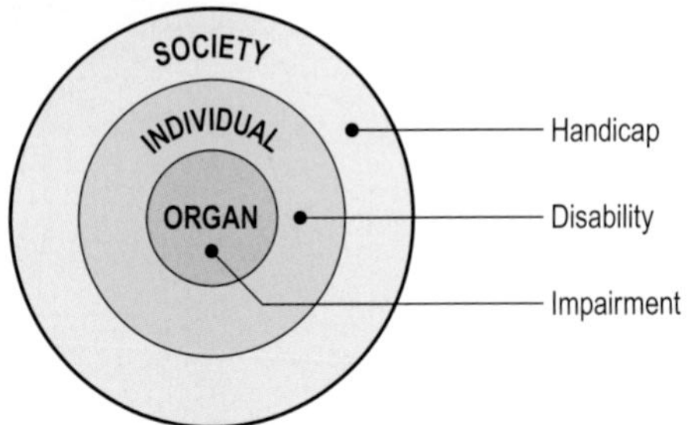

Figure 17.1 • Definitions of impairment, disability and handicap according to biopsychosocial level.

are rarely very useful in individual clinical practice, as there can be wide variations in presentation within any particular IQ range. Assumptions about functioning made because of such labelling can be handicapping to an extent that exceeds the effect of an individual's impairment. In addition, a multiplicity of relatively small impairments in a number of functional areas may result in considerable disability and handicap. Although there may statistically be an increased risk of other impairments (such as sensory impairments and mobility problems) with increasing 'retardation', this is only an association. It is particularly important in assessment to consider the whole person and his or her environment.

Also included in ICD-10 is a section on 'Disorders of psychological development' (F80–89; Table 17.2). These disorders have in common:

- onset invariably during infancy and childhood
- impairment or delay in functions strongly related to the biological maturation of the central nervous system
- steady course (i.e. remissions and relapses do not occur).

They are included here because, although they start in childhood, they can have disabling implications throughout life.

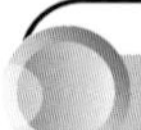

Definitions

- It is important to distinguish impairment (abnormality of structure or function) from disability (the limitations imposed by the impairment) and handicap (the sociocultural disadvantage).
- For those with a disability, societal stigma is an additional handicap, which is only temporarily lessened by changing labels.

Epidemiology

This section can be divided into:

- epidemiology of impairment
- epidemiology of specific syndromes
- epidemiology of psychiatric and psychological aspects of disability arising from the above.

Impairment and disability

The 1992 General Household Survey in the UK recorded 36.5% of people surveyed as describing themselves suffering from a serious disease or disability. Clearly, not all of these disorders will confer a level of impairment to produce 'disability' as the term is normally used in the general population. However, this figure supports pressure groups and professionals who argue for people with more obvious disabilities being seen as part of continuum within the population ('everyone is not so good at something').

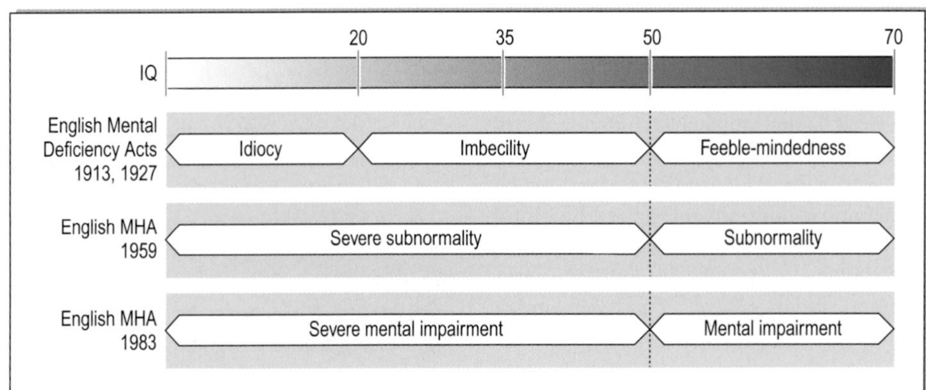

Figure 17.2 • Terms used for learning disability in successive legislation in England and Wales.

Table 17.1 ICD-10 and DSM-IV-TR classifications: (F70–79 and 317–319) Mental retardation

F70 Mild mental retardation (*DSM-IV 317*)
IQ range 50–69
Delayed understanding and use of language
Possible difficulties in gaining independence
Work in practical occupations
Any behavioural, social and emotional difficulties are similar to the 'normal'
F71 Moderate mental retardation (*DSM-IV 318.0*)
IQ range 35–49
Varying profiles of abilities
Language use and development variable (may be absent)
Often associated with epilepsy, neurological and other disability
Delay in achievement of self-care
Simple practical work
Independent living rarely achieved
F72 Severe mental retardation (*DSM-IV 318.1*)
IQ range 20–34
More marked motor impairment than F71 often found
Achievements lower end of F71
F73 Profound mental retardation (*DSM-IV 318.2*)
Severe limitation in ability to understand or comply with requests or instructions
IQ difficult to measure but <20
Little or no self-care
Mostly severe mobility restriction
Basic or simple tasks may be acquired (e.g. sorting and matching)
Mental retardation, severity unspecified (*DSM-IV 319*)
In ICD-10 a fourth character may be used to specify extent of associated behavioural impairment:
F7×.0 No, or minimal, impairment of behaviour
F7×.1 Significant impairment of behaviour requiring attention or treatment
F7×.8 Other impairments of behaviour
F7×.9 Without mention of impairment of behaviour
In ICD-10, child and adolescent psychiatric disorders may be classified multiaxially with the above designated Axis Three: Intellectual level in DSM-IV mental retardation is coded in Axis Two with personality disorder (if present).

Table 17.2 ICD-10 classification: F80–89 Disorders of psychological development

F80 Specific developmental disorders of speech and language
F80.0 Specific speech articulation disorder
F80.1 Expressive language disorder
F80.2 Receptive language disorder
F80.3 Acquired aphasia with epilepsy (Landau–Kleffner syndrome)
F80.8 Other developmental disorders of speech and language
F80.9 Developmental disorder of speech and language, unspecified
F81 Specific developmental disorders of scholastic skills
F81.0 Specific reading disorder
F81.1 Specific spelling disorder
F81.2 Specific disorder of arithmetical skills
F81.3 Mixed disorder of scholastic skills
F81.8 Other developmental disorders of scholastic skills
F81.9 Developmental disorder of scholastic skills, unspecified
F82 Specific developmental disorder of motor function
F83 Mixed specific developmental disorders
F84 Pervasive developmental disorders
F84.0 Childhood autism
F84.1 Atypical autism
F84.2 Rett's syndrome
F84.3 Other childhood disintegrative disorder
F84.4 Overactive disorder associated with mental retardation and stereotyped movements
F84.5 Asperger's syndrome
F84.8 Other pervasive developmental disorders
F84.9 Pervasive developmental disorder, unspecified
F88 Other disorder of psychological development
F89 Unspecified disorder of psychological development

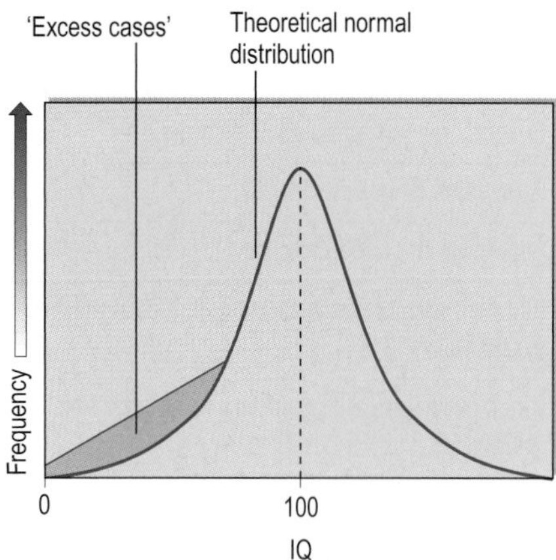

Figure 17.3 • Frequency distribution in intelligence quotients.

When IQ is used to define those with learning disabilities (LD), the assumption of normal variation in the population does not entirely determine the prevalence found, i.e. if one defines LD as an IQ of less than 70, the prevalence is 2.2% whereas the actual prevalence is 3.7% (Figure 17.3). For severe LD (IQ<50), the prevalence is approximately 0.4%. The skew to the left in Figure 17.3 is due to a combination of 'statistical' low IQ with those individuals with genetic/chromosomal abnormalities. Those with an IQ between 50 and 70 rarely have an obvious cause for their impairment, whereas individuals with an IQ below 50 frequently do have a more obvious aetiology such as a genetic abnormality.

There is a high correlation between different impairments (see Figure 17.5). A third of children with cerebral palsy are also found to have severe LD (but conversely this means that two-thirds are above this IQ level). A study of residential hospital admissions showed that 38% of those with severe LD also had cerebral palsy (with the majority having spastic paralysis of all four limbs). This latter figure must be viewed with caution, as the likelihood of hospital admission was increased by greater disability, even when the emphasis was not on care in the community. When children with LD were admitted to residential hospital, a third of the hospital population were found also to have epilepsy. Although the same reservations about a hospital population as above must apply, similar figures have been found in Swedish community studies (Table 17.3).

Specific syndromes

The frequencies of a number of the more common or well-known conditions are shown in Figure 17.4.

Table 17.3 Levels of coexistence of different impairments

	Severe mental retardation (%)	Mild mental retardation (%)
Cerebral palsy	App. 20	App. 8
Epilepsy	30–37	12–18
Hydrocephalus	5–6	2
Severe visual impairment	6–10	1–9
Severe hearing impairment	3–15	2–7
One or more major impairments	40–52	24–30

For Down's syndrome there is a clear correlation between affected births and increasing maternal age (Figure 17.5). It must be noted, however, that the majority of children with Down's syndrome are not born to women over the age of 35, despite the risk being so much greater. The figures for cytogenetic analysis of amniotic fluid at 15–16 weeks' gestation show an even higher incidence of trisomy 21 than shown in Figure 17.5, suggesting a significant fetal loss rate.

Psychiatric and psychological aspects of disability

The Isle of Wight study of psychiatric disorder in nine to 12-year-olds, carried out in the 1970s, found that the prevalence of psychiatric disorder was:

- doubled when there was physical disorder not affecting the brain
- increased fivefold by the presence of brain damage
- increased tenfold when there was also epilepsy.

Comparing studies examining the frequency of mental disorder in a learning-disabled population requires careful consideration of the definitions of both mental disorder and LD and also the population studied. Hospital studies have found prevalences of psychiatric disorder of between 32% and 59% in the learning-disabled population. In a study comparing hospital and community populations, significant psychiatric disorder was found in 31% of the former but only 13% of the latter. If minor personality quirks and behavioural 'problems' were added in, the figures were 52% and 41% respectively.

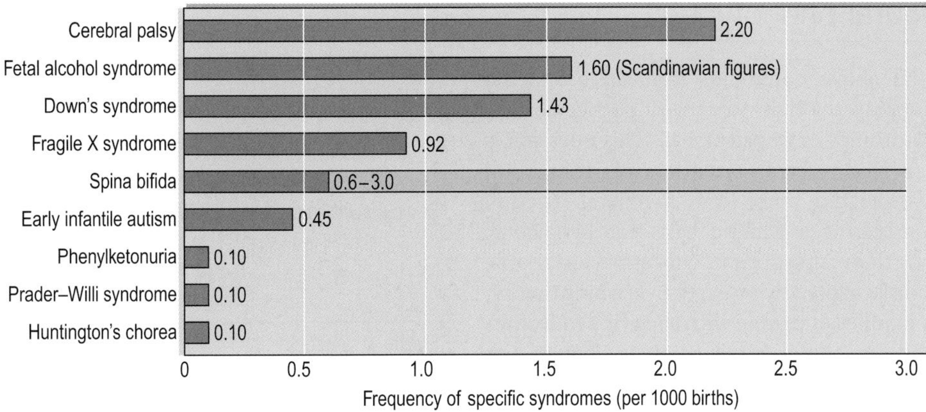

Figure 17.4 • Frequencies of specific syndromes (per 1000 births).

Corbett studied learning-disabled adults in Camberwell, south London, and found a prevalence of schizophrenia of 3.5%. This is very similar to the figures for hospital populations of adults with learning disabilities. He also found a further 3% with a previous history of schizophrenia. In the same study, he diagnosed 25% of the learning-disabled group as suffering from 'personality disorder' of varying types (see Chapter 15 for a discussion of the issues relating to such diagnoses). In a study of adults over the age of 50 with LD, 11.4% were found to be suffering from a psychiatric disorder, and 11.4% from dementia (combined figure 21%.)

In the Isle of Wight study, five out of the 38 severely learning-disabled children identified were also diagnosed as having a 'neurotic disorder' (13%). The equivalent figure in Camberwell was 4%. In more recent community studies in Scotland and Australia, around 40% of children with severe learning disability were found to have significant psychiatric disorder.

For bipolar mood disorders, the hospital point prevalence in a learning-disabled population was found to be 1.2%. A community study found that 1.5% of people older than 16 in contact with a LD service had a bipolar disorder, and a further 2% had depression.

Severe self-injurious behaviour is almost always associated with profound LD and occurs in 1.7% of the LD population. Milder stereotyped behaviours occur in 10–15% of children and adults.

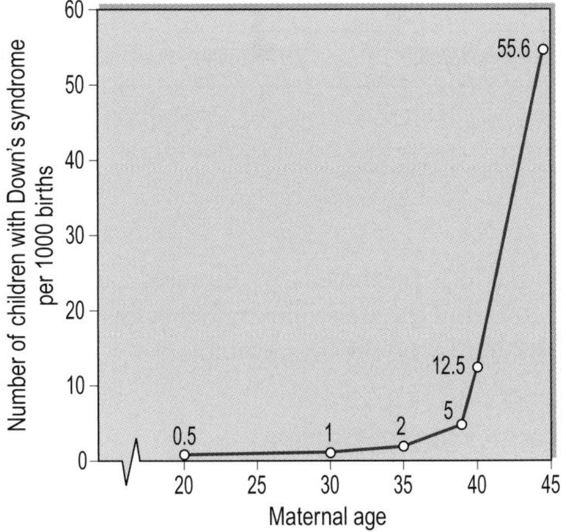

Figure 17.5 • Incidence of Down's syndrome with increasing maternal age.

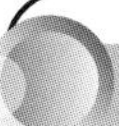

Epidemiology

- There is an increased frequency of psychiatric disorder in people with disability.
- A much higher frequency is associated with brain damage and epilepsy.

Clinical features

It would be far too simplistic to try to derive clinical features that apply to all, or even the majority of, people with impairment or disability. This has been attempted in the past for certain groups (e.g. 'the epileptic personality'), but it has subsequently been found that the features derived were more to do with the common environmental experiences of individuals (most notably the effects of institutionalization) than with their impairments. However, there are issues that are appropriate to consider when discussing the psychiatry of disability.

Behavioural phenotypes

Despite the above comments, are there specific behavioural patterns that occur with particular conditions, syndromes or impairments? This question is receiving revived research attention following a lull that was associated with, first, a general reaction against considering a genetic basis for behaviour, and second, the vast strides in education for people with disability enabled by research in learning theory. However, families of people with specific syndromes have found anecdotal similarities in behaviours between their affected family members, and this has been supported by research. Some of these findings are summarized in Table 17.4.

Table 17.4 Behavioural phenotypes: summary of associations of behaviour to specific syndromes

Angelman syndrome	Happy disposition; laughing at minimal provocation; hand-flapping; inquisitiveness
Down's syndrome	Common obsessionality and stubbornness; 25% have attention-deficit disorder in childhood
Fragile X syndrome	Idiosyncratic linguistic and interpersonal styles; disagreement about whether close association with autism
Klinefelter's syndrome	Passive and compliant in childhood; aggressive and antisocial post puberty
Lesch–Nyhan syndrome	Compulsive severely mutilating self-injurious behaviour
Sanfilippo syndrome (a mucopolysaccharidosis)	Prominent sleep disorder
Noonan's syndrome	Common problems in peer relations; stubbornness and perseverative behaviour
Prader–Willi syndrome	Insatiable appetite (diagnostic); sleep abnormalities; frequent temper tantrums; self-injury through skin picking
Rett syndrome	Reduced interest in play in early infancy followed by autistic-like symptoms; stereotypic hand movements; self-injury; anxiety and depression common
Tuberous sclerosis	75% autism, hyperactivity or both

(Derived from O'Brien G 1992 Behavioural phenotypy in developmental psychiatry. European Child and Adolescent Psychiatry Suppl No. 1.)

Challenging behaviour and self-injury

As mentioned above, there is an increased incidence of 'behavioural disturbance' shown by people with disabilities. More recently the terminology has changed to emphasize the interactional and contextual nature of most behaviours, from 'problem' behaviours to 'challenging' behaviours. This then begs the question 'challenging to whom?'. Complaints about a person's behaviour will vary between contexts and from person to person. It is also more often the case that behaviour is rarely 'challenging' to the persons themselves (although self-injurious behaviour may be an exception). A challenging behaviour seen in interactional terms may be a communication of, for example, boredom, irritation, frustration, anger or joy. Table 17.5 lists the more common 'challenging' behaviours.

Self-esteem

People with disabilities frequently show low self-esteem and negative self-concepts. This can result in a spiral of self-perpetuating behaviours. The low self-esteem is a result of frequent experiences of failure (perhaps due to inappropriately high or low expectations); negative societal attitudes (encapsulated in the question 'Does he take sugar?' to the person accompanying a disabled person); or comparison of self with 'non-disabled' family members. If such experiences are repeated and consistent, they can be incorporated into an individual's self view. Behaviour that conforms to this is then more likely to become the norm, and thus difficult to reverse. Striking exposition of such dilemmas are portrayed by 'disabled' artists, poets and actors, but these also illustrate that low self-esteem is a risk but by no means inevitable.

Family relationships

The realization of impairment and disability can occur at different stages in the life cycle. Similarly, identification of carrier status, now possible in an increasing

Table 17.5 Common challenging behaviours

Violence to self or others	Biting Hitting Spitting Headbanging Scratching Pinching Tantrums Property damage
Behaviours out of usual context	Shouting Undressing Running away Masturbation Urination Defecation Sexual behaviours towards others Vomiting Passivity and oppositional behaviour
Generally inappropriate behaviours	Rocking Flapping Stealing Kleptomania

number of inherited conditions, can be distressing for potential parents. With the wide range of antenatal diagnostic approaches now available, pre-knowledge of chromosomal and other congenital abnormalities provides the potential for termination of affected pregnancies. This can lead to moral, ethical and religious dilemmas, which, in turn, can provide the basis for discord, distortion of family relationships, parenting difficulties and frank psychiatric symptomatology.

Whether congenital or acquired, impairment and disability can produce a wide range of responses in the relatives and carers of those affected. Anger, misery and guilt are all seen, and may be fitted into a framework of the bereavement response, grieving for the loss of the expected unaffected child. Different family members will go through this process at varying rates. Less involvement with the affected individual may slow the process. In Western cultures, this is more frequently seen in fathers. As continued expression or sharing of grief may not be acceptable, pathological bereavement responses may be seen, some of which may be seen as 'healthy' by wider society (Figure 17.6).

Olshansky has coined the term 'chronic sorrow' for the second-hand experience of impairment and disability. Each new stage of development presents its challenges and its losses for the family and, with increasing self-awareness, for the individuals themselves. It used to be said that 'a handicapped person means a handicapped family'. However, although there may be difficulties to overcome, very many families with a disabled member take strong exception to this assumption. Indeed, taking the definition of handicap at the beginning of this chapter, it may be seen that the family being 'handicapped' is also a sociocultural phenomenon, and need by no means necessarily be so. Research shows that, for example, where a marriage breaks down following the birth of a disabled child, there has almost invariably been pre-existing marital discord. In other partnerships the relationship is reported to be strengthened and enhanced by such a challenge. The evidence regarding the effect on siblings is equivocal. Some studies show increased disturbance, whereas others do not; the influencing factors are many. On the whole, although some families have considerable problems many others cope admirably.

Ricks has pointed out that normal parental responses to impaired children may be maladaptive. This may be bewildering for parents, especially if they are trying hard to be as 'normal' as possible for the child. An example given by Ricks is of the child with ataxia who needs a great deal of confidence to attempt weight bearing, but who needs to practise to compensate for poor tone and balance. The natural response of parents is to hover nearby and grab the child to prevent a fall. Unfortunately, this distracts the gaze and concentration on balance and undermines confidence, leading to a greater likelihood of falling and increased parental anxiety. It is potentially distressing for carers to realize that they may have to behave against their normal parenting practice in order to give their child the opportunity to progress. Multiagency support, integrated services and the availability of 'short breaks' can all help parents.

Adolescence

In Western culture, adolescence is a time of increasing independence from parents, with greater relating to the peer group. A disabled young person may be further handicapped by the lack of facilities and opportunities for such individuation. However, there is still likely to be a reduction in the unquestioning acceptance of adult authority, together with increased size and possibly strength. Challenging behaviour can result.

Sexual feelings may be misunderstood or, in the case of physical disability, more difficult to express. An individual may be handicapped by inappropriate

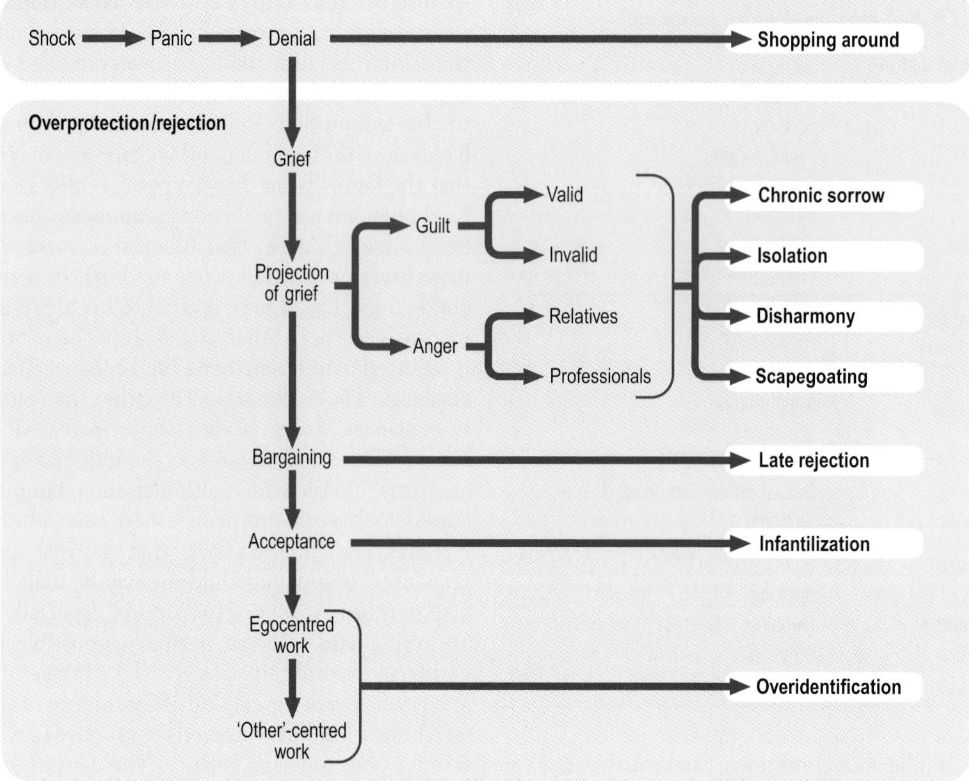

Figure 17.6 • Psychological processes in families with an impaired or disabled member. (Reproduced with permission from Bicknell J 1983 British Journal of Medical Psychology 56: 167.)

sex education, or by the reluctance of adults to consider that they might normally be exploring their sexuality at this stage of development (the concept of 'mental age' can be particularly handicapping in this respect). An increased frequency of masturbation or masturbation in inappropriate social settings (often where alternative activity is lacking) may be seen as 'challenging behaviour'.

Young people with disabilities may find themselves struggling more overtly with the issues of independence and individuation than their more able peers because of the need for more help to achieve these developmental objectives.

Living in the community

Community care legislation and practice in the UK means that most people with disabilities, however profound, now live in community accommodation of one type or another. Problems of social isolation, exploitation, psychiatric disorder and/or socially unusual or problematic behaviours are the main challenges for social and health care agencies. In particular, the 'forensic' subspecialty of disability psychology and psychiatry has become more important.

If a disabled person is living with their family, particular crises may occur with the increasing infirmity and eventual death of family carers. Planning for this inevitability is something that can be put off until it is too late. Grief may be expressed in ways unfamiliar to both wider family and professionals, or it may be suggested that a disabled person 'does not understand'. There are now many books and programmes available that may help these circumstances.

Modification of psychiatric symptomatology

Just as distress may be shown in different ways, so psychiatric symptomatology may be altered by impairment or disability. Where speech is absent, details of delusions, hallucinations and other psychotic phenomena may be impossible to elicit. However, important information and clues may be obtained by careful observation carried out in consultation with those who know the individual best. Similarly, those with impaired mobility may not show the level of activity changes seen in some psychiatric disorders (e.g. mania, depression), but sleep disturbance may still be evident, together with mood changes.

Where there is impairment of social communication (e.g. autism), variations in social relatedness, such as may occur in depression and schizophrenia, may not be so apparent. If there is a combination of physical, sensory and learning disabilities then the diagnosis of psychiatric disorder can be very difficult indeed (see Management, below). Differential 'diagnosis' of a change in a disabled person's functioning can be extremely wide.

Specific conditions

The reader is referred to other textbooks (see Further reading) for detail of the clinical features of specific conditions. However, the features of childhood autism, Down's syndrome and fragile X syndrome are shown in Figures 17.7–17.9.

Clinical features

- There is evidence that some behavioural patterns have a constitutional or syndrome-related basis (behavioural phenotypes).
- The realization of disability in a family may be experienced as a loss akin to, but more complicated than, a bereavement. The associated grieving process may become pathological.
- Pre-existing family or marital discord may be brought to the fore in families with a disabled member (as may pre-existing strengths).
- Behaviour found 'challenging' in one context may not be so in others.
- Normal parental responses may be maladaptive for a disabled child.

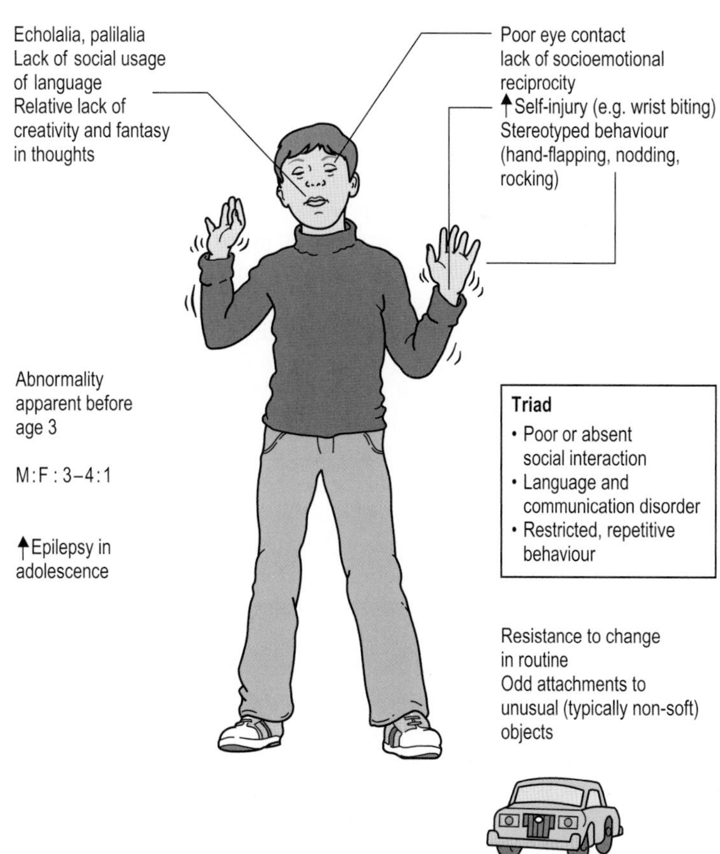

Figure 17.7 • Clinical features of childhood autism (F84.0) (Kanner's syndrome).

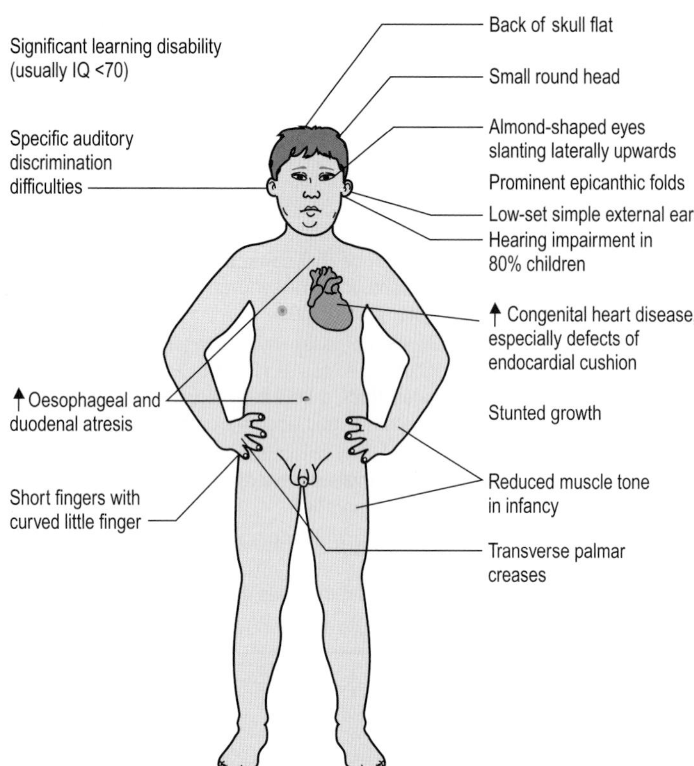

Figure 17.8 • Clinical features of Down's syndrome (trisomy 21).

Aetiology

Impairment may occur for a wide range of reasons. These are often categorized into prenatal, perinatal and acquired (Table 17.6). However, as noted in the introduction, virtually any medical condition, being by definition a pathological change in physical state, can produce impairment and disability. The reversibility or otherwise of this may have an important bearing on the degree of handicap. Western medicine and society have evolved the phenomena of 'patient' and 'sick role', which are useful in acute reversible disorders, but may not be so helpful in chronic conditions (see Chapter 4).

For people with LD, the severity of the impairment is related to the predominant aetiology. That is, for severe and profound LD the predominant aetiologies are organic, whereas in mild, and to a lesser extent moderate, LD the main causes are social and environmental. This may be usefully viewed as a continuum (Figure 17.10). Increased research in molecular genetics means that more and more links between genetic influences and impairment are being made.

Whether a psychiatric disorder develops in a person with a disability will depend on the same factors as described under the relevant heading for individuals without a prior impairment. However, particular predisposing factors, such as brain damage, may be more common in those with disability. Similarly, social and family disadvantages may be more frequent.

Aetiology

- Virtually any medical condition, producing as it does a change in physical state, may be disabling, at least on a temporary basis.
- Responses to disability, whether permanent or temporary, may be handicapping.

Management

The health and social needs of people with disabilities are wide ranging and may therefore require the involvement of a number of different professionals and agencies: the *multidisciplinary team*. Multiple disciplines may well impinge on a person and their

Figure 17.9 • Clinical features of fragile X syndrome.

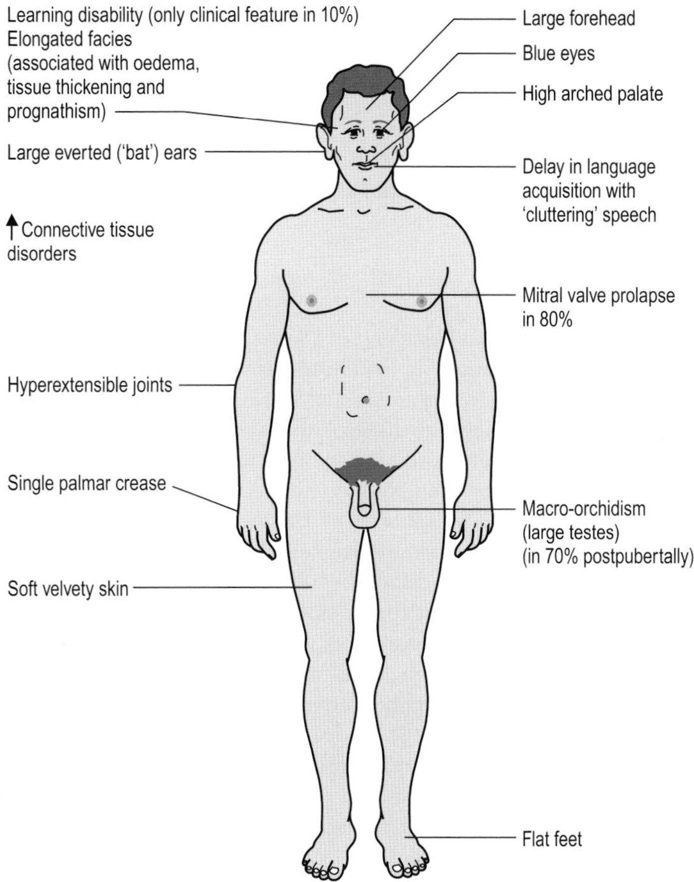

Table 17.6 Aetiology of disability

Prenatal	Perinatal	Postnatal
Inborn errors of metabolism	Asphyxia/hypoxia at birth	Meningitis/encephalitis
Chromosomal abnormalities	Mechanical birth trauma	Head injury (accidental or inflicted)
Congenital infections (rubella, cytomegalovirus, syphilis, HIV, toxoplasma)	Small babies Hyperbilirubinaemia (kernicterus) Hyperoxia (iatrogenic)	Lead poisoning (and other heavy metals)
Irradiation	Hypoglycaemia	Malnutrition
Drugs (e.g. thalidomide) Maternal alcohol intake Malnutrition, including vitamin deficiencies	Prematurity (intraventricular haemorrhage etc.)	Other infections (e.g. whooping cough) Environmental chemicals

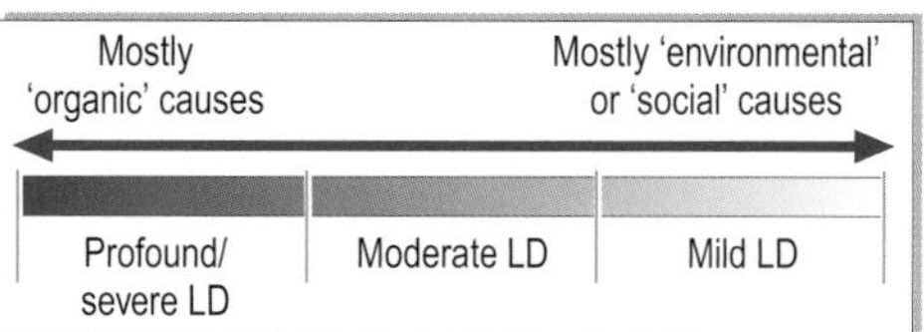

Figure 17.10 • Continuum of aetiology in learning disability.

wider network without being part of a team. This can be an additional source of handicap, as agencies may duplicate services to a person and/or the family. Alternatively, agencies may disagree about responsibilities, or simply not coordinate their activities, so that the client and/or the family do not receive the appropriate input. The concept of the *keyworker* through whom interventions are channelled has arisen in order to avoid the above difficulties. Even with such an arrangement, contact with professionals and others can be extremely time-consuming. Any design of services needs to take such issues into account in order to minimize the extra burden imposed, while maximizing the benefit to the service user.

To provide appropriate resources, *care management* has been introduced in the UK (and similar schemes elsewhere). A care manager is designated to commission appropriate social, accommodation and care inputs for disabled people in consultation with the individuals and their families.

The development of self-help and mutual support groups has promoted the involvement of users in determining the shape and development of services. Where people with disability would find it extremely difficult, if not impossible, to put forward their views (e.g. in profound mental and physical impairment with sensory disability), then *advocacy schemes* have been developed in which others, not involved in the service provision, act as advocates.

The development of a multidisciplinary approach has meant that the psychiatrist, who in the case of LD might previously have supervised the whole of the health service provision to a disabled population (particularly when that population resided in a large hospital), has now a more focused part to play. This includes:

- diagnosis and treatment of mental disorder
- identification (with other medical specialists) of the physical components of impairment and in particular their possible contribution to psychological morbidity
- provision (with others) of support, counselling and therapy where appropriate to families and their wider network
- development (according to individual skills and with others) and coordination of health services to those with impairment and disability.

Specific psychiatric treatments

Treatment interventions must always be preceded by appropriate levels of assessment. As mentioned previously, psychiatric and behavioural presentations in people with disability can occur for a wide range of reasons. Excessive reliance on any particular approach to treatment can have adverse consequences (see Case histories).

Consent is a particularly tricky issue for those with disability, particularly learning disability. No adult may give consent for another adult except in a judicial context. Legal advice may often be required where there is a doubt about capability to consent to a particular treatment option.

Behavioural treatments

Behavioural approaches can be very effective in reducing psychological and behavioural morbidity, and in increasing alternative appropriate skills. They require skilled management and supervision in order, first, to be effective, and, second, to avoid being abusive. Aversive stimuli or withdrawal of privileges are now regarded as unethical (and are not particularly effective anyway).

The helpfulness of cognitive behavioural approaches will depend as always on the level or stage of motivation, and also will need to be modified according to cognitive deficits, strengths and distortions.

Family and systemic therapy

Work with parents and/or carers is important in all cases. The degree to which this is regarded as formal 'therapy' will very much depend on the circumstances (e.g. symptoms appear related to family relationships). As noted above, issues of consent and confidentiality are no less important in this area than in other areas of medicine.

Sometimes professionals in disability teams will be specifically involved in working explicitly with the systems of carer organizations (*systemic therapy*). Negotiation of roles, tasks, aims and responsibilities are particularly crucial in these circumstances.

Psychotherapy

It has been argued that those with LD do not have the cognitive apparatus to benefit from psychotherapy, which has been seen as a white, vocal, middle-class preserve. However, more recently even those with severe LD have been shown to be able to use suitably modified individual and group approaches. Those with other disabilities also require approaches and access arrangements according to their needs (e.g. a person with hearing impairment would require a model of communication that is familiar to them). Cognitive analytical therapy has been specifically recommended by some. Art, music, drama and multisensory therapies may be more appropriate or acceptable for some.

Pharmacotherapy

Drug prescription for those with disabilities should occur only when there is a specific indication. However, it has frequently been reported that overprescribing occurs. For those with brain damage the potential for neurotoxicity is increased. In addition, the side-effects of antipsychotic drugs, such as akathisia, may be confused with the stereotypic behavioural patterns seen in people with LD.

An additional problem for those patients with LD is that the side-effect of sedation seen with some antipsychotic drugs may produce a reduced learning ability or a loss of skills. Those with brain damage may also show an increased sensitivity to the epileptogenic propensities of some antipsychotics (such interactions can promote polypharmacy where the prescriber is not aware of this, as epilepsy is more common in those with brain damage anyway).

Despite the above, psychotropic medication can be extremely helpful for some individuals with disabilities and psychiatric or behavioural disorders, for example:

- drugs prescribed for properly diagnosed psychiatric disorder
- drugs with specific effects on behaviour (e.g. haloperidol for self-injurious behaviour in autism).

Some research has demonstrated high levels of psychophysiological arousal in those with self-injurious behaviour that is decreased by 'antipsychotic' medication. More specifically, dopamine D_1 receptor antagonists and opiate antagonists (e.g. naltrexone) have been found to reduce severe self-injurious behaviour in some individuals. However, the level of research in this area is limited.

The limited evidence base means that most decisions about medication use in patients with disabilities are made by extrapolating from findings in 'non-disabled' populations. As noted above, this is not always a successful approach, so extra care is required until better evidence becomes available.

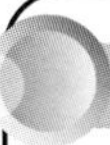

Management

- Disability confers an additional layer of complexity onto the diagnosis and treatment of mental disorder.
- A multidisciplinary, multiagency approach is required, with care being taken to avoid this process itself becoming handicapping.
- The full range of psychiatric treatments, suitably modified, may be helpful for people with disability.

Prognosis

Studies examining the prognosis of psychiatric disorder in people with disabilities show no particular differences in outcome from those without such disabilities. Problems arise, however, in considering this, as (1) it may be more difficult to diagnose psychiatric disorders accurately in disabled people, and (2) the prevalence of psychiatric disorder in such a population is higher. So that the prognosis for people with a disability because of missed or incorrect diagnosis is not made worse, it is important that they have at least equal access to appropriate services.

Mortality increases when there are significant mobility problems. The presence of one major anomaly is likely to be accompanied by another, which itself may be life-threatening (e.g. cardiac abnormalities).

There is a significantly increased incidence of Alzheimer's-type presenile dementia in Down's syndrome and also hypothyroidism (which, together with depression, may be a differential diagnosis of dementia in this population). The excess of dementia in the LD population is not, however, attributable to the coexistence of Down's syndrome and LD.

Case history A: severe learning disability

Alan, a 17-year-old with severe LD, was referred to a community LD team by his GP because of his family's concerns about his tendency to run off when out shopping. A psychiatric registrar visited the family at home and met Alan and his mother. The doctor was told that the running away occurred approximately twice a month when the family went shopping, and that Alan tended to strip off his clothes as he ran. The family were concerned on two counts; embarrassment, and fear that Alan would run out into the road in his agitation.

There was a previous long-standing history of tantrums, which the family had managed effectively by sending Alan to his room. This had not been a problem for three years prior to the referral. The tendency for Alan to run off when out if he did not get his own way had always been present, but had been managed previously by keeping a firm grip on his hand. This was no longer possible as Alan was now able to slip out of the grip of either of his parents.

Further discussions with the family and Alan himself showed that in many areas of social behaviour Alan was capable of adequate performance, but that he rarely had the opportunity to demonstrate this. A series of home-based family sessions discussed options for increasing Alan's autonomy and independence. Liaison with Alan's local social education centre increased his sphere of outside activities. Alan revealed that he disliked the hurly burly of shopping trips, and the family agreed that his need to participate in these was not essential.

The frequency of Alan's running away decreased to extremely sporadic examples, which caused greater furore in the family and the wider system because of their relative scarcity. The family were relieved by Alan's increasing enthusiasm for weekends away at a local hostel.

Case history B: moderate learning disability

Melanie, a 34-year-old woman with moderate LD but no mobility problems, who lived with her parents, presented with withdrawal, episodes of talking to herself and outbursts of aggressive behaviour, to her mother in particular. A careful and lengthy mental state examination by a senior registrar in the psychiatry of disability revealed, in addition, delusions of illness and apparent self-denigratory auditory hallucinations. The episodes of withdrawal occurred at a time of increased social pressure from peers because of her poor self-care. A diagnosis of depressive disorder was made and antidepressant medication started. In the course of the next month Melanie became increasingly disturbed and disinhibited in her behaviour. Her parents reported rather angrily that her condition was 'worse since the pills were started'. A further careful history and examination revealed that Melanie's mood had lifted but had continued to elevate, and that she was now in a hypomanic state.

Compulsory admission to hospital was arranged. Treatment with lithium and tranquillizing medication resulted in a stabilization of mood over the course of a few weeks. Unfortunately, Melanie's parents then decided that they could no longer accommodate her. A lengthy hospital stay followed, during the course of which Melanie's mood fluctuated markedly. She was eventually rehabilitated to a local staffed hostel where she was able, with continued psychiatric monitoring, to lead a more independent life. She progressed from the hostel to sharing a flat with a friend.

Further reading

Dickinson, M., Singh, I., 2010. Learning disability psychiatry. In: Puri, B.K., Treasaden, I. (Eds.), Psychiatry: an evidence-based text. Hodder Arnold, London.

Fraser, W., Kerr, M. (Eds.), 2003. Seminars in the psychiatry of learning disability. second ed. Gaskell, London.

Talbot, P., Astbury, G., Mason, T., 2010. Key concepts in learning disabilities. Sage, London.

Eating disorders

Eating disorders traditionally include anorexia nervosa, bulimia nervosa, obesity and psychogenic vomiting. In the USA over recent years 'binge eating disorder' has been added to this list. There has also been more interest in the feeding disorders of infancy (see Chapter 16). These conditions have evoked intense medical interest because they exemplify the interaction between psychological and somatic symptomatology.

Definitions and diagnostic criteria

The ICD-10 and DSM-IV-TR requirements for diagnoses of anorexia nervosa and bulimia nervosa are shown in Table 18.1. Although anorexia nervosa and bulimia nervosa are distinguished in ICD-10, the other diagnoses of 'atypical anorexia nervosa' and 'atypical bulimia nervosa' recognize that it is by no means agreed that they are distinct entities. In ICD-10 it is noted that patients with anorexia nervosa can progress to bulimia nervosa and vice versa. The situation is further confused by the suggestion by some researchers that it is appropriate to distinguish between patients with anorexia nervosa who maintain a low weight by restricting caloric intake ('restrictors') and those who use restriction together with the symptoms also seen in bulimia nervosa (vomiting, purging, excessive exercise, use of appetite suppressants and/or diuretics).

In childhood, in addition to the feeding disorders, an extreme regression – termed 'total refusal syndrome' – has been identified in a very small group of children. In this, a child not only refuses to eat, but also declines all other activity, including appropriate elimination.

Anorexia nervosa and bulimia nervosa

Epidemiology

The incidence and prevalence of eating disorders depends as always on the definition used and the population being considered. Generally speaking, anorexia and bulimia nervosa are disorders of white Caucasian young adult females of a higher social class and above-average academic achievement. The peak incidence for anorexia nervosa is around the age of 18; that for bulimia nervosa is slightly higher.

The incidence of anorexia nervosa is about eight cases per 100 000 per year, being highest in 15–19-year-old females. A two-stage screening survey showed a prevalence of anorexia nervosa of between 0.2% and 0.8%, with a higher prevalence in the upper social classes. A study of UK adolescent schoolgirls showed a prevalence of 1–2%, with the higher prevalence in private-school girls. In addition to those with a full diagnosis, a further 5% in these surveys show some features of anorexia nervosa.

The incidence of bulimia nervosa is about 12 cases per 100 000 per year. The prevalence of bulimia nervosa by current criteria is about 1%, and between 2% and 4.5% of school and college girls. Until the 1970s bulimia nervosa was thought of as a subvariant of anorexia nervosa, and so some of the earlier studies deflated figures because of this.

Table 18.1 ICD-10 and DSM-IV-TR classifications of eating disorders

ICD-10 criteria for eating disorder (F50)

F50.0 Anorexia nervosa

- Body weight maintained 15% below expected for age and height
- Weight loss self-induced by
  - — restriction of intake
  - — self-induced vomiting
  - — self-induced purging
  - — excessive exercise
  - — use of appetite suppressants or diuretics
- Morbid dread of fatness (overvalued idea)
- Self-set low weight threshold
- Disturbance of endocrine function to produce amenorrhoea in women and loss of sexual interest and potency in men (in prepubertal onset there is delay of puberty and growth restriction)

F50.1 Atypical anorexia nervosa

- Some of the above, or
- Above features to a mild degree

F50.2 Bulimia nervosa

- Bingeing, with preoccupation with food and craving of the same
- Attempts to counteract excess calorie intake by
  - — self-induced vomiting
  - — self-induced purging
  - — alternating periods of starvation
  - — use of appetite suppressants, diuretics, thyroid preparations or, in diabetes, neglect of insulin treatment
- Morbid dread of fatness
- Self-set low weight threshold
- Possible history of anorexia nervosa or atypical anorexia nervosa

F50.3 Atypical bulimia nervosa

- Some of the above (but not if predominant symptomatology is depressive, when a diagnosis of depression should be made)

F50.4 Overeating associated with other psychological disturbances

- Obesity from overeating as a reaction to stressful events where the overeating is the predominant symptom
- Excludes distress because of obesity and drug-induced obesity

F50.5 Vomiting associated with other psychological disturbances

- Psychogenic vomiting where no other mental disorder is diagnosed (includes psychogenic hyperemesis gravidarum)

DSM-IV-TR classification for eating disorder (307)

307.1 Anorexia nervosa *Specify type:* Restricting type; binge eating/purging type

307.51 Bulimia nervosa *Specify type:* Purging type/non-purging type

307.50 Eating disorder NOS

NOS, not otherwise specified.

Research criteria for binge eating disorder (classified under 307.50 above):

- Two or more episodes of binge eating over six or more months
- No recurrent purging, exercising or fasting

Continued

Table 18.1 ICD-10 and DSM-IV-TR classifications of eating disorders—cont'd

- Subjective sense of loss of control over binge eating
- PLUS three or more of the following signs. Eating
  - — more rapidly than usual
  - — large quantities of food when not physically hungry
  - — alone due to embarrassment
  - — until uncomfortably full and feeling self disgust

The male:female ratio for anorexia nervosa is 1:10, although there have been some suggestions that the incidence of anorexia nervosa in males is increasing. In prepubertal patients the sex ratio, although still predominantly female, is not so marked. For bulimia nervosa the male:female ratio is between 1:5 and 1:10.

Anorexia has been reported in patients of all ethnic origins, but it is still relatively rare in non-Caucasians. It is said to be increasing in cultures such as Japan, which are becoming more 'Westernized'.

The predominance of higher social classes is not so marked in young adolescents.

Definitions and epidemiology

- Eating disorders are most common in the young female population of the Western world.
- ICD-10 separates anorexia and bulimia nervosa as diagnostic entities, although there is a degree of overlap. Common to both is the 'morbid dread of fatness'.

Clinical features

Although the weight loss in anorexia nervosa may be rapid (particularly in exacerbations and later relapses), family members or colleagues do not usually notice the initial onset. Thus, there is usually a history of at least several weeks and often several months prior to presentation. Individual patients will often report some particular remark or event that triggered their restrictive eating. In anorexia nervosa this may initially consist of limiting the types of food taken, with a progressive diminution in the range eaten. The individual may take to eating separately and secretively. Some patients may take a particular interest in the preparation and presentation of food to others. Individuals may take to wearing baggy clothes that have the effect of disguising their weight loss.

Paradoxically, certainly in the initial stages the young person may appear more cheerful and, to outsiders, be working extra hard in school or employment. Individuals describe a satisfaction in 'control of weight', which may explain the sense of confidence displayed.

With dieting and progressive weight loss, apart from increasing cachexia, various bodily changes occur as a direct result (Figure 18.1). Profound effects on hormonal balance return hypothalamic–pituitary–gonadal hormones to a prepubertal pattern. In prepubertal

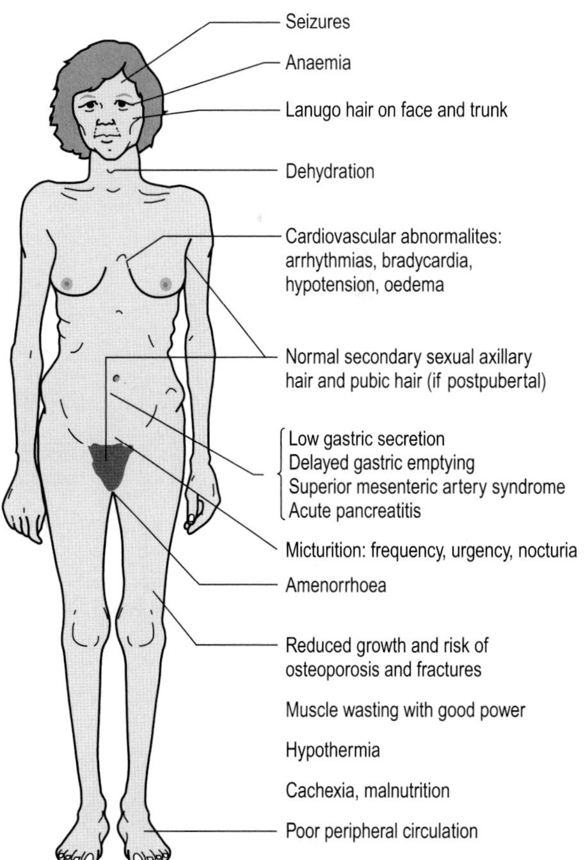

Figure 18.1 • Physical features associated with anorexia nervosa.

patients menarche is delayed. Effects on growth hormones produce a slowing or cessation of normal growth. If low weight is maintained for long enough, then final height may be stunted.

Amenorrhoea is usually related to reduction below a certain weight, although not infrequently it precedes the weight loss and may be maintained once an adequate weight is regained. In bulimia nervosa, and also in those with anorexia nervosa who use vomiting, purging, etc. to reduce their weight, a wide variety of menstrual irregularities can occur, including amenorrhoea.

In bulimia nervosa, extra medical complications occur in relation to the vomiting, purging and/or use of diuretics (Figure 18.2).

In anorexia nervosa, activity level is not a reliable indicator of the level of physical complications, as high levels of activity (including exercise, which may be used to further reduce weight) are often maintained at astonishingly low weights. Individuals may well increase their activity levels as their weight reduces.

At low weight sleep is disturbed, with difficulty settling, waking in the night and early morning wakening. Some weight-restrictive activities may be carried out secretly during periods of wakefulness.

It was recognized very early on that the use of the term anorexia (meaning loss of appetite) was a misnomer in anorexia nervosa, as the majority of sufferers will admit to extreme feelings of hunger and preoccupation with food, although this is often not admitted in the early stages to those close to them, and in some patients it is incorporated in a general pattern of denial of bodily sensation.

Low mood is very prominent in patients with anorexia nervosa and bulimia nervosa, particularly at low weight in the former. The symptoms can include the full biological array of symptoms (see Chapter 9), including sleep loss as mentioned above. In the majority of cases, the low mood resolves with return to normal weight. It must be noted that suicidal ideation and behaviour can occur in the context of this low mood. In bulimia nervosa, suicidal attempts and self-mutilation can be significant features.

Anorexia nervosa is distinguished from primary depressive disorder with its loss of appetite, loss of weight and low mood, and by the phenomenon variously described as 'morbid fear of fatness', 'weight phobia' and 'body image disturbance'. Although various experiments using distorting mirrors etc. have been used to demonstrate the apparent 'body-image' disturbance as a perceptual distortion, this phenomenon may be more accurately characterized as an overvalued idea regarding ideal weight. Such beliefs

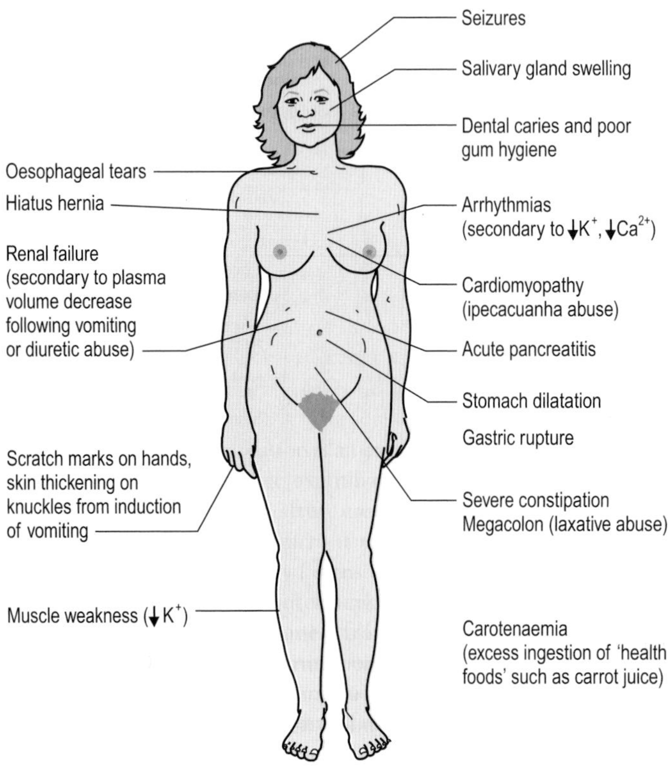

Figure 18.2 • Complications of vomiting, purging and diuretic abuse.

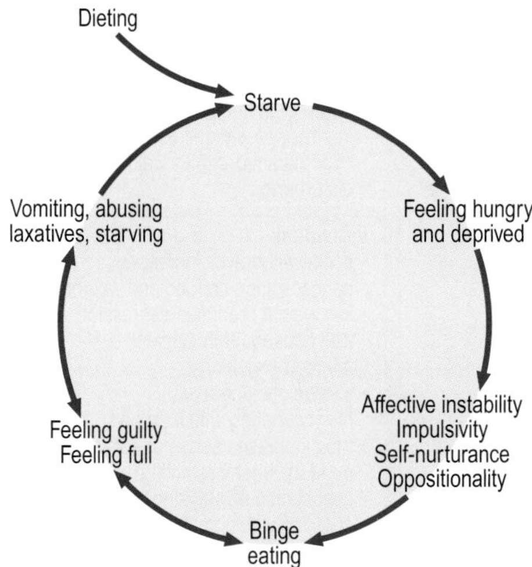

Figure 18.3 • Typical cycle in bulimia nervosa. (After Garfinkel PF, Garner DM 1982 Anorexia nervosa: a multidimensional perspective. Brunner Mazel, New York.)

may sometimes be held with almost delusional intensity. Studies of perceptual distortion are, at best, equivocal: it appears that overestimation of bodily dimensions is not pathognomonic of either anorexia or bulimia nervosa. In addition to the fear of fatness, there may also be self-denigration of bodily image and a low self-esteem. It is unclear whether this is related to 'body image' as such.

In bulimia nervosa, there is often a history of anorexia nervosa, and occasionally anorexia nervosa can be preceded by bulimic-type symptomatology. A typical cycle in bulimia nervosa is shown in Figure 18.3. It must be noted that there are very prominent psychological triggers and perpetuating factors that maintain the cycle.

'Bulimic' symptoms occur in 4–16% of patients with anorexia nervosa. It appears that there is a difference in attitude to hunger between those with anorexia, who may be described as 'restrictors', and those who may be termed 'bulimic'. In restrictors, there is a tendency to cherish the experience of hunger and associate it with a sense of mastery. There is also an ability to ignore the sensations of hunger. In those with bulimic symptoms, hunger makes them irritable and restless. Bingeing, used initially to control weight in bulimia nervosa, may later be associated with the relief of distressing emotions such as depression, guilt or anxiety.

The differential diagnosis of anorexia nervosa and bulimia nervosa is shown in Table 18.2.

Table 18.2 Differential diagnosis of anorexia nervosa and bulimia nervosa

Psychiatric	Depression Obsessive–compulsive disorder Personality disorder
Physical	Chronic debilitating disorders Neoplasia Thyroid disorder Intracranial space-occupying lesions Malabsorption syndromes Intestinal disorders, including Crohn's disease

Clinical features

- Patients with bulimia nervosa have normal or slightly above average weights.
- Those with anorexia nervosa are significantly underweight and have associated physical and psychological concomitants, most notably amenorrhoea and low mood.
- Bingeing and vomiting are dangerous activities because of their effect on the body electrolytes.

Aetiology

The aetiology of eating disorders can usefully be viewed using the biopsychosocial model (see Figure 18.4). From a development perspective these factors can also be divided according to whether they predispose, precipitate or perpetuate the symptomatology.

Low self-esteem is often observed clinically in both anorexia and bulimia, but this feature is one for which it is difficult to discriminate cause and effect. Low self-esteem also interacts with adverse life events or trauma (such as sexual abuse or bereavement), and is confounded with poor family relationships. The observations regarding family functioning (Figure 18.4), although purported to be aetiologically significant, may also be attributable to the very stressful experience of living with someone who is presenting an (apparently) self-imposed life-threatening disorder. Indeed, these features are also seen in families who have members with other 'psychosomatic' disorders.

In addition to the studies showing an increased incidence of eating disorders in first-degree relatives, it has also been observed that there are increased frequencies of mood disorder, and psychoactive and

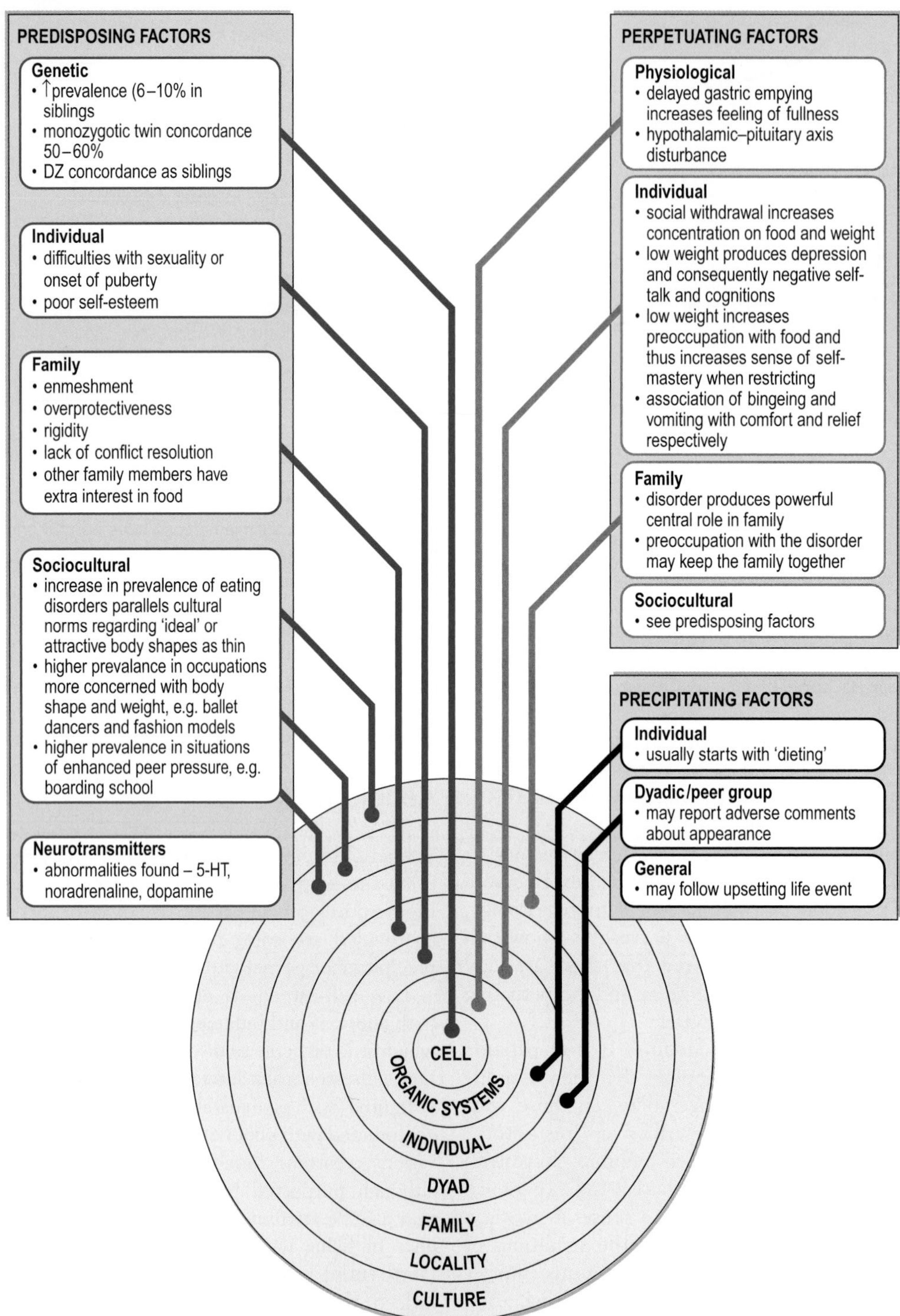

Figure 18.4 • Multifactorial aetiology of eating disorders.

substance misuse in the families of those with eating disorders. A disturbance of the hypothalamic–pituitary axis has been put forward as a causative factor. However, although such a disturbance is present, it is also seen in people who are of low weight for other reasons; therefore, it is more likely that hormonal changes are perpetuating rather than predisposing or precipitating factors.

A study of US male conscripts who entered a study on the effects of starvation rather than participate in military service is often quoted to illustrate the physical and psychological effects of significant weight reduction. The 36 men involved developed a preoccupation with food after a few weeks, and subsequently symptoms of depression, including sleep disturbance, low mood, lethargy and loss of libido. One even had to be hospitalized because of self-mutilation. Subjects reported indecision about whether to eat their reduced meals voraciously or to eat each morsel as slowly as possible. In the rehabilitation phase, bingeing behaviour and continued preoccupation with food was reported. These symptoms persisted for up to a year. However, it is possible to criticize this study on the basis of the self-selection of the subjects and the small number involved. Also, its relevance can be questioned given that the majority of those with eating disorders are female.

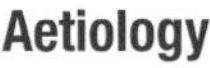

Aetiology

- The aetiology of eating disorders is still being researched, but is at present thought to be multifactorial, being a combination of cultural pressures, family attitudes, individual psychodynamics and genetic and biochemical susceptibility.
- Aetiological factors interact so that a self-perpetuating process or cycle occurs.

Management

Patients with eating disorders present a great challenge to professionals and often require lengthy, staff-intensive involvement.

Assessment

It is more than usually essential that a therapeutic relationship is established with the patient and family in which there is a degree of partnership and shared expectations. The young person is likely to be somewhat ambivalent about professional involvement, and in some circumstances may be overtly hostile. They may only be attending at the behest of concerned relatives or friends. This is particularly the case with the younger patient, and in anorexia nervosa. Thus, although the following paragraphs emphasize the information to be gained, more important is the assessment of motivation and the enhancement of engagement. A 'motivational' interviewing style (see Further reading) includes the five effective elements found in brief interventions. These are encompassed in the acronym FRAMES

- objective **f**eedback
- acceptance of personal **r**esponsibility for change
- direct **a**dvice
- a **m**enu of alternative treatments
- **e**mpathy
- **s**elf-efficacy.

This will allow some idea of the stage of motivation reached. Confrontation at any stage is likely to result in passive, if not active, resistance to change, and thus should be avoided if possible.

It is important to see the patient and the family both together and separately. The order in which this is done is a judgement that should be made in consultation after the initial introductions and explanations. The older the patient, the more appropriate it is to see them first and for longer.

Attitudes to weight, shape and eating should be carefully elicited, paying attention to the various means of weight restriction (these are often not proffered spontaneously). Eating patterns, and changes in such patterns, should be asked about as well as any adverse experiences or possible triggers. Family relationships should be explored, both in the individual interviews and when the family are seen together, and any pressures or conflicts identified together with family attitudes to eating and family history of psychiatric disorder.

A personal development history should be taken, with any earlier feeding problems noted. School progress is classically exemplary but this is by no means always the case, and so an educational history is important in order to avoid unwarranted assumptions, which might lead to later mistakes in management (e.g. using school attendance as an incentive for weight gain in someone who would really rather not go there). The view of the school (obtained with the patient's permission) can be helpful in gauging countertherapeutic pressures from the peer group or curriculum (such as the use of fat thickness callipers in physical education lessons!).

In all interviews it is advisable to avoid any comments about personal appearance as these are frequently misinterpreted (e.g. 'You look well' could lead to all sorts of soul searching about what you might be referring to).

In the mental state examination the presence of depressive symptomatology, including suicidal thoughts, should be carefully assessed. Obsessive–compulsive symptomatology should also be routinely enquired about.

A thorough physical examination should be carried out, including the patient's undressed weight and height, noting those features that confirm or deny the differential diagnosis. This may be done by the psychiatrist or arranged with another physician.

Investigations should particularly include the plasma electrolytes if there is a history of vomiting and purging. Care should be taken that the abnormalities in hormone levels associated with low weight are distinguished from those due to other causes.

Treatment

The primary aims in both anorexia and bulimia nervosa are to achieve functioning and attitudes of food, weight, shape and eating, which are 'healthy', or at least not physically, socially or psychologically handicapping. These end points are difficult to ascertain, given the sociocultural variation and the possible aetiological significance of such factors (e.g. a level of preoccupation with body shape that is to be expected in a fashion model may be incongruous in a bus driver). An essential intermediate aim in anorexia nervosa is weight restoration. In bulimia nervosa, the equivalent aims are to achieve a regular pattern of eating without bingeing, vomiting, purging or periods of extreme restriction.

It is important once the diagnosis is established to clearly state this and explore the implications, both real and imagined. Guilt and feelings of self-blame in the patient, family and friends can be significant barriers to progress, and can lead to extreme sensitivity to even implied criticism. This requires a degree of empathy with the patient and his or her confidants, so that potentially distressing emotions such as anger or fear can be examined and acknowledged.

Weight restoration in anorexia nervosa is achieved by controlled re-feeding. This is often a difficult and lengthy process. Outsiders can often greatly underestimate how frightening this process is for the young person involved. In order to regain weight, an above-average ratio of caloric intake to energy use must be achieved. This may be up to 3500 kcal per day, which is equivalent to the average daily intake of a healthy male manual worker. Problems arise because the increased bulk involved, combined with the delayed gastric emptying, which occurs at low weight, leads to complaints of feelings of fullness and an increased urge to vomit. Smaller, more frequent meals, a gradual increase in caloric intake and the use of high-calorie dietary supplements to a normal diet can at least partially circumvent this. The supplements have been criticized for their high cost and the possibility that they may be incorporated into a later distorted eating pattern.

There is no consensus among clinicians and researchers regarding:

- the advisability of determining a target weight
- how to do it
- whether it is better to specify a particular weight or a range of weights
- whether the weight should be set unilaterally or by negotiation.

Target weights may be derived from: tables of average weights for height and age; from tables that relate height to the weight at which menstruation should be resumed (on the basis that this is indicative of resumption of normal hormonal balance); or may be determined as the average weight for the age at which the eating disorder commenced (on the basis that the patient has to return to face the conflicts that were being avoided at that stage by losing weight).

Advice from a dietician can be beneficial, especially in the early stages of involvement. Those patients with bulimia can be helped to plan their intake to be more regular and ordered.

The multifactorial aetiology of eating disorders suggests a multicomponent treatment programme, and indeed most specialist centres recommend this. There is variation between centres in the particular emphasis placed on particular treatment modalities, perhaps reflecting the relative lack of consensus and research regarding the most effective approaches. It is important to be aware of the differences between individual patients in deciding the most appropriate combination of treatments. The range of treatments used is illustrated in Figure 18.5.

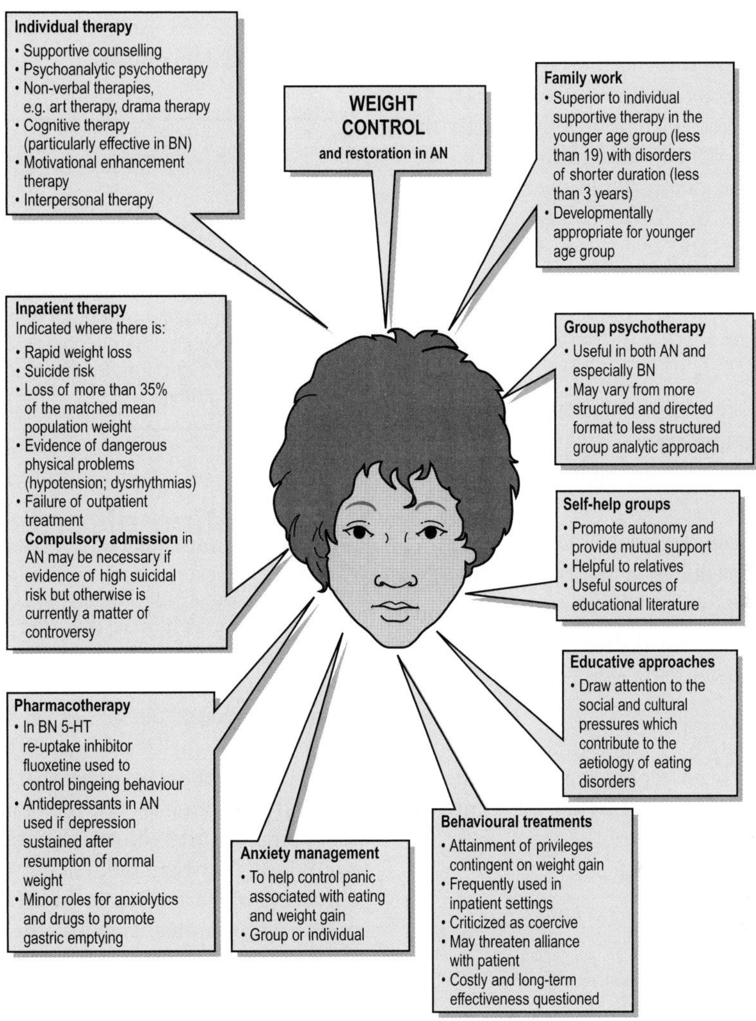

Figure 18.5 • Treatment of eating disorders.

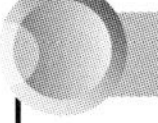

Management

- Negotiation of the treatment approach requires careful discussion with all the parties involved, but especially with the patient.
- Treatment may involve both group and individual therapies, including educational and self-help approaches.
- Inpatient treatments are still frequently employed but are increasingly being reserved for the more severe or complicated cases.

Prognosis

Morbidity

Outcome studies are hampered by high failure-to-trace rates and the increased likelihood of non-cooperation in those still suffering an eating disorder. At five to 15 year follow-up, 24–82% of patients with anorexia have recovered (meta-analysis), whereas a German study found that 70% of bulimia patients had recovered after inpatient treatment at 12-year follow-up.

Mortality

Follow-up studies have shown a mortality in anorexia of up to 5% over four to five years and may reach 20% over 20 years. Longer term follow-up shows that more patients improved, but also more died (although the rate of death diminishes with time). Just over two-thirds of deaths are a result of the effects of starvation, and one-third are by suicide. There are some recent data that suggest that competent treatment reduces mortality significantly. The following factors are predictors for death in anorexia:

- body mass <35 kg at presentation
- > one inpatient admission
- history of psychiatric hospitalization for anorexia
- psychoactive substance misuse
- longer duration of illness at treatment start
- poor social adjustment
- hospitalization for a mood disorder
- suicidality associated with comorbid psychiatric disorder.

An increase in mortality of six times the normal population risk has been reported for anorexia and nine times for bulimia. Predictors for poor outcome in bulimia include

- psychoactive substance misuse
- poor impulse control
- premorbid obesity
- lifetime history of anorexia nervosa
- older age at illness onset
- comorbid mood disorder
- poor social adjustment.

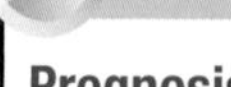

Prognosis

- Eating disorders have a high continued morbidity, which is often concealed.
- There is a mortality of around one in 20 for eating disorders. Approximately one-third of deaths are by suicide and two-thirds from the complications of disordered eating.

Binge eating disorder

In DSM-IV-TR, this has recently been identified as a separate psychiatric disorder (see Table 18.1). In a general US community sample, a prevalence of 1.8% was found, with a prevalence of 8% in a subgroup designated obese. In a weight reduction programme the incidence was 30%.

Although proponents argue that there are clinically meaningful differences between bulimia nervosa and binge eating disorder, others argue that both are part of a continuum between bulimia nervosa and obesity.

Successful treatments include behavioural weight control programmes, cognitive behavioural therapy and interpersonal therapies. In most studies, however, there is a high drop out from treatment, thus overestimating success rates.

Case history: anorexia nervosa

Janine, aged 17, attended with her younger sister Brigid, 15, and her parents, with a four-month history of slow weight loss from 57 kg to 46 kg, followed by a recent rapid weight loss to 40 kg in the course of the previous three weeks. She wore a large baggy jumper with 'Foods of the World' on it and looked sullen but alert as her parents anxiously recounted the background. Janine was a hard-working, high-achieving pupil who had taken to eating her meals in her room a year previously, 'so she could have longer with her books', and around this time had also announced that she was vegetarian.

The family had not noticed the weight loss at first, although they had remarked on her slender appearance on the family summer holiday (and had been irritated by her insistence on wearing a baggy T-shirt over her swimsuit). The parents had taken Janine to the family GP when, having found rotting food in the shrubbery below her windows, they had confronted her and she had collapsed in tears, expressing her sorrow at 'wasting good food'. The parents were particularly upset as they prided themselves on their closeness to their children.

All the family were either thin or of average build. When seen alone, Janine confirmed that she felt she was fat and feared gaining weight as she 'knew what it was to be obese'. Her dieting had started after a 'health

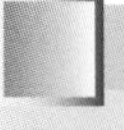

Case history: anorexia nervosa—cont'd

education' lesson in which she had been the guinea pig in a demonstration of triceps skinfold callipers – the male teacher had joked about the measurement. She had stopped menstruating three months previously. She denied bingeing, vomiting or purging, but had been exercising in her room when she could not sleep at night. She expressed annoyance at being brought along to see the psychiatrist but had been pleasantly surprised at being addressed in her own right for a long interview. No suicidal ideation was elicited, but Janine admitted to a sustained low mood and wished for help with this.

Janine expressed a preference for being seen alone but agreed that her family would also require some support, so individual sessions were arranged on a weekly basis, with slightly less frequent family meetings (with a different therapist). Careful attention was paid to explaining the physical and psychiatric complications of low weight. A re-feeding regime was instituted, which, although initially resisted, produced a reduction in the rate of weight loss, a levelling out and then a gradual increase in, weight. A weight for height was calculated at Janine's request, but led to repeated arguments with her family and therapist. Eventually, Janine withdrew from treatment saying she was 'misunderstood', and cited her therapist quoting something said by another patient as an example of 'not being regarded as an individual'. A follow-up appointment six months later was attended only by Janine's parents, who reported that she was still low in weight but no longer losing.

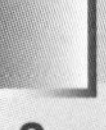

Case history: bulimia nervosa

Charlotte, 23, contacted a specialist service for those with eating disorders complaining of bingeing and vomiting over four years. The behaviour was worse at times of increased stress, such as after her marriage to a leading businessman four years previously, and following the recent death of her father. She had chosen to consult her GP when she had received a letter from her bank manager regarding an unauthorized overdraft on her personal account, which had followed a series of orders from 'Dial-a-pizza' outlets near her home. There had been a series of rows with her husband and mother-in-law.

She presented as well-dressed but slightly overweight for her height. She was tearful and remorseful, and expressed feelings of worthlessness. On direct questioning she admitted to having taken a small overdose of paracetamol a year previously, which she had 'slept off' without telling anyone. Charlotte said she still occasionally felt like harming herself after a large binge. She complained of continuing marital discord.

Charlotte was not agreeable to pursuing the suggested group treatment programme, but agreed to see an individual therapist to look at the cycle of bingeing and dieting in which she found herself. After six sessions she was still preoccupied with food but her bingeing and vomiting occurred only once every three weeks or so. She suffered a relapse after having successfully negotiated a separation from her husband. However, with further therapy, which focused on issues related to self-esteem, she regained a more ordered eating pattern. She withdrew from treatment because of 'pressure of work' in her newly established Cordon Bleu catering company.

Further reading

Bowman, G., 2006. Thin: a memoir of anorexia and recovery. Penguin, London.

Cooper, P.J., 2009. Overcoming bulimia nervosa and binge-eating: a self-help guide using cognitive behavioral techniques, third ed. Robinson, London.

Crisp, A.H., 1995. Anorexia nervosa: let me be. Lawrence Erlbaum Associates, Hove.

Freeman, C., 2009. Overcoming anorexia nervosa: a self-help guide using cognitive behavioral techniques, second ed. Robinson, London.

Garner, D.M., Garfinkel, P.E. (Eds.), 1997. Handbook of treatments for eating disorders. Guilford, New York.

Treasure, J.L., 1997. Escaping from anorexia nervosa. Psychology Press, Hove.

Webb, K., Zadeh, E., Mountford, V., Lacey, J.H., 2010. Eating disorders. In: Puri, B.K., Treasaden, I. (Eds.), Psychiatry: an evidence-based text. Hodder Arnold, London.

Cultural psychiatry

This chapter considers the presentation of psychiatric disorders in non-Western populations, including immigrants to Western countries. This is followed by a brief description of specific disorders that occur in certain non-Western countries, known as *culture-bound syndromes*.

Culture has been defined as describing the sum of learned knowledge and skills, including religion and language, which distinguishes one community from another and passes on in a recognizable form from generation to generation. Ethnic minorities share a cultural heritage and may experience discrimination. Ethnicity should be self-assigned and not based on country of birth.

Presentation of psychiatric disorders

Depression

A number of cultures do not have a word for our modern day term, depression. Although depression is widespread, its symptomatology varies between countries. Christian cultures show more guilt and suicidal ideas, whereas other cultures show more paranoia (e.g. some African and South American cultures). The lifetime prevalence of depression has been found to vary widely in different groups. For example, studies published during the first decade of the 21st century have reported a lifetime prevalence of 5.5% in American Indian tribes, 6.9% in Los Angeles Chinese Americans, 8.0% in Mexican-Americans (living in the USA), 10.4% in white Americans and 21% in Chinese American women.

Immigrants to Western countries who are of non-Western origin may not tell their doctor that they feel depressed or low when they are suffering from depression. Afro-Caribbean men, for example, may instead complain of erectile dysfunction or reduced libido. Those from the Indian subcontinent often somatize their depressive symptoms, talking instead of stomach pains, for example.

It is clearly important to have a low threshold for identifying an underlying depressive illness in such cases. Appropriate investigations of physical illnesses that can cause low mood, such as tuberculosis, should be carried out when a depressed mood has been uncovered.

Suicide rates may be low among those who adhere to particular religious beliefs that condemn suicide (e.g. Judaism, Roman Catholicism and Islam), although there may be an otherwise increased acceptance of some specific forms of ceremonial or other suicide acts, for example dowry suicides among Hindus when dowries cannot be met. Historical examples include Hindu suttee, when the widow throws herself on her husband's funeral pyre, and Japanese hara-kiri (seppuku) (disembowelment) among Japanese soldiers.

Schizophrenia

The prevalence of schizophrenia is similar throughout the world when standardized interviewing techniques are used (e.g. the present state examination

(PSE)), despite apparent local higher rates. In the past in the USA, schizophrenia was diagnosed in cases where UK psychiatrists would have diagnosed mood (affective) disorder, and in Russia a diagnosis of slow schizophrenia was applied to cases, which in the UK would have been labelled personality disorder. However, high rates (two to three times the national rate) have been reported for isolated populations in northern Sweden and for parts of Finland. Interestingly, Norwegian immigrants in the USA have been reported as having higher rates of psychotic symptoms.

Transient hallucinations, unsystematized (often paranoid) delusions, excitement and confusion have been found to be more common in Africa, and catatonic symptoms are more common in India. The outcome of schizophrenia in terms of symptoms and social functioning has been found to be better in developing countries, which may reflect the differing demands placed on patients and the way they are supported.

Some people of Afro-Caribbean origin believe in voodoo and the like, so that the expression of such beliefs does not necessarily imply that they are delusional. It is very helpful in such cases to speak to an informant from the subject's community, in order to ascertain whether the beliefs of the subject are out of keeping with those of that community. A similar consideration relates to religious beliefs in general.

In the UK much controversy has arisen over the veracity of studies showing a ninefold increase in psychosis among Afro-Caribbeans in the UK, especially among those of second-generation immigrants, compared with white British people. There is no such increase in their country of origin (e.g. the West Indies), i.e. it is not genetic. (A sixfold increase in psychosis in black African immigrants in the UK has also been found reported.) Controversy also surrounds why Afro-Caribbean individuals are more likely to be detained in psychiatric hospitals, especially in secure forensic facilities. Reasons given include: stress resulting from racial discrimination, including the consequent increase in unemployment; a greater stigma attached to mental disorders, leading to later presentation; differing sources of referral for psychiatric care (whites via GPs and Afro-Caribbeans via the police and courts); and being more likely to reside in more deprived, high-crime areas of the UK, leading to more law involvement and increased identification of mental illness as a result. Others have suggested misdiagnosis or diagnostic disagreements between Jamaican and British psychiatrists.

Other psychiatric disorders

Anorexia and bulimia nervosa are more common in developed Western countries, whereas dissociative (conversion) disorders and organic mental disorders resulting from infections and nutritional problems are more common in developing countries.

Multiple personality disorder is being increasingly diagnosed in the USA, but appears to be still very rare in the UK. This may reflect a culture-specific syndrome or even an iatrogenic disorder induced by the style of working of US psychiatrists and psychotherapists. Childhood hyperkinetic (attention-deficit) disorder is also diagnosed and treated more frequently in the USA than in the UK.

Migration

Overall, migrants tend to have an increased incidence of psychiatric disorder, but this is not invariable as shown by Indian immigrants to the UK. The impact of migration may vary depending on whether such individuals move of their own free will or are refugees. Mental illness may cause sufferers to migrate (social selection), but so may being a bright, energetic, go-ahead individual. Migration itself may result in stress, which precipitates mental illness. After arrival social and cultural conflicts may arise in a new society and, together with discrimination and minority status, lead to mental disorder (social causation).

Acculturation conflicts occur over having to reconcile parental traditions with the demands and opportunities of a new environment. Such conflicts may be more important in precipitating mental disorder than socioeconomic differences and relative deprivation of migrants compared with the host country. Among first-generation immigrants suicide rates are generally low, reflecting positive immigration selectivity and country of origin rates. Later generations have rates that converge to or even exceed local rates due to host country effects and acculturation conflicts. Such effects may be compounded by geographical isolation and low rates of help seeking among particular immigrant groups.

Culture-bound syndromes (Figure 19.1)

Amok

In this condition, which is seen in south-east Asia, there is an outburst of aggressive behaviour following a depressive episode. The patient literally 'runs amok' (the Malay word means to engage furiously in battle), and the situation may only come to an end after the patient has killed himself or has been killed by others, often after having killed others first.

Koro

Koro is seen in south-east Asia, particularly in Malaysians of Chinese extraction, and in parts of China. It occurs in men, who have an overwhelming fear that their penis is retracting into the abdomen and that death will occur immediately thereafter. Patients exhibit an acute anxiety state and may resort to tying a string around the penis or trying to clamp it. Koro is not a psychotic disorder but is instead considered to be an anxiety disorder and culture-based belief.

Latah

This occurs in the Far East and North Africa, and is a dissociative state in which patients exhibit echolalia, echopraxia and automatic obedience.

Piblokto or Arctic hysteria

This is a dissociative state seen among the Eskimo, more often in women. During attacks, typically lasting up to two hours, the patient begins to scream and cry and tear off her clothing. She may run wildly on the ice and risk her life from the low temperature. Following the episode there is usually amnesia for the attack and the patient may appear normal again.

Susto or Espanto

This condition occurs in the high Andes. Patients suffer from a prolonged depressive episode, which is believed by them to result from supernatural agencies.

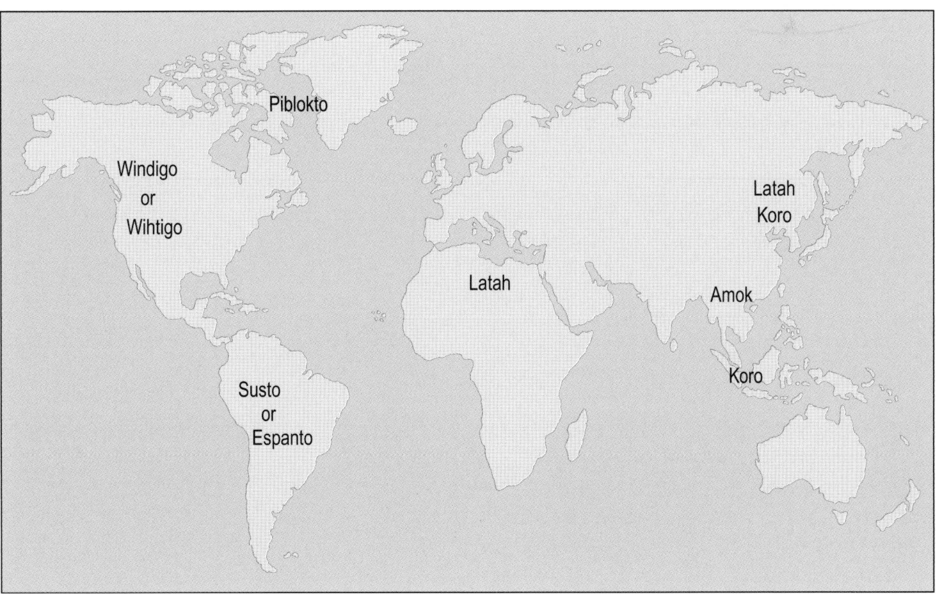

Figure 19.1 • Culture-bound syndromes.

Windigo or wihtigo

This occurs in North American Indian tribes. While suffering from a depressed mood, patients believe they have mutated into cannibalistic monsters.

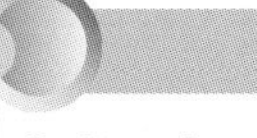

Cultural psychiatry

- Cultural psychiatry is the study of the differences between prevention, detection and management of psychiatric disorders and the maintenance of mental health in varied cultures.
- Depressive symptomatology varies between cultures, e.g. Christian cultures show more guilt and suicidal ideas.
- Although the prevalence of schizophrenia is similar throughout the world, its presentation differs, e.g. transient hallucinations, unsystematized delusions

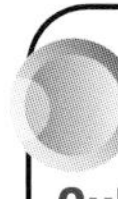

Cultural psychiatry—cont'd

and excitement are more common in Africa; catatonic symptoms are more common in India.
- Schizophrenia is more common in many immigrant groups to Western countries.
- Schizophrenia tends to have a better prognosis in Third World countries.
- Anorexia nervosa and bulimia nervosa are more common in Western countries.
- Dissociative (conversion) disorders and organic mental disorders caused by infectious and nutritional problems are more common in the Third World.
- Multiple personality disorder and childhood hyperactive disorders are more commonly diagnosed in the USA compared to the UK.
- Certain syndromes are 'culture-bound' or unique to specific population groups.

Further reading

Bhugra, D., Bhui, K. (Eds.), 2007. Textbook of cultural psychiatry. Cambridge University Press, Cambridge.

Bhugra, D., Cross, S., 2010. Cultural psychiatry. In: Puri, B.K., Treasaden, I. (Eds.), Psychiatry: an evidence-based text. Hodder Arnold, London.

Leff, J., 1988. Psychiatry around the globe: a transcultural view. Gaskell, London.

Lipsedge, M., Littlewood, R., 1979. Transcultural psychiatry. In: Granville-Grossman, K.L. (Ed.), Recent advances in clinical psychiatry3, Churchill Livingstone, Edinburgh.

Lipsedge, M., Littlewood, R., 1997. Aliens and alienists: ethnic minorities and psychiatry, third ed. Routledge, London (or Taylor & Francis, e-book).

is antipsychotic medication, which should be given in low doses. It is also important in such patients to try to overcome their social isolation by involving social services and, for example, encouraging them to attend a day hospital and engage in appropriate group activities.

Medication

The side-effects of medication to be taken by elderly patients should be carefully considered before they are prescribed. For example, those that cause postural hypotension (e.g. antipsychotics and tricyclic antidepressants) may cause the patient to fall and suffer a fracture.

Many elderly patients take more than one drug already, for example diuretics and non-steroidal anti-inflammatory drugs. The risks of side-effects increase with polypharmacy, and a careful review should be carried out to determine whether all the drugs are absolutely necessary in a given case.

Sedatives and anxiolytics, including benzodiazepines, are overprescribed to the elderly in many countries. In addition to the problems of dependency (see Chapter 3), increased sensitivity in this age group leads to an increased risk of postural instability, hangover sedation and impairment of cognitive and psychomotor performance.

Antidepressants

There are particular problems with the use of tricyclic antidepressants in the elderly. With advancing years, impairment of the functions of important organs results in changes in bioavailability, distribution and clearance, which, in turn, may lead to an increased elimination half-life of antidepressants, a lower volume of distribution and reduced clearance. This, in turn, may cause significantly higher steady-state plasma concentrations. Therefore, lower doses of tricyclic antidepressants, including their starting doses, should generally be used in the elderly.

Antimuscarinic (anticholinergic) side-effects of tricyclic antidepressants worsen pre-existing somatic problems in the elderly, and so diminish their quality of life. In addition, they can lead to poor compliance.

Antidepressants that cause postural hypotension may lead to falls in the elderly. The side-effect of dry mouth may make it difficult for elderly patients to wear dentures. Urinary retention may lead to anuria. Cardiovascular side-effects may cause myocardial or cerebral infarction. Central antimuscarinic side-effects such as impaired concentration, loss of memory and delirium are dangerous in the elderly.

Drug interactions are more common in the elderly owing to polypharmacy and can be dangerous.

Selective serotonin reuptake inhibitors (SSRIs) and the reversible inhibitors of monoamine oxidase (RIMAs) moclobemide are generally tolerated better than tricyclic antidepressants in the elderly. In the cases of citalopram, escitalopram and paroxetine, however, the maximum daily dose recommended for the elderly is lower than that which is recommended in younger adults. In the case of escitalopram, initially half the younger adult dose should be used, and a lower maintenance dose may suffice.

Psychiatry of the elderly

- There is an increasing elderly population in most countries.
- Twenty-five per cent of people over the age of 65 suffer from a psychiatric disorder, with dementia and depression being particularly common.
- Psychiatric services for the elderly should offer domiciliary assessment, community nursing, day hospital care, respite inpatient admissions and liaison with physicians.
- Depressive pseudodementia is an important differential in the diagnosis of dementia.
- The management of dementia may include support for carers, occupational therapy, reality orientation, reminiscence therapy and sheltered accommodation or long-stay inpatient admission.
- Depression may present atypically.
- There is a high risk of suicide in elderly socially isolated depressed patients.
- Paraphrenia is associated with social isolation and sensory deprivation.
- Medication should be used with care in the elderly and polypharmacy avoided whenever possible.

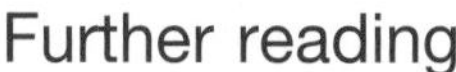

Further reading

Ames, D., O'Brien, J., Burns, A. (Eds.), 2010. Dementia. fourth ed. Hodder Arnold, London.

Baldwin, R.C., 1991. Depression: under-diagnosed and under-treated. Geriatric Medicine 21, 15.

Benjamin, B., Burns, A., 2010. Old-age psychiatry. In: Puri, B.K., Treasaden, I. (Eds.), Psychiatry: an evidence-based text. Hodder Arnold, London.

Bennett, G., 1994. Alzheimer's disease and other confusional states. Optima, London.

Jacoby, R., Oppenheimer, C. (Eds.), 2002. Psychiatry in the elderly. third ed. Oxford University Press, Oxford.

Pitt, B., 1988. Psychogeriatrics: an overview. Health Visit 61, 247.

Forensic psychiatry

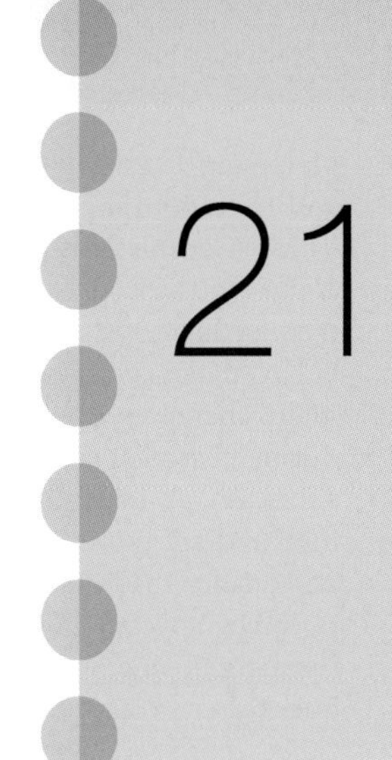

Introduction

Forensic psychiatry is the application of psychiatric knowledge to issues related to the courts and law. The principal work of forensic psychiatrists is the assessment of and preparation of psychiatric reports for the court on mentally abnormal offenders and their treatment. In practice, however, nearly all general psychiatrists will have to undertake such work on their own or new patients from time to time. In addition, forensic psychiatrists are also asked to provide advice on the management of aggressive and other severely behaviourally disturbed patients, who may not have been formally charged with offences or reached the court, for example very aggressive inpatients in ordinary psychiatric hospitals.

Forensic psychiatrists in the UK are most often based in secure psychiatric hospitals, such as Medium Secure Units or Special Hospitals, such as Broadmoor, but they frequently undertake work in prisons to provide reports for the courts on those on remand in prison awaiting trial and to advise the prison medical service on the psychiatric management of particular inmates. Forensic psychiatrists have characteristically undertaken specialist forensic psychiatry training and are not formally legally trained. However, they are often more familiar than most lawyers with the legal issues surrounding the field of mentally abnormal offenders.

The term 'forensic' comes from the Roman forum where offenders were tried. The Romans took the view that the mad were punished enough by their madness and should not be additionally punished (Satis Furore Punitor). The Bethlem Hospital in London was given cash from the early 19th century to take mentally disordered offenders, but due to the resulting stigma associated with such patients, which persists today, they were eventually placed in a new facility, the State Criminal Lunatic Asylum, which opened in 1863, following the Criminal Lunatics Asylums Act of 1860, and which was later renamed Broadmoor Hospital, the first of the special hospitals.

Special hospitals

In the UK, as constituted under the National Health Service Act of 1977, special hospitals are for individuals subject to detention who also require treatment under conditions of special (i.e. maximum) security on account of their 'violent, dangerous or criminal propensities'. Such patients are an immediate and grave danger to others, either to the public or to staff and patients in hospital. The level of security in special hospitals is equivalent to that of a security Category B prison in terms of preventing a patient escaping, but not in terms of preventing people breaking in to obtain an individual's release, as in Category A prisons.

The three special hospitals in England are Broadmoor Hospital in Berkshire, Rampton Hospital in Nottinghamshire and Ashworth Hospital in Liverpool. Rampton Hospital provides for all English female special hospital cases. Rampton and Broadmoor Hospitals also currently have dangerous and severe personality disorder (DSPD) units, but these are to be run down. These hospitals have the advantage of having large sites, facilitating greater freedom and therapeutic activities than less secure units.

Most admissions to special hospitals in the UK come via the courts. Some patients are transferred from ordinary psychiatric hospitals, where they have behaved dangerously, but may not have been formally charged with offences. Others are transferred during custodial sentences from prison. Women are admitted at least five times less frequently than men and are more likely to be civilly detained, have personality disorder and be suicidal.

Such special hospitals and their equivalents throughout the world have in the past been frequently criticized concerning their physical conditions, repressive regimes and the maltreatment of patients by staff. They have often tended to develop in isolation from the developments of practice in ordinary psychiatric facilities. A number of official enquiries have commented on the abuse of patients in such facilities, which have arisen due to the combination of poorly trained staff and a difficult-to-manage patient population among other factors. In the UK, the Fallon Inquiry in 1999 severely criticized the lack of control in a special unit for those with personality disorder in Ashworth Special Hospital. Such hospitals have been described as being in a 'no-win' situation, being criticized for keeping patients in too long, or letting the wrong ones out who, on occasions, may kill or otherwise behave dangerously again, often many years later. However, the latter may have more to do with the patients' subsequent situation or their psychiatric follow-up than with decisions made by the hospitals themselves. It can be difficult, in any case, to assess whether a patient will be dangerous in the community while he is still in a secure, single-sex ward without access to, for instance, alcohol, drugs or potential victims. The risk of re-offending is, however, long term. Nonetheless, such hospitals clearly fulfil a need in many countries, with the demand for admissions often exceeding capacity. Of relevance is Penrose's law, which was based on a 1936 study of different European countries and states that a higher national homicide rate correlates with a lower national number of psychiatric hospital beds.

Medium secure units

These were set up in England on a regional basis (hence the previous term Regional Secure Units) following the Butler and Glancy Reports of 1975 in response to an unmet need for secure care. This arose from the open-door policy since the early 1950s of ordinary psychiatric hospitals, overcrowding in special hospitals and increasing numbers of mentally abnormal offenders in prisons needing inpatient psychiatric treatment. Mentally abnormal offenders were sent by the courts to ordinary psychiatric hospitals after conviction; they would then abscond and reoffend, but not so dangerously as to require special hospital admission. They would end up in prison again, and the vicious cycle of admission and reoffending continued.

Medium secure units were set up for those whose severely disruptive and/or dangerous behaviour requires psychiatric treatment in conditions of medium security, i.e. more than that available in ordinary hospitals but less than that in special hospitals, and who also have a prospect of responding to secure care within about 18 months. However, provisions for longer stay patients in medium secure units have now also been developed. Many patients have committed dangerous offences such as homicide, rape and arson. The majority suffer from severe (psychotic) mental illness, mainly schizophrenia. Aggressive psychopaths are not considered suitable for such units, as there is no definite evidence that they are amenable to treatment within the maximum recommended duration of admission. The severely mentally handicapped are also excluded, as they can generally be managed within locked units of hospitals for the mentally handicapped.

In general, patients admitted to medium secure units are detained under the 1983 Mental Health Act. The largest number (at least 40%) come via the courts, having dangerously offended. Most, up to 90%, are male, but more recently women's enhanced medium secure (WEMS) units have been developed, the 'enhanced' referring to the therapeutic input rather than level of security. Such units have allowed chronic behaviourally disturbed females to be transferred from special hospitals.

Over a third of patients have been transferred from special hospitals as a graded step in their rehabilitation to conditions of less security and, ultimately, the community. Some patients are admitted from prison, either while on remand awaiting trial or after becoming mentally ill during a custodial sentence. Others are transferred from ordinary psychiatric hospital facilities. Most patients admitted to medium secure units are either discharged to the community, often to supervised hostels, or transferred to ordinary psychiatric facilities. A few require transfer to a special hospital.

The National Adolescent Forensic Network in the UK has now developed medium secure units for 12–18-year-olds with severe mental illness who have committed serious offences (five in number to date).

The number of places available in specialized secure psychiatric facilities is limited compared to the large number of mentally abnormal offenders. Thus, most mentally abnormal offenders continue to be dealt with by ordinary psychiatric hospitals as either in- or outpatients.

Low secure units often admit, under locked conditions, chronic behaviourally disturbed, sometimes violent, patients who have less seriously offended. Locked psychiatric intensive care units are usually for acutely mentally ill individuals who are violent, destructive or suicidal and length of admission is usually short (less than two months).

Community forensic psychiatry

Forensic psychiatry services have historically been institutionally based and for mentally disordered individuals who present substantial or a persistent risk to others. However, increasingly, specific forensic psychiatry outpatient services are being developed, which should offer specialist skills not available to non-forensic teams, e.g. anger management and specific brief treatments. These services may be either parallel to those of adult general psychiatry services or integrated with them, and have had a duty to cooperate with Multi-Agency Public Protection Arrangements (MAPPAs) since 2003.

Crime and psychiatry

Psychological motives for crime can be found in nearly all offenders, and this has led to psychiatric and, in particular, psychoanalytic interest since the time of Freud. The problem has been that this has not led to successful psychological treatments for offenders in general. Crime is now increasingly seen as a sociological phenomenon, better explained by sociological theories than by individual psychological ones. Psychiatric explanations for an offence, although providing understanding of the offender, do not necessarily provide an excuse for, nor remove legal responsibility from, him or her, although this is often perceived by the public to be the case. Psychiatrists are trained to detect the presence or absence of psychiatric disorder: they are not especially equipped to assess a defendant's responsibility for his actions, which is a legal concept. It is, of course, a philosophical question as to whether an individual in fact has complete free will: our response to events is due to the combination of our genes, previous experience and the current stresses in our life. There is also a tension between the legal system's attempt to clarify whether an individual offender is either mad and therefore in need of psychiatric treatment, or bad and in need of punishment, and the often multifactorial psychiatric explanations of behaviour. Offending is not a characteristic symptom of any mental disorder, and an offender's behaviour may arise from a combination of mental illness, premorbid personality difficulties and background.

The courts are in general, however, sympathetic to offers of psychiatric treatment as an alternative to other sentences, particularly custodial ones which are generally known to be ineffective, although guaranteeing that an individual will not offend for the period of sentence. Occasionally, the court can be dismissive of psychiatric evidence, especially as this may be perceived as being based largely on the history obtained from the individual (e.g. whether or not he says he hears voices).

A psychiatric assessment is particularly likely to be requested if there is no apparent motive for an offence, if the offender is female rather than male, and in cases of sexual offending. Even where the psychiatrist does not consider that an individual suffers from a specific mental disorder or is amenable to psychiatric treatment, the court may be assisted in sentencing by the psychological understanding provided by a psychiatric assessment.

For instance, although a theft may appear to be committed for financial gain, it will rarely be the entire explanation and other motivations, such as excitement, may be important. For example, those with personality difficulties may be unable to sustain relationships or work, and find life generally unrewarding and meaningless; they may obtain 'kicks' not only from alcohol and drug abuse, but also from the excitement of offending. One reason burglars may urinate in the homes they enter is such excitement, sometimes compounded by alcohol abuse, which itself may have given them the courage to offend. Such behaviour may also be an act of defilement. Burglars may also find it exciting creeping around while the owners are at home and asleep and, on occasions, the excitement generated may lead to a serious offence such as rape. At a deeper unconscious psychological level, offenders may, for instance, be standing up to their parents or stealing to obtain symbolic affection.

Aspects of criminology

Crime is socially determined and varies between societies and over time. In the past in the UK, both suicide and certain homosexual acts were illegal. Hence the saying that the major cause of crime is the law. Studies indicate that almost everyone commits a crime at some time in their life. Thus, there is a less clear cut-off between offenders and non-offenders than is generally assumed. Most crime goes undetected and crime statistics may merely reflect changes in detection rates, or a reduced tolerance of the public to a particular behaviour and/or increased police recording of offending, rather than, for instance, a real increase in crime. Increasing police numbers is thus likely to increase the number of offences detected and recorded. Currently, about 60% of offending in the UK is motor vehicle-related. The British Crime Survey collects information independently from the police and suggests nearly twice as much crime may be committed (over 10 million crimes per year) than is reported to the police (about five million crimes). The best deterrent appears to be the certainty of arrest rather than the severity of punishment.

Although certain categories of crime may have increased over the last 25 years, it is likely that the public's perception that we live in a less law-abiding society than formerly is misplaced. The term 'hooligan' may originate from the name of an Irish gang leader in Victorian London involved in what would now be termed mugging. Even in the early 20th century in the UK, public house brawls were common and sometimes observed by several hundred individuals at a time as entertainment. Industrial and political violence were also more common in the early part of the 20th century than at present.

The peak age of offending in the UK is 14 years for girls and 17–18 years for boys (Figure 21.1). Studies in inner London have shown that up to one in five boys have at least one conviction by the age of 21. Half the indictable crimes (more serious and eligible for trial by jury) are committed by persons under the age of 21, and 30% of males have been convicted of such an offence by the age of 30. Crime, in general, decreases with age as personality matures, except for a small peak for women aged 40–50, around the

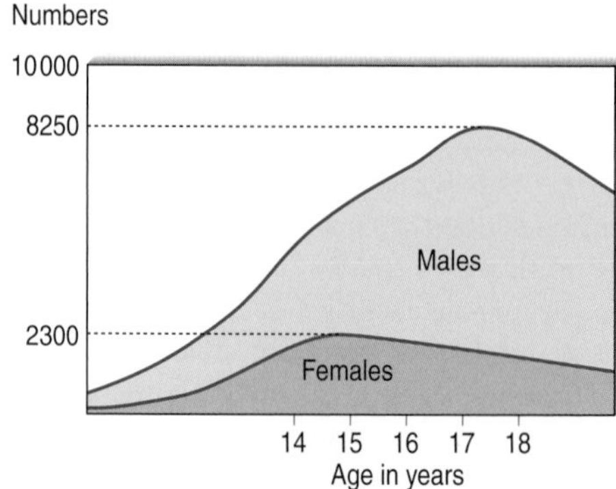

Figure 21.1 • Persons found guilty or cautioned for indictable offences in England and Wales.

menopause. With the falling numbers of those aged 14–15 in the UK, i.e. the peak age of committing crime, there has been a corresponding fall in the rates of certain offences.

Sexual differences in offending rates

In the UK, convicted males outnumber females by five to one, although this preponderance is only half of what it was 25 years ago. The excess may be due, among other factors, to the strength of males in general for repetitive violence (females tend to commit only isolated offences of violence), opportunity at work, for example fraud (although this is an area where females are also increasingly being convicted), the psychology of the male as 'bread winner' and females being generally more conforming in behaviour. A female offender generally comes from a more damaged background and is otherwise more psychologically and behaviourally disturbed than a male who has committed the same offence. This, in turn, is reflected in the fact that females in prison tend to be more behaviourally and psychiatrically disturbed than their male counterparts. Females are also reported less frequently for crimes, particularly by male police, yet are up to three times more likely to go to prison for their first offence than males.

In the past it was argued that the female equivalent to male delinquency was promiscuity, but evidence suggests that delinquent males are equally likely to be promiscuous. Some offences are by definition more common in women (e.g. those related to prostitution). Economic motives are commonly given as a rationalization for prostitution, although prostitutes as a group show an excess of mental disorder, self-harm, alcohol or drug abuse, physical disorders, personality disorders and bisexuality.

Premenstrual tension and crime

There is evidence that women premenstrually are more likely to offend, be violent in an institution or harm themselves than at other times during the menstrual cycle. Indeed, some women have successfully used premenstrual tension as a defence to a charge of homicide. It is most likely, however, that premenstrual tension is only an exacerbating factor in such individuals, and it does not imply that women in general are overall 'less responsible' at that time of the month.

Mens rea and UK forensic psychiatry hospital facilities

- Some offences require specific guilty intent (*mens rea*) as well as an unlawful act (*actus rea*), e.g. murder, rape, arson. Other offences do not require proof of guilty intent, e.g. motoring offences.
- Most mentally abnormal offenders are dealt with by ordinary psychiatric hospital facilities as out- or inpatients.
- Special hospitals treat those with mental disorder who are considered to be an immediate and grave danger to the public if they were to abscond, and who cannot be managed under conditions of medium security.
- Medium secure units in England and Wales provide psychiatric treatment under conditions of medium security, greater than ordinary hospitals but less than special hospitals.

Juvenile delinquency

Delinquency is defined as law-breaking behaviour. *Juvenile delinquency* usually means such behaviour committed by 10–21-year-olds. The majority of boys under the age of 17 may commit a delinquent act. Up to one in five males in London have a conviction by the age of 21 and half of all indictable crimes (the more serious offences eligible for trial by jury) are committed by individuals under 21. Five males are convicted for every one female. Recidivism (chronic offending) is associated with an earlier age at first offence and with both loss of life experience and institutionalization due to repeated custodial sentences.

Aetiology

This is multifactorial and is not associated with an established psychiatric disorder. Some such individuals do have personality disorders but opportunity may be more important. For those with personality disorders, the aetiology of their offending is likely to be that of their personality disorder. There is evidence that adult criminality may have an inherited genetic predisposition, especially for acquisitive crime, but this is not definitely so for juvenile delinquency.

Sociological theories include *delinquent subcultures* and associated *peer pressure*, *differential association* and *social protest theories* of the 'have nots'. Differences in juvenile delinquency rates have also been related to residence in large towns and even particular bad schools. There is also evidence of *labelling* effects, i.e. those labelled as delinquent by conviction in court are more likely to continue with such behaviour than if they are not apprehended and convicted.

Individual developmental factors

Studies of children with *conduct disorder* show that 28% grow up to be psychopathic adults, compared to 4% of those with neurotic disorder and 2% of controls.

The factors summarized in Figure 21.2, if present, are associated with the development of delinquency. If three of these five factors are present, there is a 40% chance of the individual showing delinquent behaviour during adolescence. Also, if troublesomeness at school is noted there is a 50% chance of later showing delinquent behaviour.

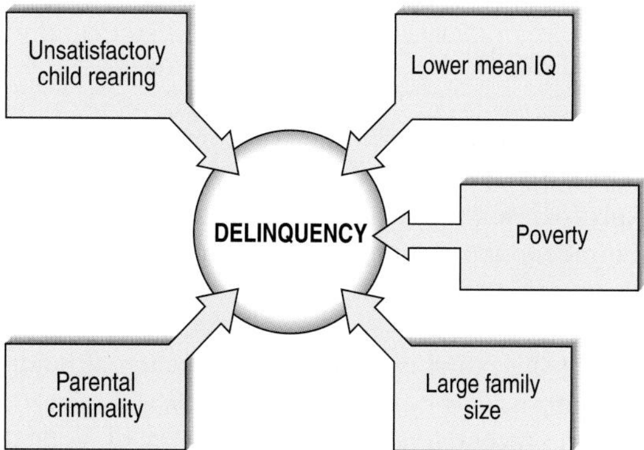

Figure 21.2 • Factors associated with the development of delinquency.

Prevention and management

Many of the factors associated with juvenile delinquency are present before birth. It might therefore be countered, for instance, by reducing family size, increasing family income to counter poverty, and countering low intelligence by special attention and remedial education. Individual counselling to improve self-esteem and counter feelings of resentment may help suitable individuals, particularly those who are of high intelligence and show good motivation, but a paternalistic, strict regime tends to be more helpful than a psychodynamically based one for those who are immature and of low intelligence.

Juvenile delinquency may be ameliorated by a good relationship with one parent or, in its absence, a counsellor, by improved emotional harmony in the home and a good experience in school, together with a good peer group. Successful employment and a good relationship/marriage also improve the prognosis as regards adult criminality.

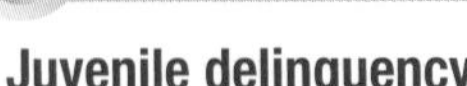

Juvenile delinquency

- Juvenile delinquency (law-breaking behaviour) is associated with:
  - low normal intelligence
  - large family size
  - poverty
  - unsatisfactory child-rearing
  - parental criminality
  - troublesomeness at school.
- Up to one in five boys may have a conviction by the age of 21, and half of indictable crimes are committed by those under 21.

Prognosis

By 19 years of age, half will have stopped their delinquent behaviour. The half who will continue are more likely to be abusing alcohol and drugs, and to gamble, to smoke and to be more sexually promiscuous. Delinquency in teenagers is also associated with criminality in adult life. The best predictor of future criminality remains the extent of previous delinquency, although offending usually ceases in the early 20s.

More recently, a 32-year follow-up of a birth cohort of 1000 New Zealanders has differentiated, apart from adult onset offenders and discontinuous offenders, life course persistent offenders and adolescence limited offenders and the implications for treatment, which is shown in Table 21.1.

Mentally abnormal offenders

It has been estimated that 1–3% of all offenders and up to one-third of those in prison suffer from a mental abnormality. Other estimates are even higher. Most suffer from personality disorder/psychopathy and/or alcohol and drug abuse or dependency. Nevertheless, there is an overrepresentation in prison of those with learning disabilities and both functional and organic mental illnesses. Imprisonment may, of course, precipitate mental illness. In the UK men outnumber women in prison by 30 to one, but female prisoners have more mental and physical disorders.

Mentally abnormal offenders have usually committed petty and minor offences. In fact, it is not certain that the mentally disordered break the law more often. Both mental illness and law-breaking are common. Up to 40% of ordinary psychiatric hospital admissions may follow threatened or actual aggression, but in most of these cases it is usually considered pointless for such individuals to be charged with their offences. When assessing offenders, it is important to bear in mind that they may become mentally ill before, or after an offence due to being in custody or to fear of the likely consequences of the offending.

After committing an offence, a mentally abnormal individual may be arrested and detained in hospital under the civil provisions of that country's Mental Health Act, or be cautioned by police, or charged. An individual must normally be charged within three days of arrest in the UK. If charged, the individual may be remanded on bail or in custody (e.g. in prison) until the court case is heard.

Forensic psychiatric assessments

Referrals to psychiatrists may be made by the court itself, the probation service and/or defence solicitors. Custom in England and Wales demands that all individuals charged with murder have reports from two psychiatrists prepared on them.

Psychiatrists are expected to assess whether an individual is fit to plead and stand trial, whether mental disorder is present, the individual's level of mental responsibility, detainability under the relevant Mental Health Act (e.g. Sections 37 and 41 of

Table 21.1 Dunedin Multidisciplinary Health and Development Study 32-year follow-up of birth cohort of 1000 New Zealanders

(A) Life course persistent offenders		
Rare, small numbers but responsible for half crime rate		
Neurodevelopment problems ↓ Temperament difficulties ↓ Disruptive behaviour ↓ Social learning poor ↓ Personality disorder, particularly antisocial personality disorder which is present in 15–25% ↓ Serious violence	 ⟶ ⟶ ⟶	 Disrupted attachments Ineffective discipline Delinquent peer influences, truanting, etc.
Victimisation of partners and children		
Poor physical, sexual and psychiatric health (especially depression)		
Substance dependence (opiates) and alcoholism		
More traumatic injuries		
Management		
Require early childhood interventions in family, but as a chronic cumulative condition requires lifelong interventions		
(B) Adolescent limited offenders		
Common		
Good neurodevelopment and also social and academic skills		
Maturation gap in period 15–25 years		
Extrovert, sensation seeking and risk taking		
Prognosis better if good partner and job		
Requires individual treatment, e.g. cognitive behavioural skills training during teen years to counteract peer influence (group treatments facilitate deviant peer networks)		
Parent management training and education useful		

the Mental Health Act 1983 in England and Wales) and to arrange any treatment recommended, on either an in- or an outpatient basis as required. Psychiatrists are also expected to give an opinion as to the degree of dangerousness of an offender, as far as they are able.

Areas to be considered in a forensic psychiatric assessment are shown in Table 21.2.

To rely solely on an offender's account may lead to an underestimate of the severity of the circumstances of the offence. For example, a paranoid psychotic patient may complain of being threatened when, in fact, the victim plausibly states that the offence was unprovoked. With incomplete information about previous convictions, a psychiatrist runs the risk of being discredited in court.

Table 21.3 outlines areas to be covered in a clinical forensic psychiatric risk assessment and management plan.

Table 21.2 A forensic psychiatric assessment

1. Full history and mental state of patient, including fantasies and impulses to offend
2. Objective account of offence, e.g. from arresting police officer or from statements (depositions) in Crown Court cases
3. Objective accounts of past offences, if any, e.g. obtain list of previous convictions
4. Additional information gathering, e.g. interviews with informants such as relatives, reading a social enquiry report from a probation officer, if prepared
5. Review of previous psychiatric records, e.g. to ascertain relationship of mental disorder to previous behaviour and response to psychiatric treatment and need for security

Multifactorial nature of offending

When assessing an offender it is important to bear in mind that no psychiatric disorder is specifically characterized by offending, and it is important to see an offence as being due to a combination of the offender, the victim and the situation/environment (Figure 21.3).

The offender

For those with a psychiatric disorder other than depression, being young and male increases the chance of committing an offence. Overall, the chronically mentally ill are more likely to commit offences than those acutely so. Those whose mental illness has relapsed and who are not compliant with treatment

Table 21.3 Clinical risk assessment and risk management planning
The aim is to get an understanding of the risk from a detailed historical longitudinal overview, obtaining information not only from the patient, who may minimize his past history, but also from informants. Ideally it should not be a 'one-off' single interview assessment.
Reconstruct in detail what happened at time of offence or behaviour causing concern
Independent information from statements of victims or witnesses or police records should be obtained where available. Don't rely on what the offender tells you or the legal offence category, e.g. arson may be of wastepaper bin in a busy ward, or with intent to kill. Possession of an offensive weapon may have been prelude to homicide.
N.B. Offence = offender × victim × circumstances.
RISK FACTORS FOR VIOLENCE
Demographic factors
Male
Young age
Socially disadvantaged neighbourhoods
Lack of social support
Employment problems
Criminal peer group
Background history
Childhood maltreatment
History of violence
First violent at young age
History of childhood conduct disorder
History of non-violent criminality

Continued

Table 21.3 Clinical risk assessment and risk management planning—cont'd
Clinical history
Psychopathy
Substance abuse
Personality disorder
Schizophrenia
Executive dysfunction
Non-compliance with treatment
Psychological and psychosocial factors
Anger
Impulsivity
Suspiciousness
Morbid jealousy
Criminal/violent attitudes
Command hallucinations
Lack of insight
Current 'context'
Threats of violence
Interpersonal discord/instability
Availability of weapons
Consider also protective factors
Practical risk assessment (history × mental state × environment) can be supplemented by standardized instruments of risk, including actuarial risk instruments based on static risk factors, e.g. Violence Risk Appraisal Guide (VRAG), and dynamic risk instruments, e.g. HCR-20 (historic, clinical and risk management -20), based on factors that can change or be managed, e.g. symptoms of mental illness and non-compliance. The psychopathy checklist-revised (PCL-R) was devised by Hare and is used to measure the presence and level of psychopathy, and has been proven to be a good predictor of risk. A short version (PCL-SV) can be used in non-forensic populations. The psychopathy checklist has two main factors (personality traits and deviancy of social behaviour). Only one-third of antisocial personality disorders reach checklist criteria for psychopathy on this scale.
In conclusion
Aim to answer how serious is the risk, i.e. its nature and magnitude, is it specific or general, conditional or unconditional, immediate, long term or volatile. Have the individuals or situational risk factors changed? Who might be at risk?
From such a risk assessment, a risk management plan should be developed to modify the risk factors and specify response triggers. This should ideally be agreed with the individual. Is there a need for more frequent follow-up appointments, an urgent care programme approach meeting or admission to hospital, detention under Mental Health Act, physical security, increased observation and/or medication required. If the optimum plan cannot be undertaken, reasons for this should be documented and a back-up plan specified.
Risk assessments and risk management plans should be communicated to others on a 'need to know' basis. On occasions, patient confidentiality will need to be breached if there is immediate grave danger to others. Police can often do little unless a specific threat is issued to an individual, whereupon they may warn or charge a subject. Very careful consideration needs to be given before informing potential victims to avoid unnecessary anxiety. Their safety is often best ensured by management of those at risk.

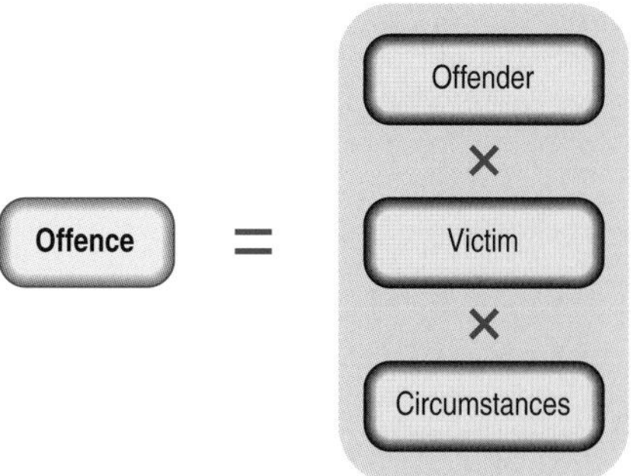

Figure 21.3 • The multifactorial nature of offending.

are also more likely to commit offences. The motivation for crime may be the same as for those who are not mentally ill (e.g. as a reaction to rejection), but may be due to delusions or hallucinations, or as a result of a deterioration in social functioning and personality due to mental illness, so that such individuals are more impulsive and have a lower stress tolerance (e.g. in schizophrenia or depressive disorder).

Those with *paranoid schizophrenia* may develop isolated paranoid delusions about particular individuals, which may go unrecognized, and they may otherwise appear to function adequately in daily life. They may plan attacks and are more effective in their execution compared to individuals with other types of schizophrenia. Specific parts of the body are more likely to be attacked by such patients (e.g. eyes).

The victim

This is most commonly a family member with whom the individual is in close proximity. This is true for victims of both the mentally disordered and 'normal' individuals. Most conflicts in any case occur within the family. Although it is important not to overrate the role of the victim, they can accidentally provoke an offence, especially if they are physically or mentally ill themselves or have been abusing alcohol or drugs. They may also not appreciate the degree of stress that a potential assailant is under. Battered children are more likely to have been temperamentally more difficult to manage.

The circumstances

These may also be important, for example in a pub, where victim and offender have both abused alcohol. Mentally ill individuals will tend to commit offences of criminal damage against public rather than private property, and in situations where they are likely to be apprehended. The availability of weapons is also important.

Outcomes of sentencing

These are given in Table 21.4. In England and Wales an individual charged with an imprisonable offence may be detained in a psychiatric hospital under Section 37 of the Mental Health Act 1983 (a six-month renewable treatment order). A Section 41 Restriction Order may be added by a Crown Court. This requires Ministry of Justice authorization for leave, transfer or conditional or absolute discharge of the individual from hospital, i.e. it removes the final decision from the patient's consultant psychiatrist and responsible clinician. The order is made 'to protect the public from serious harm' and allows for conditional discharge subject to conditions such as place of residence and compliance with psychiatric treatment.

Under English law a depressed shoplifter would be found guilty, but might be placed on a Community Rehabilitation (the old Probation) Order with a condition of psychiatric outpatient treatment. An individual suffering from schizophrenia who smashed shop windows would be found guilty of criminal damage and might then be admitted to a psychiatric hospital under a hospital order (e.g. Section 37 of the Mental Health Act 1983 in England and Wales). In cases where, for instance, an individual with schizophrenia committed a dangerous offence, a Section 41 Restriction Order (to protect the public from serious harm) may be added by a Crown Court to a Section 37 Hospital Order. Under Section 41, a patient may not go on leave or be transferred without Ministry of Justice agreement but may be conditionally discharged with specified conditions with, for example,

Table 21.4 Outcome of sentencing of mentally abnormal offenders

- The law takes its course, e.g. a fine, prison
- Conditional or absolute discharge, possibly with voluntary psychiatric treatment
- Community Rehabilitation (old Probation) Order, with or without condition of psychiatric treatment
- Detention under the Mental Health Act (e.g. under Section 37 with or without a Section 41 Restriction Order under the Mental Health Act 1983 of England and Wales)

of the court, e.g. instead of a custodial sentence, the individual may be placed on a community rehabilitation (old probation) order with or without a condition of in- or outpatient psychiatric treatment or be detained in hospital under Section 37 ± Section 41 of the Mental Health Act 1983. In other countries such mentally abnormal offenders are not legally convicted.

In certain uncommon cases the offender offers evidence of his mental disturbance either:

(a) to excuse his being tried (not fit to plead), or

(b) to agree to having done the act but not to have been fully responsible at the time (insane or diminished responsibility or automatism or infanticide).

Thus, in these cases the psychiatric evidence is presented as part of the arguments to the court and is heard before conviction.

Criminal Procedure (Insanity and Unfitness to Plead) Act 1991

(a) Unfit to plead

A mentally disordered offender may plead that he is unfit to plead (under 'disability' in relation to trial). This refers to the time of trial.

He would have to prove, using medical evidence, in a Crown Court hearing that he was not fit to do at least one of the following (based on the original test used in 1836 in R. v. Pritchard):

(1) instruct counsel ('so as to make a proper defence')

(2) appreciate the significance of pleading

(3) challenge a juror

(4) examine a witness

(5) understand and follow the evidence of Court procedure.

N.B. The defendant does not have to be fit to give evidence himself. There are current proposals to make this a more specific decision making capacity-based defence i.e. dependent on the ability to understand, remember and use relevant information to make, and to be able to tell their lawyer, their decisions.

If raised by the judge or the prosecution, this must be proved beyond reasonable doubt, but if raised by the defence, this only has to be proved on the balance of probabilities. This is a very rare plea and is only likely to be successful in cases such as severe mental impairment or for patients who are extremely paranoid, e.g. about the court or their legal representatives. In psychotic patients, unfitness to plead is significantly related to thought disorder and delusional thinking. Physical illness, e.g. pneumonia, may also result in unfitness to plead and stand trial.

If found unfit to plead, a decision for a Crown Court judge since the Domestic, Violence, Crime and Victims Act 2004, there is a provision for a trial of the facts. If found unfit to plead, this results in discretionary sentencing, including detention in hospital, a guardianship order, a supervision and treatment order or absolute discharge.

Historically the concept originates from dealing with deaf mutes. In medieval times defendants were pressed under weights to give a plea, without which they could not be convicted, executed or their property given to the Exchequer. Hence, the phrase 'press for an answer'.

In Scotland, individuals are found unfit to plead more commonly, including in cases where in England they would be convicted and detained under a Section 37 hospital order. Fitness to plead is also often a major issue in the USA where the term 'competency' is used.

(b) Not guilty by reason of insanity ('special verdict') (insanity defence) (McNaughton rules)

Historically, this defence arose from the case of McNaughton in 1843. McNaughton, believing himself to be poisoned by Whigs, attempted to shoot the Prime Minister Robert Peel, missed (or alternatively misidentified) and shot and killed Peel's Secretary. Because McNaughton was deluded and insane, he was acquitted but this caused a great deal of argument in the country, which included Queen Victoria ('Insane he may be, but not guilty he is not'), and the Law Lords were asked to issue guidance for the courts in response to five questions. Their guidance is known as the McNaughton Rules.

In this defence the offender is arguing that he is not guilty (not deserving of punishment) by reason of his insanity. It has to be proven to a court, on the balance of probabilities, that at the time of the offence, the offender laboured under such defect of reason that he met the McNaughten Rules, i.e.

(1) that by reason of such defect from disease of the mind, he did not know the nature or quality of his act (this means the physical nature of the act), or

(2) not know that what he was doing was wrong (forbidden by law)

(3) if an individual was suffering from a delusion, then his actions would be judged by their relationship to the delusion, i.e. if he believed his life to be immediately threatened, then he would be justified in striking out, but not otherwise.

Technically, this plea may be put forward for any offence, but in practice it is usually only put forward for murder or other serious offences. In fact, such a plea is rare.

Evidence from two or more medical practitioners, one approved under Section 12 of the Mental Health Act 1983, is required before return of the verdict 'Not Guilty by Reason of Insanity'.

Such a verdict implies lack of intent. However, legally, a psychiatrist can only give evidence regarding an individual's capacity to form intent (a legal concept), not the fact of intent at the time of the offence.

Under the Criminal Procedure Act 1991, if found Not Guilty by Reason of Insanity, the Judge has freedom to decide on the sentencing and disposal of defendant, i.e. discretionary sentencing, including detention in hospital under forensic treatment orders of the Mental Health Act 1983.

Criticism of McNaughten rules

These rules are now almost obsolescent. Points against them are:

(1) Hardly anybody is mad enough to fit the rules. Even McNaughten would not have been.

(2) It assumes a doctrine that mind is made up of separate independent compartments of which cognition is most important (a Victorian view).

(3) The rules are too unfair, as abnormal mental states do not fit into rigid categories.

(4) It ignores the importance of emotional disturbance and failure of will, when cognition is normal.

Homicide by mentally disordered offenders in England and Wales

Definition

Homicide is the killing of another human being. It is not necessarily unlawful.

Epidemiology

There have been around 500–600 homicides each year in England and Wales in this decade. These figures include for 2003 the 172 victims of Dr Harold Shipman, an English general practitioner who killed his elderly patients. Around a third of all homicide victims are female (half killed by their partners). This compares with around 16000 externally caused deaths each year (of these, half are suicides, others are due to misadventure, accidents, etc.).

Legal classification in England and Wales

Homicide may be lawful or unlawful.

Lawful homicide

Lawful homicide may be:

- justifiable, e.g. on behalf of the state, such as actions taken by people in the army or the police
- excusable, e.g. a pure accident or an honest or reasonable mistake.

Unlawful homicide

Unlawful homicide is defined in England and Wales as the unlawful killing of any reasonable creature in being and under the Queen's (or King's) Peace. Types of unlawful homicide include:

- murder
- manslaughter
- child destruction
- genocide
- causing death by dangerous driving
- suicide pacts
- infanticide.

Clinical categories of homicide

Parricide, the killing of near relatives, is disproportionately committed by males in late adolescence and includes patricide (killing of one's father), matricide (killing of one's mother), which in the United Kingdom is more common than patricide and tends to be committed by those with schizophrenia, perhaps reflecting the psychological difficulty of normally doing so, uxoricide (killing of one's wife) and filicide (the killing of one's child).

Serial killing involves killing individuals over time, spree killings involve killing individuals in different locations during one episode and mass killing involves killing multiple individuals at the same time and same location.

Murder

Murder is an offence at common, as opposed to statute (Parliament passed), law in England and Wales. It is defined as an unlawful killing with *malice aforethought*. Malice aforethought requires either an intention to kill or cause grievous bodily harm. Murder, like any other crime requiring proof of intent, involves proof of a subjective state of mind on the part of the accused. The *actus reus* of murder consists of both of the following:

- an unlawful act
- the act causes the death of another human being.

Murder results in a mandatory life custodial sentence in England and Wales. On average 11.5 years is served in prison, and then the prisoner is released on life licence. A few murderers do serve life.

Manslaughter

Manslaughter may be categorized into three groups, namely:

- voluntary manslaughter
- involuntary manslaughter
- corporate liability.

The third of these will not be considered further here.

Voluntary manslaughter

There are cases of homicide in which the defendant would be guilty of murder if it were not for the availability of one of the following partial defences

Diminished responsibility

As a reaction against the fact that mentally disordered people who had killed were still being hanged, given the then-mandatory death sentence for murder, which was abolished in the UK in 1965, despite other defences, such as not guilty by reason of insanity (the McNaughton Rules), a movement was created to bring in a defence of diminished responsibility, i.e. the responsibility of the offender is not totally absent because of mental abnormality but is only partially impaired; therefore, the offender would be found guilty but the sentence modified. This was made law under Section 2 of the Homicide Act 1957 and applies only to a charge of murder. The murder charge is reduced to manslaughter on the grounds of diminished responsibility.

Diminished responsibility is a defence against the charge (only) of murder; the offender may plead that at the time of the offence, he (or she) had diminished responsibility. Now, following the Coroners and Justice Act 2009, an individual is considered to have the partial defence to murder of diminished responsibility if he has an abnormality of mental functioning arising from a recognized medical condition, which substantially impaired the defendant's ability to understand the nature of the defendant's conduct, form a rational judgement and/or exercise self-control, and the abnormality of mental functioning provides an explanation for the defendant's acts.

'Abnormality of mental functioning' is left to the defendant (or his or her medical advisors) to define and is not synonymous with mental disorder as defined in the Mental Health Act 1983.

'Substantially' is also undefined and is left to the jury to decide, although the doctors may give their opinions.

The effect of a successful plea of diminished responsibility is to reduce the charge from murder to manslaughter. The verdict 'unties the judge's hands'. Murder carries a statutory sentence of life imprisonment, but the court is free to make any sentence at all with regard to manslaughter, including a hospital or community rehabilitation (probation) order or, indeed, a life prison sentence, in which case research has shown that such individuals may spend longer in custody than those convicted of murder. This may reflect concern that although abnormality of mind was identified in these cases of diminished responsibility, no ameliorating treatment is undertaken, for example in hospital, if the individual received a life prison sentence.

In addition to a report supporting the plea of diminished responsibility, the psychiatrist may also, if appropriate, wish to arrange for the appropriate hospital treatment and offer the appropriate Mental Health Act 1983 section (detention) recommendations to the court to help them with their sentencing.

The diminished responsibility defence has been used where a defence of insanity would have no hope of success. Examples include:

- mercy killing
- when the subject kills his or her spouse in a state of reactive depression

- individuals who kill in jealous frenzies
- individuals who are subject to an 'irresistible impulse' to kill (cited more often in the USA)
- subjects who kill and who are 'deranged' by psychopathic disorder.

The diminished responsibility defence has largely replaced the insanity defence in England and Wales for those charged with murder.

The most important points in favour of diminished responsibility are that:

- it allows for an overall assessment of the person
- it leads to more flexible sentencing.

Against diminished responsibility are the following points:

- There is a problem of balancing the concept of responsibility with 'determinism', e.g. does a greater propensity to lose one's temper imply less responsibility?
- It assumes that a distinction can be made between psychopathy and wickedness in terms of moral or criminal responsibility.
- Does diminished responsibility mean less power to resist temptation? If so, should the irresponsible be punished less than the responsible?
- Does an irresponsible act in a normally responsible person indicate a greater aberration of mind than irresponsible behaviour in the irresponsible?
- If a person is found to have diminished responsibility, then it may mean that the court will return such a person to society faster than a responsible offender.

Provocation. Provocation is the sudden or temporary loss of control under provocation that might make a normal person kill. Whether this occurred is for the jury to decide, although a psychiatrist's opinion may be requested. More recently, psychiatric evidence about the propensity of individuals with certain vulnerable personalities or conditions, such as learning disability, to be provoked has been accepted as admissible.

Following criticism that this defence is used inappropriately by those who kill after losing their temper and that it is not sufficiently tailored to those who kill out of fear of serious violence, e.g. those subject to prolonged domestic violence, this defence has been replaced in the Coroners and Justice Act (2009) with a new partial defence for those who kill in response to (a) fear of serious violence and/or (b) have a justified sense of being seriously wronged.

Killing in pursuance of a suicide pact (which the offender has to prove) (Section 4 Homicide Act 1957): a suicide pact is defined as being a common agreement between two or more persons, having for its object the death of all of them, whether or not each is to take his or her own life.

Involuntary manslaughter

Involuntary manslaughter refers to cases of homicide without malice aforethought. It can take several forms including:

- an unlawful and dangerous act – 'constructive manslaughter': the *actus reus* consists of an unlawful act that is dangerous and causes death
- gross negligence: the *actus reus* consists of a breach of a duty of care that the accused owes to the victim, with the result that this breach leads to the victim's death.

Infanticide

Under the Infanticide Acts 1922 and 1938 (Section 1), infanticide is defined as having occurred when a woman by any wilful act caused the death of her child under the age of 12 months, but at the time of the act or omission the balance of her mind was 'disturbed by reason of her not being fully recovered from the effect of giving birth to the child or the effect of lactation consequent upon the birth of the child'. This is technically an offence rather than a defence.

The grounds for this plea, as an alternative to murder, are less stringent than those for diminished responsibility (i.e. there is no need to prove abnormality of mental functioning); nor does it require proof of a mental disorder, e.g. mental illness. It is the policy of the Director of Public Prosecution and the Crown Prosecution Service to use this plea for such mothers. It does not apply to adopted children or to any child other than the youngest (otherwise a manslaughter plea has to be used), as it is possible to give birth on two occasions within one year.

When this plea was introduced, many such mothers had acute organic confusional puerperal psychoses. Nowadays, infanticide is rather an historical anachronism; only about one in six of such mothers have functional puerperal psychoses, the remainder being not dissimilar from those who batter their children. A conviction for infanticide usually results in a sentence of a community rehabilitation (old probation) order, often with a condition of psychiatric treatment (outpatient or inpatient).

Amnesia

Between 40% and 50% of people charged with homicide claim amnesia for the actual act.

Amnesia is not in itself a defence; the underlying condition may be, for example, a post-traumatic state, epileptic fits or acute psychosis. In the 1959 Podola Appeal case in England and Wales (Podola's amnesia was, in fact, not genuine), it was ruled that even if amnesia is genuine, it is no bar to trial.

Amnesia may be feigned by lying or caused by:

- hysterical amnesia (denial)
- failure of memory registration owing to overarousal (comparable to 'exam phobia')
- alcohol
- other psychoactive drugs
- head injury.

Drugs and alcohol

It has always been considered in England and Wales that a person is fully responsible for their actions if they knowingly used drugs or alcohol (voluntary intoxication). It is assumed that everyone knows that drunkenness is associated with aggressive and irresponsible behaviour and therefore one is responsible for not becoming drunk. The same rule applies to drug abuse. This would not apply if an individual were 'slipped' drugs or alcohol or if their doctor did not inform them of side-effects and interactions (e.g. with alcohol) of prescribed medication.

Successful defences have been based on:

- being so drunk as to be incapable of forming intent in offences requiring specific intent
- developing a mental illness, e.g. psychosis, as a result of the ingestion of a drug or alcohol (as in delirium tremens)
- where the use of a drug, which might be quite legitimate, produces a mental state abnormality that could not have been anticipated by the subject, e.g. hypoglycaemia after the use of insulin.

Thus, overall, successful defences following consumption of alcohol or drugs are based on either (i) involuntary intoxication or (ii) if intoxicated voluntarily, lack of specific intent where offences, such as murder, require this.

Automatism

A rare plea generally restricted (though not entirely) to cases of homicide. The defendant pleads that at the time of the offence his behaviour was automatic (no *mens rea*). The law uses this term to mean a state almost near unconsciousness. It refers to unconscious, involuntary, non-purposeful acts where the mind is not conscious of what the body is doing. There is a separation between the will and the act, or the mind and the act ('Mind does not go with what is being done'. Bratty v. A.G. in N. Ireland, 1961).

This is an extremely rare plea and has been successfully pleaded, particularly in cases of homicide, for offences occurring during hypoglycaemic attacks, sleepwalking or sleep, e.g. fighting tigers and snakes in dreams (theoretically this should be during night terrors in slow wave sleep, as in dreams one should be paralysed in REM sleep, but it has been argued that such offences may occur as an individual wakes from a dream). Such must be the degree of automatism that there is no capacity to form any intent to kill or any capacity to control actions.

In certain cases, e.g. offending while sleepwalking, the man has walked free from the court on the understanding that he will always lock his bedroom door.

In the past, where a defence of sane automatism is put forward, the subject is hoping to receive a total acquittal. However, the law has become aware that some automatism states are really the result, in the legal sense, of a disease of the mind, e.g. epilepsy, which may recur, and therefore in such cases the jury may be invited to consider that the defence of automatism should be regarded as evidence of insanity (Insane Automatism) and to return the Special Verdict, i.e. Not Guilty by Reason of Insanity, which would allow for discretionary sentencing, including detention in hospital.

Although, historically, sleepwalking and night terrors have been accepted as automatisms and led to acquittal, case law (Lord Justice Lawton) now differentiates sane automatism, due to external causes (extrinsic factors), e.g. hypoglycaemia due to insulin, from insane automatism, due to disease of the mind caused by mental illness or brain disease (intrinsic factors), e.g. diabetes, epilepsy and even hysterical dissociative fugue states, where the Special Verdict (Not Guilty by Reason of Insanity) should be returned.

N.B. *Pathological intoxication* (ICD-10): Sudden onset of aggression and often violent behaviour, not typical of an individual when sober, very soon after drinking amounts of alcohol (only) that would not produce intoxication in most people.

Case history: manslaughter on grounds of diminished responsibility – homicide by a male suffering from paranoid schizophrenia

A 32-year-old man, Mr A., living in England, had suffered from paranoid schizophrenia for 5 years. This was characterized by paranoid delusions about his father being in collusion with the police and members of the government to prevent Mr A. finding employment or forming a stable relationship with a woman. Due to Mr A. mental illness, there was both a deterioration in his social functioning, so that he became less able to sustain himself in the community, and a deterioration in his personality, so that he began to behave more impulsively and lost his temper more frequently under stress. He had had three previous compulsory admissions to psychiatric hospitals in the past 5 years. He responded well to inpatient treatment with antipsychotic medication, but upon discharge he complied poorly with medication, which he both resented and felt he did not need when his mental illness was in remission, in spite of advice to the contrary.

Mr A. s mental illness relapsed with a re-emergence of paranoid delusions about his father 3 months after he was last in hospital, after he had again stopped his medication. Over the course of the next month he became increasingly verbally and physically aggressive to his father and others, culminating in his using a hammer one evening to kill his father. He then immediately went next door to tell his neighbours what he had done. He waited for the police to arrive, was arrested, charged with murder and remanded to prison, where he was assessed by psychiatrists.

At the time of his trial Mr A. was considered *fit to plead and stand trial*. As at the time of the offence he knew what he was doing and that it was legally wrong, and he was not then subject to delusional beliefs that his life was in immediate danger, he was not considered not guilty by reason of insanity, i.e. he did not meet the criteria of the McNaughten Rules. However, he was considered to have been suffering from paranoid schizophrenia at the time of the offence which was affecting his perception of the situation, his judgement and the voluntary control of his actions, and, on the basis of oral and written evidence by two consultant forensic psychiatrists, a Crown Court accepted that Mr A. suffered from such an abnormality of mental functioning at the time of the offence that his responsibility was substantially impaired. The court therefore accepted the plea, made on legal advice, of *not guilty to murder, but guilty to manslaughter on the grounds of diminished responsibility.*

As Mr A. clearly continued to suffer from mental disorder, the severe mental illness of paranoid schizophrenia and required inpatient psychiatric treatment, the court further agreed to his being sentenced to be detained in a Medium Secure Unit (although it might have been a special hospital) under Section 37 of the Mental Health Act 1983 of England and Wales, on the basis of the legally required two psychiatrists' written recommendations to this end. In addition, after oral evidence had been given by one consultant forensic psychiatrist, the judge ordered that Mr A. be made subject to restrictions under Section 41 of the Mental Health Act 1983, 'to protect the public from serious harm' and also to facilitate his long-term psychiatric management, including, when he was again ready to return to the community, by specifying his place of residence and mandatory attendance for psychiatric outpatient follow-up and supervision by a probation officer or social worker.

Mr A. made good progress on depot injection antipsychotic medication. He developed good insight into the nature of his mental illness, its direct relationship to the killing of his father and his own need for antipsychotic medication for the foreseeable future. He was conditionally discharged from hospital under Section 41 of the Mental Health Act 1983 after 18 months. The conditions were that he continued to reside in a supervised hostel and that he complied with his psychiatric treatment. In fact, Mr A. remained compliant with antipsychotic medication and thus psychiatrically well. His compliance was reinforced by his realization that if he did not so comply, he would be subject to recall to hospital under the restrictions on his conditional discharge.

Mute defendants

Rarely, one may be asked to help the court decide whether an offender who appears to be mute (i.e. no speech at all) is being mute 'by malice or a visitation of God'. If mute 'by malice', the case proceeds with a not guilty plea entered on defendant's behalf. If 'by visitation of God', e.g. if deaf and dumb, the question of fitness to plead will arise with a view to disposal under the Criminal Procedure (Insanity and Unfitness to Plead) Act 1991.

Mentally disordered offenders involved with the police and courts

Following an offence, an individual may be admitted informally to a psychiatric hospital, compulsorily detained under civil sections of the Mental Health Act 1983 (e.g. Section 2, 3, 4 or 136), be cautioned by the police, which the individual has to voluntarily accept, or he may be charged. If charged, the individual may be remanded on bail or in custody (e.g. prison) until the court case. The police may also check if the person is an absconding detained patient and return him to hospital under Section 18 or Section 138.

Under the Police & Criminal Evidence Act 1984 (PACE), there is a code of practice that covers detention, treatment and questioning of persons by the police officer. If the individual is suspected to be mentally disordered by a police officer, an 'appropriate adult' must be informed and asked to come to the police station. This should ideally be an individual trained or experienced in dealing with mentally disordered people rather than an unqualified relative. An appropriate adult should be present while the individual is told their rights and can advise the person being interviewed, observe the fairness of the interview and facilitate communication with the interviewee. They may also require the presence of a lawyer.

If a decision is taken by the police to prosecute, the case is passed to the Crown Prosecution Service, who will also consider the public interest and likely adverse effects of prosecution of a mentally disordered individual.

Police and court liaison

Terminology

Diversion or early diversion

Transfer to the healthcare system of a mentally disordered individual in police custody or at first court hearing.

Diversion or police or court diversion schemes

Specific psychiatric services are provided to the police and/or courts, usually to the Magistrates Court where 98% of offenders are tried. Such services reduce time on remand in custody for the mentally ill, but may not affect the long-term risk of offending. However, it is unlikely that serious offenders, e.g. those charged with murder, will be suitable for such diversion.

Psychiatric issues relevant to police and court liaison

- Evidence of mental disorder.
- Need for out- or inpatient psychiatric treatment.
- Urgency if inpatient psychiatric treatment required.
- Nature of alleged offence and risk to others.
- Fitness to remain in police custody.
- Fit to be interviewed by police.
- Fit to plead if to appear in court.

N.B. Remember, the technical legal offence may not reflect the actual risk. For example, arson may be of a wastepaper bin in front of others on a busy hospital ward, or committed with intent to endanger the lives of others in a tower block. Similarly, possession of an offensive weapon may have been with a view to seriously harming others.

Fitness to remain in police custody

- No legal definition.
- An individual may be unfit to remain in police custody due to physical illness or psychiatric disorder.
- Serious and immediate risk to an individual's health will usually make an individual unfit to remain in police custody. Detention under a civil section of the Mental Health Act may then be indicated.

Fitness to be interviewed by police

- No legal definition.
- Individuals should be able to understand the police caution after it has been explained.
- Full orientation to time, place and person is required.
- Fitness may be questioned if an individual is likely to give answers due to his/her mental disorder that may be wrongly interpreted by the court.
- If an individual is fit to be interviewed but has a history of mental disorder, then an appropriate adult should be present. Such individuals can be provided by Appropriate Adult Schemes.

False confessions

Three types have been described.

(a) Voluntary

For instance, due to depression or morbid guilt.

(b) Coerced-compliant

Due to being pressurized during interrogation. Often such false confessions are retracted after interrogation.

(c) Coerced-internalized

Confused by interrogation and comes to believe false story. Particularly seen in learning disability.

In cases of possible suggestibility and false confessions:

- assess intellectual level
- Use Gudjonnson Suggestibility Scale.

Table 21.5 Psychiatric expert evidence

1. Fitness to plead
2. Mental responsibility, e.g., not guilty by reason of insanity, diminished responsibility
3. Mental disorder, e.g., mental illness, learning disability, personality disorder
4. Is client treatable?
5. Have arrangements been made for such treatment? e.g., For example, community rehabilitation (old probation) order with condition of outpatient treatment, or inpatient treatment under section 37 of Mental Health Act 1983
6. Is client dangerous? e.g., need for section 41 Mental Health Act 1983, placement in a special hospital
7. Suggestions about non-psychiatric management, e.g., community rehabilitation (old probation) order, supervised hostel

The areas of psychiatric expert evidence and psychiatric court reporting are summarized in Tables 21.5 and 21.6.

Homicide followed by suicide

This outcome, which, of course, precludes a criminal trial, occurred in around 7% of such offences between 1966 and 2004 in England and Wales. The rates of homicide followed by suicide have probably been higher in England and Wales in the past, with estimates of up to a half attempting suicide and a third succeeding in the 1960s, at a time when most homicides were domestic with an over-representation of female offenders and child victims, thus perhaps having more psychologically difficult consequences.

Psychodynamic aspects

Most individuals who have killed do not regard themselves as typical murderers and many resent the implications of the word 'manslaughter'. Nevertheless, although murderous thoughts can be normal, acting on them is not. Homicide can be seen as preventing something even more psychologically difficult for the individual. As a result of psychological defence mechanisms, following a homicide, some individuals can appear callously indifferent, idolize the victim or claim amnesia as the act is too painful to think or talk about.

In England and Wales the annual number of homicides due to mental disorder rose from under 50 in 1957 to above 100 in the 1970s but has now returned to the earlier low levels, whereas other homicides have continued to rise. The initial rise in homicide by the mentally disordered was attributed to the same factors responsible for the increase in other homicides, e.g. substance misuse and increased availability of weapons, and the subsequent decline to the improved awareness of, services for and treatment of mental disorder.

Internationally, the rate of homicide by the mentally ill is related to the prevalence of mental illness, which itself is fairly constant in all countries. In countries with high homicide rates, this is due to high numbers of non-mentally ill offenders, their violence being related to criminal activities, drug dealing and subcultural and economic factors. As a consequence, these countries with high homicide rates had a lower proportion of mentally ill homicide offenders.

There is thus no evidence of significantly increasing rates of homicide by mentally ill people in England and Wales, in spite of the perception by the media and the public, which, in turn, probably reflects only increasing awareness. Homicides by mentally ill people have a negligible effect on public safety in England and Wales compared with other factors, such as road traffic accidents.

Violence and mental illness

Violence is multifactorially caused and is a bio-psycho-social-environmental phenomenon. Clearly all behaviour has a biochemical basis, but although biochemical abnormalities can cause psychological symptoms, including aggression, there is also increasing evidence that psychological events, e.g. severe abuse in childhood and severe psychological trauma in adulthood, may cause neurobiological abnormalities such as in serotonin metabolism in adults. This, in turn, is associated with aggression, which is usually inhibited by serotonin. Models of violence are shown in Table 21.7. No one model can adequately explain all violence, thus different models may better explain different situations.

Aggression, using the biological definition, is intraspecific fighting. Normal aggression is seen in all members of a species, whereas pathological aggression or violence is either excessive in degree and/or arises from mental disorder. Almost all forms of mental disorder can be associated with aggression

Table 21.6 Court reporting

1. A report may be requested

(a) by a court (magistrates, Crown or higher court), usually through the probation service. Written authorization by the court must be given
(b) by the defence solicitors, in which case the patient's written permission is required before giving a report to the solicitor, which remains his/her property to use or not in court

2. Information required for a report includes

(a) information about the charge
(b) a social enquiry report from a probation officer
(c) list of previous convictions
(d) previous medical hospital records
(e) previous reports (social and medical)
(f) depositions where available, e.g. Crown Court, but not magistrate cases

3. The history will be taken from the patient and, if possible, a relative or friend

4. The client should be examined fully physically

5. The questions the court or solicitor will be particularly interested in, are

(a) has he a mental disorder?
(b) is it susceptible to or requiring specific treatment?
(c) can arrangements be made for such treatment (hospital, outpatients, etc)
(d) is the client dangerous?
(e) have you any suggestions as to his management apart from the psychiatric aspects?

6. After interview and examination of other reports etc., one can valuably discuss the case again with the probation officer or others, e.g. other psychiatrists involved in the case

(a) discuss particularly your findings and compare them with other professionals' observations, which may reveal gross discrepancies
(b) discussion may reveal unexpected channels for disposal or unforeseen difficulties

7. The general principles of the written report are

(a) it should be in clear English and technical terms should be avoided if possible. If they are used, an explanation of them should be given, e.g. paranoid (persecutory) delusions (false beliefs), auditory and visual hallucinations (voices and visions)
(b) use the report to help the court reach the most appropriate disposal for the patient
(c) the report is a recommendation to the court. The court may have other psychiatric opinions that oppose yours and may itself be unconvinced by your opinion. Thus, the onus is on you to provide the evidence in the report for your opinion
(d) the onus is also on the reporting doctor to make all the necessary medical arrangements for the disposal and management of the patient
(e) be accurate, complete and brief. The court is extremely busy and will resent a turgid, over-written report. For Magistrates, Courts, which may deal with dozens of cases a day, around two pages will suffice and, even then, only the opinion may be read

8. People use different forms for their report, but the following is suggested. Paragraph numbers and headings can be used for clarity

Para 1. Introduction

Inform the court of when and where the patient was seen, at whose request, what information was available, who were the informants, and sometimes what information was not available. State the current offence(s) for which charged and its date(s), and plea if known, i.e. guilty or not guilty

Para 2. Past medical history

Inform the court of this and of the result of medical examination, e.g. 'Physical examination revealed no abnormality'

Continued

Table 21.6 Court reporting—cont'd

Para 3. Family history
Report the important, relevant points, including family history or not of psychiatric disorder and criminality
Para 4. Personal history
Report the important points of his physical development, e.g. birth and milestones, early development, e.g. bedwetting (enuresis), schooling, e.g. truancy, and occupational history, which will include difficulties with a job, e.g. sackings or in sustaining employment, or with colleagues or supervisors at work
Para 5. Sexual history
Be reasonably discreet. The report may be read in open court
Para 6. Previous personality
Report details of personality in terms of social interaction, emotions, and habits, e.g. drinking, gambling, drugs
Para 7. Past forensic history
Technically, past convictions should not be admissible before conviction but are admissible when report is to assist sentencing. In practice, usually only one psychiatric report is prepared for both trial and sentencing
Para 8. Past psychiatric history
Report dates, diagnosis, relevant details and relationship of mental disorder and treatment to offending
Para 9. Circumstances surrounding index offence(s)
Report circumstances leading to current offence(s) and defendant's state of mind at the time of the offence, sticking to the phenomena reported, e.g. 'for the time of the offence he gives a history of tearfulness, loss of hope, poor sleeping' etc., 'these are symptoms of a depressive mental illness' etc.
Para 10. Interview
Report the result of the interview: 'he showed/did not show evidence of mental illness'. Then give a brief outline of the evidence, e.g. 'he muttered to himself and looked around the room as though hearing voices (auditory hallucinations)' etc., or list symptoms and say, e.g. 'these are symptoms of the severe mental illness of schizophrenia' etc.
Information in Paragraphs 1–10 should be factual, verifiable and ideally agreed by all, even if others' opinions differ from your own.
Para 11. Opinion
The final paragraph should express your opinion. The court will be interested particularly in your opinion as to
(a) is he fit to plead and stand his trial? (b) is he suffering from a mental disorder as defined in the Mental Health Act 1983? (c) where appropriate, comment on issues of responsibility, e.g. not guilty by reason of insanity, diminished responsibility in cases of homicide (d) if so, can arrangements be made for his treatment (fix this up if you can). Make suggestions to the court about which disposal would be appropriate, e.g. Section 37 hospital order with or without a Section 41 restriction order, outpatient psychiatric treatment as a condition of a Community Rehabilitation (old probation) Order
For example 'This man is fit to plead and stand trial In my opinion he suffers from a mental disorder as defined in the Mental Health Act 1983, the severe mental illness of schizophrenia, characterized by delusions (false beliefs) of passivity (being externally controlled) and auditory hallucinations (voices) talking about him in a derogatory way in the third person

Continued

Table 21.6 Court reporting—cont'd

In my opinion, at the time of the alleged offence of murder, Mr X was suffering from an abnormality of mental functioning, due to the severe mental illness of paranoid schizophrenia, affecting his perception, judgement and voluntary control of his actions, as substantially impaired his responsibility for his acts I consider he would benefit from treatment in a psychiatric hospital. I have made arrangements for a bed to be reserved for him at X hospital under Section 37 of the Mental Health Act 1983 if the court considers that this would be appropriate I recommend, if the court so agrees, that he additionally be made subject to restrictions under Section 41 of the Mental Health Act 1983 to protect the public from serious harm and to facilitate his long-term psychiatric management, including by specifying the conditions of his discharge from hospital, e.g. of residence, and compliance with outpatient treatment, and by providing the ability to recall him to hospital should his mental state or behaviour deteriorate or he otherwise gives rise to concern'
OR, as an alternative 'In my opinion this man does not suffer from mental disorder and is not detainable in hospital under the Mental Health Act 1983. He has an immature personality and requires considerable support and would benefit from group psychotherapy as an outpatient. If the court is prepared to consider an alternative to a custodial sentence in this case, I would recommend that, subject to the probation service's agreement, he be made subject to the direction of a Community Rehabilitation (old probation) order with a condition that he attend an outpatient group under my direction at X Mental Health Unit'
Comment on any *mitigating* circumstances, e.g. marital or work stress, and on the *prognosis*
Express any doubts you may have as to the likelihood of benefit from or risks associated with treatment in this man's case
If you have no psychiatric recommendation, say so, e.g. 'I have no psychiatric recommendation to make in this case'
Finally, if essential information is lacking or if time is not sufficient to make the necessary arrangements for a hospital bed, then do not hesitate to state your findings to date, state what you would like to do, and ask for a further period of remand

and violence (Table 21.8), although anyone can become violent. There has been a debate about whether aggression is an instinct, i.e. genetically determined but called out by the environment, or learnt. Probably there is a normal inborn assertiveness, with aggression being secondary to early developmental deprivation and insults and/or mental disorder, rather than a primary drive.

Aggression often follows frustration and threat, e.g. to a low self-esteem, and increasing tension. Aggression may, of course, be displaced from the original object onto a symbolic representation of it, e.g. arson or anger towards mother displaced onto women in general. Aggression can also be a social phenomena, e.g. in altruistic aggression and war.

Violence is action, whereas dangerousness is a potential and a matter of opinion. The term risk is now used in professional practice in preference to dangerousness. Risk is, ideally, a matter of statistical fact. It emphasizes a continuum of levels of risk, varying not only with the individual but also with the context. It may change over time and, in principle, should be based on objective assessment. Dangerousness tends to imply an all-or-none phenomenon and a static characteristic of an individual. However, clearly, risk assessment is less important than risk management, although risk management does not imply risk elimination.

Risk factors include dispositional factors, such as demographic factors, historical factors, including past violence; constitutional factors, including stress and social support; and clinical factors, including diagnoses, symptoms and substance abuse. Risk may change rapidly over time.

In the past, factors associated with violence were said to be the same, regardless of whether the offender was mentally ill, i.e. personality disorder, impulsivity, anger, violent family background and substance abuse. However, since 1992, studies have shown that having a diagnosis of mental illness is associated weakly with violence due to a subgroup with specific types of symptoms such as paranoid (persecutory) delusions (false beliefs) and delusions of passivity (being under external control). Thus, it is certain symptoms, and not particular psychiatric diagnoses alone, that are associated with violence. Nevertheless, the risk of violence is still better predicted by being a young male than by having a diagnosis of schizophrenia.

Psychiatrists are better than chance or lay people in predicting violence and better still at assessing situations where there is no risk; however, they tend to underestimate the risk of violence in females.

Table 21.7 Models of, and factors in, violence

Biological factors	"Fight or flight" response Males and the young more violent Testosterone levels Reduced serotonin levels in brain
Alcohol and drugs	50 % violent offences follow alcohol abuse in UK Disinhibits behaviour
Psychological models	
Instrumental aggression	Learn to achieve ends by violence
Cognitive model	Look at world aggressively
Behavioural model	Inconsistent, erratic parental punishment
Social learning	Peer pressure/modelling (Bandura)
Status	Status of being violent
Psychodynamic models	
Freudian	Originally primary drive due to frustration. Later, primary drive libido, aggression secondary drive
Kleinian	Annihilation anxiety
Kohut	Secondary to developmental insults or deprivations
Object relations school (Winnicott)	Creative of another
Attachment theory	Insecurely attached infant, e.g., deprived or abused, relates to others with hostility
Family factors	Physical abuse as child Parental discord and violence Parental irritability, usually due to depression
Social models	Subcultural norm, e.g. Hell's Angels, pub brawls Sporting, political and industrial violence Relative poverty and inequality Comparative anthropology, e.g. Mead's studies
Environmental factors	Avoidance of frustration by well structured and staffed milieu and non-provocative regime

Professionals also underestimate the high background base rates of violence in the community in general, e.g. up to 40% of males in a London sample had been seriously violent by the age of 32 years. The majority of violence never results in criminal charges. This also applies to inpatients who are violent, where formal charges may often be seen as serving little purpose if the patient is to remain in hospital.

Among individuals with mental illness, affective disorders are underrepresented in forensic psychiatric facilities. Violence is, however, increased in people with schizophrenia, especially those who have drifted out of treatment, and in young males with acute schizophrenia compared with those with chronic schizophrenia. Violence may arise directly from positive psychotic symptoms of mental illness, such as delusions (false beliefs) and hallucinations (e.g. voices). Mental illness, especially schizophrenia, may, however, lead indirectly to violence through associated deterioration in social functioning and personality, so that such individuals become more antisocial and impulsive and develop a lower tolerance to stress. This sometimes leads to disputes in court about the disposal of such individuals with few or no positive psychotic symptoms, who have killed, with such individuals sometimes being given, wrongly, an additional diagnosis of personality disorder to explain their violence. A mentally ill individual may also behave violently for 'normal' emotional reasons, such as fear and anger, and then experience accompanying corresponding psychotic symptoms, e.g. hallucinations of aggressive content. Violence, law involvement and imprisonment may themselves precipitate mental illness.

For a mentally ill person, the key issue is whether the individual has a delusion of a content on which he or she might act dangerously, e.g. of persecution or infidelity, but even then not all morbidly jealous

Table 21.8 Violence and psychiatric disorder

(a) Non-psychiatric causes
Social
Economic
Criminal, e.g., drug dealing
Cultural, e.g., subcultures
(b) Psychiatric causes
Violence or threats of violence in 40% pre-admission
Schizophrenia – paranoid and non-paranoid
Mania, hypomania but also depression
Alcohol abuse and withdrawal
Drug abuse and withdrawal
Hallucinogens, PCP
Benzodiazepine withdrawal
Organic mental disorder and brain damage, epilepsy, especially TLE, dementia.
Personality disorder, particularly antisocial, impulsive and borderline
Learning disability
Child and adolescent behaviour disorders
Post-traumatic stress disorder
Dissociative states
(c) Intra-familial
Spousal abuse
Child abuse
Elder abuse

individuals, for instance, assault their spouse. Twenty per cent of people presenting to hospital with their first episode of schizophrenia have threatened the lives of others, but, among these, half have already been ill for a year. Overall, however, it is unusual for a person with schizophrenia to present for the first time with serious violence, including homicide. One established period of higher risk is within a few months of discharge from hospital. People with both schizophrenia and substance abuse have higher rates of violence than those with substance abuse alone, who, in turn, have higher rates than those with schizophrenia alone.

Research has generally shown, but not universally, a consistent association between violence and delusions, particularly of threat/control override content, e.g. persecutory delusions, thought insertion and other passivity delusions. These findings are in keeping with social psychology theory that violence in general is associated with an individual feeling under threat or losing control of his/her situation.

The Royal College of Psychiatrists in 1996, in their booklet *Assessment and Clinical Management of Risk of Harm to Other People*, detailed 'warning signs' that professionals should be aware of. These were:

- beliefs of persecution or control by external forces
- previous violence or suicide attempts
- social restlessness
- poor compliance with medication or treatment
- substance abuse
- hostility, suspiciousness and anger
- threats.

Psychiatric patients tend to peak for violent offending at a later age than the general population. It is important to be aware that the oft-quoted 'best predictor of future behaviour is past behaviour' is based on non-psychiatric populations and, in any case, accounts for only 5% of the variance. A history of previous violence is, of course, required for this to be relevant in any case. Among severely (psychotic) mentally ill people, delusions of threat/control override appear to be better predictors than past behaviour.

Among all individuals, including mentally ill people, a history of expressed threats (as opposed to generalized anger), substance misuse and a history of personal deprivation and/or abuse are all associated with violence. Indeed, it has been suggested that homicide rates in general may be reduced in the UK by coordinated multiagency responses and more policy and educational initiatives targeted specifically at countering domestic violence, child abuse, alcohol abuse and the carrying of knives and other weapons.

Law-breaking behaviour in general, and violence in particular, usually decreases when the basic needs of an individual are met. For instance, an individual with schizophrenia who kills often has a characteristic history of not only non-compliance with medication, leading to relapse of his or her mental illness, but also of being in a situation of social isolation and poor home conditions. Some individuals may even offend to remove themselves from their situation in the community to the security of prison or hospital. The risk of self-harm or suicide is, however, greater for people with schizophrenia, even if they have behaved seriously violently, than homicide or serious harm to others.

In summary, although no mental illness is characterized by serious violence, including homicide, the existing evidence suggests that there is a link between mental illness and violence. Mental illness is a risk factor, but not a large one, and the risk is increased by substance abuse.

Developments in brain scanning may elucidate this area further. Our research group has found evidence, using 31-phosphorus magnetic resonance spectroscopy, of increased cerebral metabolism in male patients with schizophrenia who have dangerously violently offended, including by homicide. In a structural magnetic resonance imaging voxel-based morphometry study, evidence of reduced grey matter volume bilaterally in Brodmann areas 39 and 40 and the cerebellum were found, as shown in Figure 21.5, in those with schizophrenia who had violently offended, including by homicide, compared to matched individuals with schizophrenia who had not offended. A strong connection has been hypothesized between the supramarginal region corresponding to Brodmann area 39/40 and Broca's area, which may

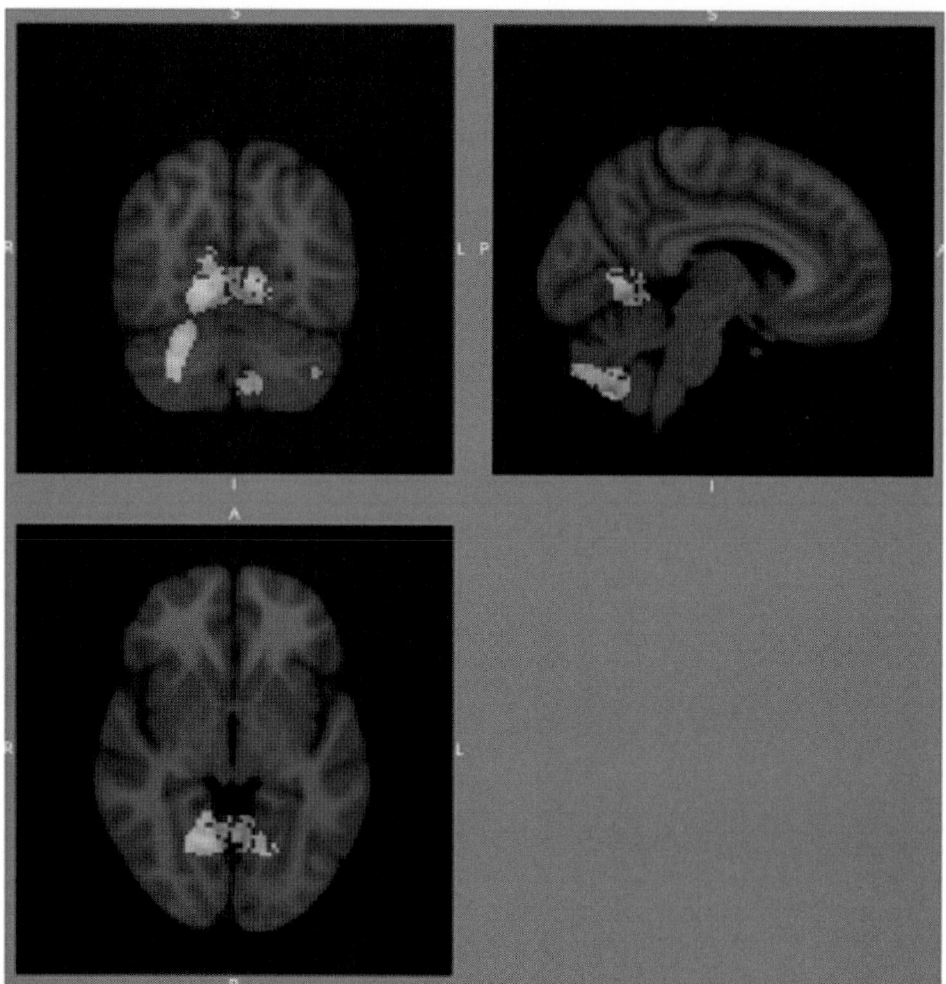

Figure 21.5 • The results of a voxel-based morphometry study of male patients with schizophrenia who had seriously dangerously offended compared with male schizophrenia patients who had not violently offended. • The *p*-value map, showing significant clusters, corrected for multiple comparisons overlaid on a standard template, shows reduced grey matter volume bilaterally in Brodmann areas 39 and 40 and in the cerebellum. (Reproduced with permission from Puri BK *et al.* 2008 BMC Psychiatry 8 Suppl 1:S6.)

correspond largely to the arcuate fasciculus, with the connectional pattern of the language regions of this model fitting the network of parietotemporal-prefrontal connections that participate in working memory. This points to the possibility of an abnormality in neural circuits involved in verbal working memory in this group of patients.

Avoidable deaths

The National Confidential Inquiry into Suicide and Homicide by People with Mental Illness, University of Manchester, England

This National Confidential Inquiry for England and Wales was set up in 1996 to collect detailed clinical information on homicides (and also suicides) by individuals in contact with mental health services. About 40–50 homicides a year are committed by such individuals.

Those with schizophrenia were responsible for 30 patient homicides a year. Half were current or recent patients, but one-third had no previous contact with services.

Those with personality disorder and a history of current or previous contact with psychiatric services were responsible for 10 cases per year.

Rates of mental disorder in all perpetrators of homicide were as shown in Table 21.9.

Fourteen per cent of homicides (seven per year) were considered 'most preventable' due to service failures, e.g. lack of adequate supervision, poor compliance.

Recommendations resulting included

Table 21.9 Rates of mental disorder in all perpetrators of homicide

Lifetime mental disorder	30%
Schizophrenia (lifetime)	5%
Contact with mental health services	18%
Contact within 12 months	9%
Mental illness at time of offence	10%

1. Ensure high-risk patients receive enhanced care planning backed up by peer review. The lack of this was considered the cause of about half of most preventable homicides.
2. Respond robustly when a care plan breaks down. Lack of response was considered to have caused 18% of the most preventable homicides. Twenty-five per cent of patient homicides were preceded by non-compliance.
3. Develop services for dual diagnosis patients, a high-risk group. Thirty-six per cent of homicide cases had dual diagnoses, i.e. mental disorder and substance abuse. Drug-induced psychosis can be just as dangerous as schizophrenia.

Inquiries into homicides by psychiatric patients

These have been mandatory in England and Wales since 1994, following a very critical and widely reported inquiry into the killing in 1992 of Jonathan Zito by Christopher Clunis, who suffered from chronic schizophrenia. Such inquiries have emphasized failures in care due to poor communication between professionals and agencies, downgrading of previous violence, failure to recognize and manage social restlessness and escalating problems, lack of contact of subjects with consultant psychiatrists, rigid catchment area practice, lack of resources, e.g. lack of acute beds and trained staff, failure to use the Mental Health Act appropriately to detain for reasons of health before violence occurs, and lack of carer involvement, although the latter may raise issues of patient confidentiality. Non-compliance with treatment in the community has been perhaps the most common major factor characterizing these cases. However, even Hippocrates noted that patients tend not to take their prescribed treatments. Also, there can, of course, be no real 'supervision' in the community in the sense of continual observation.

Overall, such inquiries have highlighted not the limitations of risk assessment, as real as these are, but failure to communicate or manage known risk. Improving community psychiatric care may thus be more useful in reducing the risk of violence than attempts at perfecting risk assessment instruments. Certainly, the use of standardized structured risk assessment instruments would not alone prevent most homicides by psychiatric patients.

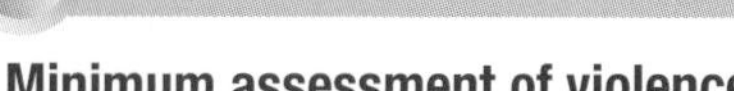

Minimum assessment of violence

- Ask informant about history of violence.
- Request previous summaries, e.g. of inpatient care, and past psychiatric and probation reports.
- Document above and otherwise keep and use proper records.
- Make plans to manage the risk and document this.
- Be particularly cautious in cases where treatment is refused, reduced or is being withheld.

Government responses to inquiry findings

The political pressure of 'something must be done' has led to the government responding with, among other initiatives, the Care Programme Approach (CPA) and the Community Treatment Order under the Mental Health Act 2007

The usefulness of the above measures remains open to question. The CPA is a process not a treatment and individuals may be unable or unwilling to comply and families may or may not wish to be involved. On the positive side, it is a needs-led multidisciplinary approach to developing a care plan, which has to be monitored and should always include a risk assessment. Drawbacks to its implementation include lack of resources, large caseloads, increase in time required for meetings and documentation, and it leading to defensive practice.

These Government responses also occur against a background of a general decline in psychiatric hospital beds, e.g. from 152 000 in 1954 to 53 700 in 1993. Those psychiatric patients who have been violent in the community, however, tend not, in fact, to be those who might have previously been on long-stay wards. However, if one closes 100 long-term hospital beds, there is an additional need for about 10 new acute beds to cope with resulting revolving door admissions and this can lead to a lack of acute beds for the emergency admission of violent patients. Increasing hospital beds alone is not the whole solution, as there is also a need for other measures such as short-term crisis community facilities. Funding has also not been related to epidemiology, e.g. in urban areas where there is an excess of schizophrenia due to social drift and where drug abuse and a younger population are also more evident, and there has otherwise been increased identification of cases, including via court and prison diversion schemes. One response by clinicians has been to increase the rates of detention under the Mental Health Act 1983, which has been most pronounced for Section 3 and for mental illness. Although there has been no significant change in the number of Section 37 hospital orders, there has been an increase in Section 41 restriction orders. Another response has been the development of assertive outreach programmes.

Habit and impulse-control disorders

Impulse-control disorders are disorders in which a person acts on an impulse that is potentially harmful and that he or she fails to resist. The impulses are usually perceived as pleasurable (egosyntonic). There is an increasing sense of wishing to commit the act with a sense of pleasure occurring once the act has been committed. These disorders have also been conceptualized as non-substance-related addictions. They do not represent personality disorders. They are described in DSM-IV-TR as impulse-control disorders, and in ICD-10 as habit and impulse disorders (see Table 21.10).

Pathological gambling, pyromania, and intermittent explosive (behaviour) disorder are more common in men, whereas kleptomania and trichotillomania are more common in women.

The offence of arson

Arson is the offence associated with fire-setting and is the unlawful and malicious (wilful) destruction of or damage to property by setting a fire. Legally, the more serious charge is arson with intent to endanger life or being reckless as to whether life was endangered. Owing to problems of detection, only 5% of cases of arson end in successful prosecution in the UK. In the UK, one school in eight is subject to arson each year.

If an individual is charged with arson, it is important to reconstruct in detail what happened at the time of the offence, for example, reading witness statements related to the case, and to not just depend on the actual legal offence category. For instance, arson may be setting fire to a wastepaper bin in a busy hospital ward in front of observing staff and fellow patients, or an impulsive or planned serious

Table 21.10 ICD-10 habit and impulse disorders

Pathological gambling	Persistently repeated gambling, which continues and often increases despite social consequences
Pathological fire-setting (pyromania)	Repeated fire-setting without any obvious motive. Intense interest in watching fires burn
	Feelings of increasing tension before the act and intense excitement immediately after it
Pathological stealing (kleptomania)	Repeated failure to resist impulses to steal objects that are not required for personal use or monetary gain
	Objects may be discarded, given away or hoarded
	Increasing sense of tension before and a sense of gratification during and immediately after the act
Trichotillomania	Noticeable hair loss due to a recurrent failure to resist impulses to pull out hair
	Hair pulling usually preceded by mounting tension and followed by sense of relief or gratification (responds to behaviour therapy or SSRI antidepressants)
Intermittent explosive (behaviour) disorder	

fire, in circumstances unlikely to be detected, with intent to kill. Of psychodynamic note is the fact that fire almost uniquely can make things disappear, including evidence. Historically, one reason individuals were burnt at the stake was to avoid spilling blood.

Epidemiology

Approximately 40% of all serious fires are started deliberately. Six per cent of fires in the UK are recorded as arson. Arson is responsible for 1% of all serious crimes in the UK. However, as the evidence is often burnt, only about a quarter of arson offences result in conviction. The peak age for arson is 17 years for men and 45 years for women. Eighty per cent of those convicted are men. There is increased incidence of arson among those with learning disabilities and those who suffer from alcohol dependence syndrome. Fifty per cent of cases of arson follow alcohol abuse, especially binge drinking of alcohol.

Clinical classification

There is no typical arsonist. Psychiatric difficulties are common, but the most common diagnoses are personality disorder and substance abuse, in up to two-thirds of cases, with about 8% suffering from a psychosis. Pure pyromania appears rare (1%) among convicted arsonists.

A clinical classification of arson is as follows:

1. Fire as a means to an end (motivated). This includes the following:
   - **(a)** Those who set few fires
     - *Psychosis*, such as schizophrenia. Such individuals may set fires, for instance, to burn out the devil or evil, or in response to hallucinatory voices.
     - *Displaced revenge, anger, or jealousy.* Rather than overt direct aggression against an individual, aggression may be displaced into setting fire to that individual's property. For instance, an employee of a warehouse or supermarket is told off by his boss, but rather than directly retaliate physically aggressively, the employee returns after business hours to set fire to his boss's property. This is the most common reason (in almost 50% of cases) found by psychiatrists among arsonists referred to them.
     - *Cover-up of other crimes*, for example homicide. Modern forensic science, however, usually overcomes such attempts at a cover-up.
     - *For insurance.* This has become increasingly common in recent years; for instance, french-fry/chip pan fires to finance the redecoration of a kitchen.
     - *Political motivation.* For example, to further their rise to power, Nazi storm troopers set fire to the Reichstag in 1932 in Berlin.
     - *Adolescent gangs.* Individuals are generally more likely to be disinhibited and behave antisocially in a group than when alone. This group is associated with a low rate of recidivism, except among gang leaders.

(b) Those who set more fires
- *Desire to be powerful or a hero.* Members of this group often have inadequate personalities. Their low self-esteem is bolstered by the sense of power they feel at the results of having set fires, e.g. the panic and the emergency services with flashing lights rushing to the scene. Sometimes this is combined with a desire to be a hero, so that after setting a fire the individual may rush into the premises and rescue pets or the elderly or infirm. On occasions they are caught owing to being seen repeatedly or even photographed, for instance, by a local newspaper at the scenes of the fires.
- *To earn money.* This occurs when part-time firemen on call-out rates set a fire. It is a particular problem in rural areas and in some countries such as France. Some individuals may be drawn to the fire service because of their fascination with fire, and psychodynamic associations have been made regarding the phallic symbolism of hoses. Anthropologists and evolutionists have suggested that females may have been impressed by the ability of males to put fires out by urinating.
- *As a cry for help.* To bring attention to a distressed emotional state.

2. Fire as a thing of interest. This includes the following:
- Pathological fire-setting (pyromania).
- Tension or depression reduction (analogous to sitting in front of a glowing coal fire)
- Sexual excitement (erotic) group. Rare. May masturbate after setting fire. Compare the symbolism of fire, e.g. 'flames of passion'

Differential diagnosis of arsonists

This includes conduct, adjustment, affective and psychotic disorders, as well as pyromania.

Comorbidity may include substance misuse, past history of sexual or physical abuse, and personality disorder, especially antisocial personality disorder. High rates of previous sexual abuse in women who set fires have been frequently described in clinical practice.

Assessment of arsonists

This depends not only on a careful, detailed history and mental state examination, but also on the gathering and study of objective information such as witness statements related to a case. It is important to determine the presence or absence of psychiatric abnormality, especially at the time of the offence, and its relationship with the offence itself. It is clearly important to determine whether there is a history of previous fire-setting and to examine precipitants.

It should be noted that suicide by fire is particularly associated with schizophrenia, perhaps explaining the choice of this most painful means of suicide. Historically, it has been described in the early 19th century among Hindu widows in India (suttee) and among monks protesting in Vietnam during the mid-20th-century war.

Management

This should clearly address any underlying or comorbid psychiatric disorders. Psychological intervention, for example, with cognitive-behavioural therapy, may be helpful.

The potential dangers of fire-raising must always be borne in mind. The fire service view is that a large fire is merely a small fire not brought under control.

In cases where an individual is charged with arson, the courts will be particularly concerned with the protection of the public and are likely to be unwilling in serious cases of arson to consider outpatient care or placement in an open psychiatric ward. Ordinary psychiatric hospitals are also inevitably reluctant to admit those who have set fires, so if hospital treatment is required it is frequently undertaken under conditions of medium or maximum security. In the absence of a psychiatric disposal, the courts usually impose a custodial sentence. In England and Wales, under the Criminal Damage Act 1971, a maximum sentence of life imprisonment can be imposed for arson (Section 1) or arson endangering life (Section 2).

Prognosis

Further offences of arson are increasingly likely if there has been a history of previous arson and if the offender continues to have an irresistible impulse to set fires or to relieve tension or obtain pleasure or sexual excitement from such fire-setting. Increased risk of further fire-setting is seen in individuals who suffer from psychosis, learning disability, or dementia. However, in an individual case, it may be difficult to tell whether that individual will reoffend. The risk of further serious offending after a period in prison or hospital is low; however, the risk of reoffending may not be apparent in the short term but only on longer follow-up, for example, 4% recidivism rate over a 20-year period.

The offence of shoplifting

The technical offence is theft, that is, from shops, an offence that, as with all offences of theft, requires the intent permanently to deprive, as well as the act, for the offence to be proved in court. Intent would clearly be indicated if an individual were seen to be hiding an object in his coat and to be looking around to make sure he was not being observed. In absent-minded shoplifting, there would theoretically be no intention to deprive.

Epidemiology

In the UK, about 5% of all shoppers shoplift. However, up to 50% of goods taken from shops may be taken by the staff of those shops, as is the case with many thefts from businesses. Sociologists have viewed shoplifting as a social disorder created by a consumer society and precipitated by the visual provocation of shop displays. Open shelves increase sales and reduce the requirement for staff, as in supermarkets, but they are associated with increased shoplifting, with such businesses having to take this into account in their business planning. Some items are left near the checkout till for impulse buying and, in addition, provide easy but inexpensive objects to be shoplifted. Objects are often taken suddenly on impulse and are of trivial value or useless. Some individuals appear to regard shoplifting as an accepted perk of shopping and may pay for other items.

Up to the early 1970s, most shoplifters in the UK were women, who then undertook more of the shopping than now, and 50% showed evidence of psychiatric disorder. Ninety per cent did not re-offend after conviction. However, the majority of shoplifters in the UK are now male and between the ages of 10 and 18 years, as reflected in signs on shops limiting the number of children allowed in at one time. Males are now more likely than females to have previous convictions. The incidence of psychiatric disorder has been reduced to about 5%, and it is questionable now whether shoplifting deserves more psychiatric attention than other thefts (90% of all offences are acquisitive). The previous predominance of female offenders coincided with the view that female offenders tended to be psychiatrically disordered, which may explain the courts' requests for psychiatric reports more often in shoplifting offences than in other, male-dominated, offences.

Classification of shoplifters

Shoplifters have been subject to lay and legal stereotyping as needy, greedy or seedy, and as professional, amateur and associated with psychiatric disorder. A useful classification is as follows.

1. Shoplifting for simple gain plus excitement, with or without associated marked antisocial attitudes

The principal motivation is excitement, and such individuals are responsible for a significant proportion of shoplifting in large cities. Individuals often feel less constrained by another country's laws when abroad. This category also includes organized gangs and those with chaotic lives who steal impulsively and commit other offences. They may come from antisocial families and be subject to relative poverty. Such shoplifting may be associated with resentment and feelings of bitterness associated with the individuals' lifestyles.

2. Shoplifting associated with psychiatric disturbance

The most common association in this group has historically been with *depression* in people of previous law-abiding personality. They may include isolated younger women with children, but they may also include middle-aged women isolated from their families, who have lost children, who have experienced the loss of a husband (including loss owing to his career), and who also may have significant physical complaints or ill-health and/or be chronically depressed. Shoplifting may be an early symptom of depression. The depression may also be associated with acute losses. Law involvement, including court appearances and associated publicity, can precipitate self-harm or suicide where offenders are depressed.

In cases of shoplifting and depression, the motivation may arise from feelings of guilt, a desire to be caught and punished, a cry for help, or represent an act of self-comfort or a treat. Other dynamics include secondary gain, e.g. in the newly poor to keep up appearances or to steal something for oneself that is not purchased with money from parents or a husband. In married female offenders, there may particularly be sexual difficulties or rejection and marital problems. Shoplifting may be an act of revenge on a husband or a partner to induce shame or punishment. For instance, it may result in the female having to be accompanied by her husband when shopping in future or alternatively in the husband having to undertake the shopping from which the wife can then opt out. For such individuals, a prison sentence may at one level be a relief from their marital or family situation.

Fewer than 5% of arrested shoplifters suffer from *kleptomania*. Figure 21.6 illustrates psychodynamic theories of this condition.

Other psychiatric disorders associated with shoplifting include anorexia and bulimia nervosa, which may reflect both hunger for food and impulsivity, and early dementia, which is associated with disinhibited behaviour, lower resistance to temptation, poor judgement and late-onset offending. Shoplifting may also occur on occasion in association with other psychotic mental illnesses, alcoholism and learning disability.

3. Absent-minded shoplifting

This implies no intent permanently to deprive and, if successfully argued in court, a not guilty verdict will result. Such shoplifting may result from undue preoccupation, distractions or harassment, e.g. caused by the shopper's own accompanying children. Other causes cited include claustrophobia in shops and various medical or psychiatric drugs that impair concentration or cause confusion. It is the prescribing doctor's responsibility to warn of such side-effects from medication. Although a defence based on medication side-effects, including the effects of benzodiazepines, is not infrequently put forward in court by shoplifters, in reality it is rarely a primary cause.

4. Shoplifting in children

This peaks around 14–15 years, with boys being predominant. Boys steal candy and books. Girls tend to steal cosmetics and clothes. The items stolen are usually of little value. The most common group is, in fact, that of 'normal' children stealing for excitement. However, child shoplifting may occur owing to subcultural standards or as an expression of emotional disturbance, e.g. as an act of defiance against parents, as a cry for help, or in association with feelings of depression, worthlessness, and a sense of guilt.

Assessment of shoplifters

An examination of the history and mental state of the individual should elucidate motives and detect any evidence of formal psychiatric disorder. The motive may often initially appear obscure, with useless objects or objects of trivial value taken suddenly on impulse, sometimes as a treat or arising from concealed resentment. Alcohol or drug abuse is often associated with shoplifting. Additional information should be obtained if possible, e.g. from the arresting police officer. It is often useful to discuss the case with the probation officer if one has been requested by the court to prepare a social inquiry report, which should also be read. It is essential to establish whether there is a history of previous convictions for shoplifting and any past psychiatric history and its relationship to offending.

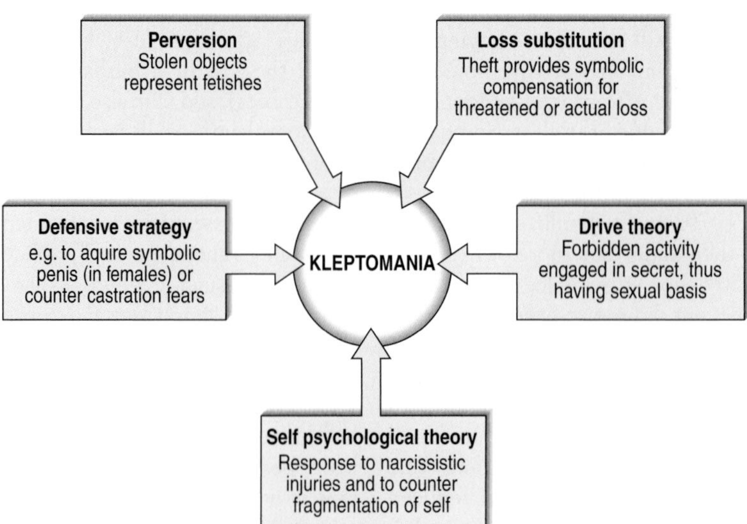

Figure 21.6 • Psychodynamic theories of kleptomania.

Management

If it is argued on psychiatric grounds that there was no intent to shoplift and the patient pleads this successfully, a finding of not guilty will result. However, individuals are often deterred from such a defence, e.g. a defence involving absent-minded shoplifting, as it will often require a number of court appearances and considerable legal expense, including payments to lawyers, to plead this successfully, and it may well involve local publicity.

Where the court accepts that intent permanently to deprive was present, the individual is legally convicted of theft. If the individual does suffer from a psychiatric disorder, including kleptomania, requiring treatment, psychiatric evidence may be used in mitigation with a view to altering the sentence, e.g. a psychiatric recommendation of outpatient psychiatric treatment may be made as part of a community rehabilitation (old probation) order.

Case history: shoplifting and depressive episode

A married, late-middle-aged female, Mrs B., whose children were grown up and had left home, lived with her husband who had become increasingly preoccupied with his career and neglectful of her. She had had a number of physical complaints since the menopause for which she had frequently attended her GP, from whose treatment, however, she considered she had obtained little benefit.

Over a period of 2 months she developed increasing feelings of sadness, which were worse in the mornings, initial insomnia and early morning wakening, and began to lose weight. One day while in a large department store doing family shopping, she stole some items of clothing. She was observed by a store detective and admitted her intent to steal when she was apprehended outside the shop. The police were called and she was charged with theft.

The police granted her bail to reside at home. She had no previous convictions and had previously been of good character. In the light of this and her apparent depression, a psychiatric report and a social enquiry report prepared by the probation service were requested by the Magistrates' court, who allowed Mrs B. continuing bail at home.

The psychiatrist considered that Mrs B. was suffering from a depressive episode and that her shoplifting was a cry for help, as well as to give herself a treat emotionally to improve her mood. At one level she acknowledged that she had had a desire to be caught to bring attention to her situation, and that her offence was, in part, an act of revenge on her husband. The legal proceedings themselves and local newspaper publicity compounded her depressive episode.

The psychiatrist discussed the case with the probation officer, who was preparing the social enquiry report and who felt that Mrs B. would benefit from the provision of emotional and practical support and direction under a community rehabilitation (old probation) order. The psychiatrist considered that Mrs B.'s depressive episode needed treatment with antidepressive medication and psychotherapy. He did not consider that she currently needed inpatient psychiatric treatment, but recommended that this should be given on an outpatient basis, as a condition of the proposed community rehabilitation (old probation) order.

When the case was finally dealt with at the Magistrates' court, Mrs B. pleaded guilty and was convicted. She was sentenced to a 2-year probation order with a condition of outpatient psychiatric treatment, to which she had to agree voluntarily.

Mrs B.'s mental state rapidly improved over the ensuing 2 months with emotional support and treatment from the psychiatrist and probation officer. The psychiatrist also saw Mrs B. together with her husband to help explore and counter some of their marital difficulties. By the end of the 2-year community rehabilitation (old probation) order Mrs B. remained psychiatrically well, had not shoplifted again and had found herself part-time clerical work.

If Mrs B. had failed to attend to see either the probation officer or the psychiatrist, or had refused psychiatric treatment, she would have been in breach of her community rehabilitation (old probation) order and its conditions and could have been taken back to court for her sentence to be reconsidered. She might then have faced a custodial sentence or an inpatient hospital treatment order.

Intermittent explosive (behaviour) disorder or episodic dyscontrol syndrome

This is included in ICD-10 under habit and impulse disorders, but not in DSM-IV-TR, and is characterized by episodes of sudden unprovoked violence. Onset is in adolescence, and males outnumber females in a ratio of 4:1. It was originally conceptualized as a form of limbic epilepsy, but this has not been borne out. The syndrome may, however, be associated with soft neurological signs and temporal lobe electroencephalogram (EEG) abnormalities, and may be helped by anticonvulsants such as carbamazepine and sodium valproate. Mood stabilizers may also be used, and lithium and selective serotonin reuptake inhibitor (SSRI) antidepressants may also help, suggesting a link to mood (affective) disorder. This disorder, in fact, usually occurs in those with a severe, often explosive, personality disorder with a propensity under stress to intemperate outbursts of anger and impulsive violence when frustrated, which equates to the emotionally unstable impulsive-type personality disorder of ICD-10 and falls within the antisocial personality disorder of DSM-IV-TR. It is of note that half of persistently aggressive offenders in general are said to have an abnormal EEG record, often an immature record (persistence of excess posterior slow-wave activity), characteristic of those with psychopathic disorder and not diagnostic of epilepsy.

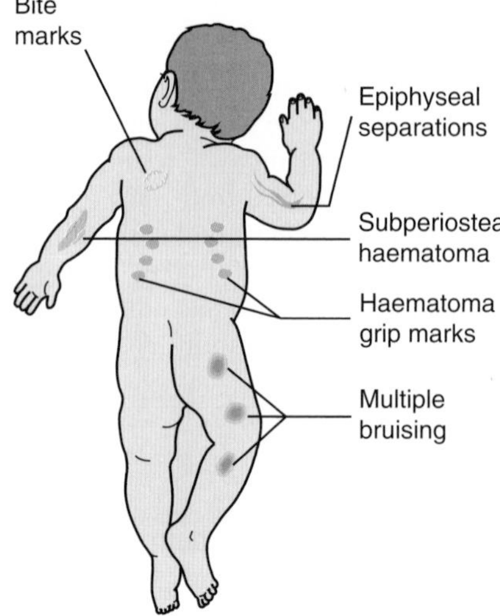

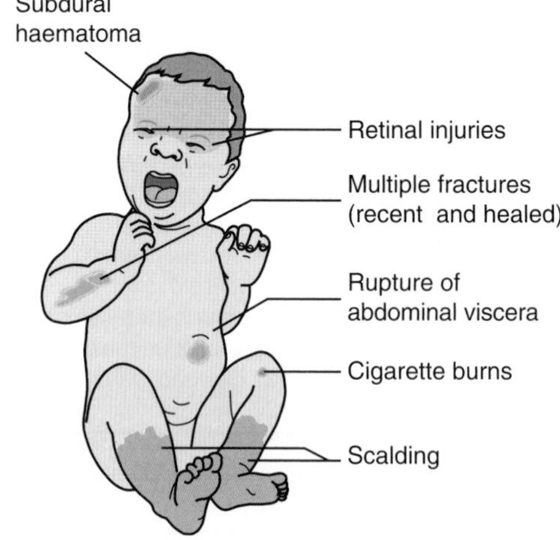

Figure 21.7 • Possible clinical features in non-accidental injury in children.

Non-accidental injury of children

This term has replaced that of 'baby battering', coined by Kempe and Kempe in 1961 as an emotive term to highlight the problem.

Characteristic features of different members of the families in which non-accidental injury of children occurs are as follows:

- Children
  - usually less than three years of age
  - failure to thrive
  - persistent crying
  - multiple injuries in time and space
  - delay in reporting and contradictory histories of injuries.

Possible clinical features are shown in Figure 21.7.

- Parents
  - often abused themselves and unhappy children
  - lower social class families
  - isolated and no support
  - marital disharmony
  - unwanted pregnancy
  - no contraception.
- Mother
  - often teenager, unmarried, neurotic and/or learning disability
  - expects love from child
  - not infrequently on diazepam (Valium).
- Father
  - in about half the cases, not biological father
  - two-thirds not married
  - often has personality disorder.
  - criminal in two-thirds of cases and one in three has conviction for violence
  - beats wife in one-quarter of cases
  - competes with the child, whom he rejects, for his wife's/partner's attention.

The incidence of psychosis in parents is low, but may be higher in severely abused cases. In the UK there are 80 child murders a year; 60 of whom are killed by their parents and 10 by strangers. The other 10 refer to individuals, not necessarily other family members, who knew the child.

Note that filicide is the killing of one's son or daughter.

Management

Early recognition of children at risk is paramount for those working in baby clinics and general practice. It depends on high professional awareness, including from health visitors and those working in nursery facilities and schools. *Child Protection Registers* are held by local authorities, which must also be able and prepared to undertake rapid emergency action (e.g. an emergency protection order). *Multidisciplinary case conferences*, with the designation of key workers, are essential in the management of such families. Special family and marital therapy may be necessary to improve the family and marital situation and to counter unrealistic expectations about, and consequent feelings of resentment towards, the child.

Homicide of infants and children

Of children killed under one year of age, 60% are killed by their mother. On occasions a mother will kill a child to spite a partner or spouse (*Medea Complex*).

There are about 20 cases per year in England and Wales of *neonatal homicide*, most within one day of life and committed by the mother. The mothers are typically of previous good behaviour, but from chaotic or dysfunctional homes. They are isolated, as reflected in their taking pregnancies to term without telling others. They may deny their pregnancy, attributing nausea to something eaten and the kicks from the baby as due to wind. Their denial, combined with psychological splitting and tendency to concealment, may result in the mother making no noise during labour. The precipitant to homicide may be the baby's first cry or a desire to kill the baby at birth before the 'beginning of life'. Alternatively, the baby may be abandoned, whereupon it may be difficult to decide if this was with intent to kill or not.

Child abduction

The relevant law is the Child Abduction Act 1984. There are three main groups

1. abduction by parents, usually in custody disputes
2. abduction of older children, usually by a man with a sexual motive
3. baby stealing, the least common group, usually carried out by women.

In the UK, in Victorian times in the 19th century, children were stolen in order to obtain their clothes. When females steal babies, in general the babies are well cared for and usually quickly recovered.

Categories of baby stealing

These include

1. comforting offences, e.g. those with learning disability who steal a baby to play with or for comfort
2. manipulative offences, where the motive may be an attempt to influence the man with whom the relationship is insecure by presenting the baby to their partner pretending the child is his, e.g. following a miscarriage of a pregnancy by him or threatened desertion
3. psychotic offences where offences are motivated by delusional ideas, e.g. that the child is a Messiah.

Spouse abuse (replaces term wife battering)/intimate partner violence

Historically in England and Wales, in the 16th century a male was not allowed to beat his wife after 10pm. In the 18th century, the Rule of Thumb applied, as a result of which a male was not legally allowed to beat his wife with a stick or implement wider than a thumb. Under the Matrimonial Causes Act 1878, a husband was allowed a free hand with his wife to the extent he could forcibly return his wife to their home.

The true incidence of spouse abuse is obscured by the hidden nature of behaviour and problems in definition, e.g. over the degree of violence. This category is responsible in England and Wales for 16% of all violent crimes and results in two homicides of females a week. Forty per cent are killed in the bedroom or kitchen. Often this is associated with psychological abuse and associated behaviours, such as excessive jealousy and control of money. In the USA it has been estimated that in 25–30% of marriages one partner would push, shove or grab the other at some point. Punches and kicks occur in 13% of marriages, and beating up or using a weapon in 5% of marriages. Surveys show that although wives attack their husbands at a not substantially lesser frequency, such attacks are much less violent and usually defensive.

Male abusers are often inarticulate, demanding and find violence empowering. Typologies include those with a frequent loss of temper and those who undertake cold deliberate assaults, as well as overcontrolled individuals who eventually 'snap' under stress. Jealousy within the relationship is a factor noted in two-thirds of cases. Half of offenders have been exposed to domestic violence as a child. Fifty per cent of assaults follow alcohol abuse. Wife battering has also been associated with gambling, unemployment and an otherwise criminal record. Offenders are often remorseful following violence. Women may be trapped in violent marriages economically, due to a lack of alternative housing, or, because of feelings of responsibility for children and/or by learned helplessness.

Battered women syndrome

This has been described as being characterized by:

- depression
- loss of self-esteem
- post-traumatic stress disorder
- substance abuse
- suicidality
- physical health problems
- sexual problems.

Intimate partner abuse mainly affects women (wives, girlfriends, female partners). If intimate partner (spouse) abuse is suspected, it can be difficult to persuade the female victim to admit that she has been physically and mentally abused. A recent Canadian screening randomized trial has found that women prefer self-completed questionnaire approaches to face-to-face questioning. Assessment of the victim must be carried out with great sensitivity. Check that the victim is not suicidal or depressed, and that she is not abusing alcohol or drugs or suffering from an anxiety disorder. The management can be difficult, particularly if the victim denies the abuse and insists on returning to the abusive partner. If there is a high risk of the abuse continuing, social services may need to be involved and the police may need to be informed. If the risk is lower, and the victim and her partner agree, then marital therapy may be arranged.

Management

- Voluntary refuges for female victims are now widely available.
- Anger management techniques can be applied to offenders.
- A non-molestation injunction can also be sought, including with attached power of arrest.
- A new multidisciplinary case conference management approach (MARAC) is developing in the UK.

Elder abuse

Estimates of up to 500 000 older people being abused a day in the UK have been made. Elder abuse includes violence, neglect or emotional abuse of elderly relatives, often surviving widowed elderly mothers. Elder abuse has replaced the term 'granny bashing'. The offender is often a son or daughter (50% over 60 years of age) of the victim and lives together with the victim. The UK prevalence rate is between 1.5% and 5.6%. Abused elders are no more physically or mentally infirm than non-abused elders.

The abuser may be otherwise under stress from marital or financial problems, be depressed, have a history of substance misuse and/or personal history of abuse themselves, and be unable to cope with the added stress of looking after the victim who may be emotionally and economically dependent. Unresolved emotional conflict is often present.

There is often a history of families being reluctant to take over the care of elder relatives but being under pressure to do so. Occasionally elder abuse arises due to equally aged spouses having to cope with/care for victims. Emotional conflict may be present between the abuser and abused. Unqualified staff in poorly managed nursing homes may also abuse the elderly.

Victim vulnerability factors, e.g. disability, dementia or paranoid illness, may be present.

N.B. Most violence is in families, i.e. where individuals are most physically and emotionally close to others.

Morbid jealousy (Othello syndrome)

Delusions of infidelity about a sexual partner can lead a sufferer to examine underwear, sexual organs of partner, etc., in an attempt to find proof of unfaithfulness, and, on occasions, to attempt to extract confessions by violence. Not infrequently, this leads to severe aggression towards, and the killing of, the sexual partner about whom the delusions are held.

This is over six times more common in males than in females (compare erotomania, which is more frequent in females), and usually commences in the 40s, after about 10 years of marriage/relationship, and is present for about four years before presenting. It is responsible for 12% of homicides due to mental illness.

Aetiology

Evolutionary theories suggest that males may be predisposed to sexual jealousy as they cannot know if it is their sperm that results in a pregnancy. Ten per cent of male birds look after offspring that are not biologically their own.

Morbid jealousy is associated with alcoholism, schizophrenia and delusional disorder. Morbid jealousy may be a forerunner of a later schizophrenic illness, this only manifesting after serious violence. Also it is associated with impotence in males. Psychodynamic theories postulate that the suspicious attitudes may be a projection of the individual's own desires for infidelity onto the victim-partner or a more internally acceptable, conscious manifestation of repressed homosexuality. Morbid jealousy is often associated with low self-esteem with resulting feelings of insecurity that the partner may not really love him and may wish to leave him for someone else.

Management

This is often difficult due to lack of insight of the subject and the sexual partner's belief that they can overcome their spouse's unjustifiable beliefs. Underlying psychiatric conditions should be adequately treated, e.g. stop alcohol abuse. Antipsychotic medication may help if compliance can be obtained. Separation may be the only answer and there is a risk of recurrence in future relationships, e.g. the case of Iliffe who killed four wives in spite of having spent periods in between in Broadmoor special hospital. It is best to work with a co-therapist, e.g. a social worker, who remains involved with the spouse, advising her of refuges, etc., while the psychiatrist concentrates on the patient.

N.B. Rivalry is where two individuals are in competition for the same object. There is no aggression to object.

Envy. One individual desires someone or something that belongs to someone else. Aggression is to the competitor or self but not to the object.

Jealousy. Fantasies of losing the object to rival. Aggression is directed not to the rival but to the object, i.e. spouse. All through history and across cultures, the main cause of female homicide has been male jealousy.

Jealousy can be normal or excessive (sometimes even in the absence of delusions, also termed morbid), i.e. for neurotic, obsessional or delusional reasons, including being secondary to affective disorder. It also arises in paranoid personalities. The boundary between normal and pathological jealousy may be indistinct. However, psychotic jealousy often responds better to treatment than neurotic jealousy.

Delusional jealousy can develop even when the spouse has, in fact, been unfaithful. The way the delusional belief develops may be more diagnostic than the pure content of the belief.

Erotomania (de Clérambault's syndrome)

This is a delusional disorder that another person, often unobtainable and of higher social status, loves the patient (usually female) intensely. It may be primary, or secondary due to a paranoid or affective disorder. It is more usually associated with schizophrenia than a pure monodelusional disorder. Only some with this disorder will display disruptive antisocial behaviour, e.g. phone calls, letter writing, following the victim, but repeated rebuttals may lead to hatred and dangerous behaviour. Gille de la Tourette, who gave his name to Tourette's syndrome, was himself killed by an erotomanic patient. Dangerousness is increased if there is a history of multiple delusional objects in the past and a premorbid antisocial personality. De Clérambault, after whom the syndrome was named, in fact shot himself while dressed in a toga and was found by Lacan, the psychotherapist.

Stalking

This is the wilful, malicious and repeated following and harassing of another person, which threatens that person's safety; 80% of victims are female. Typologies of the stalker include:

- *The rejected stalker* who acts through a mixture of revenge and desire for reconciliation. As a group they tend to be more assaultative but more likely to respond to judicial sanctions.

- *Intimacy seeking*. These include the deluded. Such individuals may stalk the famous and mental health professionals.
- *Incompetent stalker/suitor*. Such individuals lack social skills and may be intellectually limited.
- *Resentful stalkers*. They often intend to cause fear.
- *Predatory stalkers*. These are rare but may have fantasies about or be intent on sexual assaults.

There may also be false victims, including those deluded that they are being stalked. Post-traumatic stress disorder occurs in over a third of victims. Fifty per cent of stalkers threaten violence, three-quarters of whom are not, however, subsequently violent or destructive of property. The risk of violence is increased if there are prior convictions and/or substance misuse. Stalking offences are now covered by the Protection from Harassment Act 1997 in England and Wales (an injunction combined with a criminal sentence), but prevention, when possible, may be most effective.

Substance misuse and crime

Association may be due to

1. altered mental states due to drug intoxication, withdrawal or long-term consequences, e.g. organic mental disorder
2. acquisitive offences to finance substance misuse
3. technical offences under misuse of drugs legislation.

Drug and alcohol abuse usually has disinhibiting effects on behaviour, impairs judgement and is associated with violence. Alcohol abuse, including acute intoxication, is present in up to one-half of individuals at the time they commit offences of violence in the UK.

Alcohol dependence syndrome is associated with an eight times higher rate of convictions for criminal offences, including especially motoring, drunkenness and acquisitive offences. There may be a history of alcohol abuse for three years before an initial offence, within three years of which the individual is often dependent on alcohol.

About half of those with a drug dependence syndrome have convictions before they become dependent.

Glue sniffers may be charged with breach of the peace or depositing rubbish, i.e. crisp bags from which they have inhaled glue and then dropped when intoxicated. Among the non-mentally ill, cannabis may be the only drug that has antiaggressive properties.

Epilepsy

The prevalence of epilepsy in prisons in England and Wales was noted to be two to four times that in the general population in an influential study in 1977, (7.2 per 1000 compared to the general population of 4.2 per 1000). However, a more recent study in 2002 has shown a prevalence of 1% in prison, which is equivalent to that in the community. Individuals with epilepsy are no more likely to be serving a custodial sentence for a violent offence than other prisoners. Violence associated with epilepsy is, in fact, rare. Ictal phenomena, including automatism, do not account for this overrepresentation. Alternative explanations include

1. underlying organic mental disorder being responsible for both epilepsy and offending
2. development of epilepsy adversely affecting the individuals' self-esteem and resulting in social rejection, which, in turn, leads to antisocial behaviour
3. adverse social circumstances leading to both epilepsy and antisocial behaviour, e.g. being a battered baby
4. a tendency to be impulsive and antisocial, leading to offending and head injuries, and thus post-traumatic epilepsy.

If linked, the most likely relationship between epilepsy and imprisonment is that such individuals show the same biosocial disadvantages.

The association between aggressive behaviour and temporal lobe epilepsy has been widely reported. There is some evidence for amygdaloid foci, but psychosocial factors obviously also are important. As a generalization, however, neurologists say that without a history of a fit, epilepsy is unlikely to be a cause of aggression.

Half of persistently aggressive offenders are said to have an abnormal EEG, often an immature record (persistence of excess posterior slow-wave theta activity) (see Figure 15.2) characteristic of those with psychopathic disorder and not diagnostic of epilepsy.

Psychiatry and prisons

The UK has a daily population of over 80 000 prisoners with about 130 000 people received each year. There are about 20 males to every one female prisoner. This equates to about one in 15 children experiencing a parent in prison at some point, or about 25 000 at one time.

Penrose's Law described an inverse relationship between the number of psychiatric inpatients and prisoners in a country. The UK has a greater proportion of both compared to the rest of Europe, bar prisoners in Turkey. However, it is true that as the UK's psychiatric hospital population has decreased, its prison population has risen. The USA, which has 5% of the world's population, has 25% of the world's prisoners, around 2 million, perhaps largely due to policies of zero tolerance to drug-related crime (60% of those in prison are there because of this). One in three of New York's Afro-Americans have been in prison or on parole.

Prisons in England and Wales may be

1. local, such as HMP Brixton and HMP Wandsworth, which are closed and for people on remand, awaiting trial or sentence, or for convicted prisoners serving less than two years, and serve local courts, or
2. training prisons, which may be open, such as HMP Ford, or closed, such as the high security HMP Belmarsh or HMP Long Lartin, and are for prisoners serving more than two years. Some are dispersal prisons for high security risk prisoners, e.g. HMP Wormwood Scrubs.

London's local prison for women is HMP Holloway, which contains a mother and baby unit. Female prisoners have higher rates of learning disability, personality disorder, neurosis and substance misuse.

All prisoners are classified on security considerations, from Category A prisoners, who are considered to require maximum security and are subject to many restrictions, down to Category D prisoners, who are suitable for open conditions.

Young Offender Institutions (HMYOI) take those aged 15 up to 21 years requiring custody, e.g. HMYOI Feltham, near London, England.

Although custodial sentences prevent re-offending during such sentences and are increasing in length in the UK, 60% of prisoners re-offend within two years.

Prison psychiatry

Psychiatrists may be requested to assess prisoners to:

- provide court reports
- provide assessments and management and advice, including for sentenced prisoners, at the request of Prison Medical Officers
- for statutory purposes, such as preparing reports for the Parole Board.

To visit a prisoner, arrangements need to be made with the Healthcare Wing of the prison. Psychiatrists may need security clearance. Assessments have to fit in with prison routine, which only allows for two to three hours in the morning or the afternoon to see a patient, and the psychiatrist will usually need to wait for prison staff escorts upon arrival.

Issues relevant to psychiatric care in prison include the following:

- prevention, i.e. of offending and imprisonment, by psychiatric care in the community
- police station/court diversion schemes
- screening should be undertaken on reception of inmates to prison (three-quarters of psychiatric cases may be missed due to inadequate screening)
- measures to counter suicide risk, which is nine times higher than in the community (highest in first two months, especially among young males on remand who are not necessarily formally mentally ill)
- return to psychiatric hospital care under the relevant Mental Health Act while on remand, by means of court sentence or during custodial sentence
- substance misuse/detox services. Abstinence may result in a medical emergency due to withdrawal. Also, high mortality rates in cases of substance misuse upon release from prison due to loss of tolerance
- Sex Offender Treatment Programmes (SOTP)
- special therapeutic community units for sentenced prisoners with personality disorder, e.g. HMP Grendon in England
- Dangerous Severe Personality Disorder (DSPD) Units at HMP Whitmoor and HMP Franklin.

The Mental Health Act does not apply in prison, but medical treatment can be administered in good faith under common law in prison where there is lack of capacity to consent and in the best interests of the individual, e.g. to prevent immediate serious risk to others or self.

The aim is that healthcare in prison should ensure an equivalence of services to NHS care outside, with 24-hour psychiatric care/inreach for remanded and sentenced prisoners, on both medical wings and ordinary locations, provided by local general or forensic mental health services.

A National Offender Management Service (NOMS) has been established to manage offenders across the criminal justice system. Healthcare services in prison have been devolved to the NHS. An Assessment, Care in Custody and Teamwork (ACCT) approach has been developed for those at suicide/self-harm risk, based on case management, individualized care planning and multidisciplinary teamwork.

Although the prevalence of mental disorder in prison populations is high, with perhaps the majority suffering from mental disorder, albeit mainly personality disorder (40–60%) and/or substance misuse, with major depression in 10–12% and psychotic illness in around 4%, the criterion for transfer to hospital under the Mental Health Act is that an individual requires detention for inpatient psychiatric treatment, not merely that the individual might benefit from psychiatric or psychological help, including in prison. However, shortage of low, medium and maximum secure beds leads to mentally ill prisoners remaining in custody for lengthy periods.

A useful guide when assessing offenders as regards to their need for psychiatric treatment is to ignore the offence and assess the need for treatment as if one were seeing them as a new outpatient case.

Sexual offending

In the UK sexual offences account for 0.6% of all offences and 3% of indictable (more serious, eligible for trial by jury) offences. Disorders of sexual preference or paraphilias are covered in Chapter 13: not all of these are illegal and this varies between countries. The age of consent for both heterosexual and homosexual intercourse also varies between countries, and with it the seriousness with which underage sex is treated (e.g. in the UK sex with a female under the age of 13 is similar to rape in seriousness).

Sexual offending occurs much more frequently in males than females. Such offending may reflect a desire for affection or to relate, as much as for orgasm. It may also have an emotional releasing cathartic function. There is also an excess of those with learning disability. It must be noted that only a proportion of individuals who commit sexual offences have a disorder of sexual preference or a gender identity disorder. Among sexual offenders it is useful to distinguish those in whom the offending has arisen from a fixed disorder of sexual preference, from those who are usually sexually well adjusted and their sexual offending represents regressed behaviour or a latent sexual deviation released by stress or due to the disinhibiting effects of substance misuse or mental illness.

Indecent exposure is the offence in the UK that corresponds to the behaviour of the disorder of sexual preference of 'exhibitionism'. The offence is of 'openly, lewdly and obscenely exposing his person with intent to insult any female' (Vagrancy Act 1824), and applies only to males.

Transsexuals and transvestites are sometimes referred for psychiatric treatment following law involvement, which is often due to accompanying personality difficulties rather than the disorder itself unless, for instance, they have stolen female clothing. They are sometimes charged with insulting behaviour likely to cause a breach of the peace, or, on occasion, soliciting or importuning in public places for immoral purposes.

Fetishism, sexual arousal from inanimate objects, may lead to conviction when there is associated theft.

Incest is an offence in most Western countries, although the exact details of what constitutes incest (i.e. which sexual relationships are proscribed) vary. Under the Sexual Offences Act 1956 of England and Wales, it is illegal for a male to have sexual intercourse with his daughter, granddaughter, mother, sister or half-sister, and for a female over the age of 16 to have sexual intercourse with her son, father, grandfather, brother or half-brother. Father–daughter incest is the most reported. Mothers may collude with this to avoid unwanted sexual involvement with the father. The offences often only come to light following family discord. Incest is said to be more common where there is a blurring of intergenerational boundaries, physical overcrowding and where a family's social and sexual activities are confined to themselves. Usually offenders make a sharp distinction between themselves and paedophile 'child molesters', although this may be regarded as a 'minimization' of the deleterious effects of their behaviour. However, it is apparent that a clear distinction cannot be made: intrafamilial abusers abuse outside the family and paedophiles may also abuse their own children. For other individuals incestuous behaviour is part of a wider sexual promiscuity.

Rape

Rape is sexual intercourse with a woman or, since 1994, in the UK with a man, without consent by fear, force or fraud. Full vaginal or anal penetration need not occur. The rare apparent examples of females 'raping' males are dealt with in the UK by using the charge of indecent assault.

Epidemiology

The true incidence of rape is unknown. Only a fraction of cases are reported and not all of these result in conviction – in England and Wales about 2000 offences are reported every year, but only about 400 are convicted of rape. Most offenders are under 25 years of age, single, are not mentally ill and have a past history of conviction for non-sexual offences, often violence; 30% of victims in England and Wales are acquaintances or neighbours of the offender. Rape is more common in the USA than in the UK. It is also more common in the city, in the first half of the night, at weekends and in the summer.

Clinical features

Offenders often enjoy the domination and degradation of the victim. They may also misperceive as consent the victim's passivity, which is often due to fear. Offences also frequently follow alcohol abuse.

Aetiology

Rape is an offence, not a psychiatric symptom; however, psychological and sociological explanations have been put forward. Rape may be seen as the *displacement of aggression*, possibly from a rejecting society or mother. It may also be a psychological *defence against homosexuality*.

Among rapists are those with *aggressive* or *sadistic personalities*, who may view women with contempt and people in general as objects to be used or defiled. *Inhibited, frustrated men* are the public stereotype of a rapist, but this type is less common.

Rape is not confined to humans and has been described in other animals (e.g. ducks). It is also seen when *normal social sanctions* are removed and new group pressures substituted (e.g. at times of war) or among certain groups (e.g. Hell's Angels).

There is a small group who suffer from learning disabilities or mental illness. In cases of mental illness, such behaviour is more likely to be due to the generally disinhibiting effects of the illness rather than arising directly from specific sexual delusions or hallucinations. Manic patients, however, are not only disinhibited but also have an increased sexual drive, which may lead to rape.

Management

Many rapists do not regard themselves as being in need of any psychiatric or psychological help. Eighty per cent of rapists in the UK are sentenced to prison, where they are generally more highly regarded by fellow prisoners than are paedophiles. Psychological treatment, when indicated and accepted, is often aimed at improving the offenders' general social functioning, for example how to take no for an answer. Where an individual has not been helped by psychological treatment and still feels at high risk of reoffending, *antilibidinal treatment*, such as cyproterone acetate (Androcur), may be useful.

Given the nature of the offence, if treatment is to be offered in a psychiatric hospital this is likely to require conditions of security. Sexual deviation alone can now be grounds for detention under England and Wales mental health legislation since 2007.

The victim will also require counselling and may suffer from subsequent post-traumatic stress disorder and sexual dysfunction. In general, the more the victim struggles, the more physical injures they sustain. However, if they do not struggle, they tend subsequently to have more depression and guilt. Victims may also have to deal with the stress of being a witness in court, possibly being shunned by family and friends, becoming pregnant by the rape and/or being infected by a venereal disease, including HIV.

Prognosis

Follow-up studies suggest that 90% of men charged with rape will not commit a second rape, although about 15% may commit a subsequent sexual assault and a similar number commit a violent offence. Of those rapists who do similarly reoffend, their apparent dangerousness is obscured in the short term by the fact this may not occur for up to and beyond a period of 15 years later.

Assessment of sex offenders

History should include an assessment of the individual's sexual fantasies and impulses and whether these are egodystonic (the individual wishes them to be absent and would like treatment) or egosyntonic. Note should be made as to whether the sexual offending is escalating over time. Formal psychiatric disorder should be excluded on the basis of the history and mental state examination.

Physical examination should ideally be undertaken, particularly of the genitalia, as there is an increased incidence of genital abnormalities among sex offenders. Information gathering should include information from depositions and statements relating to the offence, a list of previous convictions, and a social inquiry report by a probation officer, if prepared.

Standardised structured risk assessments for sex offenders may be of use, as may *penile plethysmography* (apparatus attached to the subject's genitalia to detect penile tumescence), which may detect sexual arousal to presented deviant stimuli, and the polygraph (lie detector), especially for monitoring paedophiles.

In the light of such information, the degree of risk can be estimated and an opinion reached on whether the individual is amenable to specific psychological or psychiatric treatment. Consideration can then be given, especially in cases of minor sex offending, as to the likelihood of such an offender benefiting from being placed on a community rehabilitation (old probation) order, with or without a condition of psychiatric treatment.

Treatment

About 80% of sex offenders do not reoffend once they have been convicted. It is the recidivist who generally seeks or who is sent for treatment. However, if an individual has committed more than two sexual offences and has had no adult sexual experience, one should assume that such offending will continue. The deterrent effect of the law may be more effective than specific treatment. In general, individuals with stable personalities who are well motivated and have adult sexual fantasies do best. Motivation may be difficult to assess accurately under the stress of pending court appearances and the prospect of a prison sentence. Sex offenders can also engender strong countertransference feelings in those being asked to offer them professional help.

Principles of treatment include:

- Treat any intercurrent mental illness.
- Tackle coexisting problems, e.g. a poor marital relationship with marital (including sexual) therapy, social skills training or adult sex education, although these alone is unlikely specifically to stop sex offending.
- Specific psychological treatments, such as individual or group psychodynamic psychotherapy, or cognitive-behavioural therapy. Aversion therapy, including shame aversion therapy in the past, and covert sensitization have been be used to reduce deviant sexual arousal. Masturbatory orgasmic reconditioning, or even the therapeutic use of surrogate individuals, has been used to increase non-deviant sexual arousal. Self-control training has also been used to prevent individuals acting on deviant sexual fantasies or impulses.
- SSRIs are now the first-line medication treatment where preoccupation and rumination over the paraphilic behaviour is apparent, e.g. for exhibitionism.
- Antilibidinal treatment reduces sexual drive but is not concerned with the direction of that drive. It is most effective where sexual activity is primarily directed towards forming a relationship (e.g. in some paedophiles), but it may adversely affect the marital sexual relationship of an offender.
- In the past castration has been used as a treatment for sex offenders but never in the UK. Oestrogens have also been prescribed, but their severe feminizing effects have limited their usefulness. Benperidol (Anquil), a butyrophenone major tranquillizer, is also used but may be no more effective than other drugs in this group.

Sexual offending

- Disorders of sexual preference are persistently preferred to normal adult sexual behaviour.
- Not all sexual offenders have a disorder of sexual preference and not all acts characteristic of those with a disorder of sexual preference are against the law.
- The most common sexual offence is indecent exposure, which is associated with the disorder of sexual preference of exhibitionism. Most such offenders are inhibited, non-violent young men who do not reoffend once convicted. A few are more psychopathic and become sexually aroused.
- Paedophile offenders may be immature adolescents, middle-aged men with marital problems, or isolated elderly men. Victims are usually known to

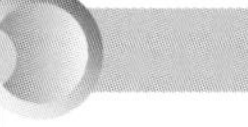

Sexual offending—cont'd

them. Paedophile offences may arise out of an affectionate relationship with the child, or alternatively the child may simply be an object of sexual gratification.

- Rape is usually an act of displaced aggression. Sadists are sexually aroused by the general infliction of pain and humiliation; rapists by forced sexual intercourse.
- Incest: sibling most common. Father–daughter most reported. Mothers may collude.

Cyproterone acetate (Androcur) is the current oral antilibidinal medication treatment most used in the UK. It inhibits the production of testosterone by enzyme block. It is a competitive antagonist of testosterone and also has an action on the hypothalamic centre and is progestogenic. It does not work in those whose sex offending is associated with alcohol abuse. It can produce gynaecomastia. It reversibly damages the germinal cells, causing the arrest of seminiferous tubules and resulting in a reduction of spermatogenesis. Leydig cells are irreversibly damaged. Medroxyprogesterone acetate is widely used in the USA. Triptorelin is a recently introduced depot injection antilibidinal depot injection.

Further reading

Treasaden, I.H., 2010. Forensic psychiatry. In: Puri, B.K., Treasaden, I. (Eds.), Psychiatry: an evidence-based text. Hodder Arnold, London.

Treasaden, I.H., 2010. Paraphilias and sexual offenders. In: Puri, B.K., Treasaden, I. (Eds.), Psychiatry: an evidence-based text. Hodder Arnold, London

Provisions for mentally abnormal offenders

The new definition of mental disorder is now more wide ranging, including sections 48, 36 and 45A now being applicable to patients with all forms of mental disorder. Restriction Orders must be indefinite, not time-limited as was possible previously. There are new provisions for sharing certain information with victims, extending this beyond those of the Domestic Violence, Crimes and Victims Act 2004.

Revised Code of Practice

This sets out five guiding principles to inform decisions under the Act, i.e. the principles of purpose, least restrictive alternative, respect, participation and effectiveness, efficiency and equity.

Mental Health Review Tribunals (MHRT)

- Independent bodies consisting of doctor, lawyer and lay person whose responsibility is to consider the justification for continued detention under the 1983 Mental Health Act.
- Chairman is a lawyer, and in the case of restricted patients is a judge.
- Patients are allowed legal aid to assist in representation, e.g. private psychiatric reports can be commissioned.
- Can order discharge or delayed discharge, and recommend (not order) transfer to another hospital or leave of absence.
- Can also order discharge or conditional discharge (i.e. with conditions such as place of residence) or deferred conditional discharge of a Section 41 restricted patient.
- Can reclassify type of mental disorder.
- See eligibility for hearings for civil and forensic Orders in Tables 22.1 and 22.2.

Patients on a 72-hour detention order have no MHRT rights, but can appeal against detention to hospital managers. There are no MHRTs in Scotland, but there is a *Mental Welfare Commission*, which safeguards the rights of both voluntary and detained patients and has the power to discharge patients. Since the Tribunals, Courts and Enforcement Act 2007, MHRTs in England and Wales are now technically First Tier Tribunals (Health, Education and Social Care Chamber) for Mental Health and there is an Upper Chamber for Appeals.

Care Quality Commission (Previously Mental Health Act Commission)

This is an independent body of part-time members (doctors, nurses, psychologists, social workers, lawyers and laypeople).

- Provides approved doctors to give second opinions on consent to treatment.
- Receives, reviews and scrutinizes detention documents and exercises a general protective function for all detained patients.
- Regularly visits psychiatric hospitals to interview detained patients and makes sure their complaints are being properly handled. Visits special hospitals monthly and other psychiatric hospitals once or twice a year.
- Responsible for Code of Practice (Section 118) on detention, treatment of all psychiatric patients (informal or detained), and consent to treatment etc., for the guidance of clinical and administrative staff in psychiatric hospitals and social workers.

Patients' rights under Mental Health Act 1983

On admission, detained patients must be advised of their legal status, their rights to appeal to Mental Health Review Tribunals, their rights in respect of consent to treatment (Table 22.3), those who have authority to discharge them, and about the Mental Health Act Commission.

Correspondence to and from informal patients cannot be interfered with. Correspondence from detained patients in ordinary psychiatric hospitals can only be withheld if the person to whom the correspondence is addressed has asked for that to

Table 22.1 Civil treatment orders under Mental Health Act 1983

Civil treatment order under Mental Health Act 1983	Grounds	Application by	Medical recommendations	Maximum duration	Eligibility for appeal to Mental Health Review Tribunal
Section 2 Admission for assessment	Mental disorder	Nearest relative or approved mental health professional (AMHP)	Two doctors (one approved under Section 12)	28 days	Within 14 days
Section 3 Admission for treatment	Mental disorder	Nearest relative or approved mental health professional (AMHP)	Two doctors (one approved under Section 12)	Six months	Within first six months. If renewed, within second six months, then every year. Mandatory every three years
Section 4 Emergency admission for assessment	Mental disorder (urgent necessity)	Nearest relative or approved mental health professional (AMHP)	Any doctor	72 hours	
Section 5 (2) Urgent detention of voluntary inpatient	Danger to self or to others		Doctor in charge of patient's care	72 hours	
Section 5(4) Nurses holding power of voluntary inpatient	Mental disorder (danger to self, health or others)	Registered mental nurse or registered nurse for mental handicap	None	Six hours	
Section 136 Admission by police	Mental disorder	Police officer	Allows patient in public place to be removed to 'place of safety'	72 hours	
Section 135	Mental disorder	Magistrates	Allows power of entry to home and removal of patient to place of safety	72 hours	

happen. Special hospitals can withhold correspondence to and from patients, except about staff and to solicitors and MPs or the Queen. (In the latter case correspondence can be sent free, as it is the Royal Mail.) Patients in any psychiatric hospital must be informed if their correspondence is withheld.

Informal inpatients have *voting rights*.

Health and social services have a duty to provide *aftercare for detained patients* when they leave hospital (Section 117).

International comparison of mental health legislation

Mental Health (Scotland) Act 2003

Section 328 defines mental disorder as any mental illness, personality disorder or learning disability.

Table 22.2 Forensic treatment orders for mentally abnormal offenders

	Grounds	Made by	Medical recommendations	Maximum duration	Eligibility for appeal to Mental Health Review Tribunal
Section 35 Remand to hospital for report	Mental disorder	Magistrates or Crown Court	Any doctor	28 days. Renewable at 28-day intervals. Maximum 12 weeks	
Section 36 Remand to hospital for treatment	Mental disorder (not if charged with murder)	Crown Court	Two doctors: one approved under Section 12	28 days. Renewable at 28-day intervals. Maximum 12 weeks	
Section 37 Hospital and guardianship orders	Mental disorder Accused of, or convicted for, an imprisonable offence	Magistrates or Crown Court	Two doctors, one approved under Section 12	Six months. Renewable for further six months and then annually	During second six months. Then every year. Mandatory every three years
Section 41 Restriction order	Added to Section 37. To protect public from serious harm	Crown Court	Oral evidence from one doctor	Without limit of time. Effect: leave, transfer, or discharge only with consent of Home Secretary	As Section 37
Section 38 Interim hospital order	Mental disorder For trial of treatment	Magistrates or Crown Court	Two doctors: one approved under Section 12	12 weeks. Renewable at 28-day intervals. Maximum six months	None
Section 47 Transfer of a sentenced prisoner to hospital	Mental disorder	Justice Secretary	Two doctors: one approved under Section 12	Until earliest date of release from sentence	Once in the first six months. Then once in the next six months. Thereafter, once a year.
Section 48 Urgent transfer to hospital of remand prisoner	Mental disorder	Justice Secretary	Two doctors: one approved under Section 12	Until trial (conviction or sentence)	Once in the first six months. Then once in the next six months. Thereafter, once a year.
Section 49 Restriction direction	Added to Section 47 or Section 48	Justice Secretary		Until end of Section 47 or 48. Effect: leave, transfer or discharge only with consent of Justice Secretary	As for Section 47 and 48 to which applied

Table 22.3 Consent to treatment under Mental Health Act 1983. Consent to treatment should be informed and voluntary (implies mental disorder, e.g. dementia, does not affect judgement)

Type of treatment	Informal	Detained
Section 62 Urgent necessity	No consent	No consent
Section 57 Irreversible, hazardous or non-established treatments, e.g. psychosurgery (e.g. leucotomy), hormone implants (for sex offenders), surgical operations (e.g. castration)	Consent and second opinion	Consent and second opinion
Section 58 Psychiatric drugs, ECT	Consent	Consent or second opinion

For first three months of treatment a detained patient's consent is not required for Section 58 medicines, but is for ECT. Patients can withdraw voluntary consent at any time.

Sexual orientation, sexual deviancy, trans-sexualism, transvestism and dependency on or use of alcohol or drugs are excluded from the definition. Under the Act, provisions exist for an RMO, an Approved Medical Practitioner (AMP) (Section 22), a Mental Health Officer (MHO) (in practice a social worker), Designated Medical Practitioners (DMPs), Mental Welfare Commission and Mental Health Tribunal. All patients have a right to advocacy (Section 259). Advanced statements are possible under Sections 275 and 276.

Part 5 of the Act details emergency detention orders, Part 6 details short-term admission orders and Part 7 community treatment orders for hospital or community.

Mental Health Act (Northern Ireland) Order 1986

Mental illness is defined in this Act as a state of mind that affects a person's thinking, perceiving, emotion or judgement to the extent that he requires care or medical treatment in his own interests or the interests of other people. Medical treatment is defined as including nursing and also care and treatment under medical supervision.

There are definitions in this Act for *mental handicap, severe mental handicap* and *severe mental impairment*. To be placed in the severe mental handicap category, there must be associated 'abnormally aggressive or seriously irresponsible conduct'.

It is stated that no person should be treated as suffering from mental disorder by reason of only a personality disorder, promiscuity or other immoral conduct, sexual deviancy or dependence on alcohol and drugs.

Part II of the Order allows compulsory admission for assessment for up to 14 days before being admitted for treatment. For the purposes of application for detention in Northern Ireland, the nearest relative can be someone living in the Republic of Ireland as well as the UK. *Temporary holding powers* are available for voluntary patients already in hospital, as with the English and Scottish Acts. These holding powers are for six hours by a professionally registered charge nurse and 48 hours by a doctor on the staff of a hospital concerned, which also includes a general hospital.

If a patient is not well enough to become a voluntary patient or to be discharged before the end of the 14-day assessment period, he may in the first instance be detained for up to six months if he is diagnosed as suffering from mental illness or severe mental impairment and he remains at high risk of serious physical harm to himself or others. The period of detention is renewable for a further six months and then annually, subject to approval, following an examination by a doctor from another hospital appointed by the Mental Health Commission.

Provisions for consent to treatment and guardianship are similar to those set out in the 1983 England and Wales Mental Health Act.

Provisions exist similar to those in the 1983 England and Wales Mental Health Act for individuals involved in criminal proceedings; for example the courts have the power to remand for examination or treatment, and interim hospital orders are also available. Hospital orders may be made regardless of the apparent availability of places, unlike in the rest of the UK, and a court may also impose a restriction order on the patient's discharge. In all hospital order cases psychiatrists are expected to give oral evidence in the court.

Individuals detained for two years are automatically referred to Mental Health Review Tribunals.

The Mental Health Commission, unlike the English equivalent, covers voluntary patients, people in guardianship and people in residential accommodation or, indeed, anybody suffering from a mental disorder. Where it upholds complaints, it has the power to hold a formal enquiry to establish facts.

At any one time Northern Ireland has fewer than about 10 patients in Britain's mainland maximum security hospitals. Northern Ireland has no maximum security hospital itself.

Therapeutic abortion is only allowed in Northern Ireland where there is undoubted grave risk to the continuing physical or mental health of the pregnant woman. This leads to women crossing from Northern Ireland to the mainland of Britain each year to have an abortion.

Mental health legislation in Eire

Mental Health Act 2001

This Act replaces the Mental Treatment Act 1945 and the Acts passed in 1953, 1961 and 1981. However, its implementation has been gradual. Section 4 details the principles underlying the Act, including the best interests of the person but with due regard to the interests of others who may be at serious harm.

Definition of mental disorder

Section 3 defines *mental disorder* as 'mental illness, severe dementia or significant intellectual impairment'. Compulsory detention should be as a result of

(a) mental disorder causing immediate and serious harm to him- or herself or to other persons

or

(b) because of the severity of the mental disorder, the judgement of the person is so impaired that if not admitted to an approved centre, this would lead to a serious deterioration

or

detention in an approved centre is likely to benefit or alleviate the condition.

Mental illness means a state of mind affecting thinking, perceiving, emotion or judgement. Significant intellectual disability means a state of arrested or incomplete development of mind, including significant impairment of intelligence and social functioning and abnormally aggressive or seriously irresponsible conduct.

Other official terms

Approved Centres include inpatient facilities or hospitals or other facilities registered with the Mental Health Commission (MHC). There are Review Tribunals and an Inspector of Mental Health Services who is a Consultant Psychiatrist appointed by the MHC.

Important sections of the Act

These include:

- application for involuntary admission (section 9)
- medical assessment (section 10)
- power of the Garda to detain and apply for involuntary admission (section 12)
- removal to an Approved Centre (section 13)
- admission to Approved Centre (section 14 and 15)
- part 4 of the Act concerns consent to treatment for patients subject to compulsion.

Table 22.4 compares the provisions for urgent civil detention under mental health legislation in the UK and the Republic of Ireland.

Table 22.5 compares the legal provisions for mentally disordered offenders in the UK and the Republic of Ireland.

Mental health legislation in Canada

Canadian courts are under provincial jurisdiction. The ten provinces and two territories also have a Court of Appeal. The highest court, the Supreme Court of Canada, is situated in Ottawa. The *Criminal Code* covers mentally abnormal offenders, but their management varies between provinces owing

Table 22.4 Comparison of urgent civil detention under mental health legislation in the UK and the Republic of Ireland

	Legislation	Out-patient	In-patient
England and Wales	Mental Health Act 1983	Section 2 or 3 should be used rather than Section 4	Section 5(2) immediately or Sections 2 or 3
Scotland	Mental Health (Care and Treatment) (Scotland) Act 2003	Part 5 if arranging; Part 6 would involve undesirable delay	Part 5 if arranging; Part 6 would involve undesirable delay
Northern Ireland	Mental Health (Northern Ireland) Order 1986	a. 4	a. 7(2) may be detained under a. 4
Republic of Ireland	Mental Health Act 2001	Sections 9 and 10	Section 2

Table 22.5 Comparison of legal provisions for mentally disordered offenders in the UK and the Republic of Ireland

	England & Wales	Scotland	Northern Ireland	Republic of Ireland
	Mental Health Act 1983	Mental Health (Care and Treatment) Scotland Act 2003	Mental Health (Northern Ireland) Order 1986	Mental Health Act 2001
Police				
Detention of mentally disordered person found in public place	Section 136	Section 297	a130	Section 12
Detention of mentally disordered person in private premises	Section 135	Section 293	a129	Section 12
Pre-trial		Criminal Procedure (Scotland) Act 1995		
Remand to hospital for assessment	Section 35	Section 52B–J	a42	–
Remand to hospital for assessment	Section 36	Section 52K–S	a43	–
Transfer of untried prisoner to hospital	Section 48	Section 52K–S	a54	–
Trial				
Criteria for fitness to plead	*R v Prichard* 1836	*HMA v Wilson Stewart v HMA* 1942	*R v Prichard*	*R v Prichard* (Section 3 CL(I) B2002)
Procedure relating to a finding of unfitness to plead	Sections 2–3 and sch 1–2 CP(IUP) A1991	Sections 54–57 CP(S)A 1995	a49 and 50A	Lunacy (Ireland) Act 1821, Juries Act 1976

Continued

Table 22.5 Comparison of legal provisions for mentally disordered offenders in the UK and the Republic of Ireland—cont'd

	England & Wales	Scotland	Northern Ireland	Republic of Ireland
Criteria for insanity at the time of the offence	*McNaughten Rules* 1843	*HMA v Kidd* 1960	CJ(NI)A 1966	*Doyle v Wicklow County Council* 1974
Procedure relating to a finding of insanity at the time of the offence	Sections 1&3 and sch 1–2 CP(IUP)A 1991	Sections 54 and 57	a50 and 50A CJ(NI)O 1996	Trial of Lunatics Act 1883
Criteria for diminished responsibility	Section 2 Homicide Act 1957	*Galbraith v HMA* 2001 Culpable Homocide	CJ(NI)O 1996	
	Mental Health Act 1983	Criminal Procedures (Scotland) Act 1995	Mental Health (Northern Ireland) Order 1986	Mental Health Act 2001
Post-conviction but pre-sentence				
Remand to hospital for assessment	Section 35	Section 52B–J Section 200	a42	–
Remand to hospital for treatment	Section 36	Section 52K–S	a43	–
Interim hospital/compulsion order	Section 38	Section 53	–	–
Transfer of untried prisoner to hospital	Section 48	Section 52B–J Section 52K–S	a54	Previous legislation applies
Sentence				
Compulsory treatment in hospital under MHA	Section 37	Section 57A	a44	–
Restriction order	Section 41	Section 59	a47	–
Hybrid order (hospital disposal with prison sentence)	Section 45A–B	Section 59A	–	–
Compulsory treatment in community under MHA	–	Section 57A	–	–
Guardianship	Section 37	Section 58(1A)	a44	–
Intervention order for incapable adult	–	Section 60B	–	–
Psychiatric probation order	sch 2 (p5) Powers of Criminal Courts (Sentencing) Act 2000	Section 230	sch 1 (p4) CJ(NI)O 1996	–
Post-sentence		Mental Health (Care and Treatment) Scotland Act 2003		
Transfer of sentenced prisoners to hospital	Section 47	Section 136	a53	Previous legislation applies
Restriction direction for transferred prisoner	Section 49	All	a55	–

to their respective mental health legislations. The Criminal Code does, however, allow a trial judge to remand an offender for psychiatric assessment under Section 543(2) and the Court of Appeal has similar provision under Section 608.2(1).

There are two maximum security hospitals in Canada, the Mental Health Centre at Penetanguishene, Ontario, and the Institut Philip Pinel in Montreal.

The Metropolitan Toronto Forensic Service (METFORS) is well known for its provision of psychiatric services to the courts and prisons. METFORS has a brief assessment unit and otherwise undertakes standard forensic psychiatric pre-trial assessments and treatments. In Ottawa there is a well-developed clinic for the treatment of and research into sexual offenders, and it has a close relationship with the probation service.

With the provinces and territories having differing mental health legislation, definitions of mental disorder vary between them. In Ontario it is defined as 'any disease or disability of the mind'. The criteria for involuntary civil committal are wide in all the provinces except Ontario, where objective evidence of potential dangerousness to self or others is required. Provinces other than Ontario have less stringent admission criteria regarding general health, welfare and safety. Most provinces require certification by two physicians prior to involuntary admission of a patient to a psychiatric facility. Periods of detention vary with the various mental health acts of the provinces. Most provinces have provision for police officers to take a person for a psychiatric examination and for judges to order that an individual charged with a criminal offence be examined, admitted and treated in a psychiatric facility.

Regarding consent to treatment, an incompetent involuntarily detained patient has the right to refuse all forms of psychiatric treatment in Nova Scotia and Ontario. If found incompetent, consent from the nearest relative is required, or, in the absence of the nearest relative, review board procedures exist to hear the case and issue treatment orders.

There is considerable variability in the roles and powers of the Mental Health Tribunals of the various provinces and territories of Canada. Persons found not guilty by reason of insanity or found unfit to proceed with a trial and who are made subject to conditions of a warrant of the Lieutenant Governor of the province of Ontario are reviewed by an advisory board, appointed by the Lieutenant Governor in Council, on at least one occasion every 12 months.

There are provisions under sections of the Criminal Code of Canada 1986 to remand a mentally abnormal offender for a psychiatric assessment for fitness to proceed with trial, if that individual is mentally ill or the balance of his mind is disturbed. The period of assessment is up to 30 days. If he is deemed not fit to plead or stand trial, a trial of fitness is ordered. If found unfit, the court orders that the person be kept in custody until the pleasure of the Lieutenant Governor of the province is known. Similarly if found not guilty by reason of insanity, the individual is also made subject to the terms of the Lieutenant Governor's warrant, and kept in a place of custody. Custody is nearly always a psychiatric facility with either maximum or medium security.

If the offence committed is minor, a probation order with a condition of psychiatric treatment may be ordered. Some correctional institutions have programmes for psychiatric treatment. If a prisoner becomes mentally ill while serving a sentence, there are provisions in the criminal code to transfer that patient to a psychiatric facility for treatment.

Mental health law in the USA

Most aspects of mental health law are delegated to the various states, so that they can enact legislation to suit local needs. Mental health legislation in the USA has been shaped by social and political forces and case law. The emphasis has always been on the least restrictive treatment. Involuntary psychiatric treatment has been considered in many ways out of keeping with the US constitution and philosophy of upholding the individual's rights of freedom, speech and behaviour.

In the past 30 years there has been a trend away from detention (certification) on grounds of need for treatment and towards increasing patients' rights and restricting involuntary treatment. This, together with a desire to reduce the number of inpatients and the cost of their care, has led to the general adoption as a criterion for detention a standard of future or potential dangerousness to themselves or others, rather than grave disability, for reasons of health alone or the client's need for treatment. Emergency hospitalization can be initiated without prior judicial approval, but subsequent commitment needs to be ordered by a judge.

Consent to treatment. Involuntary patients have the right to refuse medication. Medication to control dangerous patients in an emergency has been sanctioned if the need to prevent violence outweighs the possibility of harm to the patient and all less restrictive alternatives have been ruled out. If the patient is not dangerous, in many states the only way medication can be enforced is to have the patient declared incompetent, whereupon treatment conditions can be made, often on the basis of what the patient would have decided were he competent to do so, rather than what might be in his best interests.

In keeping with the idea of the least restrictive treatment, orders allowing outpatient committal to psychiatric treatment have emerged in nearly all states. This assists the large number of patients who have been discharged from hospital in the USA who are clearly incapable of coping with the outside world and meeting their basic needs. Such community commitment orders have been legally challenged on the grounds that if an individual is well enough to live outside an institution, it is hard to justify such a restriction of their constitutional liberty. American states are widely divided on this issue. Some have developed a new lower threshold for involuntary outpatient care.

The ruling in the case of Tarasoff versus Regents of University of California in 1974–76 (a duty to warn in 1974 modified to a duty to protect in 1976) has led many American psychotherapists to acknowledge that patient confidentiality can be violated, in view of the court's assertion that 'protected privilege ends where community peril begins'.

Mental health legislation in Australia and New Zealand

Each of the six states of Australia and its territories has its own separate mental health act and its own judicial system. Australian law is derived from the common law of England, but is not identical to it. Australian and UK mental health services and laws are, however, similar. Much Australian psychiatric care is privately based, with state provision concentrating on those with severe (psychotic) mental illness. Mental health legislation in Australia has been under constant review over recent years, with new Acts drafted and frequent amendments made to earlier Acts. The Mental Health Act 1986 of the State of Victoria included a community treatment order. This Act, together with the Mental Health Act 1990 of New South Wales, has had a significant influence on the development of legislation throughout Australia.

New Zealand has one Mental Health Act, which also has provisions for the compulsory treatment of patients in the community.

Civil legal aspects, Mental Capacity Act 2005 and ethics of psychiatry

23

Psychiatric opinions in civil law (civil capacity)

The Burden of Proof in such matters is on the balance of probabilities.

A. Issues of mental fitness

1. Contracts

Contracts require free full consent. If an individual is of unsound mind (not equivalent to mental disorder as defined by nor to being detainable under the Mental Health Act 1983) at the time of making a contract, that contract is regarded as void. However, the 'mentally incapable' are bound by contracts unless the other party or parties to the contract knew or should have known of the individual's incapacity. Under employment law an individual can be dismissed only for behavioural effects of mental disorder, not for mental disorder itself.

2. Testamentary capacity

This is the ability to make a valid will. To do this in the UK, individuals must be over the age of 18 and not be of 'unsound mind'.

This becomes an issue either at the time an individual makes a will, where a solicitor may ask for medical, including psychiatric, advice, or after that individual's death. Accurately assessing the capacity of a person to make a will would prevent the current high levels of litigation in this area.

If a patient decides to make a will, he may ask the doctor attending him to witness it, particularly if he is seriously ill. Doctors should be aware they will be regarded in law as not acting as mere lay witnesses. If a doctor does agree to do so, he is said to have 'attested the will', which implies he considers the patient to be of 'sound disposing mind and memory'. This is most often undertaken by a general medical practitioner rather than a psychiatrist. If the will is subsequently contested, the doctor may be required to appear in court to give evidence about the patient's mental state at the time he made the will.

Although not specifically defined in law, to have a 'sound disposing mind' by custom (based on Banks versus Goodfellow (1870)) the individual must:

1) know the nature and extent of his property, though not necessarily the details,

2) know all persons and their names having a claim on his bounty, and the relative strength of their claim (e.g. bearing on the distribution between persons),

3) have no morbid state of mind that might distort his natural feelings and influence his decisions,

4) have the ability to realize the nature of a will and its consequences, and

5) be able to express himself clearly and without ambiguity.

The presence of mental disorder, such as mild dementia, does not necessarily affect testamentary capacity, although clearly if the will is complex, it may do so. Testamentary capacity, however, may be severely affected if the individual has paranoid delusions about an individual who would normally be considered to have a claim on his property. The 1826 case of Dew v. Clark established, however, that even if one was deluded (in this case believing he was being pursued by evil spirits), this does not necessarily preclude an individual having testamentary capacity.

If you die having left a will, then you die 'testate' and a grant of probate enables your executor or trustee to administer the will. Wills must be in writing, save if on 'actual military service'. Wills must be made without force, fear, fraud, nor undue influence. A person making a will is either a testator or testatrix. The similarity of such words to testes is not by chance. The ancient Romans swore oaths by placing their fingers on the testes. The relevant law is the Administration of Estates Act 1982.

3. Marriage

Marriage is a contract, so that if an individual has a mental disorder at the time so as not to appreciate the nature of the contract, that contract is 'voidable' (not void). Lack of valid (competent) consent is rare, as most mentally disordered individuals appreciate the nature of marriage.

A marriage may be annulled if:

- One partner has a mental disorder at the time of the marriage so as not to appreciate the nature of the contract.
- One partner did not disclose that he or she suffered from epilepsy or a communicable venereal disease.
- Either party was under 16 years at the time of marriage.
- Pregnancy by another male at the time of marriage was not disclosed.
- There was non-consummation (no intromission of the penis).
- One of the partners was forced to agree to the marriage under duress.

Marriage continues until successfully challenged in the courts by one of the parties, resulting in the marriage being deemed 'voidable'.

Legal capacity to marry is different to the legal capacity to have sexual relations.

Apart from an inability to give valid competent consent, to marry an individual may be deemed, even if they can give valid consent, as unable to marry due to 'unfitness for marriage', i.e. having a mental disorder in terms of the definition of the Mental Health Act 1983 resulting in an incapacity to carry out the ordinary duties of marriage (not just be difficult to live with). For a marriage to be 'voidable' on such grounds, the individual must be incapable of living in a married state or carrying out the ordinary duties of marriage. Psychiatric grounds must be substantial. A Registrar will only rarely refuse to marry on the basis of unfitness for marriage, but will more commonly do so on the basis of incapacity to consent. Any person, including a doctor, may enter a 'caveat' pre-marriage with a Superintendent Registrar, who must then investigate it.

4. Sexual relationships between inpatients

(1) Article 8 European Convention on Human Rights secures the right of all to respect for private and family life, which is taken to include sexual relationships between patients.

In practice, competent detained inpatients are not precluded from marriage, but secure hospitals, such as Special Hospitals in the UK, e.g. Broadmoor Hospital, have, on the basis of need for rules governing inpatients, successfully resisted to date the right of such inpatients to have provisions made for sexual relations between them.

(2) U.N. Declaration of Rights of Mentally Retarded Persons (1971) gives the right of the mentally handicapped to live with their own family. It does not specifically refer to sexual relations, but is taken to imply this.

(3) It is illegal for male staff to have a sexual relationship with a patient, a male guardian with a subject of a guardianship order and anyone with a patient with 'severe mental handicap' in the UK.

5. Divorce

This is covered by the Matrimonial Causes Act 1973. Mental disorder may affect the capacity to consent to divorce. Non-consensual divorce is achievable only on the basis of behaviour as specified in the Matrimonial Causes Act. Thus, mental disorder is the basis for divorce only when it results in the relevant legal behaviour, i.e. adultery, unreasonable behaviour (which replaced the term cruelty), desertion, and living apart for more than two years if the respondent consents or for five years without consent (irretrievable breakdown). 'Quickie' divorces are based on filing affidavits, in contrast to divorces which are defended in court. Mental disorder most often leads to divorce by causing an irretrievable breakdown in marriage due to unreasonable behaviour.

Issues relating to the children of marriage following divorce are governed by *'supremacy of the interest of the child'*. Separation/divorce usually results in residence, which replaced the term custody, of the children with the mother, unless, for example, mental disorder, among other factors, 'affects her capacity to love and care for the child'. Contact has replaced the term access and the Child Support Agency has taken over many of the past roles of lawyers contesting financial issues related to child care in court.

A *Care Order (Children and Young Persons Act 1989)* is taken out where a parent or parents cannot safely care for the child, i.e. on grounds of actual, or risk of, serious harm and this is attributable to care. Objective, especially current, behavioural evidence carries more weight in court than predicted behaviour.

6. Tort

This is a civil wrong to a person, a reputation or the estate of an individual, e.g. libel, slander, fraud, trespass, negligence and breach of copyright. Mentally disordered individuals are considered incapable of committing a tort unless the disorder does not preclude them understanding the nature or probable consequences of their acts. Defamation, which covers slander (spoken) and libel (written, but also includes spoken word on TV, film or video), is not eligible for legal aid and is heard and adjudicated, e.g. regarding the amount of damages, by a jury. Hence, the occasional huge damages in such cases awarded by a jury. Defences include 'justification', 'fair comment', and 'mere vulgar abuse'.

7. The mentally disordered as witnesses

Mentally disordered individuals may give evidence in court or make a written statement, but it is for the magistrates or the judge to determine whether they are fit to do so and can understand the nature and obligation of the oath. To this end, medical evidence may be called for and the jury will have to consider how much weight to attach to the witness's evidence.

8. Guardianship and Appointeeship

Guardianship may be useful to help someone over age 16 years having difficulty looking after themselves.

Appointeeship. An appointee is someone authorized by the Department of Social Security in England and Wales to receive and administer benefits on behalf of someone else.

Mental Capacity Act 2005

The main provisions are as follows:

- Designated decision makers for those who lack capacity
- Lasting Power of Attorney (LPA). Like the prior Enduring Power of Attorney (EPA) but can make healthcare and welfare decisions
- Court Appointed Deputies. Replaces Receivership in the Court of Protection. Can make decisions on welfare, healthcare and financial matters, but cannot refuse consent to life-sustaining treatment.

Two new public bodies

- A new Court of Protection
- A new Public Guardian
  - Will register LPA and deputies
  - Supervise deputies
  - Be scrutinized by a Public Guardian Board.

Three Provisions to protect vulnerable people:

- Independent Mental Capacity Advocate (IMCA)
- Advance decisions to refuse treatment, including, if expressly stated, 'even if life is at risk'
- New criminal offence of ill treatment or neglect of person who lacks capacity.

1. Introduction into law

- The Independent Mental Capacity Advocacy service (IMCAs) became available on 1 April 2007.
- The Code of Practice and the criminal offence of ill treatment and wilful neglect became law in April 2007.
- From October 2007, all other elements of legislation, including the new Court of Protection, Public Guardian and the Office of the Public Guardian, became operational.
- Deprivation of Liberty Safeguards (MCA DOLS) became law in April 2009.

2. Scope of the act: exclusions under section 27

No decision on the following to be made on behalf of a person under the Mental Capacity Act 2005:

- Consent to marriage, a civil partnership or sexual relations.
- Consent to divorce/dissolution of a civil partnership on the basis of two years' separation.
- Consent to a child being placed for adoption or making of an adoption order.
- Discharging parental responsibilities in matters not relating to a child's property.
- Consent under the Human Fertilisation and Embryology Act 1990.
- Treatment of detained patients under Mental Health Act 1983 is separate from Mental Capacity Act.
- Mental Health Act 1983 consent to treatment provisions.

3. Capacity

A person may lack capacity if:

- at the material time
- he is unable to make a decision for himself in relation to the matter
- because of an impairment of, or a disturbance in the functioning of, the mind or brain (s.2)
- it does not matter whether the impairment or disturbance is permanent or temporary.

'Impairment or disturbance'

'The impairment or disturbance may occur in a wide range of situations. . .people who are affected by

- alcohol or drug misuse
- delirium
- following head injury
- mental illness
- dementia
- learning disabilities
- long-term effects of brain damage
- grave physical conditions producing confusion, drowsiness or loss of consciousness including as a result of treatment'.

(From Code of Practice.)

Able to make decision?

Under Section 3 individuals should be able to:

- understand information relevant to the decision, including potential consequences of different decisions
- retain that information for long enough to make a decision – not permanently
- use that information to make a decision
- communicate the decision, including by gesture or sign language.

A surprising or unwise decision does not of itself indicate lack of capacity.

4. Statutory principles

Under Section 1(1):

1. Everyone is assumed to have capacity unless shown otherwise.
2. No one is to be treated as unable to make a decision unless all practicable steps to assist have failed.
3. A person is not to be treated as lacking capacity only because he makes an unwise decision.
4. Any act or decision on behalf of someone who lacks capacity must be done in his best interests.
5. Before any act, there must be consideration whether the objective can be as well achieved in a less restrictive way.

Section 4: Best Interests

One must consider all the relevant circumstances, in particular

1. Involve the person if possible in any decision.
2. Other wishes/beliefs, made with capacity, or values that indicate preference.
3. Anyone already nominated, or any carers etc., e.g. Lasting Power of Attorney or Court Appointed Deputy.
4. Likely to regain capacity? If so, when?
5. Not to seek the subject's death where the decision relates to life-sustaining treatment; consider whether it is in the best interests of the person concerned. ('Life-sustaining treatment' is treatment which the provider clinician considers necessary to sustain life.)

Section 4(a): A reasonable belief

- There is sufficient compliance with the best interests requirements if (having complied with the requirements of section 4) the person making the determination reasonably believes that what s/he does or decides is in the best interests of the person concerned.

5. New Processes for Making Decisions

- Advance Decision (AD).
- Lasting Power of Attorney (LPA).
- Section 5.
- Court of Protection or Court Appointed Deputy (CAD).

a. Advance Decisions (ADs) (Section 24)

A decision made by an adult with capacity that if:

- at a later time a specified treatment is proposed to be carried out by a person providing health care, and
- at that time he lacks capacity to consent to that treatment, then the specified treatment is not to be carried out or continued.

An Advance Decision (AD) is not necessarily binding if the following tests are met:

Capacity test: if the person still has capacity to consent to treatment proposed

Validity test: if s/he withdrew the AD at any time when able to do so, or has done anything clearly inconsistent with the AD

Applicability test:

- not the treatment specified in the AD
- any specified circumstances are absent; or
- reasonable grounds for believing that important unforeseen circumstances exist, not anticipated at time of the AD.

Life sustaining threshold: An AD is not applicable to life-sustaining treatment unless it is verified by a statement to the effect that it is to apply to that treatment even if life is at risk, and the decision is in writing, signed and witnessed.

b. Lasting Power of Attorney (LPA) (Section 9)

An LPA is a power under which the donor confers on a donee or donees authority to make decisions about:

- his personal welfare or specific aspects thereof, and
- his property and affairs specified aspects thereof
- and which includes authority to make such decisions in circumstances where he no longer has capacity.

LPA limitations

The authority conferred by an LPA is subject to:

- any conditions or restrictions specified in the document
- the provisions of the Mental Capacity Act and, in particular Section 1, Principles, and Section 4 Best Interests.

c. Section 5: liability for care or treatment

Where the section 5 conditions are satisfied, someone who does an act 'in connection' with an incapacitated person's care or treatment will only incur legal liability if the act would have been unlawful if it was done with consent: as an example, negligent acts are not protected.

Section 5 conditions

- The act is 'in connection with' care or treatment.
- The person doing it takes reasonable steps to establish whether the subject has capacity.
- S/he reasonably believes that the subject lacks capacity.
- S/he reasonably believes that the act is in the subject's best interests.
- If restraint is used, s/he reasonably believes BOTH
  - that it is necessary to do the act in order to prevent harm to the subject, and
  - that the act is a proportionate response to the likelihood of their suffering harm and the seriousness of that harm.

Restraint is both the use, or threat of use, of force to achieve an outcome, or restriction of liberty of movement, whether or not resisted.

d. The Court of Protection and its elements

The court is assisted by

- the Public Guardian
- the Court Appointed Deputies (CADs)
- the Court of Protection Visitors.

Section 16 Powers of the Court

Where a matter concerns personal welfare or property and affairs, and a person lacks capacity in relation to it, then the court may decide the matter or appoint a deputy (CAD) to make decisions about where to live, contact with others, or medical treatment.

Powers of the Court over property and affairs include:

- managing, buying and selling property
- trade, profession, business and partnership matters
- contracts and debts
- wills and trust powers
- legal proceedings.

6. Advocacy & Independent Mental Capacity Advocacy Service (IMCAs) (Section 35)

The appropriate authority must arrange for Independent Mental Capacity Advocates to be available to support persons to whom decisions proposed under sections 37, 38 and 39 relate.

- Section 37: serious medical treatment.
- Section 38: accommodation: NHS.
- Section 39: accommodation: local authority.

Exceptions include where there is:

- a person nominated by the subject (in whatever manner) to be consulted in matters affecting his interests, or
- a donee of a lasting power of attorney (LPA) created by the subject, or
- a deputy appointed by the court (CAD) for the subject, or
- a donee of an enduring power of attorney (EPA) created by the subject under earlier legislation
    - In such circumstances the duty to consult an IMCA in relation to decisions under sections 37–39 does not apply.

7. Deprivation of Liberty Safeguards

The Mental Health Act 2007, as well as updating the Mental Health Act 1983, was used as a vehicle for introducing the deprivation of liberty safeguards into the Mental Capacity Act 2005. The new safeguards provide a framework for the lawful deprivation of liberty of those people who lack capacity to consent to arrangements made for their care or treatment in either a hospital or care home, and who need to be deprived of liberty in their own best interests to protect them from harm.

The Mental Capacity Act 2005 Deprivation of Liberty Safeguards (MCA DOLS) are a response to a European Court of Human Rights (ECtHR) judgement in October 2004 in the Bournewood case of HL v UK. The court found that a man with autism and a learning disability, who lacked the capacity to decide about his residence and medical treatment, and who had been admitted informally to Bournewood Hospital, was unlawfully deprived of his liberty in breach of Article 5 of the European Convention on Human Rights (ECHR).

The MAC DOLS was a remedy to the breach of the ECHR and is perceived as a major big step towards better protecting the rights of vulnerable individuals in hospitals and care homes. It is hoped that it will make a big difference to the people in care who have no or limited choice about their life. However, there is no doubt that implementing the safeguards is challenging for care homes, PCTs and the NHS Trust.

In the main, the people covered by the safeguards will be those with severe learning disabilities, older people with one of a range of dementias, or people with neurological conditions such as brain injuries. The safeguards only apply to those people not covered by the Mental Health Act 1983.

The safeguards apply to people in hospitals, and independent hospitals and care homes registered under the Care Standards Act 2000, whether they have been placed there by a PCT, a local authority or through private arrangements.

The MCA DOLS apply to people in hospitals and care homes who meet all of the following criteria. A person must:

- be aged 18 or over
- have a mental disorder such as dementia or a learning disability
- lack capacity to consent to arrangements made for their treatment and/or care
- need to have their liberty taken away in their own best interests to protect them from harm.

B. Issues of psychiatric damage

Normal ordinary emotional reactions, e.g. grief, are not eligible for compensation, but 'psychiatric damage' (legal term 'nervous shock') is. Issues regarding psychiatric damage have arisen in cases of post-concussional syndrome, accident and compensation neurosis, malingering, victims of torture, pathological grief and, since 1989, post-traumatic stress disorder, following the sinking in the English Channel of the ferry Herald of Free Enterprise. The vulnerability of the complainant is not relevant, e.g. an 'egg shell skull' is no defence and the defendant must take the plaintiff as he finds him. Dissociative (conversion) disorders constitute psychiatric damage but malingering does not, although, in practice, there is a spectrum between these conditions and it is thus important to assess the degree of unconscious production of symptoms. Symptoms in general persist longer, the longer it takes to settle a case whether there are issues of compensation or not.

Cases arising from the Hillsborough football stadium fire in Sheffield, England in 1988 led to rulings that symptoms are eligible for compensation if they result from the individual being directly subjected to the trauma, from seeing in real life a close relative (first-degree) being killed but not a distant relative (such as nephew or fiancé), from seeing the killing of a close relative broadcast on television and from hearing about this from a third person such as a policeman. Symptoms attributed to news about those not related, e.g. learnt from the radio or from watching a recording of the disaster on a television programme, did not lead to compensation. In fact, police officers attending the scene were compensated before these cases were heard.

For psychiatric damage, an individual must have a psychiatric illness.

Psychiatric damage can be:

- secondary to physical sequelae, e.g. after loss of a limb
- primarily psychological
- psychological, but secondary, e.g., to witnessing the fate of another, e.g. a lecturer having a heart attack.

A psychiatrist must define the mental disorder and give a prognosis, which is very important in cases of damage. The Court then puts a 'tariff tag' on the disorder and prognosis.

C. Psychiatric negligence (a tort)

There are three elements:

- A duty of care to a 'neighbour' (with whom the defendant has a natural relationship). This applies to the National Health Service (NHS) in the UK. If under private care, an individual can also sue for breach of contract as well.
- Breach of duty of care, includes technical and advice errors.
- Damage to other party results, i.e. foreseeable and would not have happened anyway.

The onus of proof is on the plaintiff to prove a breach of duty of care caused damage.

An individual is usually judged by the standards of his professional peers or by a professional standard. Costs may result from nervous shock, cost of care and loss of work.

Common causes of psychiatric negligence in order of frequency, according to UK medical defence societies are:

1. Suicide or attempted suicide (50%)

   This is due to failure of assessment or management. Proper care should have been present. If suicide is not prevented, the presence of good operational suicide policies, documentation of suicide risk, management plan to counter it documented in the medical records, and the informing of all relevant staff, such as nursing staff, of the suicide risk will be defences.
2. Negligent use of drugs (30%)

   This arises from the wrong drug being prescribed, the patient not being properly monitored or not properly warned, or no proper consent procedure.

   This particularly arises where drug toxicity results, e.g. for lithium:
   - delays in laboratory telling doctor result
   - failure to check thyroid and renal functioning
   - failure to monitor blood levels
   - most due to use of diuretics.
3. Misdiagnosis, especially failure to diagnose organic disorders.

Other causes include homicide by a patient, sexual misconduct of a doctor, breach of confidentiality, and lack of supervision (advice, instruction, monitoring and control), e.g. by a consultant of trainee. In practice, a doctor should never have a relationship with even an ex-patient.

Cases are scrutinized to see if 'reasonable care' compared to professional peers was present, i.e. the clinician used reasonable clinical judgement to weigh up risks, i.e. risk of illness, treated and untreated, risks of treatments and also alternative treatments and their risks.

An error of judgement or mistake becomes negligent if an individual did not exercise reasonable care. Psychiatrists as a speciality consult medical defence associations frequently, but are not among the medical specialties at high risk of litigation.

Negligence arises from the dereliction of duty directly causing damage to plaintiff (4Ds of USA law)

- cases of negligence arise from a bad outcome plus bad feelings, e.g. guilt, rage, grief, surprise.

It remains likely that, in spite of the current litigious culture, psychiatry is no different from other medical specialties in that, for every case of negligence brought, many more meritorious cases are not.

Medical records

If a risk is identified and documented, it is incumbent on the psychiatrist to manage that risk and record a management plan, e.g. tell staff of risk. The importance of good medical records are rightly emphasized as a way of countering litigation, e.g. 'if it's not recorded, it didn't occur'. However, psychiatrists will often have the opportunity to expand on their written records, e.g. if cross-examined in court. Merely recording the patient as saying he is 'not homicidal' or 'not suicidal' in the records would not prevent successful litigation if other evidence suggested otherwise, e.g. a suicidal patient may deny being at risk of suicide, but clearly be at risk of doing so on the basis of admitted symptoms of severe depression. NHS medical continuation sheets have letters and numbers at the base of the page, which give some indication of the age of the sheet, and this can sometimes reveal when entries are inappropriately made after an adverse event.

Medical, including psychiatric, negligence

Three main elements:

(1) duty of care to a 'neighbour'
(2) breach of duty of care
(3) damage to other party results.

Also:

- behaviour below standard required by law
- reasonably foreseeable damage
- actual casual connection
- Bolam Principle – if care in keeping with a body of recognized opinion, it is usually defendable, but courts act as a safety net and may disagree.

The overlap of legal and ethical considerations in psychiatry

Ethics

Ethics is a branch of philosophy. It is the science of the philosophy of morals. Ethics is concerned with which actions are right, which ends are good, is the rightness of actions inferable from the consequences and is virtuousness of motives inferred from rightness of actions etc., e.g. is it less bad to shoplift from a supermarket than from a corner shop, or for a man who repeatedly loses his temper to kill compared to one of previously good character who does so?

Ethics originates from the Greek ethos (nature or disposition) and morals from the Latin moris, the generic form of mos (custom). Though used synonymously, ethics is the science of the philosophy of morals, morals the practice or enactment of ethics. (Latin terms usually refer to real everyday matters, whereas Greek terms refer to an idealized theoretical understanding.) Thus, ethics involves the analysis of universal principles on which decisions are made, whereas morals regulate day-to-day judgement and refer to particular actions and beliefs. The law is 'silent' on many matters. Theoretically, morals should override political and legal requirements. The term moral is, however, also tainted by association with immorality and sexual misconduct.

The interest in ethical aspects of psychiatry has rapidly increased in the last 20 years, especially concerning the rights of patients, particularly in their dealings with psychiatrists, and in the USA. This concern led directly to the Code of Practice being established as prescribed in the Mental Health Act 1983 of England and Wales.

Ethics may where there is uncertainty and in obtaining the best quality judgements. It can help distinguish facts from values and is elucidating roles and duties. Law may follow ethics or ethics follow law.

The four principles of ethical medical practice are:

1. autonomy (respecting the patient's wishes)
2. beneficence (doing good)
3. non-maleficence (avoiding doing harm)
4. justice (fairness in the provision of care).

In practice, these principles often conflict and a balance has to be drawn. In medical ethics there is often a central conflict between the autonomy of the patient (e.g. avoiding concerning consent) and the duty of care of a doctor (e.g. negligence). Ethical dilemmas cannot, therefore, usually be solved by an algorithm.

Ethics of detaining patients

Patients may have a right to be treated even against their will. In some countries, e.g. particular states of the USA, it is more difficult to detain patients compared to the UK.

Ethics of consent

It is assumed, unless contested, that every adult has the right and the capacity (legal concept) (competence) to decide whether or not he/she will accept medical treatment, even if refusal risks permanent injury to health or premature death.

It is illegal to treat without consent unless in an emergency in good faith or under the Mental Health Act 1983 Part IV. Legally, if a patient is 'medically touched' without consent, this would constitute battery. Consent should be informed and voluntary, which implies that mental disorder, such as dementia, does not affect judgement. In practice, a lower threshold for capacity is made for those who consent to treatment compared to those who refuse. Refusal is not the same as lack of capacity to consent. Never threaten to impose treatment if a patient refuses and also ensure a patient is not just consenting for a quiet life. However, there is a distinction to be made between coercion and a patient's acceptance of the reality of his situation.

Valid ethical consent requires:

1. competence + information resulting in understanding
2. understanding + voluntariness can then result in an affirmative decision.

Regarding consent being based on sufficient information, to date the standard applied to this in the UK has been predominantly profession based, i.e. giving the level of information normally given by the profession in that medical situation based on the duty of care. The alternative standard is patient-based, i.e. the level of information necessary in order to allow a patient to operate his or her autonomy. Information should refer to alternative treatments and advice about substantial or unusual risks. No, or very little, information given may result in the professional being liable to a charge of battery. Inadequate information may result in a doctor being held liable and in a complaint of negligence (breach of duty of care). The term 'informed consent' is a USA one, not specifically enshrined in UK law.

A decision to consent may vary over time and different messages may be given by a patient in different modalities.

A consent form is only evidence as to consent and does not amount to the fact of consent.

To avoid negligence, even if following a 'responsible body' of medical opinion, a doctor needs to convince the court that the amount of information given or omitted can be defended.

Courts are reluctant to put a percentage figure of risk that a patient should be warned of, as the individual significance of injury to the individual is also important. Always put a note of warnings given to a patient in the notes and in a letter to GP (not on the consent form).

Individuals under 16 years can give valid consent if there is sufficient understanding. Parental consent is valid for individuals between the ages of 16 and 18 years who do not understand. Table 1 summarises what is considered sufficient information for valid consent.

Consent in English Law for Adults (aged 18 years or over)

Competent

- May refuse any, including life-saving, treatment (otherwise battery).
- Should be given information about nature of procedure, serious side-effects, likely benefits and alternatives (otherwise negligence).

Incompetent

- Doctors should act in the best interests of patients.
- Relatives and friends cannot give or withhold consent (they can only assent), but may be sources of information regarding best interests.

Minors and consent

- A person under 18 years should not be allowed to come to serious harm on the grounds that the minor and/or parents refuse consent to necessary and urgent treatment.

Table 1 Sufficient information for valid consent
The standard is now closer to the US law, i.e. OBJECTIVE PRUDENT PATIENT TEST (What a reasonable patient should be told), mainly due to changing GMC guidelines, rather than the REASONABLE DOCTOR MEDICAL TEST (PROFESSION BASED)
N.B. Case Law from England and Wales
(1) SIDAWAY vs. BOARD OF GOVERNORS OF BETHLEM ROYAL + MAUDSLEY HOSPITAL (1985) The majority of the five Law Lords supported the doctor-based standard of not telling of risk of 1% damage to spinal cord, after a neurosurgical procedure on cervical vertebrae. However, the judgement suggested if doctors were lax in informing patients, the courts may intervene.
(2) BOLAM vs. FRIERN HOSPITAL MANAGEMENT COMMITTEE (1957) 'Bolam Test'. Doctor is required to exercise the ordinary skills of a competent practitioner in field (Profession-based standard).
(3) MAYNARD vs. WEST MIDLANDS R.H.A. (1985) Even if the body of opinion is a minority, this is still defendable.
(4) BOLITHO vs. HACKNEY HEALTH AUTHORITY (1997) Even if following a 'responsible body' of medical opinion, a doctor needs to be able to convince a court that the amount of information given or omitted can be defended.

- 16–17 years olds are presumed by statute to have capacity to give consent unless the contrary is shown.
- A child under 16 who does have capacity (Gillick competent – common law) can give consent, but, if such a child refuses, consent can be overridden by those with parental responsibility or a court.
- Courts are unlikely to consider that those aged 13 or under have capacity.
- For children not Gillick competent, those with parental responsibility give consent, but have a legal obligation to act in the child's best interests.

Although psychiatric disorders can affect judgement and therefore capacity to consent, this can also occur in medical disorders, albeit less often.

The House of Lords have ruled that doctors have a common law duty (justification of necessity) to act in the best possible interests of the patient, e.g. if physically ill and not competent, e.g. unconscious, or if an individual is permanently unable to consent, e.g. due to severe learning disability, to treatments not covered by the Mental Health Act 1983.

Patients detained under the Mental Health Act may be able to give free valid consent to treatment, providing they are not complying merely to get out of hospital. Patients should know the nature and consequences of the proposed treatment, as well as the consequences of not having the treatment, and also the risks of treatment.

Although some doctors argue that it would be negligent in the case of patients not consenting to not test for medical conditions suspected (i.e. duty of care), this is not accepted legally. Undertaking an HIV/AIDS test without the patient knowing the nature of such a test and its personal and social implications constitutes assault, even if the patient consented to give blood for unspecified or other tests.

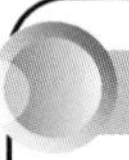

Consent

Requires:-

- information (knowing) to either profession or patient-based standard
- competency
- voluntariness
  1. competence + information → understanding
  2. understanding + voluntariness → decision.

N.B. Competence is not an absolute quality and no longer considered global

- not statutorily defined.
- depends on functioning, e.g. IQ, and purpose, e.g. complexity of issue, i.e. 'action specific'
- incompetent = incapable of giving valid consent (N.B. capacity is a legal concept)
- Mental Health Act 1983 competence is 'knowing nature, purpose and likely effects of treatment'
- treatment without consent = battery. Harm is presumed and does not have to be proven

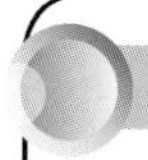

Consent (continued)

- detention without consent is false imprisonment
- consent by proxy (assent) not legal.

Exceptions to usual requirements for consent:

- Implied consent
  - By fact of consultation.
  - Patient's consent unavailable, but reasonable man would consent, e.g. unconscious patient post overdose.
- Necessity
  - Some level of patient incompetence and serious harm/death likely to occur.
  - Doctor owes duty of care.
- Emergency
  - To prevent serious harm to patient or other
- Post-suicide attempt
  - Can reverse effects of suicide attempt (anachronism as suicide was a crime), but not stop suicidal patient leaving hospital if not detainable under Mental Health Act 1983
  - Detention under Mental Health Act 1983.

Capacity (legal concept)/ competency (clinical concept, occasionally used legally)

This is the ability to know and understand the nature and consequence of legal processes and proceedings, including for medical purposes.

Assessment of capacity

This is required in many branches of medicine, including psychiatry.

- Old Age Psychiatry
  - testamentary capacity
  - power of attorney
  - finances
  - social care, e.g. sheltered home
- Forensic psychiatry
  - Fitness to plead and stand trial
- Liaison psychiatry
  - Treatment refusal
  - Leaving hospital without medical consent.

Capacity may vary over time, e.g. in delirium.

Legal principles relating to capacity

- An imprudent decision is not itself grounds for incapacity (analyse way decision made, not decision itself).
- Capacity is function specific not global.
- Standard of proof is on the balance of probabilities.

Three stages of assessing capacity (Re C [1994] All ER 819)

a) comprehension and retention of relevant information

b) ability to believe information (e.g. no delusion interfering)

c) weigh information and make decision.

Approaches to making decision for incompetent patients

Best interests

- proxy
- advance directive (living wills)
  - available in New Mental Capacity Act 2005
- substituted judgements (e.g. if patient became competent, what treatment would he choose).

BMA and Law Society Guidelines (1994) on Assessing Capacity

- Can understand nature and purpose of procedure/ treatment and why it is being proposed.
- Understands principle benefits, risks, alternatives and their risks and consequences of not being treated.
- Does not depend on detainability under Mental Health Act 1983.
- Takes into account patient's anxiety, language problems and cultural and education background.
- No relation to clinical reality, e.g. severity of illness if treatment refused.

The M.B. Test for Capacity (1997) (Needle phobia)

(1) Comprehend and retain information.

(2) Weigh information in balance and reach decision.

Patient attempts suicide and then refuses treatment in A & E Department

Theoretically, if competent, such a patient can refuse treatment. However, Medical Defence organizations in the UK have argued competence can always be questioned if an individual has harmed him/

herself, so defendable to intervene. The common law justification of 'necessity' allows reasonable interventions, including medical treatments, reasonable to the circumstances, where competence of individual unknown. Competence does not remove liability for detention under the Mental Health Act 1983 if the individual suffers from mental disorder and there is a risk to self, others or health. Section 5 (2) of the Mental Health Act 1983 allows urgent detention of a patient, including on a medical or surgical ward, but not in an A&E Department.

Confidentiality

The BMA and the Royal College of Psychiatrists state that the ideal ethical position is that doctors must protect information acquired in the course of a doctor–patient relationship. The GMC accepts that this is not an absolute position and that doctors can reveal such information if there is an immediate grave risk to the patient or others ('risk of death or serious harm'). In other circumstances a doctor should not reveal information until forced to do so, e.g. by a court order. Issues regarding confidentiality to third parties may also arise.

Incapacity to drive a motor vehicle

The patient should be advised that if he doesn't inform the Driver Vehicle Licensing Authority (DVLA) about a relevant condition, the doctor is obliged to do so. The only absolutely prescribed psychiatric disability is severe mental handicap. For lesser degrees of mental handicap, to be able to drive, the individual would need to demonstrate adequate functional ability at the wheel.

N.B. Always read carefully and consider with great care completing and signing any document given to you, e.g. regarding fitness to drive, because legal or professional proceedings may arise if you do not.

All have strict narrow criteria for information that can be divulged.

- Warrant.
- Data Protection Act 1984 (For computer stored clinical data).
- Venereal Diseases Regulations 1974 (Applies to Health Authority employees).
- Human Fertilisation and Embryology Act 1990 and amendment of 1992.

Disclosure allowed

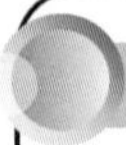

Confidentiality

General duty and guidelines, e.g. GMC.

Exceptions

- Court Order
- Statute: By law for legal proceedings
  (1) Misuse of Drugs Law: Notification of addicts.
  (2) Road Traffic Act 1988: Identification of drivers in RTAs.
  (3) Police and Criminal Evidence Act 1984.
  (4) Preventing Terrorism.

- If public interest – Public Interest Disclosure Act 1998; whistleblowing procedures
- with consent
- without identification.

In the UK, a patient or his lawyer can easily gain access to their medical records on the basis of:

- Supreme Court Act 1981 (for Personal Injury Claims).
- Access to Medical Records Act 1988 (for Reports).
- Access to Health Records Act 1990 (from 1/11/90).

Human Rights Act 1998

This incorporated the European Convention on Human Rights to UK law with full effect from October 2000. Relevant Articles to mental health care include:

Article 2: Right to life.

Article 3: Inhuman treatment.

Article 5: Right to liberty.

Article 5 (1) of European Convention on Human Rights protects patients' autonomy (no one to be detained save in specified cases as prescribed by law).

Article 5 (1) (e) concerns lawful detention of persons only if reliably shown to be of 'unsound mind', which equates to, but is not referred to as, incapacity.

Article 5 (4) guarantees the right to a speedy court review of a person's detention.

Article 6: Right to a fair trial (Includes MHRTs).

Article 8: Right to privacy, including private and family life and correspondence.

Ethics of genetic screening

Ethical debate often proceeds on the basis of either assumptions about what the patient wants or what doctors care about, e.g. it was widely assumed in the case of genetic screening for Huntington's disease that it would be harmful to the patient if the tests were positive, and thus such testing would be unethical (the principle of non-maleficence). Clinical experience has shown this to be not infrequently untrue.

Euthanasia

Treatment for depression rarely alters the attitude of patients considering this, which is often settled, considered, rational and fixed.

Methods of ethical reasoning

Most ethical dilemmas in psychiatry and, indeed, medicine, are due to one of the following issues:

- consent
- autonomy
- rationality
- confidentiality.

The following are three methods of ethical reasoning:

1. Principles

This approach offers a top-down approach to tackling ethical problems, i.e. from a general theory to particular cases, e.g. the 'Four Principle' perspective.

1. autonomy (respecting the patient's wishes)
2. beneficience (doing good)
3. non-maleficence (avoiding doing harm)
4. justice (fairness in the provision of care).

These principles, however, may conflict in individual cases, e.g. respecting the patient's wishes (autonomy) to have a detailed explanation of his condition may be at the expense of time spent with other patients (unjust). Autonomy may include the patient asking the doctor to decide for him.

2. Paradigms (Casuistry – case-based reasoning)

This offers a bottom up approach starting from cases and emphasizes two questions:

1. What changes to the case would make it clearer what to do?
2. What related situations would be less problematic ethically?

For example, how to manage the risk of death in an individual with mild learning disability pathologically water drinking. If one alters the scenario, e.g. to an overdose, the ethical issues become clearer.

Its advantages include the real-life case method and practical solutions. It is, however, professionally centred and can be biased by prejudices.

3. Perspectives

This is based on the practical skill of the capacity to view problems not only from a professional's perspectives, but also from that of the patient, the patient's relatives and other members of the multidisciplinary team. It is thus patient- and knowledge-centred, but may have the disadvantage of relativism.

Ethical theories

1. Substantive (concerned with establishing particular ethical conclusions)
   - **a.** deontological (rule-based). These theories emphasize rights, duties and responsibilities regardless of consequences, e.g. Kant's 'Categorical Imperatives'
   - **b.** consequentialist (teleology). These theories emphasize the importance of evaluating the consequences of actions, e.g. utilitarianism of John Stuart Mill.

For example, on confidentiality, consequentialist reasoning emphasizes the consequences if patients cannot trust their doctors, whereas deontological reasoning emphasizes the patient's right to privacy. Similarly, in a case where one Siamese twin must die to allow the other to live or both will die, or indeed the oft-quoted example of seven men in a boat but with only provisions for six, deontologists would say one should not kill, whereas consequentialists would emphasize the need for the greatest good.

2. Virtue Ethics. Rather than making binding, often rather negative, rules and duties, virtue ethics emphasizes changing people's attitudes to embrace the virtues, e.g. compassion, trustworthiness, integrity, conscientiousness and good relationships.
3. Analytic (concerned with the meaning of value terms and general logical form of ethical argument).

Multiple-Choice Questions

For each multiple-choice question, please choose the best answer out of the five options given.

Chapter 1: Introduction

1. Which of the following is best associated with the study of the way in which past experiences and current ways of relating result in present symptoms?
A. Cognitive therapy
B. Descriptive phenomenology
C. Health psychology
D. Psychodynamics
E. Sociology

The correct answer is D. Please refer to Table 1.1.

2. Which of the following psychoactive substances is most commonly misused in the Western world?
A. Alcohol
B. Cannabis
C. Ecstasy
D. Haloperidol
E. LSD

The correct answer is A. There is a very considerable influence of psychoactive substance use disorders (most notably alcohol dependence) on medical practice. The 1998 General Household Survey in England recorded that 27% of men and 14% of women drink alcohol at a level known to be harmful

3. In the Western world, practitioners of which of the following need to be medically qualified?
A. Art therapy
B. Cognitive behavioural therapy
C. Psychiatry
D. Psychotherapy
E. Psychology

The correct answer is C. Psychiatry is a branch of medicine. Practitioners in all the other options do not require a medical qualification; some of them may be designated 'Doctor' as a result of having obtained a PhD in psychology, for example.

4. Which of the following group of drugs was first introduced for clinical use in the 1950s?
A. Phenothiazines
B. Second-generation antipsychotics
C. SNRIs
D. SSRIs
E. Z-hypnotics (zaleplon, zolpidem and zopiclone)

The correct answer is A. The phenothiazine group of first-generation antipsychotics, such as chlorpromazine, were synthesized and introduced starting in the 1950s. The other groups of drugs given as options were introduced long after the 1950s. (SNRIs and SSRIs are groups of antidepressants.)

Chapter 2: The life net

1. Which of the following psychiatric disorders occurs in the youngest group of patients?
   A. Anorexia nervosa
   B. Bulimia nervosa
   C. Encopresis
   D. Personality disorders
   E. Schizophrenia

   The correct answer is C. This refers to faecal soiling.

2. Postnatal or puerperal depression occurs in what proportion of mothers?
   A. <1%
   B. 1–2%
   C. 10–20%
   D. 30–40%
   E. >50%

   The correct answer is C.

Chapter 3: Classification, aetiology, management and prognostic factors

1. The presence of which of the following symptoms would not, on their own, be consistent with a psychosis?
   A. Auditory hallucinations in the third-person
   B. Delusions of grandeur
   C. Catatonic behaviour
   D. Loss of insight
   E. Social phobia

   The correct answer is E.

2. In which year was the DSM-IV-TR published?
   A. 1970
   B. 1980
   C. 1990
   D. 2000
   E. 2010

   The correct answer is D.

3. First-generation antipsychotic drugs cause extrapyramidal side-effects as a result of antidopaminergic actions on which of the following?
   A. Dorsolateral prefrontal cortex
   B. Mesolimbic system
   C. Nigrostriatal system
   D. Retinal pathways
   E. Tuberoinfundibular system

   The correct answer is C.

4. With which of the following orally administered antipsychotic drugs does regular haematological monitoring need to take place?
   A. Chlorpromazine
   B. Clozapine
   C. Olanzapine
   D. Risperidone
   E. Paliperidone

   The correct answer is B. Important side-effects of clozapine are neutropenia and potentially fatal agranulocytosis. As a result, patients taking this medication must undergo regular haematological monitoring.

5. Which of the following is not a second-generation antipsychotic?
   A. Aripiprazole
   B. Fluphenazine
   C. Paliperidone
   D. Quetiapine
   E. Zotepine

   The correct answer is B. This is commonly administered in the form of a depot preparation of fluphenazine decanoate.

6. Which of the following is more likely to be a side-effect of lithium seen early in treatment rather than as a result of long-term treatment?
   A. Cardiac arrhythmia
   B. Fine tremor
   C. Memory impairment
   D. Nephrotoxicity
   E. Thyroid function disturbance

The correct answer is B. The other options are all side-effects that can occur following long-term treatment with lithium salts.

7. To which of the following classes does duloxetine belong?
   A. NARI
   B. NaSSA
   C. RIMA
   D. SNRI
   E. SSRI

The correct answer is D. It is a selective noradrenaline and serotonin reuptake inhibitor.

8. Which of the following medications is least likely to be used to treat alcohol dependence?
   A. Acamprosate
   B. Chlordiazepoxide
   C. Clomethiazole
   D. Disulfiram
   E. Lofexidine

The correct answer is E. This is used for the alleviation of symptoms in patients undergoing opioid withdrawal. It appears to act centrally (on α-adrenergic receptors) and may have a sedative effect.

9. Cognitive behavioural therapy has been found to be of benefit in which of the following?
   A. Depression
   B. Eating disorders
   C. Marital problems
   D. Obsessive–compulsive disorder
   E. All of the above

The correct answer is E.

Chapter 4: Doctor–patient communication

1. A man who enjoys fires and has an unconscious wish to be a fire-setter becomes a fireman. This might illustrate the operation of which of the following defence mechanisms?
   A. Displacement
   B. Identification
   C. Introjection
   D. Sublimation
   E. Undoing

The correct answer is D. This is the way in which the pleasure principle is satisfied by means of socially acceptable gratifications.

2. Which of the following is not considered to be a defence mechanism?
   A. Countertransference
   B. Denial
   C. Isolation
   D. Projective identification
   E. Reaction formation

The correct answer is A.

Chapter 5: History taking and clinical examination

1. In using the CAGE questionnaire, which of the following questions might you use to address the 'E' in CAGE?
   A. Have people annoyed you by criticizing your drinking?
   B. Have you ever felt guilty about your drinking?
   C. Have you ever felt that drinking is becoming too expensive?
   D. Have you ever felt you should cut down on your drinking?
   E. Have you ever had a drink first thing in the morning to steady your nerves or get rid of a hangover?

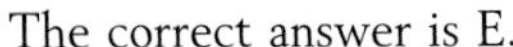

The correct answer is E.

2. You are asked to interview a 39-year-old male patient for the first time. Before speaking to him you immediately notice that he shows evidence of a lack of personal cleanliness; some of his clothes are dirty and his hair is unkempt. On the basis of these observations, which of the following diagnoses is least likely to apply in his case?
A. Dementia
B. Depression
C. Obsessive–compulsive disorder
D. Psychoactive substance use disorder
E. Schizophrenia

The correct answer is C.

3. The presence of which of the following signs is most likely to be consistent with a diagnosis of bulimia nervosa?
A. Ambitendency
B. Lanugo hair
C. Relatively fixed unchanging facies
D. Russell's sign
E. Waxy flexibility

The correct answer is D. It is caused by the use of the fingers to stimulate the gag reflex in self-induced vomiting.

4. Which of the following is not a feature of psychiatric stupor?
A. Immobility
B. May be associated with depression
C. May be associated with mania
D. Mutism
E. Unconsciousness

The correct answer is E. The patient is fully conscious.

5. Which of the following is not a Schneiderian feature of formal thought disorder?
A. Fusion
B. Distractibility
C. Drivelling
D. Omission
E. Substitution

The correct answer is B. The missing feature is derailment.

6. A patient has a persistent irrational fear of travelling by public transport. From which of the following types of phobia is she most likely to be suffering?
A. Acrophobia
B. Agoraphobia
C. Claustrophobia
D. Simple phobia
E. Social phobia

The correct answer is B. There may be elements of other phobias involved too.

7. Which of the following is not a passivity phenomenon?
A. Delusional perception
B. Made action
C. Made feeling
D. Thought withdrawal
E. Somatic passivity

The correct answer is A.

8. You see a young female inpatient with schizophrenia during the psychiatric ward round. She says she is troubled by using the lavatory because, typically, whenever she flushes the toilet, she hears voices commenting on her. What type of hallucination is this likely to be?
A. Extracampine
B. Functional
C. Hypnagogic
D. Reflex
E. Trailing phenomenon

The correct answer is B. Here, the stimulus causing the hallucination is experienced in addition to the hallucination itself.

9. A patient is unable to name, recognize or point on command to parts of his body. Which of the following is this known as?
A. Agraphaesthesia
B. Anosognosia
C. Astereognosia
D. Autotopagnosia
E. Simultanagnosia

The correct answer is D.

Chapter 6: Organic psychiatry

1. Which of the following is least likely to be a prodromal symptom of delirium?
A. Agitation
B. Amnesia
C. Hypersensitivity to light
D. Hypersensitivity to sound
E. Perplexity

The correct answer is B.

2. Which of the following is least likely to be associated with primary hypoadrenalism?
A. Buccal pigmentation
B. Depression
C. Loss of body hair
D. Vitiligo
E. Weight gain

The correct answer is E.

3. Which of the following is least likely to be associated with Cushing's syndrome?
A. Buffalo hump
B. Depression
C. Pathological fractures
D. Postural hypotension
E. Striae

The correct answer is D. This is more closely associated with Addison's disease (primary hypoadrenalism). Cushing's syndrome is more likely to be associated with hypertension.

4. Hypothyroidism may present in a young non-pregnant non-postpartum woman with which of the following?
A. Amenorrhoea
B. Lactation
C. Menorrhagia
D. Oligomenorrhoea
E. All of the above

The correct answer is E.

5. Which of the following is least likely to be associated with hyperthyroidism?
A. Bradycardia
B. Conjunctive oedema
C. Depression
D. Pretibial myxoedema
E. Proximal myopathy

The correct answer is A. Tachycardia is more likely to occur than bradycardia. Note that symptoms of the mood disorder depression are relatively common in hyperthyroidism.

6. With which of the following is the Klüver–Bucy syndrome not usually associated?
A. Alzheimer's disease
B. Hyperorality
C. Hyperphagia
D. Hyposexuality
E. Placidity

The correct answer is. D. It tends to be associated with hypersexuality.

7. Choose the incorrect option. Lewy body dementia is associated with:
A. A good symptomatic response to antipsychotic medication
B. Marked fluctuating cognitive impairment over weeks or months affecting memory

C. Marked fluctuating cognitive impairment over weeks or months affecting higher cortical functions
D. Mild spontaneous extrapyramidal symptoms
E. Visual hallucinations

The correct answer is A. Antipsychotic drugs should be avoided (or only used with extreme caution under specialized care). Their use in Lewy body dementia is associated with neuroleptic sensitivity syndrome, in which marked extrapyramidal symptoms may occur; life-threatening neuroleptic malignant syndrome may also occur.

8. Which of the following features of Huntington's disease is least likely to be correct?
A. Half the children, on average, of a patient with Huntington's disease can develop this disease
B. It is a polyglutamine disorder
C. Males and females are equally affected
D. The basal ganglia tend to be particularly affected by atrophy
E. There is a positive family history of Huntington's disease in affected cases

The correct answer is E. Although Huntington's disease is an autosomal dominant disorder, it is often the case that newly presenting patients do not give a positive family history. This may be because the Huntington's disease is a result of spontaneous mutation in the new case. In many countries it is perhaps even more likely to be the result of the fact that the patient was given away for adoption soon after birth.

9. A patient suffering from frontal lobe damage is wearing three pairs of spectacles, one on top of the other. Of which of the following phenomena is this most likely to be an example?
A. Aspontaneity
B. Disinhibition
C. Palilalia
D. Poor eyesight
E. Utilization behaviour

The correct answer is E. Objects are used repeatedly.

10. Which of the following is not a characteristic feature of Gerstmann's syndrome?
A. Agraphia
B. Dyscalculia
C. Finger agnosia
D. Prosopagnosia
E. Right–left disorientation

The correct answer is D. This usually results from non-dominant parietal or temporal lesions.

11. Kayser–Fleischer rings are most commonly associated with which of the following disorders?
A. Acute intermittent porphyria
B. AIDS
C. Cerebral abscess
D. Dementia pugilistica
E. Hepatolenticular degeneration

The correct answer is E.

Chapter 7: Psychoactive substance use disorders

1. Which of the following options is defined by the WHO as a pattern of psychoactive substance use causing damage to health?
A. Acute intoxication
B. Harmful use
C. Physical dependence
D. Psychological dependence
E. Tolerance

The correct answer is B.

2. Which of the following does not contain one unit of alcohol?
A. Beer – one pint

B. Brandy – one single measure
C. Sherry – one glass
D. Table wine (not a strong type) – one glass
E. Whisky – one single measure

The correct answer is A. This contains two units (or even more in the case of strong lagers).

3. According to the Royal College of Physicians, which of the following is the maximum recommended limit for a low-level consumption of alcohol by non-pregnant women?
A. 14 units/week
B. 21 units/week
C. 35 units/week
D. 50 units/week
E. 60 units/week

The correct answer is A. During pregnancy, abstinence or minimal consumption is recommended.

4. Which of the following is least likely to be a feature of fetal alcohol syndrome?
A. Cardiac murmurs
B. Microcephaly
C. Ocular hypertelorism
D. Short upper lip with a wide vermilion border
E. Strabismus

The correct answer is D. A long upper lip with a narrow vermilion border is more likely to be seen.

5. Which of the following is least likely to be a feature of Wernicke's encephalopathy?
A. Ataxia
B. Clouding of consciousness
C. Cortical sensory loss
D. Nystagmus
E. Peripheral neuropathy

The correct answer is C.

6. Which of the following is least likely to be a clinical feature of chronic opioid dependence in a young man?
A. Chronic diarrhoea
B. Erectile dysfunction
C. Malaise
D. Miosis
E. Tremor

The correct answer is A. Constipation is a more characteristic feature. Diarrhoea typically occurs as a withdrawal symptom.

Chapter 8: Schizophrenia and delusional (paranoid) disorders

1. Schneiderian first-rank symptoms of schizophrenia do not include which of the following?
A. Auditory hallucinations in the form of a running commentary
B. Auditory hallucinations discussing the patient in the third person
C. Derailment
D. Somatic passivity
E. Thought insertion

The correct answer is C.

2. Catatonic behaviour does not typically include which of the following?
A. Negativism
B. Posturing
C. Stupor
D. Tics
E. Waxy flexibility

The correct answer is D.

3. According to ICD-10, which of the following is more likely to be a feature of hebephrenic schizophrenia than paranoid schizophrenia?
A. Delusions of persecution
B. Delusions of reference

C. Hallucinatory voices of a threatening nature
D. Non-verbal auditory hallucinations
E. Rambling and incoherent speech

The correct answer is E.

4. Which of the following symptoms of schizophrenia is most likely to be part of Liddle's disorganization syndrome?
A. Auditory hallucinations
B. Decreased spontaneous movement
C. Flat affect
D. Inappropriate affect
E. Poverty of speech

The correct answer is D.

5. Which of the following features of schizophrenia is not true?
A. It has an earlier onset in females
B. It is more common in lower social classes
C. There is a genetic component
D. There is an increased relapse rate in those who live with families having high expressed emotion
E. Ventricular enlargement is often a feature of chronic schizophrenia seen using structural brain imaging

The correct answer is A. The onset tends to be earlier in males.

6. Which of the following is not typically a feature of tardive dyskinesia?
A. Chewing movements
B. Clenching
C. Cogwheel rigidity
D. Grimacing
E. Tongue protrusion

The correct answer is C. This is a characteristic feature of parkinsonism.

7. A middle-aged female patient is convinced that her youngest son has been replaced by 'a photocopy'. She is adamant that the person who looks like her son is not he. With which of the following disorders is this symptom most consistent?
A. A querulant delusion
B. Capgras syndrome
C. Cotard's syndrome
D. De Clérambault's syndrome
E. Fregoli syndrome

The correct answer is B.

Chapter 9: Mood disorders, suicide and parasuicide

1. Which of the following is not a biological symptom of depression?
A. Amenorrhoea
B. Constipation
C. Diurnal variation of mood
D. Early morning wakening
E. Hunger

The correct answer is E. Patients tend to suffer from reduced appetite and weight loss.

2. Select one incorrect option regarding depression:
A. Carbohydrate craving is often a feature of SAD
B. Cognitive behavioural therapy can be administered in a self-help format
C. Depressed mood is always a feature of depression
D. Depression is more common in females than males
E. SSRIs may increase the risk of suicide

The correct answer is C. Depressed patients may not always present with a depressed mood, but may instead present with somatic or other complaints.

3. Which of the following mental-state examination findings is least consistent with a diagnosis of mania?

A. Appearance – flamboyantly dressed
B. Speech – pressure of speech
C. Thoughts – flight of ideas
D. Perceptions – auditory hallucinations
E. Insight – fully present

The correct answer is E. Insight tends to be absent during manic episodes. Note that auditory hallucinations, when they occur, may confirm the patient's grandiose delusions.

4. Which of the following is more common in males than in females?
A. Bipolar disorder
B. Cyclothymia
C. Dysthymia
D. Parasuicide
E. Suicide

The correct answer is E.

5. Select one incorrect statement regarding the suicide rate in England and Wales:
A. It increased during the stress of First and Second World Wars
B. It is higher in the unemployed
C. It is higher in the unmarried
D. It is increased in schizophrenia
E. It shows a seasonal variation

The correct answer is A. The suicide rate fell during the First and Second World Wars.

Chapter 10: Neurotic and other stress-related anxiety disorders

1. Generalized anxiety disorder is characteristically associated with:
A. Avoidance
B. Long-standing free-floating anxiety
C. Evidence of acute panic lasting up to ten minutes
D. Agoraphobia
E. Improvement in performance when generalized anxiety disorder is of mild or moderate degree

The correct answer is B. Contrasts with phobic disorders where little anxiety may be experienced in absence of phobic stimulus.

2. Panic attacks are:
A. Characteristic of generalized anxiety disorder
B. Typically occur after exposure to a phobic stimulus
C. SSRI antidepressants are contraindicated
D. May lead to patients feeling they are dying
E. Can usually be 'sat out'

The correct answer is D, due to autonomic somatic anxiety symptoms.

3. Phobic disorder is:
A. Characterized by a prudent fear of a situation
B. Characterized by avoidance of feared situation but little anxiety otherwise in daily life.
C. Agoraphobia is rarely associated with panic disorder
D. Social phobia is more common in women
E. SSRI antidepressants are an effective standard treatment of specific animal phobias

The correct answer is B, for all phobias. Such patients manage their anxiety by avoidance of phobic situations

4. Post-traumatic stress disorder (PTSD):
A. Symptoms develop immediately after or during the day of the trauma
B. Avoidance, increased arousal and repetitive re-experiencing of trauma through flashbacks, hallucinations and/or illusions are characteristic
C. Comorbid substance abuse is uncommon
D. Head injury incurred at time of trauma will present with symptoms different from PTSD

E. Symptoms do not usually exceed 6 months duration from the stressful event

The correct answer is B.

5. In obsessive-compulsive disorder (OCD):
   A. Obsessions characteristically lead to avoidance
   B. Obsessions are egodystonic and insight into their irrationality is usually maintained
   C. Compulsions/rituals increase anxiety
   D. When considering the differential diagnosis, obsessional symptoms are infrequently seen in depressive disorder
   E. CBT (exposure therapy and response prevention) is rarely effective.

The correct answer is B, unlike impulses, which are often egosyntonic.

Chapter 11: The dissociative (conversion) and hypochondriasis and other somatoform disorders

1. Regarding dissociative (conversion) disorders:
   A. Conversion disorder is characterized by multiple neurological symptoms not explained by known organic disease
   B. Dissociative disorders do not require evidence of psychological causation for diagnosis
   C. A diagnosis of dissociative disorder should not be made if there is evidence of a physical or another psychiatric disorder that may explain the symptoms
   D. Conversion is a term from behavioural psychology that describes the process where psychic conflict is transferred into physical symptoms
   E. In dissociation following stress, integration of the functions of consciousness, memory, identity and movement are maintained

The correct answer is C.

2. In those presenting with medically unexplained symptoms:
   A. Those with hypochondriacal disorder believe they have a serious and often progressive undiagnosed physical disease
   B. Those with somatization disorder have the biological vegetative physical symptoms of depression
   C. In body dysmorphic disorder, patients have a delusional belief that they have a defect in their appearance
   D. In factitious disorders, symptoms are unconsciously produced
   E. In factitious disorders, patients are focussed on an external gain

The correct answer is A.

3. Dissociative (conversion) disorder:
   A. In conversion disorder, there is no loss or change in bodily function.
   B. In conversion disorder, the autonomic nervous system is predominantly affected
   C. The primary gain is the attention of others
   D. Symptoms are poorly tolerated
   E. Symptoms may be symbolic of an intrapsychic conflict or modelled on others

The correct answer is E.

4. Regarding somatoform disorders:
   A. In ICD10, these include somatization disorder, hypochondriacal disorder and persistent pain disorder
   B. Those with hypochondriacal disorder are not especially sensitive to normal physical signs and sensations
   C. Hypochondriacal disorder is the most common cause of hypochondriacal symptoms
   D. Those with somatization disorder have first-degree male relatives with an increased incidence of this disorder
   E. Both somatization disorder and hypochondriacal disorder occur primarily in females

The correct answer is A. DSM IV also includes conversion disorder and body dysmorphic disorder.

5. The following statements regarding physical symptoms are true:
A. The expression and experience of the majority of physical symptoms are uninfluenced by psychological factors
B. The onset of multiple physical symptoms late in life is usually due to physical illness
C. Munchaüsen by proxy is a factitious disorder where patients repeatedly present with feigned symptoms suggestive of serious physical illness
D. The term psychosomatic refers to psychological symptoms presumed to be caused by physical disease
E. The sick role refers to the way symptoms are perceived and acted on by an individual

The correct answer is B. This contrasts with somatization disorder, which has a characteristic onset in early adult life.

Chapter 12: Psychiatry of menstruation and pregnancy

1. Which of the following in women is more common during the premenstrual period?
A. Accidents
B. Migraine
C. Poor academic performance
D. Suicide
E. All of the above

The correct answer is E.

2. Select one incorrect statement regarding puerperal psychosis:
A. It is particularly associated with first pregnancy
B. Its incidence is up to around 1 in 200 births
C. The commonest type is an organic psychosis
D. There is an increased risk of infanticide
E. There is an increased risk of suicide

The correct answer is C.

3. Select one incorrect statement. Compared with postpartum maternity blues, postnatal depression:
A. Is more common
B. Is more likely not to have fully resolved at one year postpartum
C. Is more likely to require treatment beyond supportive psychotherapy
D. Peaks later
E. Tends to start later

The correct answer is A.

Chapter 13: Psychiatry of sexuality

1. Select one incorrect statement regarding the usual sexual response in women.
A. During the plateau phase there is areolar enlargement
B. During the resolution phase the cervix is lowered to the vaginal floor and there is some gaping of the cervical os
C. Four phases were identified by Masters and Johnson
D. The excitement phase immediately precedes the orgasm phase
E. There tends not to be a refractory period following orgasm

The correct answer is D. The plateau phase usually immediately precedes the orgasm phase.

2. Which of the following disorders of sexual preference is not correctly defined?
A. Exhibitionism – Recurrent or persistent tendency to expose the genitalia to strangers or to people in public places
B. Fetishism – Wearing of opposite-sex clothes for sexual excitement
C. Frotteurism – Rubbing up against people for sexual stimulation in crowded public places
D. Telephone scatalogia – Making of obscene telephone calls

E. Voyeurism – Recurrent or persistent tendency to look at people engaging in sexual or intimate behaviour such as undressing

The correct answer is B. The definition given is that of fetishistic transvestism. Fetishism is the reliance on some non-living object as a stimulus for sexual arousal.

3. Which of the following features is more common in Type 2 indecent exposure offenders than in Type 1 offenders?
   A. Comprise the majority of cases of indecent exposure offenders
   B. Derive little pleasure from the act
   C. Expose a flaccid penis
   D. Show little guilt
   E. The intention is not usually to have sexual intercourse with the victims

The correct answer is D.

4. A married couple is being treated with sex therapy for premature ejaculation. During which phase of their homework assignment would they use the stop–start technique?
   A. Genital sensate focus
   B. Non-genital sensate focus
   C. Premature sensate focus
   D. Vaginal containment
   E. Vaginal containment with movement

The correct answer is A.

Chapter 14: Sleep disorders

1. In which stage of normal sleep are K complexes characteristically seen in the EEG?
   A. Stage 1
   B. Stage 2
   C. Stage 3
   D. Stage 4
   E. REM

The correct answer is B. Sleep spindles also occur during this stage of sleep, as can be seen in Figure 14.1.

2. During which stage of normal sleep is the cardiac rate characteristically raised?
   A. Stage 1
   B. Stage 2
   C. Stage 3
   D. Stage 4
   E. REM

The correct answer is E. This is shown in Figure 14.1.

3. Which of the following hypnotics is particularly associated with the side-effect of taste disturbance in some patients?
   A. Melatonin
   B. Nitrazepam
   C. Zaleplon
   D. Zolpidem
   E. Zopiclone

The correct answer is E.

4. Which of the following features is more likely to be associated with narcolepsy than with hypersomnia?
   A. Attacks rarely occur in unusual places
   B. Nocturnal sleep tends to be prolonged and deep
   C. The duration of an attack is typically greater than one to two hours
   D. The onset is sudden
   E. Usually worse in the morning

The correct answer is D.

5. Which of the following features is more likely to be associated with night terrors than with nightmares?
   A. They are associated with alcohol withdrawal
   B. They are associated with β-blocker treatment
   C. They are associated with hypnotic withdrawal
   D. They tend to occur during middle and late sleep

E. They tend to take place during stages 3 and 4 of sleep

The correct answer is E. They tend to occur during REM sleep (or occasionally during stages 1 and 2 of sleep).

Chapter 15: Personality disorders

1. Which of the following types of personality disorder belongs to cluster A (withdrawn)?
A. Anxious
B. Dependent
C. Histrionic
D. Passive-aggressive
E. Schizoid

The correct answer is E.

2. Which of the following is a characteristic feature of an anankastic personality disorder?
A. Emotional coldness
B. Emotionally unstable
C. Irresponsibility
D. Oversensitivity
E. Perfectionism

The correct answer is E. It may help to recall that anankastic personality disorder is also known as obsessive–compulsive personality disorder.

3. Which of the following is not a characteristic feature of psychopathic disorder?
A. Affectionless
B. Criminal motivation
C. Egocentric
D. Impulsive
E. Lacks empathy

The correct answer is B.

Chapter 16: Child and adolescent psychiatry

1. Select one incorrect statement regarding attention-deficit hyperactivity disorder:
A. A cardinal feature is impaired attention
B. A cardinal feature is impulsivity
C. A cardinal feature is overactivity
D. It does not occur in adulthood
E. It may respond to stimulant medication

The correct answer is D.

2. Which of the following types of behaviour is not considered to be a part of conduct disorder?
A. Absconding from home
B. Defiance
C. Fighting or bullying
D. Isolated episodes of dissocial behaviour
E. Severe destructiveness to property

The correct answer is D.

3. Which of the following treatments has been successfully used in non-organic enuresis?
A. Desmopressin
B. Pad and buzzer
C. Star chart
D. All of the above
E. None of the above

The correct answer is D.

Chapter 17: Psychiatry of disability

1. What is the approximate lower bound of the range of IQs that corresponds to moderate mental retardation in ICD-10?
A. 15
B. 20
C. 35

D. 50
E. 70

The correct answer is C.

2. Which of the following is not a typical clinical feature of fragile X syndrome?
A. Delayed language acquisition
B. High arched palate
C. Large everted ears
D. Micro-orchidism
E. Mitral valve prolapse

The correct answer is D. Macro-orchidism is common.

3. Which of the following is not a typical clinical feature of childhood autism?
A. Abnormality apparent before the age of three years
B. Echolalia and palilalia
C. Increased congenital heart disease
D. Poor or absent social interaction
E. Restricted and repetitive behaviour

The correct answer is C. This is much more likely to be seen in Down's syndrome.

Chapter 18: Eating disorders

1. Which of the following is not a typical feature of postpubertal anorexia nervosa in a woman?
A. Absent secondary sexual axillary hair and pubic hair
B. Amenorrhoea
C. Cardiovascular abnormalities
D. Lanugo hair on her face and trunk
E. Poor peripheral circulation

The correct answer is A.

2. Skin thickening on the knuckles (Russell's sign) may be seen in bulimia nervosa. What is the most likely cause of this sign?
A. Anaemia
B. Hypokalaemia
C. Infection
D. Poor connective tissue growth
E. Self-induced vomiting

The correct answer is E.

Chapter 19: Transcultural psychiatry

1. Select one incorrect statement regarding cultural psychiatry:
A. Depressed adult immigrants in the Western world originating from the Indian subcontinent often somatize their depressive symptoms
B. Depressed Afro-Caribbean adult male immigrants in the Western world often complain of erectile dysfunction or reduced libido rather than of feeling low
C. High rates of schizophrenia have been reported for isolated populations in northern Sweden and for parts of Finland
D. The lifetime prevalence of depression is approximately equal in different groups worldwide
E. The rate of psychosis in Afro-Caribbeans in the UK, especially in second-generation immigrants, is much higher than that in white British people

The correct answer is D. The lifetime prevalence of depression has been found to vary widely in different groups.

2. Which of the following culture-bound syndromes affecting men is characterized by patients having an overwhelming fear that their penis is retracting into the abdomen and that death will occur immediately thereafter?
A. Amok
B. Koro
C. Latah
D. Piblokto
E. Susto

The correct answer is B.

Chapter 20: Psychiatry of the elderly

1. Which of the following cognitive enhancers is an NMDA antagonist?
   A. Donepezil
   B. Galantamine
   C. Memantine
   D. Rivastigmine
   E. None of the above

The correct answer is C. The other three, donepezil, rivastigmine and galantamine, are anticholinesterase inhibitors.

Chapter 21: Forensic psychiatry

1. In England and Wales, regarding a defendant charged with a serious violent but non-fatal offence
   A. The defendant will not be found guilty if aged 13 years
   B. Not guilty by reason of insanity (McNaughton Rules) refers to the mental state of the defendant at the time of the trial
   C. If the defendant has an abnormality of mental functioning substantially impairing his responsibility, he will be eligible for a defence of diminished responsibility
   D. A diagnosis of schizophrenia will result in a not guilty verdict
   E. Fitness to plead refers to the time of the trial

The correct answer is E. An individual may be unfit to plead at the time of the trial but fully responsible for his actions at the time of the offence, and vice versa.

2. In an adult suffering from schizophrenia, the risk of violence is not increased by:
   A. Delusions of passivity (of external control)
   B. Substance abuse
   C. The availability of a weapon
   D. Morbid jealousy (Othello syndrome)
   E. Comorbid obsessive–compulsive disorder

The correct answer is E. Although obsessions of a violent content may be present, these are resisted and seldom acted on in obsessive–compulsive disorder

Chapter 22: Mental Health Legislation

1. In the Mental Health Act 1983 of England and Wales, as amended by the Mental Health Act 2007
   A. A single definition of mental disorder has replaced the legal categories of mental illness, mental impairment and psychopathic disorder
   B. Alcohol dependence constitutes a mental disorder under the Act
   C. Sexual deviancy alone is not regarded as a mental disorder under the Act
   D. Allows for the compulsory detention and treatment of physical disorders
   E. Detention depends on an assessment of loss of capacity to consent to psychiatric treatment

The correct answer is A, since the amending Mental Health Act 2007.

2. Under the Mental Health Act 1983 for England and Wales
   A. A doctor approved under Section 12 (2) of the Mental Health Act 1983 and an Approved Mental Health Practitioner (AMHP) (not necessarily a social worker) are required to detain a patient under Section 3
   B. Section 5 (2) (Urgent detention of a voluntary inpatient-doctors' holding power) can be applied to a patient in a medical or surgical ward
   C. A patient may not be restrained and medicated unless he is detained under the Mental Health Act 1983
   D. Section 3 is an order for compulsory treatment and lasts 1 year
   E. Section 136 allows the Police to remove a mentally disordered patient from their home to a place of safety

The correct answer is B, but this does not apply to patients attending an A&E Department.

Chapter 23: Civil legal aspects, the Mental Capacity Act 2005 and ethics of psychiatry

1. Regarding capacity to consent to essential treatment for physical illness

A. Adults are assumed to have the capacity to refuse such treatment, even if it results in death, unless proven otherwise on the balance of probabilities

B. Patients with positive psychotic symptoms, such as delusions or hallucinations, of schizophrenia lack the capacity to consent to such treatment

C. The nearest relative of a patient lacking capacity to consent may consent on their behalf

D. Where a patient makes an imprudent decision to refuse life-saving treatment, a doctor has a duty to act in the patient's best interests whatever the patient says

E. Lasting powers of attorney under the Mental Capacity Act 2005 do not allow the attorney to make health decisions for those who lack capacity

The correct answer is A.

Appendix I: Summary of psychiatric classification: ICD-10

Organic, including symptomatic, mental disorders

- F00 Dementia in Alzheimer's disease
- F01 Vascular dementia
- F02 Dementia in other diseases classified elsewhere
- F03 Unspecified dementia
- F04 Organic amnesic syndrome, not induced by alcohol and other psychoactive substances
- F05 Delirium, not induced by alcohol and other psychoactive substances
- F06 Other mental disorders due to brain damage and dysfunction and to physical disease
- F07 Personality and behavioural disorders due to brain disease, damage and dysfunction
- F09 Unspecified organic or symptomatic mental disorder

Mental and behavioural disorders due to psychoactive substance use

- F10 Mental and behavioural disorders due to use of alcohol
- F11 Mental and behavioural disorders due to use of opioids
- F12 Mental and behavioural disorders due to use of cannabinoids
- F13 Mental and behavioural disorders due to use of sedatives or hypnotics
- F14 Mental and behavioural disorders due to use of cocaine
- F15 Mental and behavioural disorders due to use of other stimulants, including caffeine
- F16 Mental and behavioural disorders due to use of hallucinogens
- F17 Mental and behavioural disorders due to use of tobacco
- F18 Mental and behavioural disorders due to use of volatile solvents
- F19 Mental and behavioural disorders due to multiple drug use and use of other psychoactive substances

Schizophrenia, schizotypal and delusional disorders

- F20 Schizophrenia
- F21 Schizotypal disorder
- F22 Persistent delusional disorders
- F23 Acute and transient psychotic disorders
- F24 Induced delusional disorder
- F25 Schizoaffective disorders
- F28 Other non-organic psychotic disorders
- F29 Unspecified non-organic psychosis

Mood (affective) disorders

- F30 Manic episode
- F31 Bipolar affective disorder
- F32 Depressive episode
- F33 Recurrent depressive disorder
- F34 Persistent mood (affective) disorders
- F35 Other mood (affective) disorders
- F39 Unspecified mood (affective) disorder

Neurotic, stress-related and somatoform disorders

F40 Phobic anxiety disorders
F41 Other anxiety disorders
F42 Obsessive–compulsive disorder
F43 Reaction to severe stress, and adjustment disorders
F44 Dissociative (conversion) disorders
F45 Somatoform disorders
F48 Other neurotic disorders

Behavioural syndromes associated with physiological disturbances and physical factors

F50 Eating disorders
F51 Non-organic sleep disorders
F52 Sexual dysfunction not caused by organic disorder or disease
F53 Mental and behavioural disorders associated with the puerperium, not classified elsewhere
F54 Psychological and behavioural factors associated with disorders or diseases classified elsewhere
F55 Abuse of non-dependence-producing substances
F59 Unspecified behavioural syndromes associated with physiological disturbances and physical factors

Disorders of adult personality and behaviour

F60 Specific personality disorders
F61 Mixed and other personality disorders
F62 Enduring personality changes not attributable to brain damage and disease
F63 Habit and impulse disorders
F64 Gender identity disorders
F65 Disorders of sexual preference
F66 Psychological and behavioural disorders associated with sexual development and orientation
F68 Other disorders of adult personality and behaviour
F69 Unspecified disorder of adult personality and behaviour

Mental retardation

F70 Mild mental retardation
F71 Moderate mental retardation
F72 Severe mental retardation
F73 Profound mental retardation
F78 Other mental retardation
F79 Unspecified mental retardation

Disorders of psychological development

F80 Specific developmental disorders of speech and language
F81 Specific developmental disorders of scholastic skills
F82 Specific developmental disorder of motor function
F83 Mixed specific developmental disorders
F84 Pervasive developmental disorders
F88 Other disorders of psychological development
F89 Unspecified disorder of psychological development

Behavioural and emotional disorders with onset usually occurring in childhood and adolescence

F90 Hyperkinetic disorders
F91 Conduct disorders
F92 Mixed disorders of conduct and emotions
F93 Emotional disorders with onset specific to childhood
F94 Disorders of social functioning with onset specific to childhood and adolescence
F95 Tic disorders
F98 Other behavioural and emotional disorders with onset usually occurring in childhood and adolescence

Unspecified mental disorder

F99 Mental disorder not otherwise specified

Appendix II: Summary of psychiatric classification: DSM-IV-TR

This is a multiaxial classification with the following five axes:

Axis I Clinical disorders
Other conditions that may be a focus of clinical attention

Axis II Personality disorders
Mental retardation

Axis III General medical conditions

Axis IV Psychosocial and environmental problems

Axis V Global assessment of functioning

In the following summary, NOS stands for 'not otherwise specified'.

Axis I: Clinical disorders; other conditions that may be a focus of clinical attention

Disorders usually first diagnosed in infancy, childhood, or adolescence (excluding mental retardation, which is diagnosed on Axis II)

Learning disorder
Motor skills disorder
Communication disorders
Pervasive developmental disorders:
- Autistic disorder
- Rett's disorder
- Childhood disintegrative disorder
- Asperger's disorder
- NOS

Attention-deficit and disruptive behaviour disorders
Feeding and eating disorders of infancy and early childhood
Tic disorders
Elimination disorders:
- Encopresis
- Enuresis

Other disorders of infancy, childhood, or adolescence

Delirium, dementia, and amnestic and other cognitive disorders

Delirium
Dementia
Amnestic disorders
Other cognitive disorders

Mental disorders due to a general medical condition

Substance-related disorders
Alcohol-related disorders
Amphetamine (or amphetamine-like)-related disorders
Caffeine-related disorders
Cannabis-related disorders
Cocaine-related disorders
Hallucinogen-related disorders
Inhalant-related disorders
Nicotine-related disorders
Opioid-related disorders

Phencyclidine (or phencyclidine-like)-related disorders
Sedative-, hypnotic-, or anxiolytic-related disorders
Polysubstance-related disorders
Other (or unknown) substance-related disorders

Schizophrenia and other psychotic disorders

Schizophrenia
Schizophreniform disorder
Schizoaffective disorder
Delusional disorder
Brief psychotic disorder
Shared psychotic disorder
Psychotic disorder due to a general medical condition
Substance-induced psychotic disorder
Psychotic disorder NOS

Mood disorders

Depressive disorders
Bipolar disorders

Anxiety disorders

Panic disorder without agoraphobia
Panic disorder with agoraphobia
Agoraphobia without history of panic disorder
Specific phobia
Social phobia
Obsessive–compulsive disorder
Post-traumatic stress disorder
Acute stress disorder
Generalized anxiety disorder
Anxiety disorder due to a general medical condition
Substance-induced anxiety disorder
NOS

Somatoform disorders

Somatization disorder
Undifferentiated somatoform disorder
Conversion disorder
Pain disorder
Hypochondriasis
Body dysmorphic disorder
NOS

Factitious disorders

Dissociative disorders
Dissociative amnesia
Dissociative fugue
Dissociative identity disorder
Depersonalization disorder
NOS

Sexual and gender identity disorders

Sexual dysfunctions
- Sexual desire disorders
- Sexual arousal disorders
- Orgasmic disorders
- Sexual pain disorders
- Sexual dysfunction due to a general medical condition

Paraphilias
- Exhibitionism
- Fetishism
- Frotteurism
- Paedophilia
- Sexual masochism
- Sexual sadism
- Transvestic fetishism
- Voyeurism
- NOS

Gender identity disorders

Eating disorders

Anorexia nervosa
Bulimia nervosa
NOS

Sleep disorders

Primary sleep disorders
- Dyssomnias
- Parasomnias

Sleep disorders related to another medical disorder
Other sleep disorders

Impulse-control disorders not elsewhere classified

Adjustment disorders

Other conditions that may be a focus of clinical attention

Axis II: Personality disorders; mental retardation

Personality disorders

Paranoid personality disorder
Schizoid personality disorder
Schizotypal personality disorder
Antisocial personality disorder
Borderline personality disorder
Histrionic personality disorder
Narcissistic personality disorder
Avoidant personality disorder
Dependent personality disorder
Obsessive–compulsive personality disorder
NOS

Mental retardation

Mild mental retardation
Moderate mental retardation
Severe mental retardation
Profound mental retardation
Mental retardation, severity unspecified

Axis III: General medical conditions

Infectious and parasitic diseases

Neoplasms

Endocrine, nutritional, and metabolic diseases and immunity disorders

Diseases of the blood and blood-forming organs

Diseases of the nervous system and sense organs

Diseases of the circulatory system

Diseases of the respiratory system

Diseases of the digestive system

Diseases of the genitourinary system

Complications of pregnancy, childbirth, and the puerperium

Diseases of the skin and subcutaneous tissue

Diseases of the musculoskeletal system and connective tissue

Congenital anomalies

Certain conditions originating in the perinatal period

Symptoms, signs, and ill-defined conditions

Injury and poisoning

Axis IV: Psychosocial and environmental problems

Problems with primary support group

Problems related to the social environment

Educational problems

Occupational problems

Housing problems

Economic problems

Problems with access to health care services

Problems related to interaction with the legal system/crime

Other psychosocial and environmental problems

Axis V: Global assessment of functioning

Appendix III: Summary of history and mental state examination

History

Reason for referral
Complaints
History of presenting illness
Family history
Family psychiatric history
Personal history
Past medical history
Past psychiatric history
Psychoactive substance use
Forensic history
Premorbid personality

Mental state examination

Appearance and behaviour

- general appearance
- facial appearance
- posture and movements
- social behaviour
- rapport

Speech

- rate and quantity
- neologisms
- accent
- form
- record a sample if abnormal

Mood

- objective
- subjective
- anxiety
- affect

Thought content

- preoccupations
- obsessions
- phobias
- suicidal and homicidal thoughts

Abnormal beliefs and interpretation of events

- referred to the environment
- referred to the body
- referred to the self

Abnormal experiences

- referred to the environment
- referred to the body
- referred to the self

Cognitive state

- orientation
- attention and concentration
- memory
- general knowledge and intelligence

Insight

Glossary

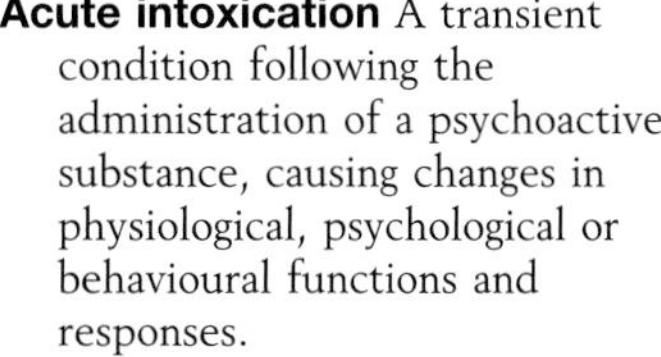

Acute intoxication A transient condition following the administration of a psychoactive substance, causing changes in physiological, psychological or behavioural functions and responses.

Affect A pattern of observable behaviours that is the expression of a subjectively experienced feeling state (emotion) and is variable over time in response to changing emotional states (DSM-III-R).

Agitation Excessive motor activity with a feeling of inner tension.

Agnosic alexia Words can be seen but not read.

Agoraphobia Literally a fear of the market-place. A generalized high anxiety level and multiple phobic symptoms occur. It may include a fear of crowds, open and closed spaces and travelling by public transport.

Alexithymia Difficulty in being aware of or describing one's emotions.

Ambitendency A series of tentative, incomplete movements carried out when a voluntary action is anticipated.

Ambivalence The simultaneous presence of opposing impulses towards the same thing.

Amnesia The inability to recall past experiences.

Amok Seen in south-east Asia. There is an outburst of aggressive behaviour in which the patient runs amok, following a depressive episode.

Anosognosia The lack of awareness of disease.

Anxiety A feeling of apprehension or tension caused by anticipating an external or internal danger.

Apathy Detachment or indifference and a loss of emotional tone and the ability to feel pleasure.

Attention The ability to focus on an activity.

Automatism An act over which a person has no control, e.g. sleepwalking.

Autoscopy (phantom mirror image) A hallucination in which one sees and recognizes oneself.

Autotopagnosia The inability to name, recognize or point on command to parts of the body.

Bereavement A term that can apply to any loss event, particularly of a negative nature, from loss of a relative by death to unemployment, divorce or even the loss of a family pet.

Blunted affect A reduction in emotional expression.

Capgras syndrome A person who is familiar to the patient is believed to have been replaced by a double.

Central (syntactical) aphasia Difficulty in arranging words in their correct sequence.

Circumstantiality Slowed thinking incorporating unnecessary trivial details. The goal of thought is finally, but slowly, reached.

Clanging Speech in which words are chosen because of their sounds rather than their meanings. It includes rhyming and punning.

Clouding of consciousness The patient is drowsy and does not react completely to stimuli. There is disturbance of attention, concentration, memory, orientation and thinking.

Coenestopathic state A localized distortion of body awareness.

Coma In deep coma there is no response to deep pain or any spontaneous movement. Tendon, pupillary and corneal reflexes are usually absent.

Compulsions or compulsive rituals Repetitive, stereotyped, seemingly purposeful behaviour that is the motor component of obsessional thoughts. Examples are checking and cleaning rituals.

Concentration The ability to sustain attention.

Concrete thinking A lack of abstract thinking, normal in childhood, and occurring in adults with organic brain disease and schizophrenia.

Confabulation Gaps in memory are unconsciously filled with false memories.

Cotard's syndrome A nihilistic delusional disorder in which, for example, the patient believes their money, friends or body parts do not exist.

Countertransference The therapist's emotions and attitudes to the patient.

Couvade syndrome A hysterical disorder in which a prospective father develops symptoms characteristic of pregnancy.

Culture-bound syndromes Specific psychiatric disorders occurring in certain non-Western countries.

Defence mechanisms Mental mechanisms that protect consciousness from the affects, ideas and desires of the unconscious.

Déjà vu The illusion of recognition of a situation.

Déjà pensé The illusion of recognition of a new thought.

Delirium A disorder of consciousness in which the patient is bewildered, disorientated and restless. There may be associated fear and hallucinations.

Delusion A false personal belief based on incorrect inference about external reality and firmly sustained in spite of what almost everyone else believes and in spite of what constitutes incontrovertible and obvious proof or evidence to the contrary. The belief is not one normally held by others of the same subculture (DSM-IV-TR).

Delusion (illusion) of doubles (l'illusion de sosies) The delusional belief that a person known to the patient has been replaced by a double; it is seen in Capgras syndrome.

Delusion of infidelity (pathological jealousy, delusional jealousy, Othello syndrome) The delusional belief that one's spouse or lover is being unfaithful.

Delusion of reference The behaviour of others, and objects and events, e.g. television broadcasts, is believed to refer to oneself in particular; when similar thoughts are held with less than delusional intensity they are ideas of reference.

Delusional perception A new and delusional significance is attached to a familiar real perception without any logical reason.

Dementia A global organic impairment of intellectual functioning without impairment of consciousness.

Denial A defence mechanism in which the subject acts as if consciously unaware of a wish or reality.

Dependence syndrome The use of psychoactive substances has a higher priority than other behaviours that once had higher value. There is a desire, often strong and overpowering, to take the substance(s) on a continuous or periodic basis.

Depersonalization One feels that one is altered or not real in some way.

Depression A low or depressed mood that may be accompanied by anhedonia, in which the ability to enjoy regular and pleasurable activities is lost. In normal grief or mourning the sadness is appropriate to the loss.

Depressive retardation A lesser form of psychomotor retardation that occurs in depression.

Derealization The surroundings do not seem real.

Disease The pathological abnormality occurring in an organism as a result of some specific noxious insult(s).

Disorders (loosening) of association (formal thought disorder) A language disorder seen in schizophrenia, e.g. knight's-move thinking and word salad.

Displacement A defence mechanism in which thoughts and feelings about one person or object are transferred on to another.

Dissociative disorder A disorder in which there is a disturbance in the normal integration of awareness of identity, consciousness, memory and control of bodily movements.

Distractibility The attention is frequently drawn to irrelevant external stimuli.

DSM-IV Diagnostic and statistical manual of mental disorders, 4th edition published by the American Psychiatric Association, Washington DC, 1994.

DSM-IV-TR Diagnostic and statistical manual of mental disorders, 4th edition, Text Revision, published by the American Psychiatric Association, Washington DC, 2000.

Dysarthria Difficulty articulating speech.

Dysphoria An unpleasant mood.

Dysthymia (depressive neurosis) A chronic depression of mood that does not fulfil the criteria for recurrent depressive disorder. Sufferers usually have periods of days or weeks when they describe themselves as well, but most of the time they feel tired and depressed (ICD-10).

Echolalia The automatic imitation of another's speech.

Echopraxia The automatic imitation of another's movements, occurring even when asked not to.

Ecstasy A feeling of intense rapture.

Ego Part of the mental apparatus that is present at the interface of the perceptual and internal demand systems. It controls voluntary thoughts and actions and, at an unconscious level, defence mechanisms.

Egomania A pathological preoccupation with oneself.

Eidetic image A vivid and detailed reproduction of a previous perception, e.g. a photographic memory.

Elevated mood A mood more cheerful than normal. It is not necessarily pathological.

Erotomania (de Clérambault's syndrome) The delusional belief that another person is deeply in love with one. It usually occurs in women, with the object often being a man of much higher social status.

Euphoric mood An exaggerated feeling of well-being. It is pathological.

Expansive mood Feelings are expressed without restraint, and one's self-importance may be overrated.

Expressive (motor) aphasia Difficulty in expressing thoughts in words while comprehension remains.

Extracampine hallucination The hallucination occurs outside one's sensory field.

Fear Anxiety caused by a recognized real danger.

Flat affect There is almost no emotional expression at all and the patient typically has an immobile face and monotonous voice.

Flight of ideas The speech consists of a stream of accelerated thoughts, with abrupt changes from topic to topic and no central direction. The connections between the thoughts may be based on chance relationships, verbal associations (e.g. alliteration and assonance), clang associations and distracting stimuli.

Formication A somatic hallucination in which insects are felt to be crawling under one's skin.

Free association The articulation, without censorship, of all thoughts that come to mind.

Free-floating anxiety Pervasive and unfocused anxiety.

Fregoli syndrome The patient believes that a familiar person, who is often believed to be the patient's persecutor, has taken on different appearances.

Freudian slips (parapraxes) Unconscious thoughts slipping through when censorship is offguard.

Fugue A state of wandering from usual surroundings and loss of memory.

Functional hallucination The stimulus causing the hallucination is experienced in addition to the hallucination.

Generalized anxiety disorder (anxiety neurosis; anxiety state; anxiety reaction) A neurotic disorder characterized by unrealistic or excessive anxiety and worry, which is generalized and persistent and not restricted to particular environmental circumstances, i.e. it is free-floating.

Global aphasia Both receptive and expressive aphasia are present at the same time.

Grief Those psychological and emotional processes, expressed both internally and externally, that accompany bereavement.

Hallucination A false sensory perception in the absence of a real external stimulus. It is perceived as being located in objective space and as having the same realistic qualities as normal perceptions. It is not subject to conscious manipulation and only indicates a psychotic disturbance when there is also impaired reality testing.

Hallucinosis Hallucinations (usually auditory) occur in clear consciousness, e.g. in alcoholism.

Harmful use A pattern of psychoactive substance use, which is causing damage to physical and/or mental health.

Health Defined by the World Health Organization as being a state of complete physical, mental and social well-being.

Health behaviour Actions taken by people who see themselves as healthy in order to prevent disease or to detect it while it is still asymptomatic.

Hemisomatognosis (hemidepersonalization) A limb is felt to be missing.

Hyperacusis An increased sensitivity to sounds.

Hyperaesthesia A sensory distortion in which sensations appear increased.

Hyperkinesis Overactivity, distractibility, excitability and impulsivity, e.g. in children.

Hypnagogic hallucination Hallucination occurring while falling asleep. It occurs in normal people.

Hypnopompic hallucination Hallucination occurring while waking from sleep. It occurs in normal people.

Hypoaesthesia A sensory distortion in which sensations appear decreased.

Hypochondriasis A preoccupation not based on real organic pathology, with a fear of having a serious physical illness. Physical sensations are unrealistically interpreted as being abnormal.

ICD-10 The tenth revision of the International classification of diseases published by the World Health Organization, Geneva, 1992.

Id An unconscious part of the mental apparatus, which is partly made up of inherited instincts and partly by acquired, but repressed, components.

Ideas of reference *see* Delusion of reference

Illness The subjective interpretation of problems that are perceived as being related to health.

Illness behaviour Actions of people who see themselves as ill, for the purpose of defining their health state and finding a remedy.

Illusion A false perception of a real external stimulus.

Inappropriate affect An affect that is inappropriate to the circumstances, e.g. appearing cheerful immediately following the death of a loved one.

Induced psychosis (folie à deux) A delusional disorder is shared by two (or more) people who are closely related emotionally. One has a genuine psychotic disorder and their delusional system is induced in the other, who may be dependent or less intelligent.

Introjection and identification Defence mechanisms by which the attitudes and behaviour of another are transposed into oneself, helping one cope with separation from that person.

Isolation A defence mechanism in which certain thoughts are isolated from others.

Jamais vu The illusion of failure to recognize a familiar situation.

Jargon aphasia Incoherent, meaningless, neologistic speech.

Knight's-move thinking Odd, tangential associations between ideas, leading to disruptions in the smooth continuity of speech.

Koro Seen in south-east Asia, particularly Malaysians of Chinese extraction, and in parts of China. Affected men have an overwhelming fear that their penis is retracting into the abdomen and that death will then occur.

Labile affect The affect repeatedly and rapidly shifts, e.g. from sadness to anger.

Latah Seen in the Far East and north Africa. It is a hysterical state in which patients exhibit echolalia, echopraxia and automatic obedience.

Learning disability (mental retardation) Classified by DSM-IV-TR and ICD-10 as an IQ of less than or equal to 70.

Logoclonia The last syllable of the last word is repeated.

Logorrhoea (volubility) Fluent and rambling speech using many words.

Macropsia Objects appear larger or nearer than they really are.

Made actions (made acts) The delusional belief that one's free will has been removed and an external agency is controlling one's actions.

Made feelings The delusional belief that one's free will has been removed and an external agency is controlling one's feelings.

Made impulses The delusional belief that one's free will has been removed and an external agency is controlling one's impulses.

Mannerisms Repeated involuntary movements that appear to be goal directed.

Mens rea A guilty state of mind at the time of a criminal offence.

Mental apparatus The id, ego and superego in psychodynamic theory.

Micropsia Objects appear smaller or farther away than they really are.

Mild mental retardation IQ of 50–70 (inclusive).

Moderate mental retardation IQ of 35–49 (inclusive).

Monomania A pathological preoccupation with a single object.

Mood A pervasive and sustained emotion that colours the person's perception of the world (DSM-IV-TR).

Mood-congruent delusion The content of the delusion is appropriate to the patient's mood.

Mood-incongruent delusion The content of the delusion is not appropriate to the patient's mood.

Mutism Total loss of speech.

Negativism A motiveless resistance to commands and attempts to be moved.

Neologism A word newly made up, or an everyday word used in a special way.

Neurosis A neurotic disorder is a psychiatric disorder in which the patient has insight into the illness, has only part of his or her personality involved in the disorder, can distinguish between subjective experiences and reality, and does not construct a false environment based on misconceptions.

Nihilistic delusion The delusional belief that others, oneself, or the world do not exist or are about to cease to exist.

Nominal aphasia Difficulty in naming objects.

Obsessions Repetitive senseless thoughts, recognized by the patient as being irrational, which, at least initially, are unsuccessfully resisted.

Overvalued idea An unreasonable and sustained intense preoccupation maintained with less than delusional intensity. The belief is demonstrably false and not normally held by others of the same subculture. There is a marked associated emotional investment.

Palilalia A word is repeated with increasing frequency.

Panic attacks Acute episodic intense anxiety attacks with or without physiological symptoms.

Pareidolia Vivid imagery occurring without conscious effort while looking at a poorly structured background.

Paramnesia A distorted recall leading to falsification of memory, e.g. confabulation, *déjà vu*, *déjà pensé*, *jamais vu*, retrospective falsification.

Parasuicide (deliberate self-harm) Any act deliberately undertaken by a patient who mimics the act of suicide, but this does not result in a fatal outcome.

Passing by the point (*vorbeigehen*) The answers to questions, although obviously wrong, show that the questions have been understood, e.g. when asked 'What colour is grass' the patient may answer 'Blue'. It is seen in the Ganser syndrome, first described in criminals awaiting trial.

Passivity phenomena The delusional belief that an external agency is controlling aspects of the self that are normally entirely under one's own control, e.g. thought alienation, made feelings, made impulses, made actions, somatic passivity.

Perseveration (of speech and movement) Mental operations carry on beyond the point at which they are appropriate.

Personality disorders Deeply ingrained and enduring behaviour patterns manifesting as inflexible responses to a broad range of personal and social situations (ICD-10).

Phantom limb Following the removal of a limb there is a continued awareness of its presence.

Phobia A persistent irrational fear of an activity, object or situation, leading to avoidance. The fear is out of proportion to the real danger and cannot be reasoned away, being out of voluntary control.

Phobic anxiety The focus of anxiety is avoided.

Physical dependence An adaptive state in which intense physical disturbance occurs when the administration of a psychoactive substance is suspended. There is a desire to take the substance to avoid the physical symptoms of the withdrawal state.

Piblokto (Arctic hysteria) A dissociative state seen in Eskimo women.

Posturing An inappropriate or bizarre bodily posture is adopted continuously over a long period.

Poverty of speech Very reduced speech, sometimes with monosyllabic answers to questions.

Premenstrual syndrome (PMS; late luteal phase dysphoric disorder) A recurrence of emotional, physical and behavioural symptoms occurring regularly during the second half of each menstrual cycle. They subside during menstruation and are completely absent between menstruation and ovulation.

Pressure of speech Increased quantity and rate of speech, which is difficult to interrupt.

Primary delusion A delusion arising fully formed without any discernible connection with previous events. It may be preceded by a delusional mood in which there is an awareness of something unusual and threatening occurring.

Profound mental retardation IQ of less than 20.

Projection A defence mechanism in which repressed thoughts and wishes are attributed to other people or objects.

Projective identification A defence mechanism in which another person is both seen as possessing and constrained to take on repressed aspects of oneself.

Pseudodementia Similar clinically to dementia, but has a non-organic cause, e.g. depression.

Pseudohallucination A form of imagery arising in the subjective inner space of the mind and lacking the substantiality of normal perceptions. It is not subject to conscious manipulation.

Psychiatry (psychological medicine) The branch of medicine dealing with mental disorder and its treatment.

Psychoactive substance A substance the administration of which can lead to relatively rapid effects on the central nervous system, including a change in the level of consciousness or the state of mind. Examples include alcohol, illicit drugs (e.g. cocaine, heroin and LSD) and licit drugs (e.g. nicotine and caffeine).

Psychological dependence A psychoactive substance produces a feeling of satisfaction and a psychological drive that requires periodic or continuous administration of the substance to produce pleasure or to avoid the psychological discomfort of its absence.

Psychology The science investigating behaviour, experience and the phenomena of mental and emotional life.

Psychomotor agitation Excess (usually unproductive) overactivity and restlessness, e.g. in agitated depression.

Psychosis A psychotic disorder is one in which the patient does not have insight, has the whole of his or her personality distorted by illness, and constructs a false environment out of subjective experiences. Delusions and/or hallucinations may occur.

Pure word deafness Words that are heard cannot be comprehended.

Rationalization A defence mechanism in which an attempt is made to explain in a logically consistent or ethically acceptable way affects, ideas and wishes the true motives of which are not consciously perceived.

Reaction formation A defence mechanism in which a psychological attitude diametrically opposed to an oppressed wish is held.

Receptive (sensory) aphasia Difficulty in comprehending word meanings.

Reduplication phenomenon Part or all of the body is felt to be duplicated.

Reflex hallucination A stimulus in one sensory field leads to a hallucination in another (*see also* Synaesthesia).

Regression A defence mechanism in which there is a return to an earlier stage of development.

Repression A defence mechanism in which there is a pushing away of unacceptable affects, ideas and wishes so that they remain in the unconscious.

Retrospective falsification False details are added to the recollection of an otherwise real memory.

Schneiderian first-rank symptoms In the absence of organic cerebral pathology the presence of any of Schneider's first-rank symptoms is indicative of, though not pathognomonic of, schizophrenia.

Sections Orders under the Mental Health Act 1983 (England and Wales), allowing the detention of patients.

Selective inattention Anxiety-provoking stimuli are blocked out.

Semicoma A semicomatose patient withdraws from the source of pain but does not show spontaneous motor activity.

Severe mental retardation IQ of 20–34 (inclusive).

Sick-role behaviour Activity by individuals who consider themselves as ill for the purpose of getting well.

Simple phobia Fear of discrete objects (e.g. spiders) or situations.

Social phobia Fear of personal interactions in a public setting, e.g. public speaking and eating in public.

Somatic passivity The delusional belief that one is a passive recipient of bodily sensations from an external agency.

Somnambulism Sleepwalking.

Somnolence A patient who is drowsy or somnolent can be awoken by mild stimuli and can speak comprehensibly, perhaps for only a short time before falling asleep again.

Stammering The flow of speech is broken by pauses and the repetition of parts of words.

Stereotypy A repeated regular fixed pattern of movement or speech that is not goal directed.

Sublimation A defence mechanism allowing unconscious wishes to be satisfied by means of socially acceptable activities.

Superego A derivative of the ego that exercises self-judgement and holds ethical and moralistic values.

Susto (Espanto) Seen in the High Andes. A prolonged depressive episode occurs that is believed to result from supernatural agencies.

Synaesthesia A stimulus in one sensory field leads to a hallucination in another (*see also* Reflex hallucination).

Systematized delusion A group of delusions united by a single theme or a delusion with multiple elaborations.

Tactile (haptic) hallucinations Superficial somatic hallucinations.

Talking past the point (*vorbeireden*) The point of what is being said is never quite reached.

Tension An unpleasant increase in psychomotor activity.

Testamentary capacity The capacity to make a legally valid will.

Thought alienation The delusional belief that one's thoughts are under the control of an outside agency, or that others are participating in one's thinking. It includes thought insertion, thought withdrawal and thought broadcasting.

Thought blocking A sudden interruption in the train of thought occurs, leaving a 'blank', after which what was being said cannot be recalled.

Thought broadcasting The delusional belief that one's thoughts are being 'read' by others, as if they were being broadcast.

Thought insertion The delusional belief that thoughts are being put into one's mind by an external agency.

Thought withdrawal The delusional belief that thoughts are being removed from one's mind by an external agency.

Tics Repeated irregular movements involving a particular muscle group.

Tolerance The desired central nervous system effects of a psychoactive substance diminish with repeated use, so that increasing doses are needed to achieve the same effects.

Trailing phenomenon Moving objects are seen as a series of discrete discontinuous images. It is associated with hallucinogens.

Transference The unconscious process in which emotions and attitudes experienced in childhood are transferred to the therapist.

Undoing (what has been done) A defence mechanism in which previous thoughts or actions are made not to have occurred.

Unit of alcohol The mass of alcohol contained in a standard measure of spirits, in a standard glass of sherry or fortified wine, a standard glass of table wine, and in half a pint of beer. It is around 8–10 g.

Visceral hallucinations Somatic hallucinations of deep sensations.

Visual asymbolia Words can be transcribed but not read.

Waxy flexibility (cerea flexibilitas) The examiner, as he or she moves part of the patient's body, has a feeling of plastic resistance as if bending a soft wax rod. The bodily part remains 'moulded' in its new position.

Windigo (Wihtigo) Seen in North American Indian tribes. A depressive disorder in which patients believe they have mutated into cannibalistic monsters.

Withdrawal state Physical and psychological symptoms, which may be complicated by delirium or convulsions, occur following absolute or relative withdrawal of a psychoactive substance after its repeated use.

Word salad (schizophasia or speech confusion) The speech is an incoherent and incomprehensible mix of words and phrases.

Zeitgebers Environmental or social cues for sleep.

Index

NB: Page numbers followed by *f* indicate figures; *t* indicate tables; *b* indicate boxes.

B

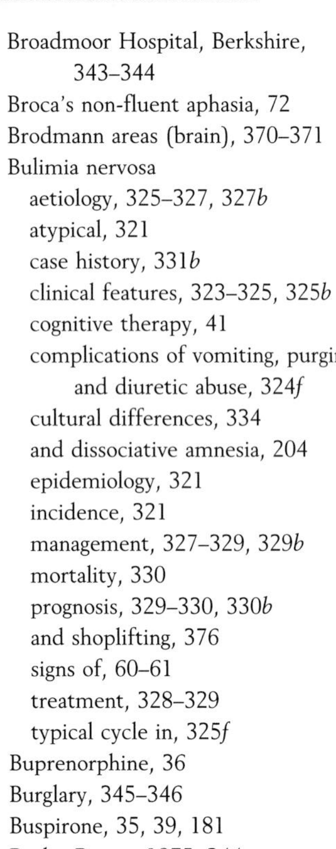

D

E

F

G

H

I

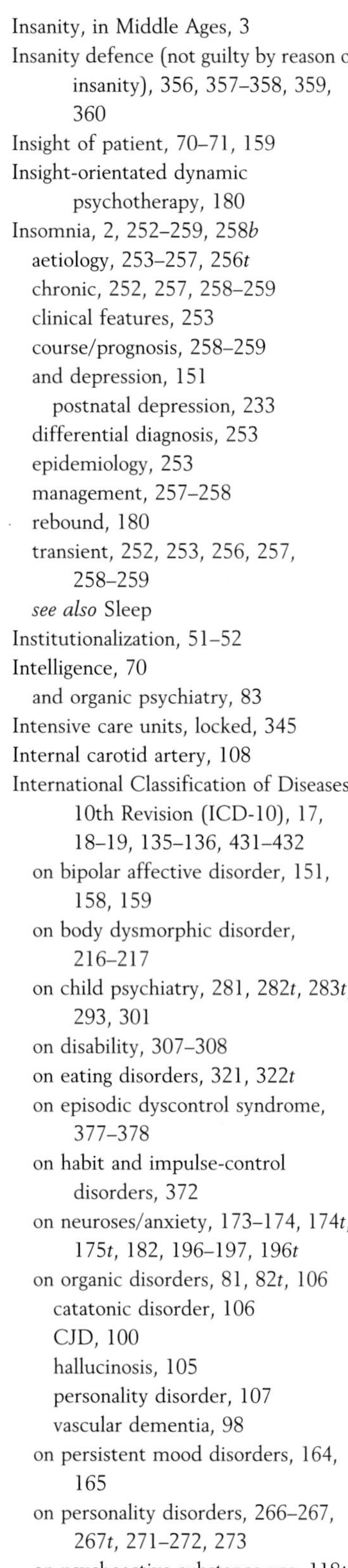

J

K

L

M

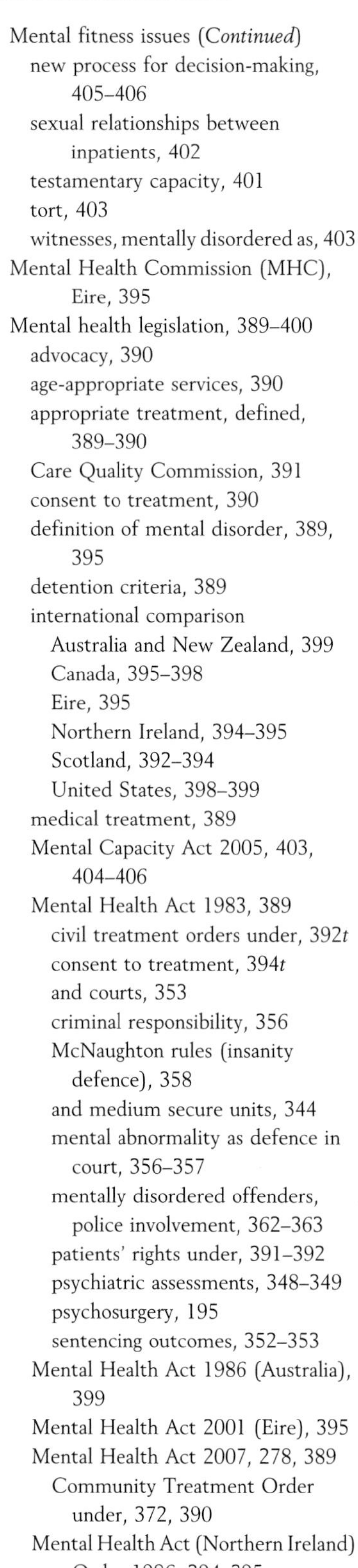

N

O

P

Q

R

S

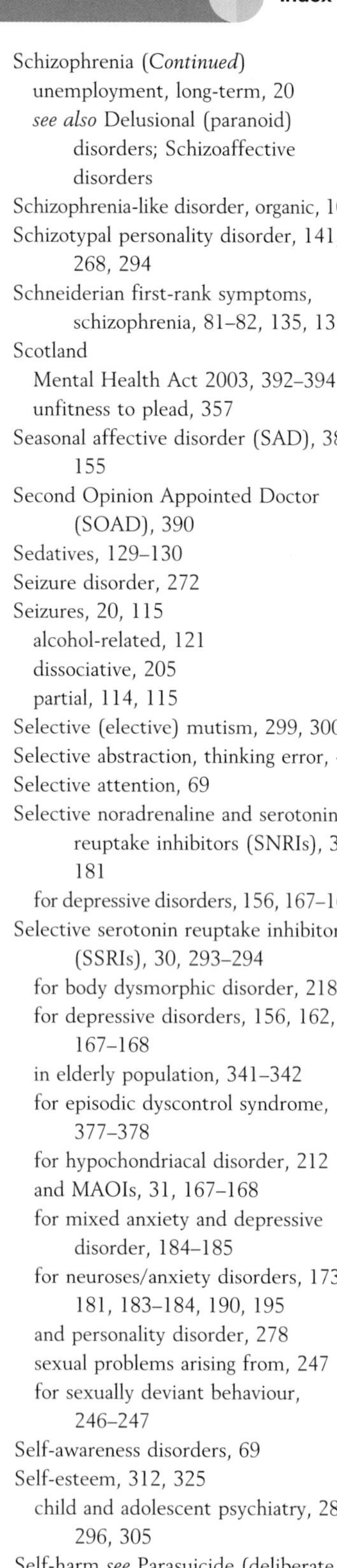

T

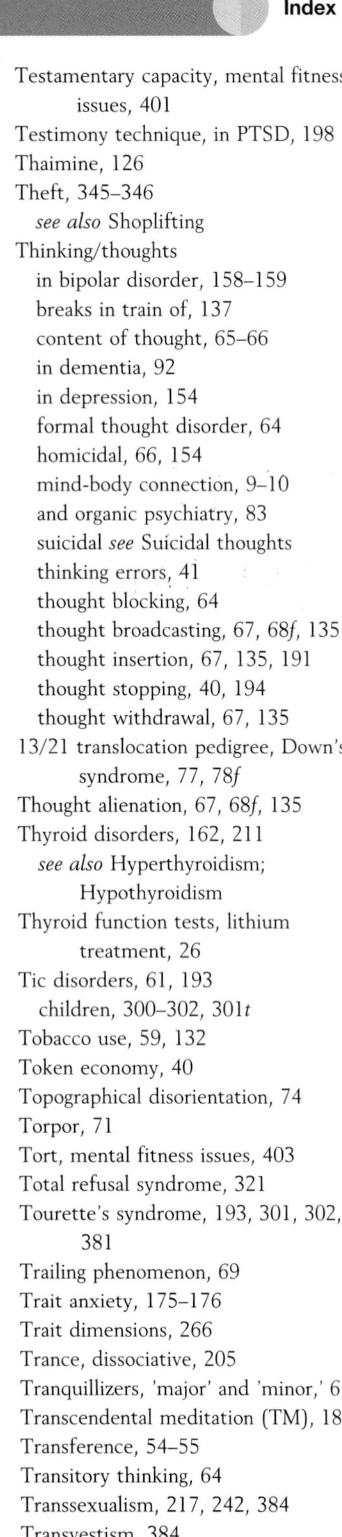

U

V

W